D0289534

The APRN's Complete Guide to Prescribing Drug Therapy

2018

Mari J. Wirfs, PhD, MN, RN, ANP-BC, FNP-BC, CNE, is a nationally certified adult nurse practitioner (ANCC since 1997) and family nurse practitioner (AANP since 1998) and certified nurse educator (NLN since 2008). Her career spans 45 years in collegiate undergraduate and graduate nursing education and clinical practice in critical care, pediatrics, psychiatric–mental health nursing, and advanced practice primary care nursing. Her PhD is in higher education administration and leadership. During her academic career, she has achieved the rank of professor with tenure in two university systems. She is a frequent guest lecturer on a variety of advanced practice topics to professional groups and general health care topics to community groups.

Dr. Wirfs was a member of the original medical staff in the establishment of Baptist Community Health Services, a community-based nonprofit primary care clinic founded post-hurricane Katrina in the New Orleans Lower Ninth Ward. Since 2002, Dr. Wirfs has served as clinical director and primary care provider at the Family Health Care Clinic, serving faculty, staff, students, and their families at New Orleans Baptist Theological Seminary (NOBTS). She is also adjunct graduate faculty, teaching Neuropsychology and Psychopharmacology, in the NOBTS Guidance and Counseling program. She is a long-time member of the National Organization of Nurse Practitioner Faculties (NONPF), Sigma Theta Tau National Honor Society of Nursing, and several other academic honor societies.

Dr. Wirfs has completed, published, and presented six quantitative research studies focusing on academic leadership, nursing education, and clinical practice issues, including one for the Army Medical Department conducted during her 8 years reserve service in the Army Nurse Corps. Dr. Wirfs has co-authored family primary care certification review books and study materials. Her first prescribing guide, *Clinical Guide to Pharmacotherapeutics for the Primary Care Provider,* was published by Advanced Practice Education Associates (APEA) from 1999 to 2014. *The APRN's Complete Guide to Prescribing Drug Therapy 2018* (launched in 2016), *The APRN's Complete Guide to Prescribing Pediatric Drug Therapy 2018* (launched in 2017), and *The PA's Complete Guide to Prescribing Drug Therapy 2018* (launched in 2017) are Springer Publishing handbook editions accompanied by the free e-book version with quarterly electronic updates.

The APRN's Complete Guide to Prescribing Drug Therapy

2018

Mari J. Wirfs, PhD, MN, RN, ANP-BC, FNP-BC, CNE

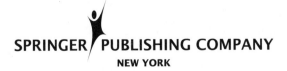

SPRINGER PUBLISHING COMPANY

NEW YORK

Copyright © 2018 Springer Publishing Company, LLC

Springer Publishing Company, LLC
11 West 42nd Street
New York, NY 10036
www.springerpub.com

Acquisitions Editor: Margaret Zuccarini
Composition: Exeter Premedia Services Private LTD.

ISBN: 978-0-8261-6658-6
e-book ISBN: 978-0-8261-6659-3

17 18 / 5 4 3 2 1

This book is a quick reference for health care providers practicing in primary care settings. The information has been extrapolated from a variety of professional sources and is presented in condensed and summary form. It is not intended to replace or substitute for complete and current manufacturer prescribing information, current research, or knowledge and experience of the user. For complete prescribing information, including toxicities, drug interactions, contraindications, and precautions, the reader is directed to the manufacturer's package insert and the published literature. The inclusion of a particular brand name neither implies nor suggests that the author or publisher advises or recommends the use of that particular product or considers it superior to similar products available by other brand names. Neither the author nor the publisher makes any warranty, expressed or implied, with respect to the information, including any errors or omissions, herein.

Library of Congress Cataloging-in-Publication Data
Names: Wirfs, Mari J., author.
Title: The APRN's complete guide to prescribing drug therapy 2018 / Mari J.
  Wirfs.
Description: New York, NY: Springer Publishing Company, LLC, [2018] |
  Includes bibliographical references and index.
Identifiers: LCCN 2017008900| ISBN 9780826166586 | ISBN 9780826166593 (ebook)
Subjects: | MESH: Drug Therapy—nursing | Advanced Practice Nursing—methods
  | Handbooks
Classification: LCC RM301 | NLM WY 49 | DDC 615.1—dc23
LC record available at https://lccn.loc.gov/2017008900

Printed in the United States of America by McNaughton & Gunn.

CONTENTS

SECTION II: APPENDICES

REVIEWERS

Kelley M. Anderson, PhD, FNP
Assistant Professor of Nursing, Georgetown University School of Nursing & Health Studies, Washington, DC

Kathleen Bradbury-Golas, DNP, RN, FNP-C, ACNS-BC
Associate Clinical Professor, Drexel University, Philadelphia, Pennsylvania
Family Nurse Practitioner, Virtua Medical Group, Hammonton and Linwood, New Jersey

Lori Brien, MS, ACNP-BC
Instructor, AG-ACNP Program, Georgetown University School of Nursing & Health Studies, Washington, DC

Jill C. Cash, MSN, APN
Nurse Practitioner, Logan Primary Care, West Frankfort, Illinois

Catherine M. Concert, DNP, RN, FNP-BC, AOCNP, NE-BC, CNL, CGRN
Nurse Practitioner—Radiation Oncology, Laura and Isaac Perlmutter Cancer Center, New York University Langone Medical Center; Clinical Assistant Professor, Pace University Lienhard School of Nursing, New York, New York

Aileen Fitzpatrick, DNP, RN, FNP-BC
Clinical Assistant Professor, Pace University Lienhard School of Nursing, New York, New York

Tracy P. George, DNP, APRN-BC, CNE
Assistant Professor of Nursing, Amy V. Cockroft Fellow 2016–2017, Francis Marion University, Florence, South Carolina

Norma Stephens Hannigan, DNP, MPH, FNP-BC, DCC, FAANP
Clinical Professor of Nursing, Coordinator, Accelerated Second Degree (A2D) Program/Sophomore Honors Program, Hunter College, CUNY Hunter-Bellevue School of Nursing, New York, New York

Ella T. Heitzler, PhD, WHNP-BC, FNP-BC, RNC-OB
Assistant Professor, Georgetown University School of Nursing and Health Studies, Washington, DC

Melissa H. King, DNP, FNP-BC, ENP-BC
Director of Advanced Practice Providers, Director of TelEmergency,
Department of Emergency Medicine, University of Mississippi Medical Center,
Jackson, Mississippi

Michael Watson, DNP, APRN, FNP-BC
Lead Family Nurse Practitioner, Wadley Regional Medical Center, Emergency
Department, Texarkana, Texas

*	single-scored tablet
**	cross-scored tablet
(II), (III), (IV), (V)	Drug Enforcement Agency (DEA) controlled substance schedule
(A), (B), (C), (D), (X)	Federal Drug Agency (FDA) pregnancy category
ABSSSI	acute bacterial skin and skin structure infection
ac	before meal
ACEI	angiotensin converting enzyme inhibitor
ALT	liver enzyme; alanine transaminase (ALT)
AM	antemeridiem, morning
APAP	acetaminophen
AST	liver enzyme, aspartate transaminase
Amp	ampule
Apo-B	apolipoprotein B
ARB	angiotensin receptor blocker
ART	antiretroviral treatment
ASE	adverse side effect
AVB	atrioventricular heart block
bid	bis in die, twice-a-day
BP	blood pressure
CAD	coronary artery disease
calib applicator	calibrated applicator
cap	capsule
CAP	community acquired pneumonia
CCB	calcium channel blocker
CFC	chlorofluorocarbon, inhaler propellant
chew tab	chewable tablet

Child-Pugh A	mild liver disease/dysfunction
Child-Pugh B	moderate liver disease/dysfunction
Child-Pugh C	severe liver disease/dysfunction
CHF	congestive heart failure
CKD	chronic kidney disease
clnsr	cleanser
conc	concentrate, concentration
conj estra	conjugated estrogen
COPD	chronic obstructive pulmonary disease
cplt	caplet
Cr	creatinine
CrCl	creatinine clearance measured in mL/min
CRI	chronic renal insufficiency
CRF	chronic renal failure
crm	cream
CVD	cardiovascular disease
DDAVP	desmopressin acetate
dL	deciliter
DM	diabetes mellitis
DMARDs	disease modifying anti-rheumatoid drugs
DVT	deep vein thrombosis
ent-coat	enteric-coated
EDTA	edatate calcium disodium
EE	ethinyl estradiol
eGFR	estimated glomerular filtration tate
EKG	electrocardiogram
EIA	exercise-induced asthma
EIAED	enzyme-inducing antiepileptic drug
EIB	exercise-induced bronchospasm

elix	elixer
emol, emol crm	emollient, emollient cream
ESA	erythropoiesis stimulating agent
ESR	erythrocyte sedimentation rate
ESRD	end stage renal disease
est	estradiol
EX, ext-rel	extended-release
g	gram
(G)	generic, generic availability
GABHS	group a beta-hemolytic streptococcus
GAD	generalized anxiety disorder
GI	gastrointestinal
gtt, gtts	drop, drops
GU	genitourinary
H_2O_2	hydrogen peroxide
HAART	highly active antiretroviral treatment
HCT	hematocrit
HCTZ	hydrochlorothiazide
HAV	hepatitis A virus
HBV	hepatitis C virus
HCV	hepatitis C virus
HDL, HDL-C	high density lipoprotein cholesterol
HFA	hydrofluoroalkane (inhaler propellent phasing in)
Hgb	hemoglobin
HgbA1c	hemoglobin A1c, the standard POC diagnostic test for diabetes
hgc	hard-gel capsule
HPV	human papillomavirus
HR	heart rate in beats per minute
HRT	hormone replacement therapy

HS	hour of sleep, bedtime
IBS-C	irritable bowel syndrome with constipation
IBS-D	irritable bowel syndrome with diarrhea
ID	intradermal
IM	intramuscular
immed-rel	immediate-release
inhal	inhalation
inj	injection
IU	international unit
IUD	intrauterine device
IV	intravenous
JRA	juvenile rheumatoid arthritis
K^+	potassium
kg	kilogram
L	liter, 1000 ml
LAA	long-acting anticholinergic
LABA	long-actine beta agonist
LAR	long-acting release
LDL, LDL-C	low density lipoprotein cholesterol
LFTs	liver function tests
Liq	liquid
lotn	lotion
LR	lactated ringers IV solution
MAOI	monoamine oxidase inhibitor
mcg	microgram
MDD	major depressive disorder
MDI	metered dose inhaler
mfr	manufacturer
mg	milligram

mg/dL	milligrams per deciliter
mg/kg/day	milligram per kilogram per day
ml, mL	milliliter
MRSA	methicillin-resistant staphylococcus aureus
MS	multiple sclerosis
MTX	methotrexate
Na$^+$	sodium
NaCl	sodium chloride
NaHCO$_3$	sodium bicarbonate
NMDA	n-methyl-d-aspartate receptor antagonist
NNRTI	nonnucleoside reverse transcriptase inhibitor
NOH	neurogenic orthostatic hypotension
non-HDL-C	non-high density lipoprotein cholesterol
norgest	norgestimate
nPEP	non-occupational post-exposure prophylaxis
NR	not rated, pregnancy category not assigned
NRTI	nucleoside reverse transcriptase inhibitor
NS	nasal spray; normal saline
NSAID	nonsteroidal anti-inflammatory drug
OA	osteoarthritis
OCD	obsessive compulsive disorder
OCP	oral contraceptive pill
ODT	orally-disintegrating tablet
Oint	ointment
ophth	ophthalmic, pertaining to the eye
orally-disint	orally-disintegrating
OTC	over-the-counter
Otic	pertaining to the ear
oz	ounce, 30 ml

pc	after meals
PBA	pseudobulbar affect
PCOS	polycystic ovarian syndrome; Stein-Leventhal Disease
Pediatric	newborn to ≤18 years-of-age
PD	Parkinson's disease
PDE5	phosphodiesterase type 5 inhibitor
PJIA	polyarticular juvenile idiopathic arthritis
PM	post-meridiem, evening
PMDD	premenstrual Dysmorphic Disorder
PMHx	past medical history
PPI	proton pump inhibitor
PO	per oral, by mouth
PO_4^{3-}	phosphate
POC	point of care
Post-op	post-operative
PR	per rectum
PRN	as needed
PTSD	post traumatic stress disorder
PUD	peptic ulcer disease
PVD	peripheral vascular disease
pwdr	powder
pwdr w. diluent	powder with diluent
q	per
qd	once daily
qHS	per hour of sleep, bedtime
qid	quater in die, four times-a-day
RA	rheumatoid arthritis
RAI	reversible anticholinesterase inhibitor
RBC	red blood cell

SC	subcutaneous
sgc	soft-gel capsule
SGOT	serum glutamic-oxaloacetic transaminase
SGPT	serum glutamic-pyruvic transaminase
SL	sublingual, under the tongue
syr	syrup
soln	solution
supp	suppository
susp	suspension
sust-rel	sustained release
SNRI	selective serotonin and norepinephrine reuptake inhibitor
SR	sustained-release
SSRI	selective serotonin reuptake inhibitor
STD	sexually transmitted disease
T1DM	type 1 diabetes mellitus
T2DM	type 2 diabetes mellitus
T3	liothyronine
T4	levothyroxine
tab	tablet
TCA	tricyclic antidepressant
TG	triglyceride
tid	ter in die, three times-a-day
TMP/SMX	trimethoprim-sulfamethoxazole
trans-sys	transdermal system
TRD	treatment-resistant depression
TSH	thyroid stimulating hormone
tsp	teaspoon, 4-5 ml
TSSRI	thienobenzodiazepine-selective serotonin reuptake inhibitor

VVC	vulvovaginal candidiasis
WBC	white blood cell
w.	with
XL	extra long-acting
XOI	xanthine oxidase inhibitor
XR	extended-release

PREFACE

The APRN's Complete Guide to Prescribing Drug Therapy is a prescribing reference intended for use by health care providers in all clinical practice settings who are involved in the primary care management of patients with acute, episodic, and chronic health problems. It is organized in a concise and easy-to-read format. Comments are interspersed throughout, including such clinically useful information as laboratory values to be monitored, patient teaching points, and safety information.

This clinical guide is divided into two sections. **Section I** presents drug treatment regimens for over 500 clinical diagnoses. Each drug is listed alphabetically by generic name, followed by the FDA pregnancy category (A, B, C, D, X, or NR if a pregnancy category has not been assigned), whether the drug is available over-the-counter (OTC), DEA schedule (I, II, III, IV, V), generic availability (G), adult and pediatric dosing regimens, brand names and available dose forms, whether tablets, caplets, or chew tabs are scored (*) or cross-scored (**), flavors of chewable, sublingual, buccal, and liquid forms, and information regarding additives (e.g., dye-free, sugar-free, preservative-free or preservative type, and alcohol-free or alcohol content).

Section II presents clinically useful information in convenient table format, including: the JNC-8 recommendations for hypertension management, the U.S. schedule of controlled substances and the FDA pregnancy categories, measurement conversions, childhood and adult immunization recommendations, brand-name drugs (with contents) for the management of common respiratory symptoms, anti-infectives by classification, pediatric dosing by weight for liquid forms, gluco-corticosteroids by potency and route of administration, and contraceptives by route of administration and estrogen and/or progesterone content. An alphabetical cross reference index of drugs by generic and brand name, with FDA pregnancy category and controlled drug schedule, facilitates quick identification of drugs by alternate names, relative safety during pregnancy, and DEA schedule.

Selected diagnoses (e.g., angina, ADHD, growth failure, glaucoma, Parkinson's disease, CMV retinitis, multiple sclerosis, cystic fibrosis) and selected drugs (e.g., anti-neoplastics, antipsychotics, anti-arrhythmics, anti-HIV drugs, and anticoagulants) are included as patients are often referred by surgeons and emergency and urgent care providers to the primary care provider for follow-up monitoring and management.

Safe, efficacious, prescribing and monitoring of drug therapy regimens require adequate knowledge about (a) the pharmacodynamics and pharmacokinetics of drugs, (b) concomitant therapies, and (c) individual characteristics of the patient (e.g., current and past medical history, physical examination findings, hepatic and renal function, and co-morbidities). Users of this clinical guide are encouraged to utilize the manufacturer's package insert, recommendations and guidance of specialists, standard of practice protocols, and the current research literature for more comprehensive information about specific drugs (e.g., special precautions, drug-drug and drug-food interactions, risk versus benefit, age-related considerations, adverse reactions) and appropriate use with individual patients.

ACKNOWLEDGMENTS

This publication, which we consider to be a "must have" for students, academicians, and practicing clinicians with prescriptive authority, represents the culmination of Springer Publishing Company's collaborative team effort. Margaret Zuccarini, Publisher, Nursing, and the Editorial Committee, shared my vision for a handy pocket prescribing reference for new and experienced prescribers in primary care. Joanne Jay, Vice President, Production and Manufacturing, designed the contents for ease and efficiency of user navigation. The production team at Exeter Premedia Services, on behalf of Springer Publishing Company, understood the critical nature of exactness in this prescribing resource, and faithfully managed the complex files as content was updated and cross-paginated for the final product. The work of the reviewers from academia and clinical practice was essential to the process and their contributions are greatly appreciated. I am proud of my association with these dedicated professionals and I thank them on behalf of the medical and advanced practice nursing community worldwide, for supporting the end goal of quality health care for all.

DRUG THERAPY BY CLINICAL DIAGNOSIS

◯ ACETAMINOPHEN OVERDOSE

ANTIDOTE/CHELATING AGENT

▷ *acetylcysteine* **(B)(G)** *Loading Dose:* 150 mg/kg administered over 15 minutes; *Maintenance:* 50 mg/kg administered over 4 hours; then 100 mg/kg administered over 16 hours
Pediatric: same as adult
    Acetadote *Vial: soln for IV infusion after dilution:* 200 mg/ml (30 ml; dilute in
    D5W (preservative-free)

Comment: *acetaminophen* overdose is a medical emergency due to the risk of irreversible hepatic injury. An IV infusion of *acetylcysteine* should be started as soon as possible and within 24 hours if the exact time of ingestion is unknown. Use a serum *acetaminophen* nomogram to determine need for treatment. Extreme caution is needed if used with concomitant hepatotoxic drugs.

◯ ACNE ROSACEA

Comment: All acne rosacea products should be applied sparingly to clean, dry skin as directed. Avoid use of topical corticosteroids.
▷ *ivermectin* **(C)** apply bid
    Soolantra *Crm:* 1% (30 g)
    Comment: **Soolantra** is a macrocyclic lactone. Exactly how it works to treat
    rosacea is unknown.

TOPICAL ALPHA-2 AGONIST

▷ *brimonidine* **(B)** apply once daily
Pediatric: <18 years: not recommended
    Mirvaso apply to affected area once daily
    Gel: 0.33% (30, 45 g tube; 30 g pump)
Comment: For persistant erythema; constricts dilated facial blood vessels to reduce redness.

TOPICAL ANTIMICROBIALS

▷ *azelaic acid* **(B)** apply bid
    Azelex *Crm:* 20% (30, 50 g)
    Finacea *Gel:* 15% (30 g); *Foam:* 15% (50 g)
▷ *metronidazole* **(B)** apply to clean dry skin
    MetroCream apply bid
    Emol crm: 0.75% (45 g)
    MetroGel apply once daily
    Gel: 1% (60 g tube; 55 g pump)
    MetroLotion apply bid
    Lotn: 0.75% (2 oz)
▷ *sodium sulfacetamide* **(C)(G)** apply 1-3 x daily
    Klaron *Lotn:* 10% (2 oz)
▷ *sodium sulfacetamide/sulfur* **(C)**
    Clenia Emollient Cream apply 1-3 x daily
    Wash: sod sulfa 10%/*sulfur* 5% (10 oz)

Clenia Foaming Wash wash affected area once <u>or</u> twice daily
Wash: sod sulfa 10%/*sulfur* 5% (6, 12 oz)
Rosula Gel apply 1-3 x daily
Gel: sod sulfa 10%/*sulfur* 5% (45 ml)
Rosula Lotion apply tid
Lotn: sod sulfa 10%/*sulfur* 5% (45 ml) (alcohol-free)
Rosula Wash wash bid
Clnsr: sod sulfa 10%/*sulfur* 5% (335 ml)

ORAL ANTIMICROBIALS

▷ *doxycycline* (D)(G) 40-100 mg bid
Pediatric: <8 years: not recommended; ≥8 years, <100 lb: 2 mg/lb on first day in 2 divided doses, followed by 1 mg/lb/day in 1-2 divided doses; ≥8 years, ≥100 lb: same as adult; *see page 572 for dose by weight*
Actilate *Tab:* 75, 150** mg
Adoxa *Tab:* 50, 75, 100, 150 mg ent-coat
Doryx *Tab:* 50, 75, 100, 150, 200 mg del-rel
Monodox *Cap:* 50, 75, 100 mg
Oracea *Cap:* 40 mg del-rel
Vibramycin *Tab:* 100 mg; *Cap:* 50, 100 mg; *Syr:* 50 mg/5 ml (raspberry-apple) (sulfites); *Oral susp:* 25 mg/5 ml (raspberry)
Vibra-Tab *Tab:* 100 mg film-coat
Comment: *doxycycline* is contraindicated <8 years-of-age, in pregnancy, and lactation (discolors developing tooth enamel). A side effect may be photosensitivity (photophobia). Do not give with antacids, calcium supplements, milk or other dairy, or within two hours of taking another drug.
▷ *minocycline* (D)(G) 200 mg on first day; then 100 mg q 12 hours x 9 more days
Pediatric: <8 years: not recommended; ≥8 years, <100 lb: 2 mg/lb on first day in 2 divided doses, followed by 1 mg/lb q 12 hours x 9 more days; ≥8 years, ≥100 lb: same as adult
Dynacin *Cap:* 50, 100 mg
Minocin *Cap:* 50, 75, 100 mg; *Oral susp:* 50 mg/5 ml (60 ml) (custard) (sulfites, alcohol 5%)
Comment: *minocycline* is contraindicated <8 years-of-age, in pregnancy, and lactation (discolors developing tooth enamel). A side effect may be photosensitivity (photophobia). Do not give with antacids, calcium supplements, milk or other dairy, or within two hours of taking another drug.

◯ ACNE VULGARIS

ANTIBACTERIAL SOAPS

Dial (OTC) wash affected area bid
Lever 2000 Antibacterial (OTC) wash affected area bid

TOPICAL ANTIMICROBIALS

Comment: All topical antimicrobials should be applied sparingly to clean, dry skin.

➤ *azelaic acid* (B) apply bid
    Azelex *Crm:* 20% (30, 50 g)
    Finacea *Gel:* 15% (30 g); *Foam:* 15% (50g)
➤ *benzoyl peroxide* (C)(G)
  Comment: *benzoyl peroxide* may discolor clothing and linens.
    Benzac-W initially apply to affected area once daily; increase to bid-tid as tolerated
      Gel: 2.5, 5, 10% (60 g)
    Benzac-W Wash wash affected area bid
      Wash: 5% (4, 8 oz); 10% (8 oz)
    Benzagel apply to affected area one or more times/day
      Gel: 5, 10% (1.5, 3 oz) (alcohol 14%)
    Benzagel Wash wash affected area bid
      Gel: 10% (6 oz)
    Desquam X⁵ wash affected area bid
      Wash: 5% (5 oz)
    Desquam X¹⁰ wash affected area bid
      Wash: 10% (5 oz)
    Triaz apply to affected area daily bid
      Lotn: 3, 6, 9% (bottle), 3% (tube); *Pads:* 3, 6, 9% (jar)
    ZoDerm apply once or twice daily
      Gel: 4.5, 6.5, 8.5% (125 ml); *Crm:* 4.5, 6.5, 8.5% (125 ml); *Clnsr:* 4.5, 6.5, 8.5% (400 ml)
➤ *clindamycin* topical (B) apply bid
  Pediatric: not recommended
    Cleocin T *Pad:* 1% (60/pck; alcohol 50%); *Lotn:* 1% (60 ml); *Gel:* 1% (30, 60 g);
      Soln w. applicator: 1% (30, 60 ml) (alcohol 50%)
    Clindagel *Gel:* 1% (42, 77 g)
    Evoclin Foam: 1% (50, 100 g) (alcohol)
➤ *clindamycin/benzoyl peroxide* topical (C) apply sparingly to clean dry skin once daily
  Pediatric: <12 years: not recommended; ≥12 years: same as adult
    Acanya (G) apply once daily-bid
      Gel: clin 1.2%/*benz* 2.5% (50 g)
    BenzaClin (G) apply bid
      Gel: clin 1%/*benz* 5% (25, 50 g)
    Duac apply daily in the evening
      Gel: clin 1%/*benz* 5% (45 g)
    Onexton Gel apply once daily
      Gel: clin 1.2%/*benz* 3.75% (50 g pump) (alcohol-free) (preservative-free)
➤ *dapsone* topical (C) apply bid
  Pediatric: <12 years: not recommended; ≥12 years: same as adult
    Aczone *Gel:* 5, 7.5% (30, 60, 90 g jar)
➤ *erythromycin/benzoyl peroxide* (C) initially apply once daily; increase to bid as tolerated
    Benzamycin Topical Gel *Gel: eryth* 3%/*benz* 5% (46.6 g/jar)
➤ *sodium sulfacetamide* (C)(G) apply tid
    Klaron *Lotn:* 10% (2 oz)

ORAL ANTIMICROBIALS

➤ *doxycycline* (D)(G) 100 mg bid
  Pediatric: <8 years: not recommended; ≥8 years, <100 lb: 2 mg/lb on first day in 2
  divided doses, followed by 1 mg/lb/day in 1-2 divided doses; ≥8 years, ≥100 lb: same
  as adult; *see page* 572 *for dose by weight*

Actilate *Tab:* 75, 150**mg
Adoxa *Tab:* 50, 75, 100, 150 mg ent-coat
Doryx *Tab:* 50, 75, 100, 150, 200 mg del-rel
Monodox *Cap:* 50, 75, 100 mg
Oracea *Cap:* 40 mg del-rel
Vibramycin *Tab:* 100 mg; *Cap:* 50, 100 mg; *Syr:* 50 mg/5 ml (raspberry-apple) (sulfites); *Oral susp:* 25 mg/5 ml (raspberry)
Vibra-Tab *Tab:* 100 mg film coat

Comment: *doxycycline* is contraindicated <8 years-of-age, in pregnancy, and lactation (discolors developing tooth enamel). A side effect may be photosensitivity (photophobia). Do not give with antacids, calcium supplements, milk or other dairy, or within two hours of taking another drug.

▶ *erythromycin base* (B)(G) 250 mg qid, 333 mg tid <u>or</u> 500 mg bid x 7-10 days; then taper to lowest effective dose
Pediatric: <45 kg: 30-50 mg in 2-4 divided doses x 7-10 days; ≥45 kg: same as adult
    Ery-Tab *Tab:* 250, 333, 500 mg ent-coat
    PCE *Tab:* 333, 500 mg

Comment: *erythromycin* may increase INR with concomitant *warfarin*, as well as increase serum level of *digoxin*, benzodiazepines and statins.

▶ *erythromycin ethylsuccinate* (B)(G) 400 mg qid x 7-10 days
Pediatric: 30-50 mg/kg/day in 4 divided doses x 7-10 days; may double dose with severe infection; max 100 mg/kg/day; *see page 574 for dose by weight*
    EryPed *Oral susp:* 200 mg/5 ml (100, 200 ml) (fruit); 400 mg/5 ml (60, 100, 200 ml) (banana); *Oral drops:* 200, 400 mg/5 ml (50 ml) (fruit); *Chew tab:* 200 mg wafer (fruit)
    E.E.S. *Oral susp:* 200, 400 mg/5 ml (100 ml) (fruit)
    E.E.S. Granules *Oral susp:* 200 mg/5 ml (100, 200 ml) (cherry)
    E.E.S. 400 Tablets *Tab:* 400 mg

Comment: *erythromycin* may increase INR with concomitant *warfarin*, as well as increase serum level of *digoxin*, benzodiazepines and statins.

▶ *minocycline* (D)(G) initially 50-200 mg/day in 2 divided doses; reduce dose after improvement
Pediatric: <8 years: not recommended; ≥8 years: same as adult
    Dynacin *Cap:* 50, 100 mg
    Minocin *Cap:* 50, 75, 100 mg; *Oral susp:* 50 mg/5 ml (60 ml) (custard) (sulfites, alcohol 5%)

Comment: *minocycline* is contraindicated <8 years-of-age, in pregnancy, and lactation (discolors developing tooth enamel). A side effect may be photosensitivity (photophobia). Do not give with antacids, calcium supplements, milk or other dairy, or within two hours of taking another drug.

▶ *tetracycline* (D)(G) initially 1 g/day in 2-4 divided doses; after improvement, 125-500 mg daily
Pediatric: <8 years: not recommended; ≥8 years, <100 lb: 25-50 mg/kg/day in 2-4 divided doses; ≥8 years, ≥100 lb: same as adult; *see page 585 for dose by weight*
    Achromycin V *Cap:* 250, 500 mg
    Sumycin *Tab:* 250, 500 mg; *Cap:* 250, 500 mg; *Oral susp:* 125 mg/5 ml (100, 200 ml) (fruit) (sulfites)

Comment: *tetracycline* is contraindicated <8 years-of-age, in pregnancy, and lactation (discolors developing tooth enamel). A side effect may be photo-sensitivity (photophobia). Do not give with antacids, calcium supplements, milk or other dairy, or within two hours of taking another drug.

TOPICAL RETINOIDS

Comment: Wash affected area with a soap-free cleanser; pat dry and wait 20 to 30 minutes; then apply sparingly to affected area; use only once daily in the evening. Avoid applying to eyes, ears, nostrils, and mouth.

Pediatric: <8 years: not recommended; ≥8 years: same as adult

▷ *adapalene* (C) apply once daily at HS
    Differin *Crm:* 0.1% (45 g); *Gel:* 0.1. 0.3% (45 g) (alcohol-free); *Pad:* 0.1% (30/pck) (alcohol 30%); *Ltn:* 0.1% (2, 4 oz)

▷ *tazarotene* (X) apply once daily at HS
  Pediatric: not recommended
    Avage Cream *Crm:* 0.1% (30 g)
    Tazorac Cream *Crm:* 0.05, 0.1% (15, 30, 60 g)
    Tazorac Gel *Gel:* 0.05, 0.1% (30, 100 g)

▷ *tretinoin* (C) apply once daily at HS
  Pediatric: <12 years: not recommended; ≥12 years: same as adult
    Atralin Gel *Gel:* 0.05% (45 g)
    Avita *Crm:* 0.025% (20, 45 g); *Gel:* 0.025% (20, 45 g)
    Renova *Crm:* 0.02% (40 g); 0.05% (40, 60 g)
    Retin-A Cream *Crm:* 0.025, 0.05, 0.1% (20, 45 g)
    Retin-A Gel *Gel:* 0.01, 0.025% (15, 45 g) (alcohol 90%)
    Retin-A Liquid *Soln:* 0.05% (alcohol 55%)
    Retin-A Micro Gel *Gel:* 0.04, 0.08, 0.1% (20, 45 g)
    Tretin-X Cream *Crm:* 0.075% (35 g) (parabens-free, alcohol-free, propylene glycol-free)

TOPICAL RETINOID/ANTIMICROBIAL COMBINATIONS

Comment: Wash affected area with a soap-free cleanser; pat dry and wait 20-30 minutes; then apply sparingly to affected area; use only once daily in the evening. Avoid eyes, ears, nostrils, and mouth.

▷ *adapalene/benzoyl peroxide* (C) apply a thin film once daily
  Pediatric: <18 years: not recommended
    Epiduo Gel *Gel: adap* 0.1%/*benz* 2.5% (45 g)

▷ *tretinoin/clindamycin* (C) apply a thin film once daily
  Pediatric: <18 years: not recommended
    Ziana Gel *Gel: tret* 0.025%/*clin* 1.2% (30, 60 g)

ORAL RETINOID

Comment: Oral retinoids are indicated only for severe recalcitrant nodular acne unresponsive to conventional therapy including systemic antibiotics.

▷ *isotretinoin* (X) initially 0.5-1 mg/kg/day in 2 divided doses; maintenance 0.5-2 mg/kg/day in 2 divided doses x 4-5 months; repeat only if necessary 2 months following cessation of first treatment course
  Pediatric: not recommended
    Accutane *Cap:* 10, 20, 40 mg (parabens)
    Amnesteem *Cap:* 10, 20, 40 mg (soy)

Comment: *isotretinoin* is *highly teratogenic* and, therefore, female patients should be counseled prior to initiation of treatment as follows: Two negative pregnancy tests are required prior to initiation of treatment and monthly thereafter. Not for use in females who are <u>or</u> who may become pregnant <u>or</u> who are breastfeeding. Two effective methods of contraception should be used for 1 month prior to, during, and continuing for 1 month following completion of treatment. Low-dose *progestin* (mini-pill) may be an *inadequate* form of contraception. No refills; a new prescription is required every 30 days and prescriptions must be filled within 7 days. Serum lipids should be monitored until response is established (usually initially and again after 4 weeks). Bone growth, serum glucose, ESR, RBCs, WBCs, and liver enzymes should be monitored. Blood should not be donated during, <u>or</u> for 1 month after, completion of treatment. Avoid the sun and artificial UV light. *Isotretinoin* should be discontinued if any of the following occurs: visual disturbances, tinnitus, hearing impairment, rectal bleeding, pancreatitis, hepatitis, significant decrease in CBC, hyperlipidemia (particularly hypertriglyceridemia).

ORAL CONTRACEPTIVES

see **Combined Oral Contraceptives** *page 487*
see **Progesterone-only Contraceptives (Mini-Pill)** *page 496*

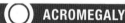 ACROMEGALY

GROWTH HORMONE RECEPTOR ANTAGONIST

▷ *pegvisomant* (B) *Loading dose:* 40 mg SC; *Maintenance:* 10 mg SC daily; titrate by 5 mg (increments <u>or</u> decrements, based on IGF-1 levels) every 4 to 6 weeks; max 30 mg/day
Pediatric: not recommended
  Somavert *Inj:* 10, 15, 20 mg
Comment: Prior to initiation of *pegvisomant*, patients should have baseline fasting serum glucose, HgbA1c, serum potassium and magnesium, liver function tests (LFTs), EKG, and gall bladder ultrasound.

Cyclohexapeptide Somatostatin

▷ *pasireotide* (C) administer SC in the thigh <u>or</u> abdomen; initial dose is 0.6 mg <u>or</u> 0.9 mg bid. Titrate dose based on response and tolerability; for patients with moderate hepatic impairment (Child-Pugh B), the recommended initial dosage is 0.3 mg twice daily and max dose 0.6 mg twice daily; avoid use in patients with severe hepatic impairment (Child-Pugh C)
Pediatric: not recommended
  Signifor LAR *Amp:* 0.3, 0.6, 0.9 mg/ml, single-dose, long-act rel (LAR) susp for inj

ACTINIC KERATOSIS

Comment: *pasireotide* is also indicated for destroying superficial basal cell carcinoma (sBCC) lesions.
▷ *diclofenac sodium* 3% (C; D ≥30 wks)(G) apply to lesions bid x 60-90 days
Pediatric: not recommended

Solaraze Gel *Gel:* 3% (50 g) (benzyl alcohol)
Comment: Contraindicated with **aspirin** allergy. As with other NSAIDs, **Solaraze Gel** should be avoided in late pregnancy (≥30 weeks) because it may cause premature closure of the ductus arteriosus.

▷ *fluorouracil* **(X)(G)** apply to lesion(s) daily-bid until erosion occurs, usually 2-4 weeks
Pediatric: not recommended
Carac *Crm:* 0.5% (30 g)
Efudex (G) *Crm:* 5% (25 g); *Soln:* 2, 5% (10 ml w. dropper)
Fluoroplex *Crm:* 1% (30 g); *Soln:* 1% (30 ml w. dropper)

▷ *imiquimod* **(B)**
Pediatric: <18 years: not recommended
Aldara (G) rub into lesions before bedtime and remove with soap and water 8 hours later; treat 2 times per week; max 16 weeks
Crm: 5% (single-use pkts/carton)
Zyclara rub into lesions before bedtime and remove with soap and water 8 hours later; treat for 2-week cycles separated by a 2-week no-treatment cycle; max 2 packs per application; max one treatment course per area
Crm: 3.75% (single-use pkts; 28/carton) (parabens)

▷ *ingenol mebutate* **(C)** limit application to one contiguous skin area of about 25 cm² using one unit dose tube; allow treated area to dry for 15 minutes; wash hands immediately after application; may remove with soapy water after 6 hours; *Face and Scalp:* apply 0.015% gel to lesions daily x 3 days; *Trunk and Extremities:* apply 0.05% gel to lesions daily x 2 days
Pediatric: <18 years: not recommended
Picato *Gel:* 0.015% (3 single-use tubes), 0.05% (2 single-use tubes)

ALCOHOL DEPENDENCE/ALCOHOL WITHDRAWAL SYNDROME

ALCOHOL WITHDRAWAL SYNDROME

Comment: Total length of time of a given detoxification regimen <u>and/or</u> length of time of treatment at any dose reduction level may be extended based on patient-specific factors, including potential <u>or</u> actual seizure, hallucinosis, increased sympathetic nervous system activity (severe anxiety, unwanted elevation in vital signs). If any of these symptoms are anticipated <u>or</u> occur, revert to an earlier step in the dosing regimen to stabilize the patient, extend the detoxification timeline and consider appropriate adjunctive drug treatments (e.g., anti-convulsants, antipsychotic agents, antihypertensive agents, sedative hypnotics agents).

▷ *clorazepate* **(D)(IV)(G)** in the following dosage schedule: *Day 1:* 30 mg initially, followed by 30-60 mg in divided doses; *Day 2:* 45-90 mg in divided doses; *Day 3:* 22.5-45 mg in divided doses; *Day 4:* 15-30 mg in divided doses; Thereafter, gradually reduce the daily dose to 7.5-15 mg; then discontinue when patient's condition is stable; max dose 90 mg/day
Tranxene *Tab:* 3.75, 7.5, 15 mg
Tranxene T-Tab *Tab:* 3.75*, 7.5*, 15*mg

▷ *chlordiazepoxide* **(D)(IV)(G)**
Librium 50-100 mg q 6 hours x 24-72 hours; then q 8 hours x 24-72 hours; then q 12 hours x 24-72 hours; then daily x 24-72 hours

Cap: 5, 10, 25 mg

Librium Injectable 50-100 mg IM <u>or</u> IV; then 25-50 mg IM tid-qid prn; max 300 mg/day

Inj: 100 mg

▶ *diazepam* (D)(IV)(G) 2-10 mg q 6 hours x 24-72 hours; then q 8 hours x 24-72 hours; then q 12 hours x 24-72 hours; then daily x 24-72 hours

Diastat *Rectal gel delivery system:* 2.5 mg

Diastat Acu Dial *Rectal gel delivery system:* 10, 20 mg

Valium *Tab:* 2*, 5*, 10*mg

Valium Injectable *Vial:* 5 mg/ml (10 ml); *Amp:* 5 mg/ml (2 ml); *Prefilled syringe:* 5 mg/ml (5 ml)

Valium Intensol Oral Solution *Conc oral soln:* 5 mg/ml (30 ml w. dropper) (alcohol 19%)

Valium Oral Solution *Oral soln:* 5 mg/5 ml (500 ml) (wintergreen-spice)

▶ *oxazepam* (C) 10-15 mg tid-qid x 24-72 hours; decrease dose <u>and/or</u> frequency every 24-72 hours; total length of therapy 5-14 days; max 120 mg/day

Cap: 10, 15, 30 mg

ABSTINENCE THERAPY

GABA Taurine Analogue

▶ *acamprosate* (C)(G) 666 mg tid; begin therapy during abstinence; continue during relapse; *CrCl 30-50-mL/min:* max 333 mg tid; *CrCl <30 mL/min:* contraindicated

Campral *Tab:* 333 mg ext-rel

Comment: **Campral** does not eliminate or diminish alcohol withdrawal symptoms.

AVERSION THERAPY

▶ *disulfiram* (X)(G)

Antabuse 500 mg once daily x 1-2 weeks; then 250 mg once daily

Tab: 250, 500 mg; *Chew tab:* 200, 500 mg

Comment: *disulfiram* use requires informed consent. Contraindications: severe cardiac disease, psychosis, concomitant use of *isoniazid, phenytoin, paraldehyde*, and topical and systemic alcohol-containing products. Approximately 20% remains in the system for 1 week after discontinuation.

Nutritional Support

▶ *thiamine* (A)(G) injectable 50-100 mg IM/IV daily (<u>or</u> tid if severely deficient)

Vial: 100 mg/1 ml (1 ml)

⭕ ALLERGIC REACTION: GENERAL

PARENTERAL ANTIHISTAMINE

▶ *diphenhydramine* (C)(G) 25-50 mg IM immediately; then q 6 hours prn

Pediatric: 1.25 mg/kg up to 25 mg IM x 1 dose; then q 6 hours prn

Benadryl Injectable *Vial:* 50 mg/ml (1 ml single-use); 50 mg/ml (10 ml multi-dose); *Amp:* 10 mg/ml (1 ml); *Prefilled syringe:* 50 mg/ml (1 ml)

Oral Drugs for Allergy, Cough, and Cold *see page* 535
Topical Corticosteroids *see page* 506
Parenteral Corticosteroids *see page* 511
Oral Corticosteroids *see page* 509

ALZHEIMER'S DISEASE

NUTRITIONAL SUPPLEMENT

▷ *L-methylfolate calcium (as metafolin)/methylcobalamin/N-acetyl cysteine* (NE) take 1 cap once daily

    Cerefolin *Cap:* metafo 5.6 mg/*methyl* 2 mg/*N-ace* 600 mg (gluten-free, yeast-free, lactose-free)

    Comment: **Cerefolin** is indicated in the dietary management of patients treated for early memory loss, with emphasis on those at risk for neurovascular oxidative stress, hyperhomocysteinemia, mild to moderate cognitive impairment with or without vitamin B-12 deficiency, vascular dementia, or Alzheimer's disease.

REVERSIBLE ANTICHOLINESTERASE INHIBITORS (RAIs)

Comment: The RAI drugs do not halt disease progression. They are indicated for early-stage disease; not effective for severe dementia. If treatment is stopped for more than several days, re-titrate from lowest dose. Side effects include nausea, anorexia, dyspepsia, diarrhea, headache, and dizziness. Side effects tend to resolve with continued treatment. Peak cognitive improvements are seen 12 weeks into therapy (increased spontaneity, reduced apathy, lessened confusion, and improved attention, conversational language, and performance of daily routines).

▷ *donepezil* (C)(G) initially 5 mg q HS, increase to 10 mg after 4-6 weeks as needed; max 23 mg/day

    Aricept *Tab:* 5, 10, 23 mg

    Aricept ODT *ODT tab:* 5, 10 mg orally-disint

▷ *galantamine* (B) initially 4 mg bid x at least 4 weeks; usual maintenance 8 mg bid; max 16 mg bid

    Razadyne *Tab:* 4, 8, 12 mg

    Razadyne ER *Tab:* 8, 16, 24 mg ext-rel

    Razadyne Oral Solution *Oral soln:* 4 mg/ml (100 ml w. calib pipette)

▷ *rivastigmine* (B)(G)

    Exelon initially 1.5 mg bid, increase every 2 weeks as needed; max 12 mg/day; take with food

      Cap: 1.5, 3, 4.5, 6 mg

    Exelon Oral Solution initially 1.5 mg bid; may increase by 1.5 mg bid at intervals of at least 2 weeks; usual range 6-12 mg/day; max 12 mg/day; if stopped, restart at lowest dose and re-titrate; may take directly from syringe or mix with water, fruit juice, or cola

      Oral soln: 2 mg/ml (120 ml w. dose syringe)

    Exelon Patch initially apply 4.6 mg/24 hours patch; if tolerated, may increase to 9.5mg/24 hours patch after 4 weeks; max 13.3 mg/24 hours; change patch daily; apply to clean, dry, hairless, intact skin; rotate application site; allow 14 days before applying new patch to same site

      Patch: 4.6, 9.5, 13.3 mg/24 hours trans-sys (30/carton)

▷ *tacrine* (C) initially 10 mg qid, increase 40 mg/day q 4 weeks as needed; max 160 mg/day

Cognex *Cap:* 10, 20, 30, 40 mg

Comment: Transaminase levels should be checked every 3 months.

N-METHYL-D-ASPARTATE (NMDA) RECEPTOR ANTAGONIST

▷ *memantine* (B)

Namenda (G) initially 5 mg once daily; titrate weekly in 5 mg/day increments; *Week 2:* 5 mg bid; *Week 3:* 5 mg AM and 10 mg PM; *Week 4:* 10 mg bid; *CrCl 5-29 mL/min:* max 5 mg bid

Tab: 5, 10 mg

Namenda Oral Solution (G) initially 5 mg once daily; titrate weekly in 5 mg increments administered bid

Oral soln: 2 mg/ml (360 ml) (peppermint) (sugar-free, alcohol-free)

Namenda Titration Pak

Cap: 7 x 7 mg, 7 x 14 mg, 7 x 21 mg, 7 x 28 mg/pck

Namenda XR (G) initially 7 mg once daily; titrate in 7 mg increments weekly; max 28 mg once daily; do not divide doses

Cap: 7, 14, 21, 28 mg ext-rel

Comment: *memantine* does not halt disease progression. It is indicated for moderate to severe dementia.

N-METHYL-D-ASPARTATE (NMDA) RECEPTOR ANTAGONIST/ACETYLCHOLIN-ESTERASE INHIBITOR COMBINATION

▷ *memantine/donepezil* (C) initiate one 28/10 dose daily in the evening after stabilized on *memantine* and *donepezil* separately; start the day after the last dose of *memantine* and *donepezil* taken separately; swallow whole or open cap and sprinkle on applesauce; *CrCl 5-29 mL/min:* take one 14/10 dose once daily in the evening

Namzaric

Cap: **Namzaric 7/10:** *mem* 7 mg/*done* 10mg
Namzaric 14/10: *mem* 14 mg/*done* 10 mg
Namzaric 21/10: *mem* 21 mg/*done* 10mg
Namzaric 28/10: *mem* 28 mg/*done* 10 mg

ERGOT ALKALOID (DOPAMINE AGONIST)

▷ *ergoloid mesylate* (C) 1 mg tid

Hydergine *Tab:* 1 mg
Hydergine LC *Cap:* 1 mg
Hydergine Liquid *Liq:* 1 mg/ml (100 ml w. calib dropper) (alcohol 28.5%)

⊙ **AMEBIASIS**

AMEBIASIS (INTESTINAL)

▷ *diiodohydroxyquin (iodoquinol)* (C)(G) 650 mg tid pc x 20 days
Pediatric: <6 years: 40 mg/kg/day in 3 divided doses pc x 20 days; max 1.95 g; 6-12 years: 420 mg tid pc x 20 days
Tab: 210, 650 mg

▷ *metronidazole* (**not for use in 1st; B in 2nd, 3rd**)(**G**) 750 mg tid x 5-10 days
Pediatric: 35-50 mg/kg/day in 3 divided doses x 10 days
> **Flagyl** *Tab:* 250*, 500*mg
> **Flagyl 375** *Cap:* 375 mg
> **Flagyl ER** *Tab:* 750 mg ext-rel

Comment: Alcohol is contraindicated during treatment with oral *metronidazole* and for 72 hours after therapy due to a possible *disulfiram*-like reaction (nausea, vomiting, flushing, headache).

▷ *tinidazole* (**not for use in 1st; B in 2nd, 3rd**) 2 g daily x 3 days; take with food
Pediatric: <3 years: not recommended; ≥3 years: 50 mg/kg daily x 3 days; take with food; max 2 g/day
> **Tindamax** *Tab:* 250*, 500*mg

Comment: Alcohol is contraindicated during treatment with oral *tinidazole* and for 72 hours after therapy due to a possible *disulfiram*-like reaction (nausea, vomiting, flushing, headache).

▷ *paromomycin* 25-35 mg/kg/day in 3 divided doses x 5-10 days
Pediatric: same as adult
> **Humatin** *Cap:* 250 mg

AMEBIASIS (EXTRAINTESTINAL)

▷ *chloroquine phosphate* (**C**)(**G**) 1 g PO daily x 2 days; then 500 mg daily x 2 to 3 weeks or 200-250 mg IM daily x 10-12 days (when oral therapy is impossible); use with intestinal amebicide
Pediatric: see mfr pkg insert
> **Aralen** *Tab:* 500 mg; *Amp:* 50 mg/ml (5 ml)

◯ AMEBIC LIVER ABSCESS

ANTI-INFECTIVES

▷ *metronidazole* (**not for use in 1st; B in 2nd, 3rd**)(**G**) 250 mg tid or 500 mg bid or 750 mg daily x 7 days
Pediatric: not recommended
> **Flagyl** *Tab:* 250*, 500*mg
> **Flagyl 375** *Cap:* 375 mg
> **Flagyl ER** *Tab:* 750 mg ext-rel

Comment: Alcohol is contraindicated during treatment with oral *metronidazole* and for 72 hours after therapy due to a possible *disulfiram*-like reaction (nausea, vomiting, flushing, headache).

▷ *tinidazole* (**not for use in 1st; B in 2nd, 3rd**) 2 g once daily x 3-5 days; take with food
Pediatric: <3 years: not recommended; ≥3 years: 50 mg/kg once daily x 3-5 days; take with food; max 2 g/day
> **Tindamax** *Tab:* 250*, 500*mg

Comment: Alcohol is contraindicated during treatment with oral *tinidazole* and for 72 hours after therapy due to a possible *disulfiram*-like reaction (nausea, vomiting, flushing, headache).

⬤ AMENORRHEA: SECONDARY

▷ *estrogen/progesterone* (X)
  Premarin (*estrogen*) 0.625 mg daily x 25 days; then 5 days off; repeat monthly
  Provera (*progesterone*) 5-10 mg last 10 days of cycle; repeat monthly
▷ *estrogen replacement* (X)
  see **Menopause** *page 264*
▷ *human chorionic gonadotropin* 5,000-10,000 units IM x 1 dose following last dose
  of menotropins
  Pregnyl *Vial:* 10,000 units (10 ml) w. diluent (10 ml)
▷ *medroxyprogesterone* (X) *Monthly:* 5-10 mg last 5-10 days of cycle; begin on the
  16th or 21st day of cycle; repeat monthly; *One-time only:* 10 mg once daily x 10 days
  Amen *Tab:* 10 mg
  Provera *Tab:* 2.5, 5, 10 mg
▷ *norethindrone* (X) 2.5-10 mg daily x 5-10 days
  Aygestin *Tab:* 5 mg
▷ *progesterone, micronized* (X)(G) 400 mg q HS x 10 days
  Prometrium *Cap:* 100, 200 mg

  Comment: Administration of *progesterone* induces optimum secretory
  transformation of the *estrogen*-primed endometrium. Administration of
  progesterone is contraindicated with breast cancer, undiagnosed vaginal
  bleeding, genital cancer, severe liver dysfunction or disease, missed abortion,
  thrombophlebitis, thromboembolic disorders, cerebral apoplexy, and pregnancy.

⬤ ANAPHYLAXIS

▷ *epinephrine* (C)(G) 0.3-0.5 mg (0.3-0.5 ml of a 1:1000 soln) SC q 20-30 minutes as
  needed up to 3 doses
  Pediatric: <2 years: 0.05-0.1 ml; 2-6 years: 0.1 ml; ≥6-12 years: 0.2 ml; All: q 20-30
  minutes as needed up to 3 doses; >12 years: same as adult
Parenteral Corticosteroids *see page 511*
Oral Corticosteroids *see page 509*

ANAPHYLAXIS EMERGENCY TREATMENT KITS

▷ *epinephrine* (C) 0.3 ml IM or SC in thigh; may repeat if needed
  Pediatric: 0.01 mg/kg SC or IM in thigh; may repeat if needed; <15 kg: not estab-
  lished; 15-30 kg: 0.15 mg; >30 kg: same as adult
  Adrenaclick *Auto-injector:* 0.15, 0.3 mg (1 mg/ml; 1, 2/carton) (sulfites)
  Auvi-Q *Auto-injector:* 0.15, 0.3 mg (1 mg/ml; 1/pck w. 1 non-active training
  device) (sulfites)
  EpiPen *Auto-injector 0.3 mg* (*epi* 1:1000, 0.3 ml (1, 2/carton) (sulfites)
  EpiPen Jr *Auto-injector 0.15 mg* (*epi* 1:2000, 0.3 ml) (1, 2/carton) (sulfites)
  Twinject *Auto-injector:* 0.15, 0.3 mg (epi 1:1000) (1, 2/carton) (sulfites)
▷ *epinephrine/chlorpheniramine* (C) epinephrine 0.3 ml SC or IM *plus* 4 tabs *chlor-
  pheniramine* by mouth
  Pediatric: infants to 2 years: 0.05-0.1 ml SC or IM; ≥2-6 years: 0.15 ml SC or IM *plus*
  1 tab *chlor;* ≥6-12 years: 0.2 ml SC or IM *plus* 2 tabs *chlor*
  Ana-Kit two 0.3 ml syringes of *epi* 1:1000 for self-injection *plus* *chlor* 2 mg
  chewable tabs x 4

ANEMIA OF CHRONIC KIDNEY DISEASE (CKD) AND CHRONIC RENAL FAILURE (CRF)

ERYTHROPOIESIS STIMULATING AGENTS (ESAs)

▷ *darbepoetin alpha* (erythropoiesis stimulating protein) (C) administer IV or SC q 1-2 weeks; do not increase more frequently than once per month; *Not currently receiving epoetin alpha:* initially 0.75 mcg/kg once weekly; adjust based on Hgb levels (target not to exceed 12 g/dL); reduce dose if Hgb increases more than 1 g/dL in any 2-week period; suspend therapy if polycythemia occurs; *Converting from epoetin alpha and for dose titration:* see mfr pkg insert
Pediatric: not recommended

    Aranesp *Vial:* 25, 40, 60, 100, 150, 200, 300, 500 mcg/ml (single-dose) for IV or SC administration (preservative-free, albumin [human] or polysorbate 80)
    Aranesp Singleject, Aranesp Sureclick Singleject *Prefilled syringe:* 25, 40, 60, 100, 150, 200, 300, 500 mcg (single-dose) for IV or SC administration (preservative-free, albumin [human] or polysorbate 80)

▷ *peginesatide* (C) use lowest effective dose; initiate when Hgb <10 g/dL; do not increase dose more often than every 4 weeks; if Hgb rises rapidly (i.e., >1 g/dL in 2 weeks or >2 g/dL in 4 weeks), reduce dose by 25% or more; if Hgb approaches or exceeds 11 g/dL, reduce or interrupt dose and then when Hgb decreases, resume dose at approximately 25% below previous dose; if Hgb does not increase by >1 g/dL after 4 weeks, increase dose by 25%; if response inadequate after a 12-week escalation period, use lowest dose that will maintain Hgb sufficient to reduce need for RBC transfusion; discontinue if response does not improve; *Not currently on ESA:* initially 0.04 mg/kg as a single IV or SC dose once monthly; *Converting from epoetin alfa:* administer first dose 1 week after last epoetin alfa; *Converting from darbepoetin alfa:* administer first dose at next scheduled dose of darbepoetin alfa
Pediatric: not established

    Omontys *Vial, single-use:* 2, 3, 4, 5, 6 mg (0.5 ml) (preservative-free); *Vial, multi-use:* 10, 20 mg (2 ml) (preservatives); *Prefilled syringe:* 2, 3, 4, 5, 6 mg (0.5 ml) (preservative-free)

ERYTHROPOIETIN HUMAN, RECOMBINANT

▷ *epoetin alpha* (C) individualize; initially 50-100 units/kg 3 x/week; IV (dialysis or nondialysis) or SC (nondialysis); usual max 200 units/kg 3 x/week (dialysis) or 150 units/kg 3 x/week (non-dialysis); target Hct 30-36%
Pediatric: <1 month: not recommended; ≥1 month: individualize; *Dialysis:* initially 50 units/kg 3 x/week IV or SC; target Hct 30-36%

    Epogen *Vial:* 2,000, 3,000, 4,000, 10,000, 40,000 units/ml (1 ml) single-use for IV or SC administration (albumin [human]; preservative-free)
    Epogen Multidose *Vial:* 10,000 units/ml (2 ml); 20,000 units/ml, (1 ml) for IV or SC administration (albumin [human]; benzoyl alcohol)
    Procrit *Vial:* 2,000, 3,000, 4,000, 10,000, 40,000 units/ml (1 ml) single-use for IV or SC administration (albumin [human]) (preservative-free)
    Procrit Multidose *Vial:* 10,000 units/ml (2 ml); 20,000 units/ml, (1 ml) for IV or SC administration (albumin [human]; benzoyl alcohol)

ANEMIA: FOLIC ACID DEFICIENCY

▷ *folic acid* (A)(OTC) 0.4-1 mg once daily

Comment: *folic acid (vitamin B-9)* 400 mcg daily is recommended during pregnancy to prevent neural tube defects. Women who have had a baby with a neural tube defect should take 400 mcg every day, even when not planning to become pregnant, and if planning to become pregnant should take 4 mg daily during the month before becoming pregnant until at least the 12th week of pregnancy.

ANEMIA: IRON DEFICIENCY

Comment: Hemochromatosis and hemosiderosis are contraindications to iron therapy. *Iron* supplements are best absorbed when taken between meals and with *vitamin C*-rich foods. Excessive *iron* may be extremely hazardous to infants and young children. All vitamin and mineral supplements should be kept out of the reach of children.

IRON PREPARATIONS

▷ *ferrous gluconate* (A)(G) 1 tab once daily

    Fergon (OTC)
        Pediatric: not recommended
        Tab: iron 27 mg (240 mg as gluconate)

▷ *ferrous sulfate* (A)(G)

    Feosol Tablets (OTC) 1 tab tid-qid pc and HS
        Pediatric: <6 years: use elixir; ≥6-12 years: 1 tab tid pc
        Tab: iron 65 mg (200 mg as sulfate)
    Feosol Capsules (OTC) 1-2 caps daily
        Pediatric: not recommended
        Cap: iron 50 mg (169 mg as sulfate) sust-rel
    Feosol Elixir (OTC) 5-10 ml tid
        Pediatric: >1 year: 2.5-5 ml tid between meals
        Elix: iron 44 mg (220 mg as sulfate) per 5 ml
    Fer-In-Sol (OTC) 5 ml daily
        Pediatric: <4 years, use drops; ≥4 years: 5 ml once daily
        Syr: iron 18 mg (90 mg as sulfate) per 5 ml (480 ml)
    Fer-In-Sol Drops (OTC)
        Pediatric: <4 years: 0.6 ml daily; ≥4 years: use syrup
        Oral drops: iron 15 mg (75 mg as sulfate) per 5 ml (50 ml)

ANEMIA: MEGALOBLASTIC/ANEMIA: PERNICIOUS

Comment: Signs of *vitamin B-12* deficiency include megaloblastic anemia, glossitis, paresthesias, ataxia, spastic motor weakness, and reduced mentation.

▷ *vitamin B-12 (cyanocobalamin)* (A)(G) 500 mcg intranasally once a week; may increase dose if serum B-12 levels decline; adjust dose in 500 mcg increments

    Nascobal Nasal Spray

Intranasal gel: 500 mcg/0.1 ml (1.3 ml, 4 doses) (citric acid, benzalkonium chloride)
Comment: **Nascobal Nasal Spray** is indicated for maintenance of hematologic remission following IM B-12 therapy without nervous system involvement. Must be primed before each use.

Ⓞ ANGINA PECTORIS: STABLE

▷ *aspirin* (D) 325 mg (range 75-325 mg) once daily
Comment: Daily ASA dose is contingent upon whether the patient is also taking an anticoagulant <u>or</u> antiplatelet agent.

CALCIUM ANTAGONISTS

Comment: Calcium antagonists are contraindicated with history of ventricular arrhythmias, sick sinus syndrome, 2nd <u>or</u> 3rd degree heart block, cardiogenic shock, acute myocardial infarction, and pulmonary congestion.

▷ *amlodipine* (C)(G) 5-10 mg daily
  Pediatric: not recommended
      Norvasc *Tab:* 2.5, 5, 10 mg

▷ *diltiazem* (C)(G)
      Cardizem initially 30 mg qid; may increase gradually every 1-2 days; max 360 mg/day in divided doses
          Pediatric: not recommended
          Tab: 30, 60, 90, 120 mg
      Cardizem CD initially 120-180 mg daily; adjust at 1- to 2-week intervals; max 480 mg/day
          Pediatric: not recommended
          Cap: 120, 180, 240, 300, 360 mg ext-rel
      Cardizem LA initially 180-240 mg daily; titrate at 2 week intervals; max 540 mg/day
          Pediatric: not recommended
          Tab: 120, 180, 240, 300, 360, 420 mg ext-rel
      Cartia XT initially 180 mg <u>or</u> 240 mg once daily; max 540 mg once daily
          Cap: 120, 180, 240, 300 mg ext-rel
      Dilacor XR initially 180 mg <u>or</u> 240 mg once daily; max 540 mg once daily
          Cap: 180, 240 mg ext-rel
      Tiazac initially 120-180 mg daily; max 540 mg/day
          Cap: 120, 180, 240, 300, 360, 420 mg ext-rel

▷ *nicardipine* (C)(G) initially 20 mg tid; adjust q 3 days; max 120 mg/day
  Pediatric: not recommended
      Cardene *Cap:* 20, 30 mg

▷ *nifedipine* (C)(G)
  Pediatric: not recommended
      Adalat CC initially 30 mg once daily; usual range 30-60 mg tid; max 90 mg/day
          Tab: 30, 60, 90 mg ext-rel
      Procardia initially 10 mg tid; titrate over 7-14 days: max 30 mg/dose and 180 mg/day in divided doses
          Cap: 10, 20 mg
      Procardia XL initially 30-60 mg daily; titrate over 7-14 days; max dose 90 mg/day
          Tab: 30, 60, 90 mg ext-rel

▷ **verapamil** (C)(G)
   Pediatric: not recommended
      Calan 80-120 mg tid; increase daily <u>or</u> weekly if needed
        Tab: 40, 80*, 120*mg
      Calan SR initially 120 mg once daily; increase weekly if needed
        Tab: 120, 180, 240 mg
      Covera HS initially 180 mg q HS; titrate in steps to 240 mg; then to 360 mg;
      then 480 mg if needed
        Tab: 180, 240 mg ext-rel
      Isoptin SR initially 120-180 mg in the AM; may increase to 240 mg in the AM;
      then 180 mg q 12 hours <u>or</u> 240 mg in the AM and 120 mg in the PM; then
      240 mg q 12 hours
        Tab: 120, 180*, 240*mg sust-rel

BETA-BLOCKERS

Comment: Beta-blockers are contraindicated with history of sick sinus syndrome
(SSS), 2nd <u>or</u> 3rd degree heart block, cardiogenic shock, pulmonary congestion,
asthma, moderate to severe COPD with FEV1 <50% predicted, patients with chronic
bronchodilator treatment.
▷ **atenolol** (D)(G) initially 25-50 mg daily; increase weekly if needed; max 200 mg
  daily
  Pediatric: not recommended
      Tenormin *Tab:* 25, 50, 100 mg
▷ **metoprolol succinate** (C)
  Pediatric: not recommended
      Toprol-XL initially 100 mg in a single dose once daily; increase weekly if
      needed; max 400 mg/day
        Tab: 25*, 50*, 100*, 200*mg ext-rel
▷ **metoprolol tartrate** (C)
  Pediatric: not recommended
      Lopressor (G) initially 25-50 mg bid; increase weekly if needed; max
      400 mg/day
        Tab: 25, 37.5, 50, 75, 100 mg
▷ **nadolol** (C)(G) initially 40 mg daily; increase q 3-7 days; max 240 mg/day
  Pediatric: not recommended
      Corgard *Tab:* 20*, 40*, 80*, 120*, 160*mg
▷ **propranolol** (C)(G)
  Pediatric: not recommended
      Inderal LA initially 80 mg daily in a single dose; increase q 3-7 days; usual range
      120-160 mg/day; max 320 mg/day in a single dose
        Cap: 60, 80, 120, 160 mg sust-rel
      InnoPran XL initially 80 mg q HS; max 120 mg/day
        Cap: 80, 120 mg ext-rel

NITRATES

Comment: Use a daily nitrate dosing schedule that provides a dose-free period of 14
hours <u>or</u> more to prevent tolerance. **aspirin** and **acetaminophen** may relieve nitrate-
induced headache. *Isosorbide* is not recommended for use in MI <u>and/or</u> CHF. Nitrate
use is a contraindication for using phosphodiesterase type 5 inhibitors: **sildenafil**
(Viagra), **tadalafil** (Cialis), **vardenafil** (Levitra).

▷ *isosorbide dinitrate* (C)
> *Pediatric:* not recommended
>> **Dilatrate-SR** 40 mg once daily; max 160 mg/day
>>> *Cap:* 40 mg sust-rel
>> **Isordil Titradose** initially 5-20 mg q 6 hours; maintenance 10-40 mg q 6 hours
>>> *Tab:* 5, 10, 20, 30, 40 mg

▷ *isosorbide mononitrate* (C)
> *Pediatric:* not recommended
>> **Imdur** initially 30-60 mg q AM; may increase to 120 mg daily; max 240 mg/day
>>> *Tab:* 30*, 60*, 120 mg ext-rel
>> **Ismo** 20 mg upon awakening; then 20 mg 7 hours later
>>> *Tab:* 20*mg

▷ *nitroglycerin* (C)(G)
> *Pediatric:* not recommended
>> **Nitro-Bid Ointment** initially 1/2 inch q 8 hours; titrate in 1/2 inch increments
>>> *Oint:* 2% (20, 60 g)
>> **Nitrodisc** initially one 0.2-0.4 mg/hour patch for 12-14 hours/day
>>> *Transdermal disc:* 0.2, 0.3, 0.4 mg/hour (30, 100/carton)
>> **Nitro-Dur** initially 0.2-0.4 mg/hour patch for 12-14 hours/day
>>> *Transdermal patch:* 0.1, 0.2, 0.3, 0.4, 0.6, 0.8 mg/hour
>> **Nitrolingual Pump Spray** 1-2 sprays on <u>or</u> under tongue; max 3 sprays/15 minutes
>>> *Spray:* 0.4 mg/dose (14.5 g, 200 doses)
>> **Nitromist** 1-2 sprays at onset of attack, on <u>or</u> under the tongue while sitting; may repeat q 5 minutes as needed; max 3 sprays/15 minutes; may use prophylactically 5-10 minutes prior to exertion; do not inhale spray; do not rinse mouth for 5-10 minutes after use
>>> *Lingual aerosol spray:* 0.4 mg/actuation (230 metered sprays)
>> **Nitrostat** 1 tab SL; may repeat q 5 minutes x 3
>>> *SL tab:* 0.3 (1/100 gr), 0.4 (1/150 gr), 0.6 (1/4 gr) mg
>> **Transderm-Nitro** initially one 0.2 mg/hour <u>or</u> 0.4 mg/hour patch for 12-14 hours/day
>>> *Transdermal patch:* 0.1, 0.2, 0.4, 0.6, 0.8 mg/hour

NON-NITRATE PERIPHERAL VASODILATOR

▷ *hydralazine* (C)(G) initially 10 mg qid x 2-4 days; then increase to 25 mg qid for remainder of first week; then increase to 50 mg qid; max 300 mg/day
> *Tab:* 10, 25, 50, 100 mg

NITRATE/PERIPHERAL VASODILATOR COMBINATION

▷ *isosorbide/hydralazine HCl* (C) initially 1 tab tid; max 2 tabs tid
>> **Bidil** *Tab:* isosorb 20 mg/hydral 37.5 mg

NON-NITRATE ANTI-ANGINAL

▷ *ranolazine* (C) initially 500 mg bid; may increase to max 1 g bid
>> **Ranexa** *Tab:* 500, 1000 mg ext-rel
>> **Comment: Ranexa** is indicated for the treatment chronic angina that is inadequately controlled with other antianginals. Use with amlodipine, beta-blocker, <u>or</u> nitrate.

ANOREXIA/CACHEXIA

APPETITE STIMULANTS

▶ *cyproheptadine* (B)(G) initially 4 mg tid prn; then adjust as needed; usual range 12-16 mg/day; max 32 mg/day
Pediatric: <2 years: not recommended; ≥2-6 years: 2 mg bid-tid prn; max 12 mg/day; 7-14 years: 4 mg bid-tid prn; max 16 mg/day; >14 years: same as adult
  Periactin *Tab: cypro* 4*mg; *Syr: cypro* 2 mg/5 ml
▶ *dronabinol* (cannabinoid) (B)(III) initially 2.5 mg bid before lunch and dinner; may reduce to 2.5 mg q HS or increase to 2.5 mg before lunch and 5 mg before dinner; max 20 mg/day in divided doses
Pediatric: not recommended
  Marinol *Cap:* 2.5, 5, 10 mg (sesame oil)
▶ *megestrol* (progestin) (X)(G) 40 mg qid
Pediatric: not recommended
  Megace *Tab:* 20*, 40*mg
  Megace ES *Oral susp (concentrate):* 125 mg/ml; 625 mg/5 ml (5 oz) (lemon-lime)
  Megace Oral Suspension *Oral susp:* 40 mg/ml (8 oz); 820 mg/20 ml) (lemon-lime)
  Megestrol Acetate Oral Suspension (G) 125 mg/ml
Comment: *megestrol* is indicated for the treatment of anorexia, cachexia, or an unexplained, significant weight loss in patients with a diagnosis of AIDS.

ANTHRAX (*BACILLUS ANTHRACIS*)

POSTEXPOSURE PROPHYLAXIS OF INHALATIONAL ANTHRAX AND TREATMENT OF INHALED AND CUTANEOUS ANTHRAX INFECTION

Immune globulin

▶ *bacillus athracis immune globulin intravenous (human)* (NE) administer via IV infusion at a maximum rate of 2 ml/min; dose is weight-based as follows, but may doubled in severe cases if weight >5 kg:
Pediatric: <16 years: not established; 5-<10 kg: 1 vial; 10-<18 kg: 2 vials; 18-<25 kg: 3 vials; 25-<35 kg: 4 vials; 35-<50 kg: 5 vials; 50-<60 kg: 6 vials; ≥60 kg: 7 vials
  Anthrasil *Vial:* (60 units) sterile solution of purified human immune globulin G (IgG) containing polyclonal antibodies that target the anthrax toxins of *Bacillus anthracis* for IV infusion
  Comment: Anthrasil is indicated for the emergent treatment of inhaled anthrax in combination with appropriate antibacterial agents
▶ *ciprofloxacin* (C) 500 mg (or 10-15 mg/kg/day) q 12 hours for 60 days (start as soon as possible after exposure)
Pediatric: <18 years: usually not recommended
  Cipro (G) *Tab:* 250, 500, 750 mg; *Oral susp:* 250, 500 mg/5 ml (100 ml) (strawberry)
  Cipro XR *Tab:* 500, 1000 mg ext-rel
  ProQuin XR *Tab:* 500 mg ext-rel
Comment: *ciprofloxacin* is contraindicated <18 years-of-age, and during pregnancy and lactation. Risk of tendonitis or tendon rupture, especially 60 years-of-age and older.

▷ *doxycycline* (D)(G) 100 mg daily bid
Pediatric: <8 years: not recommended ≥8 years, <100 lb: 2 mg/lb on first day in 2 divided doses, followed by 1 mg/lb/day in a single or divided doses; ≥8 years, ≥100 lb: same as adult; *see page 572 for dose by weight*
  Actilate *Tab:* 75, 150**mg
  Adoxa *Tab:* 50, 75, 100, 150 mg ent-coat
  Doryx *Tab:* 50, 75, 100, 150, 200 mg del-rel
  Monodox *Cap:* 50, 75, 100 mg
  Oracea *Cap:* 40 mg del-rel
  Vibramycin *Tab:* 100 mg; *Cap:* 50, 100 mg; *Syr:* 50 mg/5 ml (raspberry-apple) (sulfites); *Oral susp:* 25 mg/5 ml (raspberry)
  Vibra-Tab *Tab:* 100 mg film-coat
Comment: *doxycycline* is contraindicated <8 years-of-age, in pregnancy, and lactation (discolors developing tooth enamel). A side effect may be photo-sensitivity (photophobia). Do not give with antacids, calcium supplements, milk or other dairy, or within two hours of taking another drug.

▷ *minocycline* (D)(G) 100 mg q 12 hours
Pediatric: <8 years: not recommended; ≥8 years, <100 lb: 2 mg/lb on first day in 2 divided doses, followed by 1 mg/lb q 12 hours x 9 more days; ≥8 years, ≥100 lb: same as adult
  Dynacin *Cap:* 50, 100 mg
  Minocin *Cap:* 50, 75, 100 mg; *Oral susp:* 50 mg/5 ml (60 ml) (custard) (sulfites, alcohol 5%)
Comment: *minocycline* is contraindicated <8 years-of-age, in pregnancy, and lactation (discolors developing tooth enamel). A side effect may be photo-sensitivity (photophobia). Do not give with antacids, calcium supplements, milk or other dairy, or within two hours of taking another drug.

TREATMENT OF INHALATIONAL, GI, AND OROPHARYNGEAL ANTHRAX

▷ *ciprofloxacin* (C) 400 mg IV q 12 hours (start as soon as possible); then, switch to 500 mg PO q 12 hours for total 60 days
Pediatric: <18 years: usually not recommended; 10-15 mg/kg IV q 12 hours (start as soon as possible); then switch to 10-15 mg/kg PO q 12 hours for 60 days
  Cipro (G) *Tab:* 250, 500, 750 mg; *Oral susp:* 250, 500 mg/5 ml (100 ml) (strawberry); *IV conc:* 10 mg/ml after dilution (20, 40 ml); *IV premix:* 2 mg/ml (100, 200 ml)
  Cipro XR *Tab:* 500, 1000 mg ext-rel
  ProQuin XR *Tab:* 500 mg ext-rel
Comment: *ciprofloxacin* is contraindicated <18 years-of-age, and during pregnancy and lactation. Risk of tendonitis or tendon rupture, especially 60 years-of-age and older. Infuse IV *ciprofloxacin* over 60 minutes.

▷ *doxycycline* (D)(G) 100 mg daily bid
Pediatric: <8 years: not recommended ≥8 years, <100 lb: 2 mg/lb on first day in 2 divided doses, followed by 1 mg/lb/day in a single or divided doses; ≥8 years, ≥100 lb: same as adult; *see page 572 for dose by weight*
  Actilate *Tab:* 75, 150**mg
  Adoxa *Tab:* 50, 75, 100, 150 mg ent-coat
  Doryx *Tab:* 50, 75, 100, 150, 200 mg del-rel
  Monodox *Cap:* 50, 75, 100 mg

Oracea *Cap:* 40 mg del-rel
Vibramycin *Tab:* 100 mg; *Cap:* 50, 100 mg; *Syr:* 50 mg/5 ml (raspberry-apple)
(sulfites); *Oral susp:* 25 mg/5 ml (raspberry)
Vibra-Tab *Tab:* 100 mg film-coat

Comment: *doxycycline* is contraindicated <8 years-of-age, in pregnancy, and
lactation (discolors developing tooth enamel). A side effect may be photo-
sensitivity (photophobia). Do not give with antacids, calcium supplements, milk or
other dairy, or within two hours of taking another drug.

▷ *minocycline* (D)(G) 100 mg q 12 hours
Pediatric: <8 years: not recommended; ≥8 years, <100 lb: 2 mg/lb on first day in
2 divided divided doses, followed by 1 mg/lb q 12 hours x 9 more days; ≥8 years,
≥100 lb: same as adult

Dynacin *Cap:* 50, 100 mg
Minocin *Cap:* 50, 75, 100 mg; *Oral susp:* 50 mg/5 ml (60 ml) (custard) (sulfites,
alcohol 5%)

Comment: *minocycline* is contraindicated <8 years-of-age, in pregnancy, and
lactation (discolors developing tooth enamel). A side effect may be photo-
sensitivity (photophobia). Do not give with antacids, calcium supplements, milk or
other dairy, or within two hours of taking another drug.

ANXIETY DISORDER: GENERALIZED (GAD)/ ANXIETY DISORDER: SOCIAL (SAD)

1ST GENERATION ANTIHISTAMINE

▷ *hydroxyzine* (C)(G) 50-100 mg qid; max 600 mg/day
Pediatric: <6 years: 50 mg/day divided qid; ≥6 years: 50-100 mg/day divided qid
Atarax *Tab:* 10, 25, 50, 100 mg; *Syr:* 10 mg/5 ml (alcohol 0.5%)
Vistaril *Cap:* 25, 50, 100 mg; *Oral susp:* 25 mg/5 ml (4 oz) (lemon)

AZASPIRONES

▷ *buspirone* (B) initially 7.5 mg bid; may increase by 5 mg/day q 2-3 days; max 60 mg/
day
Pediatric: <6 years: not recommended; 6-17 years: same as adult
BuSpar *Tab:* 5, 10, 15*, 30* mg

BENZODIAZEPINES

Comment: If possible when considering a benzodiazepine to treat anxiety, a short-
acting benzodiazepines should be used only prn to avert intense anxiety and panic
for the least time necessary while a different non-addictive antianxiety regimen (e.g.,
SSRI, SNRI, TCA, **buspirone**, beta-blocker) is established and effective treatment goals
achieved. Benzodiazepines have a high addiction potential when they are chronically
used and are common drugs of abuse. *Benzodiazepine withdrawal syndrome* may
include restlessness, agitation, anxiety, insomnia, tachycardia, tachypnea, diaphoresis,
and may be potentially life threatening depending on the benzodiazepine and the
length of use. Symptoms of withdrawal from short-acting benzodiazepines, such as
alprazolam (Xanax), *oxazepam*, *lorazepam* (Ativan), *triazolam* (Halcion), usually

appear within 6-8 hours after the last dose and may continue 10-14 days. Symptoms of withdrawal from long-acting benzodiazepines, such as *diazepam* (Valium), *clonazepam* (Klonopin), *chlordiazepam* (Librium), usually appear within 24-96 hours after the last dose and may continue from 3-4 weeks to 3 months. People who are heavily dependent on benzodiazepines may experience *protracted withdrawal syndrome* (PAWS), random periods of sharp withdrawal symptoms months after quitting. A closely monitored medical detoxification regimen may be required for a safe withdrawal and to prevent PAWS. Detoxification includes gradual tapering of the benzodiazepine along with other medications to manage the withdrawal symptoms.

Short Acting

▷ *alprazolam* (D)(IV)(G)
Pediatric: <18 years: not recommended
   Niravam initially 0.25-0.5 mg tid; may titrate every 3-4 days; max 4 mg/day
      Tab: 0.25*, 0.5*, 1*, 2*mg orally-disint
   Xanax initially 0.25-0.5 mg tid; may titrate every 3-4 days; max 4 mg/day
      Tab: 0.25*, 0.5*, 1*, 2*mg
   Xanax XR initially 0.5-1 mg once daily, preferably in the AM; increase at intervals of at least 3-4 days by up to 1 mg/day. Taper no faster than 0.5 mg every 3 days; max 10 mg/day. When switching from immediate-release *alprazolam*, give total daily dose of immediate-release once daily.
      Tab: 0.5, 1, 2, 3 mg ext-rel
▷ *oxazepam* (C)(IV)(G) 10-15 mg tid-qid for moderate symptoms; 15-30 mg tid-qid for severe symptoms
Pediatric: not recommended
Cap: 10, 15, 30 mg

Intermediate Acting

▷ *lorazepam* (D)(IV)(G) 1-10 mg/day in 2-3 divided doses
Pediatric: not recommended
   Ativan *Tab:* 0.5, 1*, 2*mg
   Lorazepam Intensol *Oral conc:* 2 mg/ml (30 ml w. graduated dropper)

Long Acting

▷ *chlordiazepoxide* (D)(IV)(G)
Pediatric: <6 years: not recommended; ≥6 years: 5 mg bid-qid; increase to 10 mg bid-tid
   Librium 5-10 mg tid-qid for moderate symptoms; 20-25 mg tid-qid for severe symptoms
      Cap: 5, 10, 25 mg
   Librium Injectable 50-100 mg IM or IV; then 25-50 mg IM tid-qid prn; max 300 mg/day
      Inj: 100 mg
▷ *chlordiazepoxide/clidinium* (D)(IV) 1-2 caps tid-qid: max 8 caps/day
Pediatric: not recommended
   Librax *Cap: chlor* 5 mg/*clid* 2.5 mg
▷ *clonazepam* (D)(IV)(G) initially 0.25 mg bid; increase to 1 mg/day after 3 days
Pediatric: <18 years: not recommended
   Klonopin *Tab:* 0.5*, 1, 2 mg

  Klonopin Wafers dissolve in mouth with or without water
   Wafer: 0.125, 0.25, 0.5, 1, 2 mg orally-disint
▷ *clorazepate* (D)(IV)(G) 30 mg/day in divided doses; max 60 mg/day
 Pediatric: <9 years: not recommended; ≥9 years: same as adult
  Tranxene *Tab:* 3.75, 7.5, 15 mg
  Tranxene SD do not use for initial therapy
   Tab: 22.5 mg ext-rel
  Tranxene SD Half Strength do not use for initial therapy
   Tab: 11.25 mg ext-rel
  Tranxene T-Tab *Tab:* 3.75*, 7.5*, 15*mg
▷ *diazepam* (D)(IV)(G) 2-10 mg bid to qid
 Pediatric: not recommended
  Diastat *Rectal gel delivery system:* 2.5 mg
  Diastat AcuDial *Rectal gel delivery system:* 10, 20 mg
  Valium *Tab:* 2*, 5*, 10*mg
  Valium Injectable *Vial:* 5 mg/ml (10 ml); *Amp:* 5 mg/ml (2 ml); *Prefilled syringe:*
  5 mg/ml (5 ml)
  Valium Intensol Oral Solution *Conc oral soln:* 5 mg/ml (30 ml w. dropper)
  (alcohol 19%)
  Valium Oral Solution *Oral soln:* 5 mg/5 ml (500 ml) (wintergreen spice)

TRICYCLIC ANTIDEPRESSANTS (TCAs)

Comment: Co-administration of TCAs with SSRIs requires extreme caution.
▷ *doxepin* (C)(G) usual optimum dose 75-150 mg/day; elderly lower initial dose and
 therapeutic dose; max single dose 150 mg; max 300 mg/day in divided doses
  Sinequan
   Pediatric: not recommended
   Cap: 10, 25, 50, 75, 100, 150 mg; *Oral conc:* 10 mg/ml (4 oz w. dropper)
Comment: Glaucoma, urinary retention, and bipolar disorder are contraindications
to *doxepin*. Separate from MAOIs by at least 14 days. Separate from *fluoxetine* by at
least 5 weeks. Avoid abrupt cessation. doxepin is potentiated by CYP2D6 inhibitors
(e.g., *cimetidine*, SSRIs, phenothiazines, type 1C antiarrhythmics).

PHENOTHIAZINES

▷ *prochlorperazine* (C)(G)
  Compazine 5 mg tid-qid
   Pediatric: not recommended
   Tab: 5 mg; *Syr:* 5 mg/5 ml (4 oz) (fruit); *Rectal supp:* 2.5, 5, 25 mg
  Compazine Spansule 15 mg q AM or 10 mg q 12 hours
   Pediatric: not recommended
   Spansule: 10, 15 mg sust-rel
▷ *trifluoperazine* (C)(G) 1-2 mg bid; max 6 mg/day; max 12 weeks
 Pediatric: not recommended
  Stelazine *Tab:* 1, 2, 5, 10 mg

SELECTIVE SEROTONIN REUPTAKE INHIBITORS (SSRIs)

Comment: Co-administration of SSRIs with TCAs requires extreme caution.
Concomitant use of MAOIs and SSRIs is absolutely contraindicated. Avoid St. John's

wort and other serotonergic agents. A potentially fatal adverse event is *serotonin syndrome*, caused by serotonin excess. Milder symptoms require HCP intervention to avert severe symptoms that can be rapidly fatal without urgent/emergent medical care. Symptoms include restlessness, agitation, confusion, tachycardia, hypertension, dilated pupils, muscle twitching, muscle rigidity, loss of muscle coordination, diaphoresis, diarrhea, headache, shivering, piloerection, hyperpyrexia, cardiac arrhythmias, seizures, loss of consciousness, coma, death. Common symptoms of the *serotonin discontinuation syndrome* include flu-like symptoms (nausea, vomiting, diarrhea, headaches, diaphoresis); sleep disturbances (insomnia, nightmares, constant sleepiness); mood disturbances (dysphoria, anxiety, agitation); cognitive disturbances (mental confusion, hyperarousal); and sensory and movement disturbances (imbalance, tremors, vertigo, dizziness, electric-shock-like sensations in the brain often described by sufferers as "brain zaps").

▷ *escitalopram* (C)(G) initially 10 mg daily; may increase to 20 mg daily after 1 week; *Elderly* or hepatic impairment, 10 mg once daily

Pediatric: <12 years: not recommended; 12-17 years: initially 10 mg once daily; may increase to 20 mg once daily after 3 weeks

Lexapro *Tab:* 5, 10*, 20*mg

Lexapro Oral Solution *Oral soln:* 1 mg/ml (240 ml) (peppermint) (parabens)

▷ *fluoxetine* (C)(G)

Prozac initially 20 mg daily; may increase after 1 week; doses >20 mg/day may be divided into AM and noon doses; max 80 mg/day

Pediatric: <8 years: not recommended; 8-17 years: initially 10-20 mg once daily; start lower weight children at 10 mg once daily; if starting at 10 mg once daily, may increase after 1 week to 20 mg once daily

Cap: 10, 20, 40 mg; *Tab:* 30*, 60*mg; *Oral soln:* 20 mg/5 ml (4 oz) (mint)

Prozac Weekly following daily *fluoxetine* therapy at 20 mg/day x 13 weeks, may initiate **Prozac Weekly** 7 days after the last 20 mg *fluoxetine* dose

Pediatric: not recommended

Cap: 90 mg ent-coat del-rel pellets

▷ *paroxetine maleate* (D)(G)

Pediatric: not recommended

Paxil initially 10-20 mg daily in AM; may increase by 10 mg/day at weekly intervals as needed; max 60 mg/day

Tab: 10*, 20*, 30, 40 mg

Paxil CR initially 12.5-25 mg daily in AM; may increase by 12.5 mg at weekly intervals as needed; max 62.5 mg/day

Tab: 12.5, 25, 37.5 mg ent-coat cont-rel

Paxil Suspension initially 10-20 mg daily in AM; may increase by 10 mg/day at weekly intervals as needed; max 60 mg/day

Oral susp: 10 mg/5 ml (250 ml) (orange)

▷ *sertraline* (C) initially 50 mg daily; increase at 1 week intervals if needed; max 200 mg daily

Pediatric: <6 years: not recommended; 6-12 years: initially 25 mg daily; max 200 mg/day; 13-17 years: initially 50 mg daily; max 200 mg/day

Zoloft *Tab:* 15*, 50*, 100*mg; *Oral conc:* 20 mg per ml (60 ml [dilute just before administering in 4 oz water, ginger ale, lemon-lime soda, lemonade, or orange juice]) (alcohol 12%)

SEROTONIN AND NOREPINEPHRINE REUPTAKE INHIBITORS (SNRIs)

▷ *venlafaxine* (C)(G)
Effexor initially 75 mg/day in 2-3 divided doses; may increase at 4 day intervals in 75 mg increments to 150 mg/day; max 225 mg/day
Pediatric: <18 years: not recommended
Tab: 37.5, 75, 150, 225 mg
Effexor XR initially 75 mg q AM; may start at 37.5 mg daily x 4-7 days; then increase by increments of up to 75 mg/day at intervals of at least 4 days; usual max 375 mg/day
Pediatric: not recommended
Tab: Cap: 37.5, 75, 150 mg ext-rel

COMBINATION AGENTS

▷ *chlordiazepoxide/amitriptyline* (D)(G)
Pediatric: not recommended
Limbitrol 3-4 tabs/day in divided doses
Tab: chlor 5 mg/*amit* 12.5 mg
Limbitrol DS 3-4 tabs/day in divided doses; max 6 tabs/day
Tab: chlor 10 mg/*amit* 25 mg
▷ *perphenazine/amitriptyline* (C)(G) 1 tab bid-qid
Pediatric: not recommended
Tab: **Etrafon 2-10:** *perph* 2 mg/*amit* 10 mg
Etrafon 2-25: *perph* 2 mg/*amit* 25 mg
Etrafon 4-25: *perph* 4 mg/*amit* 25 mg

APHTHOUS STOMATITIS (MOUTH ULCER, CANKER SORE)

ANTI-INFLAMMATORY AGENTS

▷ *dexamethasone* elixir (B) 5 ml swish and spit q 12 hours
Pediatric: not recommended
Elix: 0.5 mg/ml
▷ *triamcinolone acetonide* 0.1% dental paste (NE)(G) press (do not rub) thin film onto lesion at bedtime and, if needed, 2-3 x daily after meals; re-evaluate if no improvement in 7 days
Oralone *Dental paste:* 0.1% (5 g)
▷ *triamcinolone* 1% in **Orabase** (B) apply 1/4 inch to each ulcer bid-qid until ulcer heals
Pediatric: not recommended
Kenalog in Orabase *Crm:* 1% (15, 60, 80 g)

TOPICAL ANESTHETICS

▷ *benzocaine* topical gel (C)(G) apply tid-qid
▷ *benzocaine* topical spray (C)(G) 1 spray to painful area every 2 hours as needed; retain for 15 seconds, then spit
Cepocal Spray (OTC), **Chloraseptic Spray** (OTC)

> *lidocaine* viscous soln (B)(G) 15 ml gargle or swish, then spit; repeat after 3 hours; max 8 doses/day
> *Pediatric:* <3 years: 1.25 ml; apply with cotton-tipped applicator; may repeat after 3 hours; max 8 doses/day
>> **Xylocaine Viscous Solution** *Viscous soln:* 2% (20, 100, 450 ml)
> *triamcinolone* (**Kenalog**) in **Orabase** (C) apply with swab

DEBRIDING AGENT/CLEANSER

> *carbamide peroxide 10%* (NE)(OTC) apply 10 drops to affected area; swish x 2-3 minutes, then spit; do not rinse; repeat treatment qid
>> **Gly-Oxide** *Liq:* 10% (50, 60 ml squeeze bottle w. applicator)

ANTI-INFECTIVES

> *minocycline* (D)(G) swish and spit 10 ml susp (50 mg/5 ml) or 1 x 100 mg cap or 2 x 50 mg caps dissolved in 180 ml water, bid x 4-5 days
> *Pediatric:* <8 years: not recommended; ≥8 years: same as adult
>> **Dynacin** *Cap:* 50, 100 mg
>> **Minocin** *Cap:* 50, 75, 100 mg; *Oral susp:* 50 mg/5 ml (60 ml) (custard) (sulfites, alcohol 5%)
>
> Comment: *minocycline* is contraindicated <8 years-of-age, in pregnancy, and lactation (discolors developing tooth enamel). A side effect may be photo-sensitivity (photophobia). Do not give with antacids, calcium supplements, milk or other dairy, or within two hours of taking another drug.
> *tetracycline* (D) swish and spit 10 ml susp (125 mg/5 ml) or one 250 mg tab/cap dissolved in 180 ml water qid x 4-5 days
> *Pediatric:* <8 years: not recommended; ≥8 years: same as adult; *see page* 585 *for dose by weight*
>> **Achromycin V** *Cap:* 250, 500 mg
>> **Sumycin** *Tab:* 250, 500 mg; *Cap:* 250, 500 mg; *Oral susp:* 125 mg/5 ml (100, 200 ml) (fruit) (sulfites)
>
> Comment: *tetracycline* is contraindicated <8 years-of-age, in pregnancy, and lactation (discolors developing tooth enamel). A side effect may be photo-sensitivity (photophobia). Do not give with antacids, calcium supplements, milk or other dairy, or within two hours of taking another drug.

ASPERGILLOSIS (*SCEDOSPORIUM APIOSPERMUM, FUSARIUM* SPP.)

INVASIVE INFECTION

> *isavuconazonium* (C) swallow cap whole; *Loading dose:* 372 mg q 8 hours x 6 doses (48 hours); *Maintenance:* 372 mg once daily starting 12-24 hours after last loading dose
> *Pediatric:* <18 years: not established
>> **Cresemba** *Cap:* 186 mg; *Vial:* 372 mg pwdr for reconstitution (7/blister pck) (preservative-free)

Comment: **Cresemba** is indicated for the treatment of invasive aspergillus and mucormycosis in patients >18-years-old who are at high risk due to being severely compromised.

▷ *posaconazole* **(D)** take with food; swallow tab whole; *Day 1:* 300 mg bid; then 300 mg once daily for duration of treatment (e.g., resolution of neutropenia or immunosuppression)
 Pediatric: <13 years: not recommended; ≥13 years: same as adult
  Noxafil *Tab:* 100 mg del-rel; *Oral susp:* 40 mg/ml (105 oz w. dosing spoon) (cherry)
  Comment: **Noxafil** is indicated as prophylaxis for invasive aspergillus and candida infections in patients >13-years-old who are at high risk due to being severely compromised.

▷ *voriconazole* **(D)(G)** PO: <40 kg: 100 mg q 12 hours; may increase to 150 mg q 12 hours if inadequate response; >40 kg: 200 mg q 12 hours; may increase to 300 mg q 12 hours if inadequate response; *IV:* 6 mg/kg q 12 hours x 2 doses; then 4 mg/kg q 12 hours; max rate 3 mg/kg/hour over 1-2 hours
 Pediatric: not recommended
  Vfend *Tab:* 50, 200 mg
  Vfend I.V. for Injection *Vial:* 200 mg pwdr for reconstitution (preservative-free)
  Vfend *Oral susp:* 40 mg/ml pwdr for reconstitution (75 ml) (orange)

⭕ ASTHMA

Parenteral Corticosteroids *see page* 511
Oral Corticosteroids *see page* 509

LEUKOTRIENE RECEPTOR ANTAGONISTS (LRAs)

Comment: The LRAs are indicated for prophylaxis and chronic treatment, only. Not for primary (rescue) treatment of acute asthma attack.

▷ *montelukast* **(B)(G)** 10 mg once daily in the PM; for EIB, take at least 2 hours before exercise; max 1 dose/day
 Pediatric: <12 months: not recommended; 12-23 months: one 4 mg granule pkt daily; 2-5 years: one 4 mg chew tab or granule pkt daily; 6-14 years: one 5 mg chew tab daily; ≥15 years: same as adult
  Singulair *Tab:* 10 mg
  Singulair Chewable *Chew tab:* 4, 5 mg (cherry) (phenylalanine)
  Singulair Oral Granules *Granules:* 4 mg/pkt; take within 15 minutes of opening pkt; may mix with applesauce, carrots, rice, or ice cream

▷ *zafirlukast* **(B)** 20 mg bid, 1 hour ac or 2 hours pc
 Pediatric: <7 years: not recommended; 7-11 years: 10 mg bid 1 hour ac or 2 hours pc; ≥12 years: same as adult
  Accolate *Tab:* 10, 20 mg

▷ *zileuton* **(C)**
 Pediatric: <12 years: not recommended; ≥12 years: same as adult
  Zyflo 1 tab qid
   Tab: 600 mg
  Zyflo CR 2 tabs bid
   Tab: 600 mg ext-rel

IGE BLOCKER (IGG1K MONOCLONAL ANTIBODY)

▷ *omalizumab* (B) 150-375 mg SC every 2-4 weeks based on body weight and pre-treatment serum total IgE level; max 150 mg/injection site
Pediatric: <12 years: not recommended; 30-90 kg + IgE >30-100 IU/ml 150 mg q 4 weeks; 90-150 kg + IgE >30-100 IU/ml or 30-90 kg + IgE >100-200 IU/ml or 30-60 kg + IgE >200-300 IU/ml 300 mg q 4 hours; >90-150 kg + IgE >100-200 IU/ml or >60-90 kg + IgE >200-300 IU/ml or 30-70 kg + IgE >300-400 IU/ml 225 mg q 2 weeks; >90-150 kg + IgE >200-300 IU/ml or >70-90 kg + IgE >300-400 IU/ml or 30-70 kg + IgE >400-500 IU/ml or 30-60 kg + IgE >500-600 IU/ml or 30-60 kg + IgE >600-700 IU/ml 375 mg q 2 weeks
  Xolair *Vial:* 150 mg pwdr for SC injection after reconstitution (preservative-free)

INHALED ANTICHOLINERGICS

▷ *ipratropium bromide* (C)(G)
  Atrovent 2 inhalations qid; additional inhalations as required; max 12 inhalations/day
    Pediatric: not recommended
    Inhaler: 18 mcg/actuation (14 g, 200 inh)
  Atrovent Inhalation Solution 500 mcg tid-qid prn by nebulizer
    Pediatric: not recommended
    Inhal soln: 0.02% (500 mcg in 2.5 ml; 25/carton)

INHALED CORTICOSTEROIDS

Comment: Instruct patient to rinse mouth after using an inhaled steroid to reduce risk of oral candidiasis. Not for primary (rescue) treatment of acute asthma attack.
▷ *beclomethasone dipropionate* (C)(G) *Previously using only bronchodilators:* initiate 40-80 mcg bid; max 320 mcg bid; *Previously using inhaled corticosteroid:* initiate 40-160 mcg bid; max 320 mcg/day; *Previously taking a systemic corticosteroid:* attempt to to wean off the systemic drug after approximately 1 week after initiating; rinse mouth after use
Pediatric: not recommended
  Qvar
    Inhal aerosol: 40, 80 mcg/metered dose actuation (8.7 g, 120 inh) metered dose inhaler (chlorofluorocarbon [CFC]-free)
▷ *budesonide* (B)
  Pulmicort Flexhaler initially 180-360 mcg bid; max 360 mcg bid; rinse mouth after use
    Pediatric: <6 years: not recommended; ≥6 years: 1-2 inhalations bid
    Flexhaler: 90 mcg/actuation (60 inh); 180 mcg/actuation (120 inh)
  Pulmicort Respules (G) adult use flexhaler
    Pediatric: <12 months: not recommended; 12 months-8 years: *Previously using only bronchodilators:* initiate 0.5 mg/day once daily or in 2 divided doses; may start at 0.25 mg daily; *Previously using inhaled corticosteroids:* initiate 0.5 mg once daily or in 2 divided doses; max 1 mg/day; *Previously taking oral corticosteroids:* initiate 1 mg/day daily or in 2 divided doses; >8 years: use flexhaler; rinse mouth after use
    Inhal susp: 0.25, 0.5, 1 mg/2 ml (30/carton)

▷ *ciclesonide* (C) initially 80 mcg bid; max 320 mcg/day; rinse mouth after use; *Previously on inhaled corticosteroid:* initially 80 mcg bid; *Previously on oral steroid:* 320 mg bid
Pediatric: <12 years: not recommended; ≥12 years: same as adult
    Alvesco
    Inhal aerosol: 80, 160 mcg/actuation (6.1 g, 60 inh)

▷ *flunisolide* (C) rinse mouth after use
    AeroBid, AeroBid-M initially 2 inhalations bid; max 8 inhalations/day; rinse mouth after use
    Pediatric: <6 years: not recommended; 6-15 years: 2 inhalations bid; ≥15 years: same as adult
    Inhaler: 250 mcg/actuation (7 g, 100 inh)
    Aerospan HFA initially 160 mcg bid; max 320 mcg bid
    Pediatric: <6 years: not recommended; 6-11 years: 80 mcg bid; max 160 mcg bid; ≥12 years: same as adult
    Inhaler: 80 mcg (5.1 g, 60 doses; 80 mcg, 120 doses)

▷ *fluticasone furoate* (C) *currently not on inhaled corticosteroid:* usually initiate at 100 mcg once daily at the same time each day; may increase to 200 mcg once daily if inadequate response after 2 weeks; max 200 mcg/day; rinse mouth after use
Pediatric: not established
    Arnuity Ellipta *Inhal:* 100, 200 mcg/dry pwdr per inhalation (30 doses)
    Comment: **Arnuity Ellipta** is not for primary treatment of status asthmaticus <u>or</u> acute asthma episodes. **Arnuity Ellipta** is contraindicated with severe hypersensitivity to milk proteins.

▷ *fluticasone propionate* (C)
    Flovent, Flovent HFA initially 88 mcg bid; *Previously using an inhaled corticosteroid:* initially 88-220 mcg bid; *Previously taking an oral corticosteroid:* 880 mcg bid; rinse mouth after use
    Pediatric: use **Flovent Diskus**
    Inhaler: 44 mcg/actuation (7.9 g, 60 inh; 13 g, 120 inh); 110 mcg/actuation (13 g, 120 inh); 220 mcg/actuation (13 g, 120 inh)
    Flovent Diskus initially 100 mcg bid; max 500 mcg bid; *Previously using an inhaled corticosteroid:* initially 100-250 mcg bid; max 500 mcg bid; *Previously taking an oral corticosteroid:* 1000 mcg bid
    Pediatric: <4 years: not recommended; 4-11 years: initially 50 mcg bid; max 100 mcg bid; rinse mouth after use; ≥12 years: same as adult
    Diskus: 50, 100, 250 mcg/inh dry pwdr (60 blisters w. diskus)

▷ *mometasone furoate* (C) 220-440 mcg once daily <u>or</u> bid; max 880 mcg/day; rinse mouth after use
    Asmanex HFA *Inhaler:* 100, 200 mcg/actuation (13 g, 120 inh)
    Pediatric: not established
    Asmanex Twisthaler *Inhaler:* 110 mcg/actuation (30 inh), 220 mcg/actuation (30, 60, 120 inh)
    Pediatric: <4 years: not recommended; 4-11 years: 110 mcg once daily in the PM; rinse mouth after use

▷ *triamcinolone* (C)
    Azmacort 2 inhalations tid-qid <u>or</u> 4 inhalations bid; rinse mouth after use
    Pediatric: <6 years: not recommended; 6-12 years: 1-2 inhalations tid <u>or</u> 2-4 inhalations bid; >12 years: same as adult
    Inhaler: 100 mcg/actuation (20 g, 240 inh)

INHALED MAST CELL STABILIZERS (PROPHYLAXIS)

Comment: IMCSs are for prophylaxis and chronic treatment, only. Not for primary (rescue) treatment of acute asthma attack.

▷ *cromolyn sodium* (B)(G)

Intal 2 inhalations qid; 2 inhalations up to 10-60 minutes before precipitant as prophylaxis; rinse mouth after use

Pediatric: <2 years: not recommended; 2-5 years: use inhal soln via nebulizer; >5 years: 2 inhalations qid via inhaler

Inhaler: 0.8 mg/actuation (8.1, 14.2 g; 112, 200 inh)

Intal Inhalation Solution 20 mg by nebulizer qid; 20 mg up to 10-60 minutes before precipitant as prophylaxis

Pediatric: <2 years: not recommended; ≥2 years: same as adult

Inhal soln: 20 mg/2 ml (60, 120/carton)

▷ *nedocromil sodium* (B)

Tilade 2 sprays qid; rinse mouth after use

Pediatric: <6 years: not recommended; ≥6 years: 2 sprays qid

Inhaler: 1.75 mg/spray (16.2 g; 104 sprays)

Tilade Nebulizer Solution 0.5% 1 amp qid by nebulizer

Pediatric: <2 years: not recommended; ≥2 years: initially 1 amp qid by nebulizer; 2-5 years: initially 1 amp tid by nebulizer; ≥5 years: same as adult

Inhal soln: 11 mg/2.2 ml (2 ml; 60, 120/carton)

INHALED BETA AGONISTS (BRONCHODILATORS)

▷ *albuterol sulfate* (C)(G)

AccuNeb Inhalation Solution 1 unit-dose vial tid-qid prn by nebulizer; ages 2-12 years only; not for adult

Pediatric: <2 years: not recommended; 2-12 years: initially 0.63 mg or 1.25 mg tid-qid; 6-12 years: with severe asthma, or >40 kg, or 11-12 years: initially 1.25 mg tid-qid

Inhal soln: 0.63, 1.25 mg/3ml (3 ml, 25/carton) (preservative-free)

Albuterol Inhalation Solution (G) not recommended

Pediatric: <2 years: not recommended; ≥2 years: 1 vial via nebulizer over 5-15 minutes

Inhal soln: 0.63 mg/3 ml (0.021%); 1.25 mg/3 ml (0.042%) (25/carton)

Albuterol Inhalation Solution 0.5% (G) not recommended

Pediatric: <4 years: not recommended; ≥4 years: same as adult

Inhal soln: 0.083% (25/carton)

Albuterol Nebules (G) 2.5 mg (0.5 ml of 5% diluted to 3 ml with sterile NS or 3 ml of 0.083%) tid-qid

Pediatric: use other forms

Inhal soln: 0.083% (25/carton)

Proair HFA Inhaler 1-2 inhalations q 4-6 hours prn; 2 inhalations 15 minutes before exercise as prophylaxis for exercise-induced asthma (EIA)

Pediatric: <4 years: not established; ≥4 years: same as adult

Inhaler: 90 mcg/actuation (0.65 g, 200 inh) (CFC-free)

Proair RespiClick 1-2 inhalations q 4-6 hours prn; 2 inhalations 15-30 minutes before exercise as prophylaxis for exercise-induced asthma (EIA)

Pediatric: not established

Inhaler: 90 mcg/actuation (8.5 g, 200 inh)

Proventil HFA Inhaler 1-2 inhalations q 4-6 hours prn; 2 inhalations 15 minutes before exercise as prophylaxis for exercise-induced asthma (EIA)

Pediatric: <4 years: use syrup; ≥4 years: same as adult

Inhaler: 90 mcg/actuation with a dose counter (6.7 g, 200 inh)

Proventil Inhalation Solution 2.5 mg diluted to 3 ml with normal saline tid-qid prn by nebulizer

Pediatric: use syrup

Inhal soln: 0.5% (20 ml w. dropper); 0.083% (3 ml; 25/carton)

Ventolin Inhaler 2 inhalations q 4-6 hours prn; 2 inhalations 15 minutes before exercise as prophylaxis for exercise-induced asthma

Pediatric: <2 years: not recommended; 2-4 years: use syrup; >4 years: same as adult

Inhaler: 90 mcg/actuation (17 g, 220 inh)

Ventolin Rotacaps 1-2 cap inhalations q 4-6 hours prn; 2 inhalations 15 minutes before exercise as prophylaxis for exercise-induced asthma (EIA)

Pediatric: <4 years: not recommended; ≥4 years 1-2 caps q 4-6 hours prn

Rotacaps: 200 mcg/Rotacaps (100 doses/Rotacaps)

Ventolin 0.5% Inhalation Solution

Pediatric: <2 years: not recommended; ≥2 years: initially 0.1-0.15 mg/kg/dose tid-qid prn; 10-15 kg: 0.25 ml diluted to 3 ml with normal saline by nebulizer tid-qid prn; >15 kg: 0.5 ml diluted to 3 ml with normal saline by nebulizer tid-qid prn

Inhal soln: 20 ml w. dropper

Ventolin Nebules

Pediatric: <2 years: not recommended; ≥2 years: initially 0.1-0.15 mg/kg/dose tid-qid prn; 10-15 kg: 1.25 mg or 1/2 nebule tid-qid prn; >15 kg: 2.5 mg or 1 nebule tid-qid prn

Inhal soln: 0.083% (3 ml; 25/carton)

▷ *isoproterenol* (B) *Rescue:* 1 inhalation prn; repeat if no relief in 2-5 minutes; *Maintenance:* 1-2 inhalations q 4-6 hours

Pediatric: <12 years: not recommended; ≥12 years: same as adult

Medihaler-ISO *Inhaler:* 80 mcg/actuation (15 ml, 30 inh)

▷ *levalbuterol tartrate* (C)(G) initially 0.63 mg tid q 6-8 hours prn by nebulizer; may increase to 1.25 mg tid at 6-8 hour intervals as needed

Pediatric: not recommended

Xopenex *Inhal soln:* 0.31, 0.63, 1.25 mg/3 ml (24/carton) (preservative-free)

Xopenex HFA *Inh:* 45 mg (15 g, 200 inh) (preservative-free)

Xopenex Concentrate *Vial:* 1.25 mg/0.5 ml (30/carton) (preservative-free)

▷ *metaproterenol* (C)(G)

Alupent 2-3 inhalations tid-qid prn; max 12 inhalations/day

Pediatric: <6 years: use syrup; ≥6 years: via nebulizer 0.1-0.2 ml diluted with normal saline to 3 ml, up to q 4 hours prn

Inhaler: 0.65 mg/actuation (14 g, 200 doses)

Alupent Inhalation Solution 5-15 inhalations tid-qid prn; q 4 hours prn for acute attack

Pediatric: <6 years: use syrup ≥6 years: via nebulizer 0.1-0.2 ml diluted with normal saline to 3 ml, up to q 4 hours prn

Inhal soln: 5% (10, 30 ml w. dropper)

▷ *pirbuterol* (C) 1-2 inhalations q 4-6 hours prn; max 12 inhalations/day
    Maxair
        Pediatric: <12 years: not recommended
        Autohaler: 200 mcg/actuation (14 g, 400 inh); *Inhaler:* 200 mcg/actuation (25.6 g, 300 inh)
▷ *terbutaline* (B) 2 inhalations q 4-6 hours prn
    Pediatric: not recommended
    Inhaler: 0.2 mg/actuation (10.5 g, 300 inh)

INHALED RACEPINEPHRINE (BRONCHODILATOR)

▷ *racepinephrine* (C)(OTC)(G) 1-3 inhalations not more than every 3 hours; max 12 inhalations/24 hours
    Pediatric: <4 years: not recommended; ≥4 years: same as adult
        Asthmanephrin Inhaler *Starter kit:* 10 x 0.5 ml vials 2.25% solution for atomized inhalation w. EZ Breathe Atomizer; *Refills:* 30 x 0.5 ml vials 2.25% solution for atomized inhalation
Comment: Inhalational epinephrine is only recommended for use during pregnancy when there are no alternatives and benefit outweighs risk.

INHALED LONG-ACTING ANTICHOLINERGIC

▷ *tiotropium (as bromide monohydrate)* (C) 2 inhalations once daily using inhalation device; do not swallow caps
    Pediatric: <12 years: not recommended; ≥12 years: same as adult
        Spiriva HandiHaler *Inhal device:* 18 mcg/cap pwdr for inhalation (5, 30, 90 caps w. inhalation device)
        Spiriva Respimat *Inhal device:* 1.25, 2.5 mcg/actuation cartridge w. inhalation device (4 g, 60 metered actuations) (benzylkonian chloride)
Comment: *tiotropium* is for prophylaxis and chronic treatment, only. Not for primary (rescue) treatment of acute attack. Avoid getting powder in eyes. Caution with narrow-angle glaucoma, BPH, bladder neck obstruction, and pregnancy. Contraindicated with allergy to *atropine* or its derivatives (e.g., *ipratropium*).

INHALED ANTICHOLINERGIC/BETA AGONIST

▷ *ipratropium bromide/albuterol sulfate* (C) 2 inhalations qid
    Combivent 2 inhalations qid; additional inhalations as required; max 12 inhalations/day
        Pediatric: not recommended
        Inhaler: ipra 18 mcg/*albu* 90 mcg/actuation (14.7 g, 200 inh)
    Duoneb 1 vial via nebulizer 4-6 times daily prn
        Pediatric: <18 years: not recommended
        Inhal soln: ipra 0.5 mg (0.017%)/*albu* 2.5 mg (0.083%) per 3 ml (23/carton)

INHALED BETA AGONIST (LONG-ACTING) (LABA)

▷ *arformoterol* (C) 15 mcg bid via nebulizer
    Pediatric: not recommended
        Brovana *Inhal soln:* 15 mcg/2 ml (2 ml; 30/carton)

Comment: *arformoterol* is indicated for the treatment of COPD but is used off-label for the treatment of asthma. It is used for prophylaxis and chronic treatment, only. Not for primary (rescue) treatment of acute attack.

▷ *formoterol fumarate* (C)

    Foradil Aerolizer 12 mcg q 12 hours

        Pediatric: <5 years: not recommended; ≥5 years: same as adult

        Inhaler: 12 mcg/cap (12, 60 caps w. device)

    Performist 20 mcg q 12 hours

        Pediatric: not recommended

        Inhal soln: 20 mcg/2 ml (60/carton)

Comment: *formoterol* is for prophylaxis and chronic treatment, only. Not for primary (rescue) treatment of acute attack. Do not mix *formoterol* with other drugs. *formoterol* off-label for asthma.

▷ *olodaterol* (C)

  Pediatric: not established

    Striverdi Respimat 12 mcg q 12 hours

        Inhal soln: 2.5 mcg/cartridge (metered actuation) (40 g, 60 metered actuations) (benzalkonium chloride)

    Comment: **Striverdi Respimat** is contraindicated in persons with asthma without use of long-term control medication.

▷ *salmeterol* (C)(G) 2 inhalations q 12 hours prn; 2 inhalations at least 30-60 minutes before exercise as prophylaxis for exercise-induced asthma; do not use extra doses for exercise-induced bronchospasm if already using regular dose

    Serevent Diskus

        Pediatric: <4 years: not recommended; ≥4 years: 1 inhalation q 12 hours prn; 1 inhalation at least 30-60 minutes before exercise as prophylaxis for exercise-induced asthma; do not use extra doses for exercise-induced bronchospasm if already using regular dose

        Diskus (pwdr): 50 mcg/actuation (60 doses/disk)

CORTICOSTEROID/INHALED LONG-ACTING BETA AGONIST (LABA)

▷ *budesonide/formoterol* (C) 1 inhalation bid; rinse mouth after use

  Pediatric: <12 years: not recommended; ≥12 years: same as adult

    Symbicort 80/4.5

        Inhaler: bud 80 mcg/for 4.5 mcg

    Symbicort 160/4.5

        Inhaler: bud 160 mcg/for 4.5 mcg

▷ *fluticasone propionate/salmeterol* (C)

    Advair HFA *Not previously using inhaled steroid:* start with 2 inh 45/21 or 115/21 bid; if insufficient response after 2 weeks, use next higher strength; max 2 inh 230/50 bid; *Already using inhaled steroid;* see mfr pkg insert; rinse mouth after use

    Advair HFA 45/21

        Pediatric: not recommended

        Inhaler: flu pro 45 mcg/sal 21 mcg/actuation (CFC-free)

    Advair HFA 115/21

        Pediatric: not recommended

        Inhaler: flu pro 115 mcg/sal 21 mcg/actuation (CFC-free)

    Advair HFA 230/21

Pediatric: not recommended
Inhaler: flu pro 230 mcg/*sal* 21 mcg/actuation (CFC-free)

Advair Diskus *Not previously using inhaled steroid:* start with 1 inh 100/50 bid; *Already using inhaled steroid:* see mfr pkg insert; rinse mouth after use

Advair Diskus 100/50
Pediatric: <4 years: not recommended; 4-11 years: 1 inhalation bid; >11 years: 1 inhalation bid
Diskus: flu pro 100 mcg/*sal* 50 mcg/actuation (60 blisters)

Advair Diskus 250/50 1 inhalation bid; rinse mouth after use
Pediatric: 4-12 years: use 100/50 strength; >12 years: same as adult
Diskus: flu pro 250 mcg/*sal* 50 mcg/actuation (60 blisters)

Advair Diskus 500/50
Pediatric: 4-12 years: use 100/50 strength; >12 years: same as adult
Diskus: fluticasone propionate 500 mcg/salmeterol 50 mcg/actuation (60 blisters)

Comment: **Advair Diskus** is not a rescue inhaler. Allow 12 hours between doses.

▷ *fluticasone furoate/vilanterol* (C) 1 inhalation 100/25 once daily at the same time each day
Pediatric: <17 years: not established

Breo Ellipta 100/25 *Inhal pwdr: flu* 100 mcg/*vil* 25 mcg dry pwdr per inhal (30 doses)
Breo Ellipta 200/25 *Inhal pwdr: flu* 200 mcg/*vil* 25 mcg dry pwdr per inhal (30 doses)

Comment: **Breo Ellipta** is contraindicated with severe hypersensitivity to milk proteins.

▷ *mometasone furoate/formoterol fumarate* (C) 2 inhalations bid; rinse mouth after use
Pediatric: not established

Dulera 100/5 *Inhaler: mom* 100 mcg/*for* 5 mcg (HFA)
Dulera 200/5 *Inhaler: mom* 200 mcg/*for* 5 mcg (HFA)

Comment: **Dulera** is not a rescue inhaler.

ANTICHOLINERGIC/INHALED LONG-ACTING BETA AGONIST (LABA)

▷ *glycopyrrolate/formoterol fumarate* (C) 2 inhalations bid (AM & PM)
Pediatric: <18 years: not established

Bevespi Aerosphere *Metered dose inhaler:* **9/4.8** *Inhal pwdr: gly 9 mcg/for 4.8 mcg* per inhal (10.7 g, 120 inh)

ORAL BETA2-AGONISTS (BRONCHODILATORS)

▷ *albuterol* (C)
Albuterol Syrup (G) *Adults:* 2-4 mg tid-qid; may increase gradually; max 8 mg qid; *Elderly:* initially 2-3 mg tid-qid; may increase gradually; max 8 mg qid
Pediatric: <2 years: not recommended; ≥2-6 years: 0.1 mg/kg tid; initially max 2 mg tid; may increase gradually to 0.2 mg/kg tid; max 4 mg tid; >6-12 years: 2 mg tid-qid; may increase gradually; max 6 mg qid; ≥12 years: same as adult
Syr: 2 mg/5 ml

Proventil 2-4 mg tid-qid prn
Pediatric: <6 years: not recommended; ≥6 years: same as adult
Tab: 2, 4 mg

Proventil Repetabs 4-8 mg q 12 hours prn
Pediatric: use syrup
Repetab: 4 mg sust-rel

Proventil Syrup 5-10 ml tid-qid prn; may increase gradually; max 20 ml qid prn
Pediatric: <2 years: not recommended; ≥2-6 years: 0.1 mg/kg tid prn; max initially 5 ml tid prn; may increase gradually to 0.2 mg/kg tid prn; max 10 ml tid; >6-14 years: 5 ml tid-qid prn; may increase gradually; max 60 ml/day in divided doses; >14 years: same as adult
Syr: 2 mg/5 ml
Ventolin 2-4 mg tid-qid prn; may increase gradually; max 8 mg qid
Pediatric: <2 years: not recommended; ≥2-6 years: 0.1 mg/kg tid prn; max initially 2 mg tid prn; may increase gradually to 0.2 mg/kg tid; max 4 mg tid; >6-14 years: 2 mg tid-qid prn; may increase gradually; max 6 mg tid
Tab: 2, 4 mg; *Syr:* 2 mg/5 ml (strawberry)
VoSpire ER 4-8 mg q 12 hours prn; max 32 mg/day divided q 12 hours; swallow whole
Pediatric: <6 years: not recommended; ≥6-12 years: 4 mg q 12 hours; max 24 mg/day q 12 hours; >12 years: same as adult
Tab: 4, 8 mg ext-rel
▷ *metaproterenol* (C)
Alupent 20 mg tid-qid prn
Pediatric: <6 years: not recommended (doses of 1.3-2.6 mg/kg/day have been used); ≥6-9 years (<60 lb): 10 mg tid-qid prn; >9-12 years (>60 lb): 20 mg tid-qid prn; >12 years: same as adult
Tab: 10, 20 mg; *Syr:* 10 mg/5 ml

METHYLXANTHINES

Comment: Check serum theophylline level just before 5th dose is administered. Therapeutic theophylline level: 10-20 mcg/ml.
▷ *theophylline* (C)(G)
Theo-24 initially 300-400 mg once daily at HS; after 3 days, increase to 400-600 mg once daily at HS; max 600 mg/day
Pediatric: <45 kg: initially 12-14 mg/kg/day; max 300 mg/day; increase after 3 days to 16 mg/kg/day to max 400 mg; after 3 more days increase to 30 mg/kg/day to max 600 mg/day; ≥45 kg: same as adult
Cap: 100, 200, 300, 400 mg ext-rel
Theo-Dur initially 150 mg bid; increase to 200 mg bid after 3 days; then to 300 mg bid after 3 more days
Pediatric: <6 years: not recommended; 6-15 years: initially 12-14 mg/kg/day in 2 divided doses; max 300 mg/day; then increase to 16 mg/kg in 2 divided doses; max 400 mg/day; then to 20 mg/kg/day in 2 divided doses; max 600 mg/day; ≥15 years: same as adult
Tab: 100, 200, 300 mg ext-rel
Theolair-SR
Pediatric: not recommended
Tab: 200, 250, 300, 500 mg sust-rel
Uniphyl 400-600 mg daily with meals
Pediatric: not recommended
Tab: 400*, 600*mg cont-rel

METHYLXANTHINE/EXPECTORANT

▷ *dyphylline/guaifenesin* (C) 1 tab qid

Lufyllin GG *Tab:* dyphy 200 mg/guaif 200 mg; *Elix:* dyphy 100 mg/guaif 100 mg per 15 ml

HUMANIZED INTERLEUKIN-5 ANTAGONIST MONOCLONAL ANTIBODY

▷ *mepolizumab* (NE) 100 mg SC once every 4 weeks in upper arm, abdomen, or thigh
Pediatric: <12 years: not recommended; ≥12 years: same as adult
Nucala *Vial:* 100 mg pwdr for reconstitution, single-use (preservative-free)
Comment: **Nucala** is an add-on maintenance treatment for severe asthma. There is a pregnancy exposure registry that monitors pregnancy outcomes in women exposed to **Nucala** during pregnancy. Healthcare providers can enroll patients or encourage patients to enroll themselves by calling 1-877-311-8972 or visiting www.mothertobaby.org/asthma.

 ATROPHIC VAGINITIS

Oral Estrogens *see Menopause page 264*

VAGINAL ESTROGEN PREPARATIONS

▷ *estradiol* (X)(G)
Vagifem Vaginal Tablet 1 tab intravaginally daily x 2 weeks; then 1 tab intravaginally twice weekly
Vag tab: 10 mcg (15 tabs w. applicators)
Yuvafem Vaginal Tablet 1 tab intravaginally daily x 2 weeks; then 1 tab intravaginally twice weekly
Vag tab: 10 mcg (15 tabs w. applicators)
▷ *estradiol* (X)
Estrace Vaginal Cream 2-4 g daily x 1-2 weeks; then gradually reduce to 1/2 initial dose x 1-2 weeks; then maintenance dose of 1 g 1-3 times/week
Vag crm: 0.01% (1 oz tube w. calib applicator)
▷ *estrogens, conjugated* (X)
Premarin Cream 2 g/day intravaginally
Vag crm: 1.5 oz w. applicator marked in 1/2 g increments to max 2 g
▷ *estropipate* (X)
Ogen Cream 2-4 g intravaginally daily x 3 weeks; discontinue 4th week; continue in this cyclical pattern
Vag crm: 1.5 mg/g (42.5 g w. calib applicator)

 ATTENTION DEFICIT HYPERACTIVITY DISORDER (ADHD)

SELECTIVE NOREPINEPHRINE REUPTAKE INHIBITOR (SNRI)

▷ *atomoxetine* (C) take one dose daily in the morning or in two divided doses in the morning and late afternoon or early evening; initially 40 mg/kg; increase after at least 3 days to 80 mg/kg; then after 2-4 weeks may increase to max 100 mg/day
Pediatric: <6 years: not recommended; ≥6 years, <70 kg: initially 0.5 mg/kg/day: increase after at least 3 days to 1.2 mg/kg/day; max 1.4 mg/kg/day or 100 mg/day (whichever is less); ≥6 years, >70 kg: same as adult

Strattera *Cap:* 10, 18, 25, 40, 60, 80, 100 mg

Comment: Not associated with stimulant or euphoric effects. May discontinue without tapering.

STIMULANTS

▷ *amphetamine sulfate* (C)(II)

Adzenys XT-ODT take with or without food; individualize the dosage according to the therapeutic needs and response; initially 6.3 mg once daily in the morning; increase in increments of 3.1 mg or 6.3 mg at weekly intervals; max recommended dose 18.8 mg once daily (6-12 years-of-age) and 12.5 mg once daily (13-17 years-of-age);
Pediatric: <6 years: not recommended; ≥6 years: same as adult
Comment: Patients taking **Adderall XR** may be switched to **Adzenys XR-ODT** at the equivalent dose taken once daily; switching from any other amphetamine products (e.g., **Adderall** immediate-release), discontinue that treatment, and titrate with **Adzenys XR-ODT** using the titration schedule (see mfr pkg insert)
ODT: 3.1, 6.3, 9.4, 12.5, 15.7, 18.8 mg orally-disint (orange) (fructose)
Dyanavel XR Oral Suspension initially 2.5 mg or 5 mg once daily in the morning; may increase in increments of 2.5 mg to 5 mg per day every 4-7 days; max 20 mg per day; shake bottle prior to administration
Pediatric: <6 years: not recommended; ≥6 years: same as adult
Oral susp: 2.5 mg/ml (464 ml)
Evekeo initially 5 mg once or twice daily at the same time(s) each day; may increase by 5 mg/day at weekly intervals; max 40 mg/day
Pediatric: <3 years: not recommended; ≥3-5 years: initially 2.5 mg once or twice daily at the same time(s) each day; may increase by 2.5 mg/day at weekly intervals; max 40 mg/day; ≥6 years: same as adult
Tab: 5, 10 mg

▷ *dextroamphetamine sulfate* (C)(II)(G) initially start with 10 mg daily; increase by 10 mg at weekly intervals if needed; may switch to daily dose with sust-rel spansules when titrated
Pediatric: <3 years: not recommended; ≥3-5 years: 2.5 mg daily; may increase by 2.5 mg daily at weekly intervals if needed; 6-12 years: initially 5 mg daily or bid; may increase by 5 mg/day at weekly intervals; usual max 40 mg/day; >12 years: initially 10 mg daily; may increase by 10 mg/day at weekly intervals; max 40 mg/day
Dexedrine *Tab:* 5*mg (tartrazine)
Dexedrine Spansule *Cap:* 5, 10, 15 mg ext-rel
Dextrostat *Tab:* 5, 10 mg (tartrazine)

▷ *dextroamphetamine saccharate/dextroamphetamine sulfate/amphetamine aspartate/amphetamine sulfate* (C)(II)(G) not indicated for adults
Adderall initially 10 mg daily; may increase weekly by 10 mg/day; usual max 60 mg/day in 2-3 divided doses; first dose on awakening; then q 4-6 hours prn
Pediatric: <6 years: not indicated; ≥6-12 years: initially 5 mg daily; may increase by 5 mg/day at weekly intervals; >12 years: same as adult
Tab: 5**, 7.5**, 10**, 12.5**, 15**mg, 3.75 mg, 20**, 30**mg
Adderall XR 20 mg by mouth once daily in AM; may increase by 10 mg/day at weekly intervals; max: 60 mg/day
Pediatric: <6 years: not recommended; ≥6 years: initially 10 mg daily in the AM; may increase by 10 mg/day at weekly intervals; max 30 mg/day; 13-17

years: 10-20 mg by mouth daily in the AM; may increase by 10 mg/day at weekly intervals; max 40 mg/day; Do not chew; may sprinkle on apple sauce
Cap: 5, 10, 15, 20, 25, 30 mg ext-rel

▷ *dexmethylphenidate* (C)(II)(G) not indicated for adults
Pediatric: <6 years: not recommended; ≥6 years: initially 2.5 mg bid; allow at least 4 hours between doses; may increase at 1 week intervals; max 20 mg/day
Focalin *Tab:* 2.5, 5, 10*mg (dye-free)
Focalin XR *Cap:* 5, 10, 15, 20, 25, 30, 35, 40 mg ext-rel

▷ *lisdexamphetamine dimesylate* (C)(II) 30 mg once daily in the AM; may increase by 10-20 mg/day at weekly intervals; max 70 mg/day
Pediatric: <6 years: not recommended; ≥6 years: same as adult
Vyvanse *Cap:* 20, 30, 40, 50, 60, 70 mg
Comment: May dissolve **Vyvanse** capsule contents in water; take immediately.

▷ *methamphetamine* (C)(II)(G) initially 5 mg once daily to bid; may increase by 5 mg/day at weekly intervals; usual effective dose 20-25 mg/day
Desoxyn Granumets
Pediatric: <6 years: not recommended; ≥6 years: same as adult
Tab: 5, 10, 15 mg sust-rel

▷ *methylphenidate (regular-acting)* (C)(II)(G)
Methylin, Methylin Chewable, Methylin Oral Solution usual dose 20-30 mg/day in 2-3 divided doses 30-45 minutes before a meal; max 60 mg/day
Pediatric: <6 years: not recommended; ≥6 years: initially 5 mg bid ac (breakfast and lunch); may increase 5-10 mg/day at weekly intervals; max 60 mg/day
Tab: 5, 10*, 20*mg; *Chew tab:* 2.5, 5, 10 mg; (grape; phenylalanine); *Oral soln:* 5, 10 mg/5 ml (grape)
Ritalin 10-60 mg/day in 2-3 divided doses 30-45 minutes ac; max 60 mg/day
Pediatric: <6 years: not recommended; ≥6 years: initially 5 mg bid ac (breakfast and lunch); may increase by 5-10 mg at weekly intervals as needed; max 60 mg/day
Tab: 5, 10*, 20*mg

▷ *methylphenidate (long-acting)* (C)(II)
Concerta initially 18 mg q AM; may increase in 18 mg increments as needed; max 54 mg/day; do not crush <u>or</u> chew
Pediatric: <6 years: not recommended; ≥6-12 years: initially 18 mg daily; max 54 mg/day; ≥13-17 years: initially 18 mg daily; max 72 mg/day <u>or</u> 2 mg/kg, whichever is less
Tab: 18, 27, 36, 54 mg sust-rel
Metadate CD (G) 1 cap daily in the AM; may sprinkle on food; do not crush <u>or</u> chew
Pediatric: <6 years: not recommended; ≥6 years: initially 20 mg daily; may gradually increase by 20 mg/day at weekly intervals as needed; max 60 mg/day
Cap: 10, 20, 30, 40, 50, 60 mg immed- and ext-rel beads
Metadate ER 1 tab daily in the AM; do not crush <u>or</u> chew
Pediatric: <6 years: not recommended; >6 years: use in place of regular-acting *methylpheni- date* when the 8-hour dose of **Metadate-ER** corresponds to the titrated 8-hour dose of regular-acting *methylphenidate*
Tab: 10, 20 mg ext-rel (dye-free)
QuilliChew ER initially 1 x 10 mg chew tab once daily in the AM
Pediatric: <6 years: not recommended; initially 10 mg daily; may gradually increase by 20 mg/day at weekly intervals as needed; max 60 mg/day
Chew tab: 20*, 30*, 40 mg ext-rel

Quillivant XR initially 20 mg once daily in the AM, with or without food; may be titrated in increments of 10-20 mg/day at weekly intervals; daily doses above 60 mg have not been studied and are not recommended; shake the bottle vigorously for at least 10 seconds to ensure that the correct dose is administered

Pediatric: <6 years: not recommended; ≥6 years: same as adult

Bottle: 5 mg/ml, 25 mg/5 ml pwdr for reconstitution; 300 mg (60 ml), 600 mg (120 ml), 750 mg (150 ml), 900 mg (180 ml)

Comment: **Quillivant XR** must be reconstituted by a pharmacist, not by the patient or caregiver.

Ritalin LA (G) 1 cap daily in the AM

Pediatric: <6 years: not recommended; ≥6 years: use in place of regular-acting *methylphenidate* when the 8-hour dose of **Ritalin LA** corresponds to the titrated 8-hour dose of regular-acting *methylphenidate*; max 60 mg/day

Cap: 10, 20, 30, 40 mg ext-rel (immed- and ext-rel beads)

Ritalin SR 1 cap daily in the AM

Pediatric: <6 years: not recommended; ≥6 years: use in place of regular-acting *methylphenidate* when the 8-hour dose of **Ritalin SR** corresponds to the titrated 8-hour dose of regular-acting *methylphenidate*; max 60 mg/day

Tab: 20 mg sust-rel (dye-free)

▷ *methylphenidate* (transdermal patch) **(C)(II)(G)** not applicable >17 years

Pediatric: <6 years: not recommended; ≥6-17 years: initially 10 mg patch applied to hip 2 hours before desired effect daily in the AM; may increase by 5-10 mg at weekly intervals; max 60 mg/day

Daytrana *Transdermal patch:* 10, 15, 20, 30 mg

▷ *pemoline* **(B)(IV)** 18.75-112.5 mg/day; usually start with 37.5 mg in AM; may increase 18.75 mg/day at weekly intervals; max 112.5 g/day

Pediatric: <6 years: not recommended; ≥6 years: same as adult

Cylert *Tab:* 18.75*, 37.5*, 75*mg

Cylert Chewable *Chew tab:* 37.5*mg

Comment: Check baseline serum ALT and monitor every 2 weeks thereafter.

CENTRAL ALPHA2A-AGONIST

▷ *guanfacine* **(B)(G)** not applicable >17 years

Pediatric: <6 years: not recommended; ≥6-17 years: initially 1 mg once daily; may increase by 1 mg/day at weekly intervals; usual max 4 mg/day

Intuniv *Tab:* 1, 2, 3, 4 mg ext-rel

Comment: Take **Intuniv** with water, milk, or other liquid. Do not take with a high-fat meal. Withdraw gradually by 1 mg every 3-7 days.

TRICYCLIC ANTIDEPRESSANTS (TCAs)

*see **Depression** page 105*

OTHER AGENTS

▷ *clonidine* **(C)(G)**

Catapres 4-5 mcg/kg/day

Pediatric: <12 years: not recommended; ≥12 years: same as adult

Tab: 0.1*, 0.2*, 0.3*mg

Kapvay not indicated for adults
Pediatric: <6 years: not recommended; ≥6-12 years: initially 0.1 mg at bedtime x 1 week; then 0.1 mg bid x 1 week; then 0.1 mg AM and 0.2 mg PM x 1 week; then 0.2 mg bid; withdraw gradually by 0.1 mg/day at 3-7 day intervals
Tab: 0.1, 0.2 mg ext-rel

AMINOKETONES (FOR THE TREATMENT OF ADHD)

▷ *bupropion HCl* (B)(G)
Pediatric: <18 years: not recommended
Wellbutrin initially 100 mg bid for at least 3 days; may increase to 375 <u>or</u> 400 mg/day after several weeks; then after at least 3 more days, 450 mg in 4 divided doses; max 450 mg/day, 150 mg/single dose
Tab: 75, 100 mg
Wellbutrin SR initially 150 mg in AM for at least 3 days; may increase to 150 mg bid if well tolerated; usual dose 300 mg/day; max 400 mg/day
Tab: 100, 150 mg sust-rel
Wellbutrin XL initially 150 mg in AM for at least 3 days; increase to 150 mg bid if well tolerated; usual dose 300 mg/day; max 400 mg/day
Tab: 150, 300 mg sust-rel

◯ BACTERIAL ENDOCARDITIS: PROPHYLAXIS

Comment: Bacterial endocarditis prophylaxis is appropriate for persons with a history of previous infective endocarditis, persons with a prosthetic cardiac valve or prosthetic material used for valve repair, cardiac transplant patients who develop cardiac valvulopathy, congenital heart disease (CHD), unrepaired cyanotic CHD including palliative shunts and conduits, completely repaired congenital heart defect(s) with prosthetic material or device, whether placed by surgery or by catheter intervention, during the first 6 months after the procedure, repaired CHD with residual defects at the site or adjacent to the site of a prosthetic patch or prosthetic device (which may inhibit endothelialization), or any other condition deemed to place a patient at high risk.

DENTAL, ORAL, RESPIRATORY TRACT, <u>OR</u> ESOPHAGEAL PROCEDURES

▷ *amoxicillin* (B)(G) 2 g PO 30-60 minutes before procedure as a single dose <u>or</u> 3 g 1 hour before procedure and 1.5 g 6 hours later
Pediatric: 50 mg/kg as a single dose <u>or</u> 50 mg/kg (max 3 g) 1 hour before procedure and (max 1.5 g) 25 mg/kg 6 hours later; ≥40 kg: same as adult; *see pages 554-557 for dose by weight*
Amoxil *Cap:* 250, 500 mg; *Tab:* 875*mg; *Chew tab:* 125, 200, 250, 400 mg (cherry-banana-peppermint) (phenylalanine); *Oral susp:* 125, 250 mg/5 ml (80, 100, 150 ml) (strawberry); 200, 400 mg/5 ml (50, 75, 100 ml) (bubble gum); *Oral drops:* 50 mg/ml (30 ml) (bubble gum)
Trimox *Tab:* 125, 250 mg; *Cap:* 250, 500 mg; *Oral susp:* 125, 250 mg/5 ml (80, 100, 150 ml) (raspberry-strawberry)
▷ *ampicillin* (B)(G) 2 g PO/IM/IV 30-60 minutes before procedure
Pediatric: 50 mg/kg PO/IM/IV 30-60 minutes before procedure

Omnipen, Principen *Cap:* 250, 500 mg; *Oral susp:* 125, 250 mg/5 ml (100, 150, 200 ml) (fruit)
Unisyn *Vial:* 1.5, 3 g

▶ *azithromycin* (B) 500 mg 30-60 minutes before procedure
Pediatric: 15 mg/kg 30-60 minutes before procedure; max 500 mg; *see page* 559 *for dose by weight*
Zithromax *Tab:* 250, 500, 600 mg; *Oral susp:* 100 mg/5 ml (15 ml); 200 mg/5 ml (15, 22.5, 30 ml) (cherry)

▶ *cefazolin* (B) 1 g IM/IV 30-60 minutes before procedure
Pediatric: 25 mg/kg IM/IV 30-60 minutes before procedure
Ancef *Vial:* 250, 500 mg; 1, 5 g
Kefzol *Vial:* 500 mg; 1 g

▶ *ceftriaxone* (B)(G) 1 g IM/IV as a single dose
Pediatric: 50 mg/kg IM/IV as a single dose
Rocephin *Vial:* 250, 500 mg; 1, 2 g

▶ *cephalexin* (B)(G) 2 g as a single dose 30-60 minutes before procedure
Pediatric: 50 mg/kg as a single dose 30-60 minutes before procedure; *see page* 568 *for dose by weight*
Keflex *Cap:* 250, 333, 500, 750 mg; *Oral susp:* 125, 250 mg/5 ml (100, 200 ml) (strawberry)

▶ *clarithromycin* (C)(G) 500 mg or 500 mg ext-rel as a single dose 30-60 minutes before procedure
Pediatric: 15 mg/kg as a single dose 30-60 minutes before procedure; *see page* 569 *for dose by weight*
Biaxin *Tab:* 250, 500 mg
Biaxin Oral Suspension *Oral susp:* 125, 250 mg/5 ml (50, 100 ml) (fruit-punch)
Biaxin XL *Tab:* 500 mg ext-rel

▶ *clindamycin* (B)(G) 600 mg PO as a one time single dose or 300 mg 30-60 minutes before procedure and 150 mg 6 hours later; take with a full glass of water
Pediatric: 20 mg/kg (max 300 mg) 1 hour before procedure and 10 mg/kg (max 150 mg) 6 hours later; take with a full glass of water; *see page* 570 *for dose by weight*
Cleocin (G) *Cap:* 75 (tartrazine), 150 (tartrazine), 300 mg; *Vial:* 150 mg/ml (2, 4 ml) (benzyl alcohol)
Cleocin Pediatric Granules (G) *Oral susp:* 75 mg/ml (100 ml)(cherry)

▶ *erythromycin estolate* (B)(G) 1 g 1 hour before procedure; then 500 mg 6 hours later
Pediatric: 20 mg/kg 1 hour before procedure; then 10 mg/kg 6 hours later; *see page* 573 *for dose by weight*
Ilosone *Pulvule:* 250 mg; *Tab:* 500 mg; *Liq:* 125, 250 mg/5 ml (100 ml)
Comment: *erythromycin* may increase INR with concomitant *warfarin*, as well as increase serum level of *digoxin*, benzodiazepines and statins.

▶ *penicillin V potassium* (B)(G) 2 g 1 hour before procedure; then 1 g 6 hours later or 2 g 1 hour before procedure; then 1 g q 6 hours x 8 doses
Pediatric: <60 lb: 1 g 1 hour before procedure; then 500 mg 6 hours later or 1 g 1 hour before procedure; then 500 mg q 6 hours x 8 doses; >12 years: same as adult; *see page* 583 *for dose by weight*
Pen-Vee K *Tab:* 250, 500 mg; *Oral soln:* 125 mg/5 ml (100, 200 ml); 250 mg/5 ml (100, 150, 200 ml)

BACTERIAL VAGINOSIS (BV; *GARDNERELLA VAGINALIS*)

PROPHYLAXIS AND RESTORATION OF VAGINAL ACIDITY

▷ *acetic acid/oxyquinolone* (C) one full applicator intravaginally bid for up to 30 days
  Pediatric: not recommended
    Relagard *Gel:* acet acid 0.9%/oxyq 0.025% (50 g tube w. applicator)

Comment: The following treatment regimens for *bacterial vaginosis* are published in the **2015 CDC Sexually Transmitted Diseases Treatment Guidelines**. Treatment regimens are presented by generic drug name first, followed by information about brands and dose forms. BV is associated with adverse pregnancy outcomes, including premature rupture of the membranes, preterm labor, preterm birth, intraamniotic infection, and postpartum endometritis. Therefore, treatment is recommended for all pregnant women with symptoms <u>or</u> positive screen.

RECOMMENDED REGIMENS

Regimen 1
▷ *metronidazole* 500 mg bid x 7 days

Regimen 2
▷ *metronidazole* gel 0.75% one full applicatorful (5 g) once daily x 5 days

Regimen 3
▷ *clindamycin* cream 2% one full applicatorful (5 g) intravaginally once daily at bedtime x 5 days

CDC Alternate Regimens

Regimen 1
▷ *tinidazole* 2 g once daily x 2 days

Regimen 2
▷ *tinidazole* 1 g once daily x 5 days

Regimen 3
▷ *clindamycin* 300 mg bid x 7 days

Regimen 4
▷ *clindamycin* ovules 100 mg intravaginally once daily at bedtime x 3 days

Drug Brands and Dose Forms

▷ *clindamycin* (B)
    Cleocin (G) *Cap:* 75 (tartrazine), 150 (tartrazine), 300 mg
    Cleocin Pediatric Granules (G) *Oral susp:* 75 mg/5 ml (100 ml) (cherry)
    Cleocin Vaginal Cream *Vag crm:* 2% (21, 40 g tubes w. applicator)
    Cleocin Vaginal Ovules *Vag supp:* 100 mg
▷ *metronidazole* (not for use in 1st; B in 2nd, 3rd)
    Flagyl *Tab:* 250*, 500*mg
    Flagyl 375 *Cap:* 375 mg
    Flagyl ER *Tab:* 750 mg ext-rel
    MetroGel-Vaginal, Vandazole *Vag gel:* 0.75% (70 g w. applicator) (parabens)

Comment: Alcohol is contraindicated during treatment with oral *metronidazole* and for 72 hours after therapy due to a possible *disulfiram*-like reaction (nausea, vomiting, flushing, headache).

▷ *tinidazole* (not for use in 1st; B in 2nd, 3rd)
   Tindamax *Tab:* 250*, 500*mg

Comment: Alcohol is contraindicated during treatment with oral *tinidazole* and for 72 hours after therapy due to a possible *disulfiram*-like reaction (nausea, vomiting, flushing, headache).

BALDNESS: MALE PATTERN

TYPE II 5-ALPHA-REDUCTASE SPECIFIC INHIBITOR

▷ *finasteride* (X)(G) 1 mg daily
   Propecia *Tab:* 1 mg

Comment: Pregnant women should not touch broken *finasteride* tabs. Use of Propecia, a 5-alpha reductase inhibitor, is associated with low but increased risk of high-grade prostate cancer.

PERIPHERAL VASODILATOR

▷ *minoxidil* topical soln (C) 1 ml from dropper or 6 sprays bid
   Pediatric: <18 years: not recommended
      Rogaine for Men (OTC) *Regular soln:* 2% (60 ml w. applicator) (alcohol 60%);
      Extra strength soln: 5% (60 ml w. applicator) (alcohol 30%)
      Rogaine for Women (OTC) Regular soln: 2% (60 ml w. applicator) (alcohol 60%)
   Comment: Do not use *minoxidil* on abraded or inflamed scalp.

BELL'S PALSY

▷ *prednisone* (C)(G) 80 mg once daily x 3 days; then 60 mg daily x 3 days; then 40 mg daily x 3 days; then 20 mg x 1 dose; then discontinue
   Deltasone *Tab:* 2.5*, 5*, 10*, 20*, 50*mg

BENIGN ESSENTIAL TREMOR

ANTI-PARKINSON'S AGENT

▷ *amantadine* (C)(G) 200 mg daily or 100 mg bid; 4 tsp of syrup once daily or 2 tsp bid
   Symmetrel *Tab:* 100 mg; *Syr:* 50 mg/5 ml (raspberry)

BETA-BLOCKER

▷ *propranolol* (C)(G)
   Inderal initially 40 mg bid; usual range 160-240 mg/day
      Tab: 10*, 20*, 40*, 60*, 80*mg
   Inderal LA initially 80 mg once daily in a single dose; increase q 3-7 days; usual range 120-160 mg/day; max 320 mg/day in a single dose

Cap: 60, 80, 120, 160 mg sust-rel
InnoPran XL initially 80 mg q HS; max 120 mg/day
Cap: 80, 120 mg ext-rel

◯ BENIGN PROSTATIC HYPERPLASIA (BPH)

ALPHA-1 BLOCKERS

Comment: Educate patient regarding potential side effect of hypotension especially with first dose. Usually start at lowest dose and titrate upward.
▷ *doxazosin* (C)
Cardura initially 1 mg daily; may double dose every 1-2 weeks; max 8 mg/day
Tab: 1*, 2*, 4*, 8*mg
Cardura XL initially 4 mg once daily with breakfast; may titrate after 3-4 weeks; max 8 mg/day
Tab: 4, 8 mg ext-rel
▷ *silodosin* (B) 8 mg once daily; *CrCl 30-50 mL/min:* 4 mg once daily
Rapaflo *Cap:* 4, 8 mg
▷ *terazosin* (C)(G) initially 1 mg q HS; titrate up to 10 mg once daily; max 20 mg/day
Hytrin *Cap:* 1, 2, 5, 10 mg

ALPHA-1A BLOCKERS

▷ *alfuzosin* (B)(G) 10 mg once daily taken immediately after the same meal each day
UroXatral *Tab:* 10 mg ext-rel
▷ *tamsulosin* (B)(G) initially 0.4 mg once daily; may increase to 0.8 mg daily after 2-4 weeks if needed
Flomax *Cap:* 0.4 mg
Comment: May take **Flomax** 0.4 mg plus **imitrex** 0.5 mg once daily as combination therapy.

TYPE II 5-ALPHA-REDUCTASE INHIBITOR

Comment: Pregnant women and women of childbearing age should not handle *finasteride*. Monitor for potential side effects of decreased libido <u>and/or</u> impotence. Low, but increased risk of being diagnosed with high-grade prostate cancer.
▷ *finasteride* (X) 5 mg once daily
Proscar *Tab:* 5 mg

TYPES I AND II 5-ALPHA-REDUCTASE INHIBITOR

Comment: Pregnant women and women of childbearing age should not handle *dutasteride*. Monitor for potential side effects of decreased libido <u>and/or</u> impotence. Low, but increased risk of being diagnosed with high-grade prostate cancer.
▷ *dutasteride* (X)(G) 0.5 mg once daily
Avodart *Cap:* 0.5 mg
Comment: May take **Avodart** 0.5 mg with **Flomax** 0.4 mg once daily as combination therapy.

TYPE I AND II 5-ALPHA-REDUCTASE INHIBITOR/ALPHA-1A BLOCKER

▷ *dutasteride/tamsulosin* (X)(G) take 1 cap once daily after the same meal each day
   Jalyn *Cap: duta* 0.5 mg/*tam* 0.4 mg

PHOSPHODIESTERASE TYPE 5 (PDE5) INHIBITORS, CGMP-SPECIFIC

Comment: Oral PDE5 inhibitors are contraindicated in patients taking nitrates.
Caution with history of recent MI, stroke, life-threatening arrhythmia, hypotension,
hypertension, cardiac failure, unstable angina, retinitis pigmentosa, CYP3A4 inhibitors
(e.g., *cimetidine*, the azoles, *erythromycin*, grapefruit juice), protease inhibitors (e.g.,
ritonavir), CYP3A4 inducers (e.g., *rifampin*, *carbamaepine*, *phenytoin*, *phenobarbital*),
alcohol, antihypertensive agents. Side effects include headache, flushing, nasal
congestion, rhinitis, dyspepsia, and diarrhea.

▷ *tadalafil* (B) 5 mg once daily at the same time each day; *CrCl 30-50 mL/min:* initially
   2.5 mg; *CrCl <30 mL/min:* not recommended; *Concomitant alpha blockers:* not recommended
   Cialis *Tab:* 2.5, 5, 10, 20 mg

 BILE ACID DEFICIENCY

BILE ACID

▷ *ursodiol* (B)
   Dissolution of radiolucent non-calcified gallstones <20 mm diameter: 8-10 mg/kg/
   day in 2-3 divided doses; *Prevention:* 13-15 mg/kg/day in 4 divided doses
   Pediatric: not recommended
   Actigall *Cap:* 300 mg
   Comment: *ursodiol* decreases the amount of cholesterol produced by the liver
   and absorbed by the intestines. It helps break down cholesterol that has formed
   into stones in the gallbladder. *ursodiol* increases bile flow in patients with
   primary biliary cirrhosis. It is used to treat small gallstones in people who cannot
   have cholecystectomy surgery and to prevent gallstones in overweight patients
   undergoing rapid weight loss. *ursodiol* is not for treating gallstones that are
   calcified.

 BINGE EATING DISORDER

CENTRAL NERVOUS SYSTEM (CNS) STIMULANT

▷ *lisdexamfetamine dimesylate* (C)(II) swallow whole <u>or</u> may open and mix/dissolve
   contents of cap in yogurt, water, orange juice and take immediately; 30 mg once daily
   in the AM; may adjust in increments of 20 mg at weekly intervals; target dose 50-70
   mg/day; max 70 mg/day; *GFR 15-<30 mL/min:* max 50 mg/day; *GFR <15 mL/min,
   ESRD:* max 30 mg/day
   Vyvanse *Cap:* 10, 20, 30, 40, 50, 60 70 mg
   Comment: **Vyvanse** is not approved <u>or</u> recommended for weight loss treatment
   of obesity.

◯ BIPOLAR I DISORDER: DEPRESSION

Comment: The cornerstone of treatment for Bipolar I Disorder: Depression is mood-stabilizers (*lithium* and *valproate*). Common adjunctive agents include antiepileptics, antipsychotics, and combination agents. Mounting evidence suggests that antidepressants aren't effective in the treatment of bipolar depression. A major study funded by the National Institute of Mental Health (NIMH) showed that adding an antidepressant to a mood stabilizer was no more effective in treating bipolar I depression than using a mood stabilizer alone. Another NIMH study found that antidepressants work no better than placebo. If antidepressants are used at all, they should be combined with a mood stabilizer such as *lithium* or *valproic acid*. Taking an antidepressant without a mood stabilizer is likely to trigger a manic episode. Antidepressants can increase mood cycling. Many experts believe that over time, antidepressant use in people with bipolar disorder has a mood destabilizing effect, increasing the frequency of manic and depressive episodes. Drugs and conditions that can mimic bipolar I disorder include thyroid disorders, corticosteroids, antidepressants, adrenal disorders (e.g. Addison's disease, Cushing's syndrome), antianxiety drugs, drugs for Parkinson's disease, vitamin B12 deficiency, neurological disorders (e.g. epilepsy, multiple sclerosis).

MOOD STABILIZERS

Lithium Salts Mood Stabilizer

▷ *lithium carbonate* (D)(G) swallow whole; *Usual maintenance:* 900-1200 mg/day in 2-3 divided doses
Pediatric: not recommended
    Lithobid *Tab:* 300 mg slow-rel
Comment: Signs and symptoms of *lithium* toxicity can occur below 2 mEq/L and include blurred vision, tinnitus, weakness, dizziness, nausea, abdominal pains, vomiting, diarrhea to (severe) hand tremors, ataxia, muscle twitches, nystagmus, seizures, slurred speech, decreased level of consciousness, coma, death.

Valproate Mood Stabilizer

▷ *divalproex sodium* (D)(G) take once daily; swallow ext-rel form whole; initially 25 mg/kg/day in divided doses; max 60 mg/kg/day; *Elderly:* reduce initial dose and titrate slowly
Pediatric: not recommended
    Depakene *Cap:* 250 mg; *Syr:* 250 mg/5 ml (16 oz)
    Depakote *Tab:* 125, 250 mg
    Depakote ER *Tab:* 250, 500 mg ext-rel
    Depakote Sprinkle *Cap:* 125 mg

ANTIEPILEPTICS

▷ *carbamazepine* (D) ext-rel oral forms should be swallowed whole; may open caps and sprinkle on applesauce (do not crush or chew beads); initially 400 mg/day in 2 divided doses; adjust in increments of 200 mg/day; max 1.6 g/day. *Elderly:* reduce initial dose and titrate slowly; oral doses are preferred; IV administration is recommended when the patient is unable to swallow an oral form (see **Carnexiv**)
Pediatric: not recommended

Carbatrol (G) *Cap:* 200, 300 mg ext-rel
Carnexiv *Vial:* 10 mg/ml (20 ml)
Comment: The total daily dose of **Carnexiv** is 70% of the total daily oral *carbamazepine* dose (see mfr pkg insert for dosage conversion table). The total daily dose should be equally divided into four 30-minute infusions, separated by 6 hours. Must be diluted prior to administration. Patients should be switched back to oral *carbamazepine* at their previous total daily oral dose and frequency of administration as soon as clinically appropriate. The use of **Carnexiv** for more than 7 consecutive days has not been studied.
Equetro (G) *Cap:* 100, 200, 300 mg ext-rel
Tegretol (G) *Tab:* 200*mg; *Chew tab:* 100*mg; *Oral susp:* 100 mg/5 ml (450 ml; citrus-vanilla)
Tegretol XR (G) *Tab:* 100, 200, 400 mg ext-rel
Comment: *carbamazepine* is indicated in mixed episodes in bipolar I disorder.

▶ *lamotrigine* (C)(G) *Not taking an enzyme-inducing antiepileptic drug (EIAED) (e.g., phenytoin, carbamazepine, phenobarbital, primidone, valproic acid):* 25 mg once daily x 2 weeks; then 50 mg once daily x 2 weeks; then 100 mg once daily x 2 weeks; then target dose 200 mg once daily; *Concomitant valproic acid:* 25 mg every other day x 2 weeks; then 25 mg once daily x 2 weeks; then 50 mg once daily x 1 week; then target dose 100 mg once daily; *Concomitant EIAED, not valproic acid:* 50 mg once daily x 2 weeks; then 100 mg daily in divided doses; then increase weekly by 100 mg in divided doses to target dose 400 mg/day in divided doses daily
Pediatric: not recommended
Lamictal *Tab:* 25*, 100*, 150*, 200*mg
Lamictal Chewable Dispersible Tab *Chew tab:* 2, 5, 25, 50 mg (black current)
Lamictal ODT *ODT:* 25, 50, 100, 200 mg
Lamictal XR *Tab:* 25, 50, 100, 200 mg ext-rel
Comment: *lamotrigine* is indicated for maintenance treatment of bipolar I disorder. See mfr pkg insert for drug interactions, interactions with contraceptives and hormone replacement therapy, and discontinuation protocol

ANTIPSYCHOTICS

Comment: Side effects of antipsychotics include drowsiness, weight gain, sexual dysfunction, dry mouth, constipation, blurred vision.

▶ *aripiprazole* (C)(G) initially 15 mg once daily; may increase to max 30 mg/day
Pediatric: <10 years: not recommended; ≥10-17 years: initially 2 mg/day in a single dose for 2 days; then increase to 5 mg/day in a single dose for 2 days; then increase to target dose of 10 mg/day in a single dose; may increase by 5 mg/day at weekly intervals as needed to max 30 mg/day
Abilify *Tab:* 2, 5, 10, 15, 20, 30 mg
Abilify Discmelt *Tab:* 15 mg orally-disint (vanilla) (phenylalanine)
Abilify Maintena *Vial:* 300, 400 mg ext-rel pwdr for IM injection after reconstitution; 300, 400 mg single-dose prefilled dual-chamber syringes w. supplies
Comment: **Abilify** is indicated for acute and maintenance treatment of mixed episodes in bipolar I disorder, as monotherapy or as adjunct to **lithium** or *valproic acid.*

▶ *asenapine* (C) allow SL tab to dissolve on tongue; do not split, crush, chew, or swallow; do not eat or drink for 10 minutes after administration; *Monotherapy:* 10 mg bid; *Adjunctive therapy:* 5 mg bid; may increase to max 10 mg bid

Pediatric: <10 years: not established; 10-17 years: *Monotherapy:* initially 2.5 mg bid; may increase to 5 mg bid after 3 days; then to 10 mg bid after 3 more days; max 10 mg bid

Saphris *SL tab:* 2, 5, 5, 10 mg (black cherry)

Comment: **Saphris** is indicated for acute treatment of manic <u>or</u> mixed episodes in bipolar I disorder, as monotherapy <u>or</u> as adjunct to *lithium* <u>or</u> *valproic acid*.

▷ *cariprazine* (NE)
Pediatric: not established

Vraylar *Cap:* 1.5, 3, 4.5, 6 mg; 7-count (1 x 1.5 mg, 6 x 3 mg) mixed blister pck

Comment: **Vraylar** is an atypical antipsychotic with partial agonist activity at D2 and 5-HT1A receptors and antagonist activity at 5-HT2A receptors. It is indicated for acute treatment of mixed episodes in bipolar I disorder. There is a **Vraylar** pregnancy exposure registry that monitors pregnancy outcomes in women exposed to **Vraylar** during pregnancy. For more information, contact the National Pregnancy Registry for Atypical Antipsychotics at 1-866-961-2388 <u>or</u> visit https://womensmentalhealth.org/clinical-and-research-programs/pregnancyregistry. Safety and effectiveness in pediatric patients have not been established.

▷ *lurasidone* (B) initially 20 mg once daily; usual range 20 to max 120 mg/day; take with food; *CrCl <50 mL/min, moderate hepatic impairment (Child Pugh 7-9):* max 80 mg/day; *Child Pugh 10-15):* max 40 mg/day
Pediatric: not established

Latuda *Tab:* 20, 40, 60, 80, 120 mg

Comment: **Latuda** is indicated for major depressive episodes associated with bipolar I disorder as monotherapy and as adjunctive therapy with *lithium* <u>or</u> *valproic* acid. Contraindicated with concomitant strong CYP3A4 inhibitors (e.g., *ketoconazole, voriconazole, clarithromycin, ritonavir*) and inducers (e.g., *phenytoin, carbamazepine, rifampin, St. John's wort*); see mfr pkg insert if patient taking moderate CYP3A4 inhibitors (e.g., *diltiazem, atazanavir, erythromycin, fluconazole, verapamil*)

▷ *quetiapine fumarate* (C)

SeroQUEL initially 25 mg bid, titrate q 2nd or 3rd day in increments of 25-50 mg bid-tid; usual maintenance 400-600 mg/day in 2-3 divided doses
Pediatric: <10 years: not recommended; ≥10-17 years: initially 25 mg bid, titrate q 2nd <u>or</u> 3rd day in increments of 25-50 mg bid-tid; max 600 mg/day in 2-3 divided doses

Tab: 25, 50, 100, 200, 300, 400 mg

SeroQUEL XR swallow whole; administer once daily in the PM; *Day 1:* 50 mg; *Day 2:* 100 mg; *Day 3:* 200 mg; *Day 4:* 300 mg; usual range 400-600 mg/day
Pediatric: <18 years: not recommended

Tab: 50, 150, 200, 300, 400 mg ext-rel

▷ *risperidone* (C) *Tab:* initially 2-3 mg once daily; may adjust at 24 hour intervals by 1 mg/day; usual range 1-6 mg/day; max 6 mg/day; *Oral soln:* do not take with cola or tea; *M-tab:* dissolve on tongue with or without fluid; *Consta:* administer deep IM in the deltoid or gluteal; give with oral *respirodone* <u>or</u> other antipsychotic x 3 weeks; then stop oral form; 25 mg IM every 2 weeks; max 50 mg every 2 weeks

Risperdal
Pediatric: <5 years: not established; 5-10 years: initially 0.5 mg once daily at the same time each day adjust at 24 hour intervals by 0.5-1 mg to target dose 1-2.5 mg/day; usual range 1-6 mg/day; max 6 mg/day; >10 years: same as adult

Tab: 0.25, 0.5, 1, 2, 3, 4 mg; *Oral soln:* 1 mg/ml (100 ml)

Risperdal Consta
Pediatric: <18 years: not established
> *Vial:* 12.5, 25, 37.5, 50 mg pwdr for long-acting IM inj after reconstitution, single-use, w. diluent and supplies

Risperdal M-Tab
Pediatric: <10 years: not established; ≥10 years: same as adult
> *Tab:* 0.5, 1, 2, 3, 4 mg orally-disint (phenylalanine)

Comment: **Risperdol** tabs, oral solution, and M-tabs are indicated for the short-term monotherapy of acute mania o̲r mixed episodes associated with bipolar I disorder, o̲r in combination with *lithium* o̲r *valproic acid* in adults
Risperdol Consta is indicated as monotherapy o̲r adjunctive therapy to *lithium* o̲r *valproic acid* for the maintenance treatment mania and mixed episodes in bipolar I disorder.

▷ *ziprasidone* (C)(G) *Adult:* take with food; initially 40 mg bid; on day 2, may increase to 60-80 mg bid; *Elderly:* lower initial dose and titrate slowly
Pediatric: not recommended
> **Geodon** *Cap:* 20, 40, 60, 80 mg

Comment: **Geodon** is indicated for acute and maintenance treatment of mixed episodes in bipolar I disorder, as monotherapy o̲r as adjunct to *lithium* o̲r *valproic acid*.

COMBINATION AGENTS

Thienobenzodiazepine/Selective Serotonin Reuptake Inhibitor Combinations

▷ *fluoxetine* (C)(G)
> **Prozac** initially *olanzapine* 5 mg pl̲us fluoxetine 20 mg daily in the PM; range *olanzapine* 5-12.5 mg pl̲us *fluoxetine* 20-50 mg; risk of hypotension, o̲r hepatic impairment, slow metabolizers, or sensitive to *olanzapine*, initially *olanzapine* 2.5-5 mg pl̲us *fluoxetine* 20 mg daily in the PM; *fluoxetine* doses >20 mg/day may be divided into AM and noon doses
> *Pediatric:* not recommended
>> *Cap:* 10, 20, 40 mg; *Tab:* 30*, 60*mg; *Oral soln:* 20 mg/5 ml (4 oz) (mint)
> **Prozac Weekly** following daily *fluoxetine* therapy at 20 mg/day for 13 weeks, may initiate
> **Prozac Weekly** 7 days after the last 20 mg *fluoxetine* dose
> *Pediatric:* not recommended

▷ *olanzapine/fluoxetine* (C) initially 1 x 6/25 cap once daily in the PM; titrate; max 1 x 12/50 cap once daily in the PM
Pediatric: <10 years: not recommended; 10-17 years: initially 1 x 3/25 cap once daily in the PM; max 1 x 12/50 cap once daily in the PM
> **Symbyax**
>> *Cap:* **Symbyax 3/25:** *olan* 3 mg/*fluo* 25 mg
>> **Symbyax 6/25:** *olan* 6 mg/*fluo* 25 mg
>> **Symbyax 6/50:** *olan* 6 mg/*fluo* 50 mg
>> **Symbyax 12/25:** *olan* 12 mg/*fluo* 25 mg
>> **Symbyax 12/50:** *olan* 12 mg/*fluo* 50 mg

Comment: **Symbyax** is indicated for the treatment of depressive episodes associated with bipolar I disorder and treatment-resistant depression (TRD).

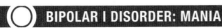

BIPOLAR I DISORDER: MANIA

Comment: The cornerstone of treatment for Bipolar I Disorder: Mania is mood-stabilizers (**lithium** and **valproic acid**). Common adjunctive agents include antiepileptics and antipsychotics. Drugs and conditions that can mimic bipolar I disorder include thyroid disorders, corticosteroids, antidepressants, adrenal disorders (e.g., Addison's disease, Cushing's syndrome), antianxiety drugs, drugs for Parkinson's disease, vitamin B12 deficiency, neurological disorders (e.g., epilepsy, multiple sclerosis).

MOOD STABILIZERS

Lithium Salts Mood Stabilizer

▷ *lithium carbonate* **(D)(G)** swallow whole; *Usual maintenance:* 900-1200 mg/day in 2-3 divided doses
Pediatric: not recommended
    Lithobid *Tab:* 300 mg slow-rel
    Comment: Signs and symptoms of **lithium** toxicity can occur below 2 mEq/L and include blurred vision, tinnitus, weakness, dizziness, nausea, abdominal pains, vomiting, diarrhea to (severe) hand tremors, ataxia, muscle twitches, nystagmus, seizures, slurred speech, decreased level of consciousness, coma, death.

Valproate Mood Stabilizer

▷ *divalproex sodium* **(D)(G)** take once daily; swallow ext-rel form whole; initially 25 mg/kg/day in divided doses; max 60 mg/kg/day; *Elderly:* reduce initial dose and titrate slowly
Pediatric: not recommended
    Depakene *Cap:* 250 mg; *Syr:* 250 mg/5 ml (16 oz)
    Depakote *Tab:* 125, 250 mg
    Depakote ER *Tab:* 250, 500 mg ext-rel
    Depakote Sprinkle *Cap:* 125 mg

ANTIEPILEPTICS

▷ *carbamazepine* **(D)** ext-rel forms should be swallowed whole; may open caps and sprinkle on applesauce (do not crush <u>or</u> chew beads); initially 400 mg/day in 2 divided doses; adjust in increments of 200 mg/day; max 1.6 g/day. *Elderly:* reduce initial dose and titrate slowly; oral doses are preferred; IV administration is recommended when the patient is unable to swallow an oral form (see **Carnexiv**)
Pediatric: not recommended
    Carbatrol (G) *Cap:* 200, 300 mg ext-rel
    Carnexiv *Vial:* 10 mg/ml (20 ml)
    Comment: The total daily dose of **Carnexiv** is 70% of the total daily oral **carbamazepine** dose (see mfr pkg insert for dosage conversion table). The total daily dose should be equally divided into four 30-minute infusions, separated by 6 hours. Must be diluted prior to administration. Patients should be switched back to oral **carbamazepine** at their previous total daily oral dose and frequency of administration as soon as clinically appropriate. The use of **Carnexiv** for more than 7 consecutive days has not been studied.
    Equetro (G) *Cap:* 100, 200, 300 mg ext-rel

Tegretol (G) *Tab:* 200*mg; *Chew tab:* 100*mg; *Oral susp:* 100 mg/5 ml (450 ml; citrus-vanilla)
Tegretol XR (G) *Tab:* 100, 200, 400 mg ext-rel
Comment: *carbamazepine* is indicated in mixed episodes in bipolar I disorder.

➤ *lamotrigine* (C)(G) *Not taking an enzyme-inducing antiepileptic drug (EIAED) (e.g., phenytoin, carbamazepine, phenobarbital, primidone, valproic acid):* 25 mg once daily x 2 weeks; then 50 mg once daily x 2 weeks; then 100 mg once daily x 2 weeks; then target dose 200 mg once daily; *Concomitant valproic acid:* 25 mg every other day x 2 weeks; then 25 mg once daily x 2 weeks; then 50 mg once daily x 1 week; then target dose 100 mg once daily; *Concomitant EIAED, not valproic acid:* 50 mg once daily x 2 weeks; then 100 mg daily in divided doses; then increase weekly by 100 mg in divided doses to target dose 400 mg/day in divided doses daily
Pediatric: not recommended

Lamictal *Tab:* 25*, 100*, 150*, 200*mg
Lamictal Chewable Dispersible Tab *Chew tab:* 2, 5, 25, 50 mg (black current)
Lamictal ODT *ODT:* 25, 50, 100, 200 mg
Lamictal XR *Tab:* 25, 50, 100, 200 mg ext-rel

Comment: *lamotrigine* is indicated for maintenance treatment of bipolar I disorder. See mfr pkg insert for drug interactions, interactions with contraceptives and hormone replacement therapy, and discontinuation protocol

➤ *topiramate* (D)(G) initially 25 mg daily in the PM; then 25 mg bid; then, 25 mg in the AM and 50 mg in the PM; then, 50 mg bid
Pediatric: <12 years: not recommended

Topamax *Tab:* 25, 50, 100, 200 mg
Topamax Sprinkle Caps *Cap:* 15, 25 mg

ANTIPSYCHOTICS

Comment: Side effects of antipsychotics include drowsiness, weight gain, sexual dysfunction, dry mouth, constipation, blurred vision.

➤ *aripiprazole* (C)(G) initially 15 mg once daily; may increase to max 30 mg/day
Pediatric: <10 years: not recommended; ≥10-17 years: initially 2 mg/day in a single dose for 2 days; then increase to 5 mg/day in a single dose for 2 days; then increase to target dose of 10 mg/day in a single dose; may increase by 5 mg/day at weekly intervals as needed to max 30 mg/day

Abilify *Tab:* 2, 5, 10, 15, 20, 30 mg
Abilify Discmelt *Tab:* 15 mg orally-disint (vanilla) (phenylalanine)
Abilify Maintena *Vial:* 300, 400 mg ext-rel pwdr for IM injection after reconstitution; 300, 400 mg single-dose prefilled dual-chamber syringes w. supplies
Comment: **Abilify** is indicated for acute and maintenance treatment of mixed episodes in bipolar I disorder, as monotherapy or as adjunct to *lithium* or *valproic acid.*

➤ *asenapine* (C) allow SL tab to dissolve on tongue; do not split, crush, chew, or swallow; do not eat or drink for 10 minutes after administration; *Monotherapy:* 10 mg bid; *Adjunctive therapy:* 5 mg bid; may increase to max 10 mg bid
Pediatric: <10 years: not established; 10-17 years: *Monotherapy:* initially 2.5 mg bid; may increase to 5 mg bid after 3 days; then to 10 mg bid after 3 more days; max 10 mg bid

Saphris *SL tab:* 2, 5, 5, 10 mg (black cherry)
Comment: **Saphris** is indicated for acute treatment of manic or mixed episodes in bipolar I disorder, as monotherapy or as adjunct to *lithium* or *valproic acid.*

▷ *cariprazine* (NE)
　　Pediatric: not established
　　　　Vraylar *Cap:* 1.5, 3, 4.5, 6 mg; 7-count (1 x 1.5 mg, 6 x 3 mg) mixed blister pck
　　　　Comment: **Vraylar** is an atypical antipsychotic with partial agonist activity at D2
　　　　and 5-HT1A receptors and antagonist activity at 5-HT2A receptors. It is indicated
　　　　for acute treatment of mixed episodes in bipolar I disorder. There is a **Vraylar**
　　　　pregnancy exposure registry that monitors pregnancy outcomes in women
　　　　exposed to **Vraylar** during pregnancy. For more information, contact the National
　　　　Pregnancy Registry for Atypical Antipsychotics at 1-866-961-2388 or visit https://
　　　　womensmentalhealth.org/clinical-and-research-programs/pregnancyregistry.
　　　　Safety and effectiveness in pediatric patients have not been established.

▷ *chlorpromazine* (C)(G) initially 10 mg tid-qid; may increase semi-weekly by 25-50
　　mg/day
　　Pediatric: ≥6 months: initially 0.25 mg/lb every 4-6 hours prn or 0.5 mg/lb rectally
　　q 6-8 hours prn
　　　　Thorazine *Tab:* 10, 25, 50, 100, 200 mg; *Spansule:* 30, 75, 150 mg sust-rel; *Syr:*
　　　　10 mg/5 ml (4 oz) (orange custard); *Oral conc:* 30 mg/ml (4 oz); 100 mg/ml (2, 8
　　　　oz); *Supp:* 25, 100 mg
　　　　Comment: *chlorpromazine* is indicated for rapid control of severe psychotic
　　　　symptoms.

▷ *lurasidone* (B) initially 20 mg once daily; usual range 20 to max 120 mg/day; take
　　with food; *CrCl <50 mL/min, moderate hepatic impairment (Child Pugh 7-9):* max 80
　　mg/day; *Child Pugh 10-15):* max 40 mg/day
　　Pediatric: not established
　　　　Latuda *Tab:* 20, 40, 60, 80, 120 mg
　　　　Comment: **Latuda** is indicated for major depressive episodes associated with
　　　　bipolar I disorder as monotherapy and as adjunctive therapy with *lithium* or
　　　　valproic acid. Contraindicated with concomitant strong CYP3A4 inhibitors
　　　　(e.g., *ketoconazole, voriconazole, clarithromycin, ritonavir*) and inducers
　　　　(e.g., *phenytoin, carbamazepine, rifampin, St. John's wort*); see mfr pkg insert
　　　　if patient taking moderate CYP3A4 inhibitors (e.g., *diltiazem, atazanavir,
　　　　erythromycin, fluconazole, verapamil*)

▷ *quetiapine fumarate* (C)
　　　　SeroQUEL initially 25 mg bid, titrate q 2nd or 3rd day in increments of 25-50
　　　　mg bid-tid; usual maintenance 400-600 mg/day in 2-3 divided doses
　　　　Pediatric: <10 years: not recommended; ≥10-17 years: initially 25 mg bid, titrate
　　　　q 2nd or 3rd day in increments of 25-50 mg bid-tid; max 600 mg/day in 2-3
　　　　divided doses
　　　　　　Tab: 25, 50, 100, 200, 300, 400 mg
　　　　SeroQUEL XR swallow whole; administer once daily in the PM; *Day 1:* 50 mg;
　　　　Day 2: 100 mg; *Day 3:* 200 mg; *Day 4:* 300 mg; usual range 400-600 mg/day
　　　　Pediatric: <18 years: not recommended
　　　　　　Tab: 50, 150, 200, 300, 400 mg ext-rel

▷ *risperidone* (C) *Tab:* initially 2-3 mg once daily; may adjust at 24 hour intervals
　　by 1 mg/day; usual range 1-6 mg/day; max 6 mg/day; *Oral soln:* do not take with
　　cola or tea; *M-tab:* dissolve on tongue with or without fluid; *Consta:* administer
　　deep IM in the deltoid or gluteal; give with oral *risperidone* or other antipsychot-
　　ic x 3 weeks; then stop oral form; 25 mg IM every 2 weeks; max 50 mg every 2
　　weeks

Risperdal
Pediatric: <5 years: not established; 5-10 years: initially 0.5 mg once daily at the same time each day adjust at 24 hour intervals by 0.5-1 mg to target dose 1-2.5 mg/day; usual range 1-6 mg/day; max 6 mg/day; >10 years: same as adult
    Tab: 0.25, 0.5, 1, 2, 3, 4 mg; *Oral soln:* 1 mg/ml (100 ml)
Risperdal Consta
Pediatric: <18 years: not established
    Vial: 12.5, 25, 37.5, 50 mg pwdr for long-acting IM inj after reconstitution, single-use, w. diluent and supplies
Risperdal M-Tab
Pediatric: <10 years: not established; ≥10 years: same as adult
    Tab: 0.5, 1, 2, 3, 4 mg orally-disint (phenylalanine)
COMMENT: **Risperdol** tabs, oral solution, and M-tabs are indicated for the short-term monotherapy of acute mania or mixed episodes associated with bipolar I disorder, or in combination with *lithium* or *valproic acid* in adults **Risperdol Consta** is indicated as monotherapy or adjunctive therapy to *lithium* or *valproic acid* for the maintenance treatment mania and mixed episodes in bipolar I disorder.

▷ *ziprasidone* (C)(G) *Adult:* take with food; initially 40 mg bid; on day 2, may increase to 60-80 mg bid; *Elderly:* lower initial dose and titrate slowly
Pediatric: not recommended
    Geodon *Cap:* 20, 40, 60, 80 mg
    COMMENT: **Geodon** is indicated for acute and maintenance treatment of mania and mixed episodes in bipolar I disorder, as monotherapy or as adjunct to *lithium* or *valproic acid*.

◯ BITE: CAT

TETANUS PROPHYLAXIS

▷ *tetanus toxoid* vaccine (C) 0.5 ml IM x 1 dose if previously immunized
    Vial: 5 Lf units/0.5 ml (0.5, 5 ml); *Prefilled syringe:* 5 Lf units/0.5 ml (0.5 ml)
    see Tetanus page 408 *for patients not previously immunized*

ANTI-INFECTIVES

▷ *amoxicillin/clavulanate* (B)(G) 500 mg tid or 875 mg bid x 10 days
    Augmentin *Tab:* 250, 500, 875 mg; *Chew tab:* 125, 250 mg (lemon-lime); 200, 400 mg (cherry-banana) (phenylalanine); *Oral susp:* 125 mg/5 ml (banana), 250 mg/5 ml (75, 100, 150 ml) (orange); 200, 400 mg/5 ml (50, 75, 100 ml) (orange) (phenylalanine)
        Pediatric: 40-45 mg/kg/day divided tid x 10 days or 90 mg/kg/day divided bid x 10 days *see page* 556 *for dose by weight*
    Augmentin ES-600 *Oral susp:* 600 mg/5 ml (50, 75, 100, 125, 150, 200 ml) (strawberry cream) (phenylalanine) every 12 hours
        Pediatric: <3 months: not recommended; ≥3 months, <40 kg: 90 mg/kg/day in 2 divided doses; ≥40 kg: not recommended
    Augmentin XR 2 tabs q 12 hours x 7-10 days
        Pediatric: <16 years: use other forms; ≥16 years: same as adult
        Tab: 1000*mg ext-rel

> *cefuroxime axetil* (B)(G) 500 mg bid x 10 days
> *Pediatric:* 15 mg/kg bid x 10 days; *see page 567 for dose by weight*
>   **Ceftin** *Tab:* 250, 500 mg; *Oral susp:* 125, 250 mg/5 ml (50, 100 ml) (tutti-frutti)
> *doxycycline* (D)(G) 100 mg bid day 1; then 100 mg daily x 10 days
> *Pediatric:* <8 years: not recommended ≥8 years, <100 lb: 2 mg/lb on first day in 2 divided doses, followed by 1 mg/lb/day in 1-2 divided doses; ≥8 years, ≥100 lb: same as adult; *see page 572 for dose by weight*
>   **Actilate** *Tab:* 75, 150**mg
>   **Adoxa** *Tab:* 50, 75, 100, 150 mg ent-coat
>   **Doryx** *Tab:* 50, 75, 100, 150, 200 mg del-rel
>   **Monodox** *Cap:* 50, 75, 100 mg
>   **Oracea** *Cap:* 40 mg del-rel
>   **Vibramycin** *Tab:* 100 mg; *Cap:* 50, 100 mg; *Syr:* 50 mg/5 ml (raspberry-apple) (sulfites); *Oral susp:* 25 mg/5 ml (raspberry)
>   **Vibra-Tab** *Tab:* 100 mg film-coat

Comment: *doxycycline* is contraindicated <8 years-of-age, in pregnancy, and lactation (discolors developing tooth enamel). A side effect may be photo-sensitivity (photophobia). Do not give with antacids, calcium supplements, milk or other dairy, or within two hours of taking another drug.

> *penicillin V potassium* (B)(G) 500 mg PO qid x 3 days
> *Pediatric:* 15-50 mg/kg/day in 3-6 divided doses x 3 days; ≥12 years: same as adult; *see page 583 for dose by weight*
>   **Pen-Vee K** *Tab:* 250, 500 mg; *Oral soln:* 125 mg/5 ml (100, 200 ml); 250 mg/5 ml (100, 150, 200 ml)

◯ BITE: DOG

TETANUS PROPHYLAXIS

> *tetanus toxoid* vaccine (C) 0.5 ml IM x 1 dose if previously immunized
> *Vial:* 5 Lf units/0.5 ml (0.5, 5 ml); *Prefilled syringe:* 5 Lf units/0.5 ml (0.5 ml)
> see *Tetanus* page 408 for patients not previously immunized

ANTI-INFECTIVES

> *amoxicillin/clavulanate* (B)(G) 500 mg tid <u>or</u> 875 mg bid x 10 days
>   **Augmentin** *Tab:* 250, 500, 875 mg; *Chew tab:* 125, 250 mg (lemon-lime); 200, 400 mg (cherry-banana) (phenylalanine); *Oral susp:* 125 mg/5 ml (banana), 250 mg/5 ml (75, 100, 150 ml) (orange); 200, 400 mg/5 ml (50, 75, 100 ml) (orange) (phenylalanine)
>   *Pediatric:* 40-45 mg/kg/day divided tid x 10 days <u>or</u> 90 mg/kg/day divided bid x 10 days *see page 556 for dose by weight*
>   **Augmentin ES-600** *Oral susp:* 600 mg/5 ml (50, 75, 100, 125, 150, 200 ml) (strawberry cream) (phenylalanine) every 12 hours
>   *Pediatric:* <3 months: not recommended; ≥3 months, <40 kg: 90 mg/kg/day in 2 divided doses; ≥40 kg: not recommended
>   **Augmentin XR** 2 tabs q 12 hours x 7-10 days
>   *Pediatric:* <16 years: use other forms; ≥16 years: same as adult
>   *Tab:* 1000*mg ext-rel

➤ *clindamycin* (B) (administer with fluoroquinolone in adult and TMP-SMX in children) 300 mg qid x 10 days
  Pediatric: 8-16 mg/kg/day in 3-4 divided doses x 10 days; *see page 570 for dose by weight*
    Cleocin (G) *Cap:* 75 (tartrazine), 150 (tartrazine), 300 mg
    Cleocin Pediatric Granules (G) *Oral susp:* 75 mg/5 ml (100 ml)(cherry)
➤ *doxycycline* (D)(G) 100 mg bid
  Pediatric: <8 years: not recommended ≥8 years, <100 lb: 2 mg/lb on first day in 2 divided doses, followed by 1 mg/lb/day in 1-2 divided doses; ≥8 years, ≥100 lb: same as adult; *see page 572 for dose by weight*
    Actilate *Tab:* 75, 150**mg
    Adoxa *Tab:* 50, 75, 100, 150 mg ent-coat
    Doryx *Tab:* 50, 75, 100, 150, 200 mg del-rel
    Monodox *Cap:* 50, 75, 100 mg
    Oracea *Cap:* 40 mg del-rel
    Vibramycin *Tab:* 100 mg; *Cap:* 50, 100 mg; *Syr:* 50 mg/5 ml (raspberry-apple) (sulfites); *Oral susp:* 25 mg/5 ml (raspberry)
    Vibra-Tab *Tab:* 100 mg film-coat
  Comment: *doxycycline* is contraindicated <8 years-of-age, in pregnancy, and lactation (discolors developing tooth enamel). A side effect may be photosensitivity (photophobia). Do not give with antacids, calcium supplements, milk or other dairy, or within two hours of taking another drug.
➤ *penicillin V potassium* (B)(G) 500 mg PO qid x 3 days
  Pediatric: 50 mg/kg/day in 4 divided doses x 3 days; ≥12 years: same as adult; *see page 583 for dose by weight*
    Pen-Vee K *Tab:* 250, 500 mg; *Oral soln:* 125 mg/5 ml (100, 200 ml); 250 mg/5 ml (100, 150, 200 ml)

BITE: HUMAN

TETANUS PROPHYLAXIS

➤ *tetanus toxoid* vaccine (C) 0.5 ml IM x 1 dose if previously immunized
  Vial: 5 Lf units/0.5 ml (0.5, 5 ml)
  Prefilled syringe: 5 Lf units/0.5 ml (0.5 ml)
  *see **Tetanus** page 408 for patients not previously immunized*

ANTI-INFECTIVES

➤ *amoxicillin/clavulanate* (B)(G) 500 mg tid or 875 mg bid x 10 days
    Augmentin *Tab:* 250, 500, 875 mg; *Chew tab:* 125, 250 mg (lemon-lime); 200, 400 mg (cherry-banana) (phenylalanine); *Oral susp:* 125 mg/5 ml (banana), 250 mg/5 ml (75, 100, 150 ml) (orange); 200, 400 mg/5 ml (50, 75, 100 ml) (orange) (phenylalanine)
      Pediatric: 40-45 mg/kg/day divided tid x 10 days or 90 mg/kg/day divided bid x 10 days *see page 556 for dose by weight*
    Augmentin ES-600 *Oral susp:* 600 mg/5 ml (50, 75, 100, 125, 150, 200 ml) (strawberry cream) (phenylalanine) every 12 hours
      Pediatric: <3 months: not recommended; ≥3 months, <40 kg: 90 mg/kg/day in 2 divided doses; ≥40 kg: not recommended

Augmentin XR 2 tabs q 12 hours x 7-10 days
  Pediatric: <16 years: use other forms; ≥16 years: same as adult
  Tab: 1000*mg ext-rel
➤ *cefoxitin* (B) 80-160 mg/kg/day IM in 3-4 divided doses x 10 days; max 12 g/day
  Pediatric: <3 months: not recommended; ≥3 months: same as adult
  Mefoxin Injectable *Vial:* 1, 2 g
➤ *ciprofloxacin* (C) 500 mg bid x 10 days
  Pediatric: <18 years: not recommended
  Cipro (G) *Tab:* 250, 500, 750 mg; *Oral susp:* 250, 500 mg/5 ml (100 ml)
  (strawberry)
  Cipro XR *Tab:* 500, 1000 mg ext-rel
  ProQuin XR *Tab:* 500 mg ext-rel
  Comment: *ciprofloxacin* is contraindicated <18 years-of-age, and during pregnancy
  and lactation. Risk of tendonitis or tendon rupture, especially 60 years-of-age and older.
➤ *erythromycin base* (B)(G) 250 mg qid x 10 days
  Pediatric: <45 kg: 30-40 mg/kg/day in 4 divided doses x 10 days; ≥45 kg: same as adult
  Ery-Tab *Tab:* 250, 333, 500 mg ent-coat
  PCE *Tab:* 333, 500 mg
  Comment: *erythromycin* may increase INR with concomitant *warfarin*, as well as
  increase serum level of *digoxin*, benzodiazepines and statins.
➤ *erythromycin ethylsuccinate* (B)(G) 400 mg qid x 10 days
  Pediatric: 30-50 mg/kg/day in 4 divided doses x 10 days; may double dose with
  severe infection; max 100 mg/kg/day; *see page 574 for dose by weight*
  EryPed *Oral susp:* 200 mg/5 ml (100, 200 ml) (fruit); 400 mg/5 ml (60, 100,
  200 ml) (banana); *Oral drops:* 200, 400 mg/5 ml (50 ml) (fruit); *Chew tab:*
  200 mg wafer (fruit)
  E.E.S. *Oral susp:* 200, 400 mg/5 ml (100 ml) (fruit)
  E.E.S. Granules *Oral susp:* 200 mg/5 ml (100, 200 ml) (cherry)
  E.E.S. 400 Tablets *Tab:* 400 mg
  Comment: *erythromycin* may increase INR with concomitant *warfarin*, as well as
  increase serum level of *digoxin*, benzodiazepines and statins.
➤ *trimethoprim/sulfamethoxazole* (D)(G) bid x 10 days
  Pediatric: <2 months: not recommended; ≥2 months: 40 mg/kg/day of *sulfamethox-
  azole* in 2 divided doses bid x 10 days; *see page 587 for dose by weight*
  Bactrim, Septra 2 tabs bid x 10 days
    Tab: trim 80 mg/*sulfa* 400 mg*
  Bactrim DS, Septra DS 1 tab bid x 10 days
    Tab: trim 160 mg/*sulfa* 800 mg*
  Bactrim Pediatric Suspension, Septra Pediatric Suspension
    Oral susp: trim 40 mg/*sulfa* 200 mg per 5 ml (100 ml) (cherry) (alcohol 0.3%)
  Comment: *trimethoprim/sulfamethoxazole* is not recommended in pregnancy or
  lactation. *CrCl 15-30 mL/min*: reduce dose by 1/2; *CrCl <15 mL/min*: not recommended

◯ BLEPHARITIS

OPHTHALMIC AGENTS

➤ *erythromycin ophthalmic ointment* (B) apply 1/2 inch bid-qid x 14 days; then q HS
  x 10 days

Pediatric: same as adult
Ilotycin *Oint:* 5 mg/g (1/2 oz)
➤ *polymyxin/bacitracin* ophthalmic ointment **(C)** apply 1/2 inch bid-qid x 14 days; then q HS
Pediatric: same as adult
Polysporin *Oint: poly B* 10,000 U/*baci* 500 U (3.75 g)
➤ *polymyxin B/bacitracin/neomycin* ophthalmic ointment **(C)** apply 1/2 inch bid-qid x 14 days; then q HS
Pediatric: same as adult
Neosporin *Oint: poly B* 10,000 U/*baci* 400 U/*neo* 3.5 mg/g (3.75 g)
➤ *sodium sulfacetamide* **(C)**
Bleph-10 Ophthalmic Solution 2 drops q 4 hours x 7-14 days
Pediatric: <2 years: not recommended; ≥2 years: 1-2 drops q 2-3 hours during the day x 7-14 days
Ophth soln: 10% (2.5, 5, 15 ml) (benzalkonium chloride)
Bleph-10 Ophthalmic Ointment apply 1/2 inch qid and HS x 7-14 days
Pediatric: <2 years: not recommended; >2 years: same as adult
Ophth oint: 10% (3.5 g) (phenylmercuric acetate)

SYSTEMIC AGENTS

➤ *tetracycline* **(D)(G)** 250 mg qid x 7 days
Pediatric: <8 years: not recommended; ≥8 years, <100 lb: 25-50 mg/kg/day in 2-4 divided doses x 7-10 days; ≥100 lb: same as adult; *see page 585 for dose by weight*
Achromycin V *Cap:* 250, 500 mg
Sumycin *Tab:* 250, 500 mg; *Cap:* 250, 500 mg; *Oral susp:* 125 mg/5 ml (100, 200 ml) (fruit) (sulfites)
Comment: *tetracycline* is contraindicated <8 years-of-age, in pregnancy, and lactation (discolors developing tooth enamel). A side effect may be photosensitivity (photophobia). Do not give with antacids, calcium supplements, milk or other dairy, or within two hours of taking another drug.

◯ BREAST CANCER: PROPHYLAXIS

ANTI-ESTROGEN AGENTS

➤ *fulvestrant* **(D)** 250 mg IM once monthly; administer 2.5 ml IM in each buttock concurrently
Faslodex *Prefilled syringe:* 50 mg/ml (2 x 2.5 ml, 1 x 5 ml)
➤ *letrozole* **(D)(G)** 2.5 mg daily
Femara *Tab:* 2.5 mg film-coat
Comment: *letrozole* is indicated for the extended adjuvant treatment of early breast cancer in postmenopausal women, who have received 5 years of adjuvant *tamoxifen* therapy.
➤ *tamoxifen citrate* **(D)(G)** 20 mg once daily x 5 years
Tab: 10, 20 mg
Comment: Cautious use of *tamoxifen* with concomitant *coumarin*-type anticoagulation therapy, history of DVT, <u>or</u> history of pulmonary embolus.

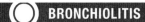

BRONCHIOLITIS

Inhaled Beta$_2$-Agonists (Bronchodilators) *see Asthma page* 29
Oral Beta$_2$-Agonists (Bronchodilators) *see Asthma page* 35
Inhaled Corticosteroids *see Asthma page* 29
Parenteral Corticosteroids *see page* 511
Oral Corticosteroids *see page* 509

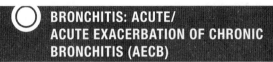

BRONCHITIS: ACUTE/
ACUTE EXACERBATION OF CHRONIC
BRONCHITIS (AECB)

Comment: Antibiotics are seldom needed for treatment of acute bronchitis because the etiology is usually viral.
Inhaled Beta$_2$-Agonists (Bronchodilators) *see Asthma page* 29
Oral Beta$_2$-Agonists (Bronchodilators) *see Asthma page* 35
Decongestants *see page* 353
Expectorants *see page* 353
Antitussives *see page* 353

ANTI-INFECTIVES FOR SECONDARY BACTERIAL INFECTION

▷ *amoxicillin* (B)(G) 500-875 mg bid or 250-500 mg tid x 10 days
  Pediatric: <40 kg (88 lb): 20-40 mg/kg/day in 3 divided doses x 10 days or 25-45 mg/kg/day in 2 divided doses x 10 days; ≥40 kg: same as adult; *see page 554 for dose by weight*
    Amoxil *Cap:* 250, 500 mg; *Tab:* 875*mg; *Chew tab:* 125, 200, 250, 400 mg (cherry-banana-peppermint) (phenylalanine); *Oral susp:* 125, 250 mg/5 ml (80, 100, 150 ml) (strawberry); 200, 400 mg/5 ml (50, 75, 100 ml) (bubble gum); *Oral drops:* 50 mg/ml (30 ml) (bubble gum)
    Moxatag *Tab:* 775 mg ext-rel
    Trimox *Tab:* 125, 250 mg; *Cap:* 250, 500 mg; *Oral susp:* 125, 250 mg/5 ml (80, 100, 150 ml) (raspberry-strawberry)
▷ *amoxicillin/clavulanate* (B)(G) 500 mg tid or 875 mg bid x 10 days
    Augmentin *Tab:* 250, 500, 875 mg; *Chew tab:* 125, 250 mg (lemon-lime); 200, 400 mg (cherry-banana) (phenylalanine); *Oral susp:* 125 mg/5 ml (banana), 250 mg/5 ml (75, 100, 150 ml) (orange); 200, 400 mg/5 ml (50, 75, 100 ml) (orange) (phenylalanine)
      Pediatric: 40-45 mg/kg/day divided tid x 10 days or 90 mg/kg/day divided bid x 10 days *see page 556 for dose by weight*
    Augmentin ES-600 *Oral susp:* 600 mg/5 ml (50, 75, 100, 125, 150, 200 ml) (strawberry cream) (phenylalanine) every 12 hours
      Pediatric: <3 months: not recommended; ≥3 months, <40 kg: 90 mg/kg/day in 2 divided doses; ≥40 kg: not recommended
    Augmentin XR 2 tabs q 12 hours x 7-10 days
      Pediatric: <16 years: use other forms; ≥16 years: same as adult
      Tab: 1000*mg ext-rel
▷ *ampicillin* (B) 250-500 mg qid x 10 days
  Pediatric: not recommended for bronchitis in children

Omnipen, Principen *Cap:* 250, 500 mg; *Oral susp:* 125, 250 mg/5 ml (100, 150, 200 ml) (fruit)

▷ *azithromycin* (B) 500 mg x 1 dose on day 1, then 250 mg daily on days 2-5 <u>or</u> 500 mg once daily x 3 days <u>or</u> 2 g in a single dose
Pediatric: not recommended for bronchitis in children
Zithromax *Tab:* 250, 500, 600 mg; *Oral susp:* 100 mg/5 ml (15 ml); 200 mg/5 ml (15, 22.5, 30 ml) (cherry); *Pkt:* 1 g for reconstitution (cherry-banana)
Zithromax Tri-pak *Tab:* 3 x 500 mg tabs/pck
Zithromax Z-pak *Tab:* 6 x 250 mg tabs/pck
Zmax *Oral susp:* 2 g ext-rel for reconstitution (cherry-banana) (148 mg Na$^+$)

▷ *cefaclor* (B)(G) 250-500 mg q 8 hours x 10 days; max 2 g/day
Tab: 500 mg; *Cap:* 250, 500 mg; *Susp:* 125 mg/5 ml (75, 150 ml) (strawberry); 187 mg/5 ml (50, 100 ml) (strawberry); 250 mg/5 ml (75, 150 ml) (strawberry); 375 mg/5 ml (50, 100 ml) (strawberry)
Pediatric: <16 years: ext-rel not recommended; ≥16 years: same as adult
Cefaclor Extended Release *Tab:* 375, 500 mg ext-rel

▷ *cefadroxil* (B) 1-2 g in 1-2 divided doses x 10 days
Pediatric: 30 mg/kg/day in 2 divided doses x 10 days; *see page 561 for dose by weight*
Duricef *Tab:* 1 g; *Cap:* 500 mg; *Oral susp:* 250 mg/5 ml (100 ml); 500 mg/5 ml (75, 100 ml) (orange-pineapple)

▷ *cefdinir* (B) 300 mg bid x 5-10 days <u>or</u> 600 mg daily x 10 days
Pediatric: <6 months: not recommended; 6 months-12 years: 14 mg/kg/day in 1-2 divided doses x 10 days; ≥12 years: same as adult; *see page 562 for dose by weight*
Omnicef *Cap:* 300 mg; *Oral susp:* 125 mg/5 ml (60, 100 ml) (strawberry)

▷ *cefditoren pivoxil* (B) 400 mg bid x 10 days
Pediatric: not recommended
Spectracef *Tab:* 200 mg
Comment: **Spectracef** is contraindicated with milk protein allergy <u>or</u> carnitine deficiency.

▷ *cefixime* (B)(G)
Pediatric: <6 months: not recommended; ≥6 months-12 years, <50 kg: 8 mg/kg/day in 1-2 divided doses x 10 days; ≥12 years, >50 kg: same as adult; *see page 563 for dose by weight*
Suprax *Tab:* 400 mg; *Cap:* 400 mg; *Oral susp:* 100, 200 mg/5 ml (50, 75, 100 ml) (strawberry)

▷ *cefpodoxime proxetil* (B) 200 mg bid x 10 days
Pediatric: <2 months: not recommended; ≥2 months-12 years: 10 mg/kg/day (max 400 mg/dose) <u>or</u> 5 mg/kg/day bid (max 200 mg/dose) x 10 days; >12 years: same as adult; *see page 564 for dose by weight*
Vantin *Tab:* 100, 200 mg; *Oral susp:* 50, 100 mg/5 ml (50, 75, 100 mg) (lemon creme)

▷ *cefprozil* (B) 500 mg q 12 hours x 10 days
Pediatric: <2 years: not recommended; 2-12 years: 15 mg/kg q 12 hours x 10 days; >12 years: same as adult; *see page 565 for dose by weight*
Cefzil *Tab:* 250, 500 mg; *Oral susp:* 125, 250 mg/5 ml (50, 75, 100 ml) (bubble gum) (phenylalanine)

▷ *ceftibuten* (B) 400 mg daily x 10 days
Pediatric: 9 mg/kg daily x 10 days; max 400 mg/day; *see page 566 for dose by weight*
Cedax *Cap:* 400 mg; *Oral susp:* 90 mg/5 ml (30, 60, 90, 120 ml); 180 mg/5 ml (30, 60, 120 ml) (cherry)

➤ *ceftriaxone* (B)(G) 1-2 g IM daily continued 2 days after signs of infection have disappeared; max 4 g/day
Pediatric: 50 mg/kg IM daily and continued 2 days after clinical stability
  Rocephin *Vial:* 250, 500 mg; 1, 2 g
➤ *cefuroxime axetil* (B)(G) 250-500 mg bid x 10 days
Pediatric: 15 mg/kg bid x 10 days; ≥12 years: same as adult; *see page 567 for dose by weight*
  Ceftin *Tab:* 250, 500 mg; *Oral susp:* 125, 250 mg/5 ml (50, 100 ml) (tutti-frutti)
➤ *cephalexin* (B)(G) 250-500 mg qid <u>or</u> 500 mg bid x 10 days
Pediatric: 25-50 mg/kg/day in 4 divided doses x 10 days; ≥12 years: same as adult; *see page 568 for dose by weight*
  Keflex *Cap:* 250, 333, 500, 750 mg; *Oral susp:* 125, 250 mg/5 ml (100, 200 ml) (strawberry)
➤ *clarithromycin* (C)(G) 500 mg <u>or</u> 500 mg ext-rel once daily x 7 days
Pediatric: <6 months: not recommended; ≥6 months: 7.5 mg/kg bid x 7 days; ≥12 years: same as adult; *see page 569 for dose by weight*
  Biaxin *Tab:* 250, 500 mg
  Biaxin Oral Suspension *Oral susp:* 125, 250 mg/5 ml (50, 100 ml) (fruit-punch)
  Biaxin XL *Tab:* 500 mg ext-rel
➤ *dirithromycin* (C)(G) 500 mg daily x 7 days
Pediatric: <12 years: not recommended; ≥12 years: same as adult
  Dynabac *Tab:* 250 mg
➤ *doxycycline* (D)(G) 100 mg bid x 10 days
Pediatric: <8 years: not recommended; ≥8 years, <100 lb: 2 mg/lb on first day in 2 divided doses, followed by 1 mg/lb/day in 1-2 divided doses; ≥8 years, ≥100 lb: same as adult; *see page 572 for dose by weight*
  Actilate *Tab:* 75, 150**mg
  Adoxa *Tab:* 50, 75, 100, 150 mg ent-coat
  Doryx *Tab:* 50, 75, 100, 150, 200 mg del-rel
  Monodox *Cap:* 50, 75, 100 mg
  Oracea *Cap:* 40 mg del-rel
  Vibramycin *Tab:* 100 mg; *Cap:* 50, 100 mg; *Syr:* 50 mg/5 ml (raspberry-apple) (sulfites); *Oral susp:* 25 mg/5 ml (raspberry)
  Vibra-Tab *Tab:* 100 mg film-coat
Comment: *doxycycline* is contraindicated <8 years-of-age, in pregnancy, and lactation (discolors developing tooth enamel). A side effect may be photosensitivity (photophobia). Do not give with antacids, calcium supplements, milk or other dairy, or within two hours of taking another drug.
➤ *erythromycin ethylsuccinate* (B)(G) 400 mg qid x 7 days
Pediatric: 30-50 mg/kg/day in 4 divided doses x 7 days; may double dose with severe infection; max 100 mg/kg/day; *see page 574 for dose by weight*
  EryPed *Oral susp:* 200 mg/5 ml (100, 200 ml) (fruit); 400 mg/5 ml (60, 100, 200 ml) (banana); *Oral drops:* 200, 400 mg/5 ml (50 ml) (fruit); *Chew tab:* 200 mg wafer (fruit)
  E.E.S. *Oral susp:* 200, 400 mg/5 ml (100 ml) (fruit)
  E.E.S. Granules *Oral susp:* 200 mg/5 ml (100, 200 ml) (cherry)
  E.E.S. 400 Tablets *Tab:* 400 mg
Comment: *erythromycin* may increase INR with concomitant *warfarin*, as well as increase serum level of *digoxin*, benzodiazepines and statins.

▷ *gemifloxacin* (C) 320 mg daily x 5 days
   Pediatric: <18 years: not recommended
      Factive *Tab:* 320*mg
   Comment: *gemifloxacin* is contraindicated <18 years-of-age, and during pregnancy
   and lactation. Risk of tendonitis or tendon rupture, especially 60 years-of-age and older.
▷ *levofloxacin* (C) *Uncomplicated:* 500 mg daily x 7 days; *Complicated:* 750 mg daily
   x 7 days
   Pediatric: <18 years: not recommended
      Levaquin *Tab:* 250, 500, 750 mg
   Comment: *levofloxacin* is contraindicated <18 years-of-age, and during pregnancy and
   lactation. Risk of tendonitis or tendon rupture, especially 60 years-of-age and older.
▷ *loracarbef* (B) 200-400 mg bid x 7 days
   Pediatric: 30 mg/kg/day in 2 divided doses x 7 days; ≥12 years: same as adult;
   see page 581 for dose by weight
      Lorabid *Pulvule:* 200, 400 mg; *Oral susp:* 100 mg/5 ml (50, 100 ml);
      200 mg/5 ml (50, 75, 100 ml) (strawberry bubble gum)
▷ *moxifloxacin* (C)(G) 400 mg daily x 5 days
   Pediatric: <18 years: not recommended
      Avelox *Tab:* 400 mg; IV soln: 400 mg/250 mg (latex-free, preservative-free)
   Comment: *moxifloxacin* is contraindicated <18 years-of-age and during pregnancy
   and lactation. Risk of tendonitis or tendon rupture, especially 60 years-of-age and older.
▷ *ofloxacin* (C)(G) 400 mg bid x 10 days
   Pediatric: <18 years: not recommended
      Floxin *Tab:* 200, 300, 400 mg
   Comment: *ofloxacin* is contraindicated <18 years-of-age and during pregnancy and
   lactation. Risk of tendonitis or tendon rupture, especially 60 years-of-age and older.
▷ *telithromycin* (C) 2 x 400 mg tabs in a singe dose daily x 5 days
   Pediatric: <18 years: not recommended
      Ketek *Tab:* 400 mg
▷ *tetracycline* (D)(G) 250-500 mg qid x 7 days
   Pediatric: <8 years: not recommended; ≥8 years, <100 lb: 25-50 mg/kg/day in 2-4
   divided doses x 7 days; ≥8 years, ≥100 lb: same as adult; *see page 585 for dose by weight*
      Achromycin V *Cap:* 250, 500 mg
      Sumycin *Tab:* 250, 500 mg; *Cap:* 250, 500 mg; *Oral susp:* 125 mg/5 ml (100,
      200 ml) (fruit) (sulfites)
   Comment: *tetracycline* is contraindicated <8 years-of-age, in pregnancy, and
   lactation (discolors developing tooth enamel). A side effect may be photo-
   sensitivity (photophobia). Do not give with antacids, calcium supplements, milk
   or other dairy, or within two hours of taking another drug.
▷ *trimethoprim/sulfamethoxazole* (D)(G) bid x 10 days
   Pediatric: <2 months: not recommended; ≥2 months: 40 mg/kg/day of
   sulfamethoxazole in 2 divided doses bid x 10 days; ≥12 years: same as adult;
   see page 587 for dose by weight
      Bactrim, Septra 2 tabs bid x 10 days
         Tab: trim 80 mg/*sulfa* 400 mg*
      Bactrim DS, Septra DS 1 tab bid x 10 days
         Tab: trim 160 mg/*sulfa* 800 mg*
      Bactrim Pediatric Suspension, Septra Pediatric Suspension
         Oral susp: trim 40 mg/*sulfa* 200 mg per 5 ml (100 ml) (cherry)
         (alcohol 0.3%)

Comment: *trimethoprim/sulfamethoxazole* is not recommended in pregnancy or lactation. *CrCl 15-30 mL/min:* reduce dose by 1/2; *CrCl <15 mL/min:* not recommended

◯ BRONCHITIS: CHRONIC/CHRONIC OBSTRUCTIVE PULMONARY DISEASE (COPD)

Oral Beta₂-Agonists (Bronchodilators) *see Asthma page 35*
Inhaled Corticosteroids *see Asthma page 29*
Parenteral Corticosteroids *see page 511*
Oral Corticosteroids *see page 509*
Inhaled Beta₂-Agonists (Bronchodilators) *see Asthma page 29*

LONG-ACTING INHALED BETA2-AGONIST (LABA)

▶ *indacaterol* (C) inhale contents of one 75 mcg cap daily
  Pediatric: not established
    Arcapta Neohaler *Neohaler Device/Cap:* 75 mcg pwdr for inhalation (5 blister cards, 6 caps/card)
  Comment: Remove cap from blister cap immediately before use. For oral inhalation with **Neohaler** device only. *indacaterol* is indicated for the long-term maintenance treatment of bronchoconstriction in patients with COPD. Not indicated for treating asthma, for primary treatment of acute symptoms, or for acute deterioration of COPD.
▶ *indacaterol/glycopyrrolate* (C) inhale the contents of one cap twice daily
  Pediatric: not established
    Utibron Neohaler *Neohaler Device/Cap:* inda 27.5 mcg/glyco 15.6 mcg pwdr for inhalation (1, 10 blister cards, 6 caps/card)
▶ *olodaterol* (C)
  Pediatric: not established
    Striverdi Respimat 12 mcg q 12 hours
      Inhal soln: 2.5 mcg/cartridge (metered actuation) (40 g, 60 metered actuations) (benzalkonium chloride)
▶ *salmeterol* (C)(G) 1 inhalation q 12 hours
  Serevent Diskus
    Pediatric: <4 years: not recommended; ≥4 years: same as adult
      Diskus (pwdr): 50 mcg/actuation (60 doses/disk)

INHALED ANTICHOLINERGICS

▶ *ipratropium bromide* (B)(G)
  Pediatric: not recommended
    Atrovent 2 inhalations qid; max 12 inhalations/day
      Inhaler: 14 g (200 inh)
    Atrovent Inhalation Solution 500 mcg by nebulizer tid-qid
      Inhal soln: 0.02% (2.5 ml)
  Comment: *ipatropium bromide* is contraindicated with severe hypersensitivity to milk proteins.
▶ *umeclidinium* (C) 1 inhalation once daily at the same time each day
  Pediatric: not established
    Incruse Ellipta *Inhal pwdr:* 62.5 mcg/inhalation (30 doses) (lactose)

Comment: **Incruse Ellipta** is contraindicated with allergy to *atropine* <u>or</u> its derivatives.

INHALED LONG-ACTING ANTI-CHOLINERGICS (LAA) (ANTIMUSCARINICS)

Comment: Inhaled LAAs are for prophylaxis and chronic treatment, only. Not for primary (rescue) treatment of acute attack. Avoid getting powder in eyes. Caution with narrow-angle glaucoma, BPH, bladder neck obstruction, and pregnancy. Contraindicated with allergy to atropine <u>or</u> its derivatives (e.g., *ipratropium*). Avoid other anticholinergic agents.

▷ *aclidinium bromide* (C) 1 inhalation twice daily using inhaler
  Pediatric: not recommended
      Tudorza Pressair *Inhal device:* 400 mcg/actuation (60 doses per inhalation device)
▷ *tiotropium (as bromide monohydrate)* (C) 1 inhalation daily using inhaler; do not swallow caps
  Pediatric: not recommended
      Spiriva HandiHaler *Inhal device:* 18 mcg/cap (5, 30, 90 caps w. inhalation device)

ANTI-CHOLINERGIC/INHALED LONG-ACTING BETA2-AGONIST (LABA)

▷ *ipratropium/albuterol* (C) 1 inhalation qid; max 6 inhalations/day
  Pediatric: not established
      Combivent Respimat *Inhal soln:* ipra 20 mcg/*alb* 100 mcg per inhalation (4 g, 120 inhal)
      Comment: **Combivent Respimat** is contraindicted with *atropine* allergy.
▷ *tiotropium/olodaterol* (C) 2 inhalations once daily at the same time each day; max 2 inhalations/day
  Pediatric: not established
      Stiolto Respimat *Inhal soln:* tio 2.5 mcg/*olo* 2.5 mcg per actuation (4 g, 60 inh) (benzalkonium chloride)
      Comment: **Stiolto Respimat** is not for treating asthma, for relief of acute bronchospasm, <u>or</u> acutely deteriorating COPD.
▷ *umeclidinium/vilanterol* (C) 1 inhalation once daily at the same time each day
  Pediatric: not established
      Anoro Ellipta *Inhal soln:* ume 62.5 mcg/*vila* 25 mcg per inhalation (30 doses)
      Comment: **Anoro Ellipta** is contraindicted with severe hypersensitivity to milk proteins.

CORTICOSTEROID/INHALED LONG-ACTING BETA AGONIST (LABA)

▷ *fluticasone furoate/vilanterol* (C) 1 inhalation 100/25 once daily at the same time each day
  Pediatric: <17 years: not established
      Breo Ellipta 100/25 *Inhal pwdr:* flu 100 mcg/*vil* 25 mcg dry pwdr per inhalation (30 doses)
      Breo Ellipta 200/25 *Inhal pwdr:* flu 200 mcg/*vil* 25 mcg dry pwdr per inhalation (30 doses)
      Comment: **Breo Ellipta** is contraindicated with severe hypersensitivity to milk proteins.

METHYLXANTHINES

Comment: Check serum theophylline level just before 5th dose is administered.
Therapeutic theophylline level: 10-20 mcg/ml.

▷ *theophylline* (C)(G)

> **Theo-24** initially 300-400 mg once daily at HS; after 3 days, increase to 400-600 mg once daily at HS; max 600 mg/day
> > *Pediatric:* <45 kg: initially 12-14 mg/kg/day; max 300 mg/day; increase after 3 days to 16 mg/kg/day to max 400 mg; after 3 more days increase to 30 mg/kg/day to max 600 mg/day; ≥45 kg: same as adult
> > *Cap:* 100, 200, 300, 400 mg ext-rel

> **Theo-Dur** initially 150 mg bid; increase to 200 mg bid after 3 days; then increase to 300 mg bid after 3 more days
> > *Pediatric:* <6 years: not recommended; ≥6-15 years: initially 12-14 mg/kg/day in 2 divided doses; max 300 mg/day; then increase to 16 mg/kg in 2 divided doses; max 400 mg/day; then to 20 mg/kg/day in 2 divided doses; max 600 mg/day
> > *Tab:* 100, 200, 300 mg ext-rel

> **Theolair-SR** *Tab:* 200, 250, 300, 500 mg sust-rel
> > *Pediatric:* not recommended

> **Uniphyl** 400-600 mg daily with meals
> > *Pediatric:* not recommended
> > *Tab:* 400*, 600*mg cont-rel

METHYLXANTHINE/EXPECTORANT COMBINATION

▷ *dyphylline/guaifenesin* (C)

> **Lufyllin GG** 1 tab qid <u>or</u> 15-30 ml qid
> > *Tab: dyphy* 200 mg/*guaif* 200 mg; *Elix: dyphy* 100 mg/*guaif* 100 mg per 15 ml

SELECTIVE PHOSPHODIESTERASE 4 (PDE4) INHIBITOR

▷ *roflumilast* (C)

> *Pediatric:* not recommended
> > **Daliresp** 500 mcg once daily
> > *Tab:* 500 mcg

Comment: *roflumilast* is indicated to reduce the risk of COPD exacerbations in severe COPD patients with chronic bronchitis and a history of exacerbations.

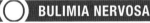 **BULIMIA NERVOSA**

SELECTIVE SEROTONIN REUPTAKE INHIBITOR (SSRI)

▷ *fluoxetine* (C)(G)

> **Prozac** initially 20 mg daily; may increase after 1 week; doses >20 mg/day may be divided into AM and noon doses; usual daily dose 60 mg; max 80 mg/day
> > *Pediatric:* <8 years: not recommended; 8-17 years: initially 10-20 mg/day; start lower weight children at 10 mg/day; if starting at 10 mg daily, may increase after 1 week to 20 mg daily
> > *Cap:* 10, 20, 40 mg; *Tab:* 30*, 60*mg; *Oral soln:* 20 mg/5 ml (4 oz) (mint)

> **Prozac Weekly** following daily *fluoxetine* therapy at 20 mg/day for 13 weeks, may initiate **Prozac Weekly** 7 days after the last 20 mg *fluoxetine* dose

Pediatric: not recommended
Cap: 90 mg ent-coat del-rel pellets

◑ BURN: MINOR

▷ *silver sulfadiazine* (C)(G) apply topically to burn 1-2 x daily
Pediatric: not recommended
Silvadene *Crm:* 1% (20, 50, 85, 400, 1000 g jar; 20 g tube)
Comment: *silver sulfadiazine* is contradicted in sulfa allergy.

TOPICAL/TRANSDERMAL ANESTHETICS

Comment: *lidocaine* should not be applied to non-intact skin.
▷ *lidocaine* burn gel (B)(G)
Pediatric: not recommended
▷ *lidocaine* cream (B)
Pediatric: not recommended
LidaMantle *Crm:* 3% (1, 2 oz)
Lidoderm *Crm:* 3% (85 g)
▷ *lidocaine* lotion (B)
Pediatric: not recommended
LidaMantle *Lotn:* 3% (177 ml)
▷ *lidocaine* 5% patch (B)(G) apply up to 3 patches at one time for up to 12 hours/24-hour period (12 hours on/12 hours off); patches may be cut into smaller sizes before removal of the release liner; do not re-use
Pediatric: not recommended
Lidoderm *Patch:* 5% (10x14 cm; 30/carton)
▷ *lidocaine* 2.5%/*prilocaine* 2.5%
Emla Cream (B) (5, 30 g)

◑ BURSITIS

Acetaminophen for IV Infusion *see Pain page* 306
Oral Prescription NSAIDs *see Pain page* 501
Other Oral Analgesics *see Pain page* 308
Topical/Transdermal NSAIDs *see Pain page* 307
Parenteral Corticosteroids *see page* 511
Oral Corticosteroids *see page* 509
Topical Analgesic and Anesthetic Agents *see page* 499

◯ CANDIDIASIS: ABDOMEN, BLADDER, ESOPHAGUS, KIDNEY

▷ *voriconazole* (D)(G) *PO:* <40 kg: 100 mg q 12 hours; may increase to150 mg q 12 hours if inadequate response; ≥40 kg: 200 mg q 12 hours; may increase to 300 mg q 12 hours if inadequate; *IV:* 6 mg/kg q 12 hours x 2 doses; then 4 mg/kg q 12 hour; max rate 3 mg/kg/hour over 1-2 hours; response
Pediatric: not recommended

Vfend *Tab:* 50, 200 mg
Vfend I.V. for Injection *Vial:* 200 mg pwdr for reconstitution (preservative-free)
Vfend *Oral susp:* 40 mg/ml pwdr for reconstitution (75 ml) (orange)

 CANDIDIASIS: ORAL (THRUSH)

ORAL ANTIFUNGALS

➤ *clotrimazole* (C) *Prophylaxis:* 1 troche dissolved in mouth tid; *Treatment:* 1 troche dissolved in mouth 5 times/day x 10-14 days
  Pediatric: <3 years: not recommended; ≥3 years: same as adult
    Mycelex Troches *Troches:* 10 mg
➤ *fluconazole* (C) 200 mg x 1 dose first day; then 100 mg once daily x 13 days
  Pediatric: >2 weeks: 6 mg/kg x 1 day; then 3 mg/kg/day for at least 3 weeks; *see page 577 for dose by weight*
    Diflucan *Tab:* 50, 100, 150, 200 mg; *Oral susp:* 10, 40 mg/ml (35 ml) (orange)
➤ *gentian violet* (NE)(G) apply to oral mucosa with a cotton swab tid x 3 days
➤ *itraconazole* (C) 200 mg daily x 7-14 days
  Pediatric: 5 mg/kg daily x 7-14 days; max 200 mg/day; *see page 570 for dose by weight*
    Sporanox *Oral soln:* 10 mg/ml (150 ml) (cherry-caramel)
➤ *miconazole* (C) One buccal tab once daily x 14 days; apply to upper gum region; hold in place 30 seconds; do not crush, chew, or swallow
  Pediatric: <16 years: not recommended; ≥16 years: same as adult
    Oravig *Buccal tab:* 50 mg (14/pck)
➤ *nystatin* (C)(G)
    Mycostatin 1-2 pastilles dissolved slowly in mouth 4-5 times/day x 10-14 days; max 14 days
      Pediatric: same as adult
      Pastille: 200,000 units/pastille (30 pastilles/pck)
    Mycostatin Suspension 4-6 ml qid swish and swallow
      Pediatric: Infants: 1 ml in each cheek qid after feedings; *Older children:* same as adult
      Oral susp: 100,000 units/ml (60 ml w. dropper)

INVASIVE INFECTION

➤ *posaconazole* (D) take with food; 100 mg bid on day one; then 100 mg once daily x 13 days; refractory, 400 mg bid
  Pediatric: <13 years: not recommended; ≥13 years: same as adult
    Noxafil *Oral susp:* 40 mg/ml (105 ml) (cherry)
    Comment: Noxafil is indicated as prophylaxis for invasive aspergillus and candida infections in patients >13-years-old who are at high risk due to being severely compromised.

CANDIDIASIS: SKIN

TOPICAL ANTIFUNGALS

➤ *butenafine* (B) apply bid x 1 week or once daily x 4 weeks
  Pediatric: <12 years: not recommended; ≥12 years: same as adult

Lotrimin Ultra (C)(OTC) *Crm:* 1% (12, 24 g)
    Mentax *Crm:* 1% (15, 30 g)
Comment: *butenafine* is a benzylamine, not an azole. Fungicidal activity continues for at least 5 weeks after the last application.

▷ *ciclopirox* (B)
    Loprox Cream apply bid; max 4 weeks
        Pediatric: <10 years: not recommended; ≥10 years: same as adult
        Crm: 0.77% (15, 30, 90 g)
    Loprox Lotion apply bid; max 4 weeks
        Pediatric: <10 years: not recommended; ≥10 years: same as adult
        Lotn: 0.77% (30, 60 ml)
    Loprox Gel apply bid; max 4 weeks
        Pediatric: <16 years: not recommended; ≥16 years: same as adult
        Gel: 0.77% (30, 45 g)
▷ *clotrimazole* (B) apply bid x 7 days
    Pediatric: same as adult
    Lotrimin *Crm:* 1% (15, 30, 45 g)
    Lotrimin AF (OTC) *Crm:* 1% (12 g); *Lotn:* 1% (10 ml); *Soln:* 1% (10 ml)
▷ *econazole* (C) apply bid x 14 days
    Spectazole *Crm:* 1% (15, 30, 85 g)
▷ *ketoconazole* (C) apply once daily x 14 days
    Nizoral Cream *Crm:* 2% (15, 30, 60 g)
▷ *miconazole* 2% (C) apply once daily x 2 weeks
    Pediatric: same as adult
    Lotrimin AF Spray Liquid (OTC) *Spray liq:* 2% (113 g) (alcohol 17%)
    Lotrimin AF Spray Powder (OTC) *Spray pwdr:* 2% (90 g) (alcohol 10%)
    Monistat-Derm *Crm:* 2% (1, 3 oz); *Spray liq:* 2% (3.5 oz); *Spray pwdr:* 2% (3 oz)
▷ *nystatin* (C)
    Nystop Powder dust affected skin freely bid-tid
        Pwdr: nystatin 100,000 U/g (15 g)

ORAL ANTIFUNGALS

▷ *amphotericin b* (B) apply tid-qid x 7-14 days
    Fungizone *Oral susp:* 100 mg/ml (24 ml w. dropper)
▷ *ketoconazole* (C) 400 mg once daily x 1-2 weeks
    Pediatric: <2 years: not recommended; ≥2 years: 3.3-6.6 mg/kg once daily
    Nizoral *Tab:* 200 mg

INVASIVE INFECTION

▷ *posaconazole* (D) take with food; 100 mg bid on day one; then 100 mg once daily x 13 days; refractory, 400 mg bid x 13 days
    Pediatric: <13 years: not recommended; ≥13 years: same as adult
    Noxafil *Oral susp:* 40 mg/ml (105 ml) (cherry)
    Comment: Noxafil is indicated as prophylaxis for invasive aspergillus and candida infections in patients >13 years old who are at high risk due to being severely compromised.

⬤ CANDIDIASIS: VULVOVAGINAL (MONILIASIS)

PROPHYLAXIS

▷ *acetic acid/oxyquinolone* (C) one full applicator intravaginally bid for up to 30 days
  Pediatric: not recommended
    Relagard *Gel: acetic acid* 0.9%/*oxyquin* 0.025% (50 g tube w. applicator)

Comment: The following treatment regimens for vulvovaginal candidiasis (VVC) are published in the **2015 CDC Sexually Transmitted Diseases Treatment Guidelines**. Treatment regimens are presented by generic drug name first, followed by information about brands and dose forms. Complicated VVC (recurrent, severe, non-albicans, or women with uncontrolled diabetes, debilitation, or immunosuppression) may require more intensive treatment and/or longer duration of treatment. VVC frequently occurs during pregnancy. Only topical azole therapies, applied for 7 days, are recommended during pregnancy.

ORAL Rx AGENT

▷ *fluconazole* 150 mg in a single dose; complicated VVC, 150 mg x 3 doses on days 1, 4, 7 or weekly x 6 months

Rx INTRAVAGINAL AGENTS

Regimen 1

▷ *butoconazole* 2% cream (bioadhesive product) 5 g intravaginally in a single dose

Regimen 2

▷ *nystatin* 100,000-unit vaginal tablet once daily x 14 days

Regimen 3

▷ *terconazole* 0.4% cream 5 g intravaginally once daily x 7 days

Regimen 4

▷ *terconazole* 0.8% cream 5 g intravaginally once daily x 3 days

Regimen 5

▷ *terconazole* 80 mg vaginal suppository intravaginally once daily x 3 days

OTC INTRAVAGINAL AGENTS

Regimen 1

▷ *butoconazole* 2% cream 5 g intravaginally once daily x 3 days

Regimen 2

▷ *clotrimazole* 1% cream intravaginally once daily x 7-14 days

Regimen 3

▷ *clotrimazole* 2% cream intravaginally once daily x 3 days

Regimen 4

▷ *miconazole* 2% cream intravaginally once daily x 7 days

Regimen 5

▷ *miconazole* 4% cream intravaginally once daily x 3 days

Regimen 6

▷ *miconazole* 100 mg vaginal suppository intravaginally once daily x 7 days

Regimen 7

▷ *miconazole* 200 mg vaginal suppository intravaginally once daily x 3 days

Regimen 8

▷ *miconazole* 1,200 mg vaginal suppository intravaginally in a single application

Regimen 9

▷ *tioconazole* 6.5% ointment 5 g intravaginally in a single application

DRUG BRANDS AND DOSE FORMS

▷ *butoconazole* cream 2% (C)
> Gynazole-12% Vaginal Cream *Prefilled vag applicator:* 5 g
> Femstat-3 Vaginal Cream (OTC) *Vag crm:* 2% (20 g w. 3 applicators); *Prefilled vag applicator:* 5 g (3/pck)

▷ *clotrimazole* (B)(OTC)
> Gyne-Lotrimin Vaginal Cream (OTC) *Vag crm:* 1% (45 g w. applicator)
> Gyne-Lotrimin Vaginal Suppository (OTC) *Vag supp:* 100 mg (7/pck)
> Gyne-Lotrimin 3 Vaginal Suppository (OTC) *Vag supp:* 200 mg (3/pck)
> Gyne-Lotrimin Combination Pack (OTC) *Combination pck:* 7-100 mg supp <u>with</u> 7 g 1% cream
> Gyne-Lotrimin 3 Combination Pack (OTC) *Combination pck:* 200 mg supp (7/pck) <u>plus</u> 1% cream (7 g)
> Mycelex-G Vaginal Cream *Vag crm:* 1% (45, 90 g w. applicator)
> Mycelex-G Vaginal Tab 1 *Tab:* 500 mg (1/pck)
> Mycelex Twin Pack *Twin pck:* 500 mg tab (7/pck) <u>with</u> 1% crm (7 g)
> Mycelex-7 Vaginal Cream (OTC) *Vag crm:* 1% (45 g w. applicator)
> Mycelex-7 Vaginal Inserts (OTC) *Vag insert:* 100 mg insert (7/pck)
> Mycelex-7 Combination Pack (OTC) *Combination pck:* 100 mg inserts (7/pck) <u>plus</u> 1% crm (7 g)

▷ *fluconazole* (C)
> Diflucan *Tab:* 50, 100, 150, 200 mg; *Oral susp:* 10, 40 mg/ml (35 ml) (orange)

▷ *miconazole* (B)
> Monistat-3 Combination Pack (OTC) *Combination pck:* 200 mg supp (3/pck) <u>plus</u> 2% crm (9 g)

Monistat-7 Combination Pack (OTC) *Combination pck:* 100 mg supp (7/pck) plus 2% crm (9 g)
Monistat-7 Vaginal Cream (OTC) *Vag crm:* 2% (45 g w. applicator)
Monistat-7 Vaginal Suppositories (OTC) *Vag supp:* 100 mg supp (7/pck)
Monistat-3 Vaginal Suppositories (OTC) *Vag supp:* 200 mg supp (3/pck)
▷ *nystatin* (C)
Mycostatin *Vag tab:* 100,000 U (1/pck)
▷ *terconazole* (C)
Terazol-3 Vaginal Cream *Vag crm:* 0.8% (20 g w. applicator)
Terazol-3 Vaginal Suppositories *Vag supp:* 80 mg supp (3/pck)
Terazol-7 Vaginal Cream *Vag crm:* 0.4% (45 g w. applicator)
▷ *tioconazole* (C)
1-Day (OTC) *Vag oint:* 6.5% (prefilled applicator x 1)
Monistat 1 Vaginal Ointment (OTC) *Vag oint:* 6.5% (prefilled applicator x 1)
Vagistat-1 Vaginal Ointment (OTC) *Vag oint:* 6.5% (prefilled applicator x 1)

INVASIVE INFECTION

▷ *posaconazole* (D) take with food; 100 mg bid on day 1; then 100 mg once daily x 13 days; refractory, 400 mg bid
Pediatric: <13 years: not recommended; ≥13 years: same as adult
Noxafil *Oral susp:* 40 mg/ml (105 ml) (cherry)
Comment: Noxafil is indicated as prophylaxis for invasive aspergillus and candida infections in patients >13-years-old who are at high risk due to being severely compromised.

CARPAL TUNNEL SYNDROME (CTS)

Acetaminophen for IV Infusion *see Pain page* 306
Oral Prescription NSAIDs *see page* 501
Other Oral Analgesics *see Pain page* 308
Topical/Transdermal NSAIDs *see Pain page* 307
Parenteral Corticosteroids *see page* 511
Oral Corticosteroids *see page* 509
Topical Analgesic and Anesthetic Agents *see page* 499

CAT SCRATCH FEVER (*BARTONELLA* INFECTION)

Comment: Cat scratch fever is usually self-limited. Treatment should be limited to severe or debilitating cases.

ANTI-INFECTIVES

▷ *azithromycin* (B)(G) 500 mg x 1 dose on day 1, then 250 mg daily on days 2-5 or 500 mg daily x 3 days or Zmax 2 g in a single dose
Pediatric: 12 mg/kg/day x 5 days; max 500 mg/day; *see page 559 for dose by weight*
Zithromax *Tab:* 250, 500, 600 mg; *Oral susp:* 100 mg/5 ml (15 ml); 200 mg/5 ml (15, 22.5, 30 ml) (cherry); *Pkt:* 1 g for reconstitution (cherry-banana)

Zithromax Tri-pak *Tab:* 3 x 500 mg tabs/pck
Zithromax Z-pak *Tab:* 6 x 250 mg tabs/pck
Zmax *Oral susp:* 2 g ext-rel for reconstitution (cherry-banana) (148 mg Na⁺)

▷ *doxycycline* (D)(G) 100 mg daily bid
Pediatric: <8 years: not recommended >8 years, <100 lb: 2 mg/lb on first day in 2 divided doses, followed by 1 mg/lb/day in 1-2 divided doses; ≥8 years, >100 lb: same as adult; *see page 572 for dose by weight*

Actilate *Tab:* 75, 150**mg
Adoxa *Tab:* 50, 75, 100, 150 mg ent-coat
Doryx *Tab:* 50, 75, 100, 150, 200 mg del-rel
Monodox *Cap:* 50, 75, 100 mg
Oracea *Cap:* 40 mg del-rel
Vibramycin *Tab:* 100 mg; *Cap:* 50, 100 mg; *Syr:* 50 mg/5 ml (raspberry-apple) (sulfites); *Oral susp:* 25 mg/5 ml (raspberry)
Vibra-Tab *Tab:* 100 mg film-coat

Comment: *doxycycline* is contraindicated <8 years-of-age, in pregnancy, and lactation (discolors developing tooth enamel). A side effect may be photo-sensitivity (photophobia). Do not give with antacids, calcium supplements, milk or other dairy, or within two hours of taking another drug.

▷ *erythromycin base* (B)(G) 500-1000 mg qid x 4 weeks
Pediatric: <45 kg: 30-50 mg in 2-4 divided doses x 4 weeks; ≥45 kg: same as adult
Ery-Tab *Tab:* 250, 333, 500 mg ent-coat
PCE *Tab:* 333, 500 mg

Comment: *erythromycin* may increase INR with concomitant *warfarin*, as well as increase serum level of *digoxin*, benzodiazepines and statins.

▷ *erythromycin ethylsuccinate* (B)(G) 400 mg qid x 4 weeks
Pediatric: 30-50 mg/kg/day in 4 divided doses x 4 weeks; may double dose with severe infection; max 100 mg/kg/day; *see page 575 for dose by weight*
EryPed *Oral susp:* 200 mg/5 ml (100, 200 ml) (fruit); 400 mg/5 ml (60, 100, 200 ml) (banana); *Oral drops:* 200, 400 mg/5 ml (50 ml) (fruit); *Chew tab:* 200 mg wafer (fruit)
E.E.S. *Oral susp:* 200, 400 mg/5 ml (100 ml) (fruit)
E.E.S. Granules *Oral susp:* 200 mg/5 ml (100, 200 ml) (cherry)
E.E.S. 400 Tablets *Tab:* 400 mg

Comment: *erythromycin* may increase INR with concomitant *warfarin*, as well as increase serum level of *digoxin*, benzodiazepines and statins.

▷ *trimethoprim/sulfamethoxazole* (D)(G) bid x 10 days
Pediatric: <2 months: not recommended; ≥2 months: 40 mg/kg/day of *sulfamethox-azole* in 2 divided doses bid x 10 days; *see page 587 for dose by weight*
Bactrim, Septra 2 tabs bid x 10 days
Tab: trim 80 mg/*sulfa* 400 mg*
Bactrim DS, Septra DS 1 tab bid x 10 days
Tab: trim 160 mg/*sulfa* 800 mg*
Bactrim Pediatric Suspension, Septra Pediatric Suspension
Oral susp: trim 40 mg/sulfa 200 mg per 5 ml (100 ml) (cherry) (alcohol 0.3%)

Comment: *trimethoprim/sulfamethoxazole* is not recommended in pregnancy or lactation. *CrCl 15-30 mL/min:* reduce dose by 1/2; *CrCl <15 mL/min:* not recommended

⬤ CELLULITIS

Comment: Duration of treatment should be 10-30 days. Obtain culture from site. Consider blood cultures.

ANTI-INFECTIVES

▷ *amoxicillin* (B)(G) 500-875 mg bid or 250-500 mg tid x 10 days
  Pediatric: <40 kg (88 lb): 20-40 mg/kg/day in 3 divided doses x 10 days or 25-45 mg/kg/day in 2 divided doses x 10 days; ≥40 kg: same as adult; *see page 554 for dose by weight*
    Amoxil *Cap:* 250, 500 mg; *Tab:* 875*mg; *Chew tab:* 125, 200, 250, 400 mg (cherry-banana-peppermint) (phenylalanine); *Oral susp:* 125, 250 mg/5 ml (80, 100, 150 ml) (strawberry); 200, 400 mg/5 ml (50, 75, 100 ml) (bubble gum); *Oral drops:* 50 mg/ml (30 ml) (bubble gum)
    Moxatag *Tab:* 775 mg ext-rel
    Trimox *Tab:* 125, 250 mg; *Cap:* 250, 500 mg; *Oral susp:* 125, 250 mg/5 ml (80, 100, 150 ml) (raspberry-strawberry)
▷ *amoxicillin/clavulanate* (B)(G) 500 mg tid or 875 mg bid x 10 days
    Augmentin *Tab:* 250, 500, 875 mg; *Chew tab:* 125, 250 mg (lemon-lime); 200, 400 mg (cherry-banana) (phenylalanine); *Oral susp:* 125 mg/5 ml (banana), 250 mg/5 ml (75, 100, 150 ml) (orange); 200, 400 mg/5 ml (50, 75, 100 ml) (orange) (phenylalanine)
      Pediatric: 40-45 mg/kg/day divided tid x 10 days or 90 mg/kg/day divided bid x 10 days *see page 556 for dose by weight*
    Augmentin ES-600 *Oral susp:* 600 mg/5 ml (50, 75, 100, 125, 150, 200 ml) (strawberry cream) (phenylalanine) every 12 hours
      Pediatric: <3 months: not recommended; ≥3 months, <40 kg: 90 mg/kg/day in 2 divided doses; ≥40 kg: not recommended
    Augmentin XR 2 tabs q 12 hours x 7-10 days
      Pediatric: <16 years: use other forms; ≥16 years: same as adult
      Tab: 1000*mg ext-rel
▷ *azithromycin* (B)(G) 500 mg x 1 dose on day 1, then 250 mg daily on days 2-5 or 500 mg daily x 3 days or **Zmax** 2 g in a single dose
  Pediatric: 12 mg/kg/day x 5 days; max 500 mg/day; *see page 559 for dose by weight*
    Zithromax *Tab:* 250, 500, 600 mg; *Oral susp:* 100 mg/5 ml (15 ml); 200 mg/5 ml (15, 22.5, 30 ml) (cherry); *Pkt:* 1 g for reconstitution (cherry-banana)
    Zithromax Tri-pak *Tab:* 3 x 500 mg tabs/pck
    Zithromax Z-pak *Tab:* 6 x 250 mg tabs/pck
    Zmax *Oral susp:* 2 g ext-rel for reconstitution (cherry-banana) (148 mg Na$^+$)
▷ *cefaclor* (B)(G) 250-500 mg q 8 hours x 10 days; max 2 g/day
  Pediatric: <1 month: not recommended; 20-40 mg/kg bid or q 12 hours x 10 days; max 1 g/day; *see page 560 for dose by weight*
    Tab: 500 mg; *Cap:* 250, 500 mg; *Susp:* 125 mg/5 ml (75, 150 ml) (strawberry); 187 mg/5 ml (50, 100 ml) (strawberry); 250 mg/5 ml (75, 150 ml) (strawberry); 375 mg/5 ml (50, 100 ml) (strawberry)
    CefaclorRExtended Release
      Pediatric: <16 years: ext-rel not recommended; ≥16years: same as adult
        Tab: 375, 500 mg ext-rel

➤ *cefpodoxime proxetil* (B) 400 mg bid x 7-14 days
  Pediatric: <2 months: not recommended; ≥2 months-12 years: 10 mg/kg/day (max 400 mg/dose) or 5 mg/kg/day bid (max 200 mg/dose) x 7-14 days; >12 years: same as adult; *see page 564 for dose by weight*
    Vantin *Tab:* 100, 200 mg; *Oral susp:* 50, 100 mg/5 ml (50, 75, 100 mg) (lemon cream)
➤ *cefprozil* (B) 500 mg q 12 hours x 10 days
  Pediatric: <2 years: not recommended; 2-12 years: 15 mg/kg q 12 hours x 10 days; >12 years: same as adult; *see page 565 for dose by weight*
    Cefzil *Tab:* 250, 500 mg; *Oral susp:* 125, 250 mg/5 ml (50, 75, 100 ml) (bubble gum) (phenylalanine)
➤ *ceftaroline fosamil* (B) administer 600 mg once every 12 hours, by IV infusion over 5-60 minutes, x 5-14 days
  Pediatric: <18 years: not established
    Teflaro *Vial:* 400, 600 mg pwdr for reconstitution, single-use (10/carton)
    Comment: **Teflaro** is indicated for the treatment of adults with acute bacterial skin and skin structures infection (ABSSSI).
➤ *ceftriaxone* (B)(G) 1-2 g daily x 5-14 days IM; max 4 g daily
  Pediatric: 50-75 mg/kg IM in 1-2 divided doses x 5-14 days; max 2 g/day
    Rocephin *Vial:* 250, 500 mg; 1, 2 g
➤ *cefuroxime axetil* (B)(G) 250-500 mg bid x 10 days
  Pediatric: <3 months: not recommended; ≥3 months: 30 mg/kg/day in 2 divided doses x 10 days; *see page 567 for dose by weight*
    Ceftin *Tab:* 250, 500 mg; *Oral susp:* 125, 250 mg/5 ml (50, 100 ml) (tutti-frutti)
➤ *cephalexin* (B)(G) 500 mg bid x 10 days
  Pediatric: 25-50 mg/kg/day in 4 divided doses x 10 days; *see page 568 for dose by weight*
    Keflex *Cap:* 250, 333, 500, 750 mg; *Oral susp:* 125, 250 mg/5 ml (100, 200 ml) (strawberry)
➤ *clarithromycin* (C)(G) 500 mg q 12 hours or 500 mg ext-rel once daily x 10 days
  Pediatric: <6 months: not recommended; ≥6 months: 7.5 mg/kg bid x 10 days; *see page 569 for dose by weight*
    Biaxin *Tab:* 250, 500 mg
    Biaxin Oral Suspension *Oral susp:* 125, 250 mg/5 ml (50, 100 ml) (fruit-punch)
    Biaxin XL *Tab:* 500 mg ext-rel
➤ *dalbavancin* (C) 1000 mg administered once as a single dose via IV infusion over 30 minutes or initially 1,000 mg once, followed by 500 mg 1 week later; infuse over 30 minutes; *CrCl <30 mL/min:* not receiving dialysis: initially 750 mg, followed by 375 mg 1 week later
  Pediatric: <18 years: not established
    Dalvance *Vial:* 500 mg pwdr for reconstitution, single-use (preservative-free)
    Comment: **Dalvance** is indicated for the treatment of adults with acute bacterial skin and skin structures infection (ABSSSI) caused by gram positive bacteria.
➤ *dicloxacillin* (B)(G) 500 mg q 6 hours x 10 days
  Pediatric: 12.5-25 mg/kg/day in 4 divided doses x 10 days; *see page 571 for dose by weight*
    Dynapen *Cap:* 125, 250, 500 mg; *Oral susp:* 62.5 mg/5 ml (80, 100, 200 ml)
➤ *dirithromycin* (C)(G) 500 mg once daily x 5-7 days
  Pediatric: <12 years: not recommended; ≥12 years: same as adult
    Dynabac *Tab:* 250 mg
➤ *erythromycin base* (B)(G) 250 mg qid or 333 mg tid or 500 mg bid x 7-10 days; then taper to lowest effective dose
  Pediatric: <45 kg: 30-50 mg in 2-4 divided doses x 7-10 days; ≥45 kg: same as adult

Ery-Tab *Tab:* 250, 333, 500 mg ent-coat
PCE *Tab:* 333, 500 mg

Comment: *erythromycin* may increase INR with concomitant **warfarin**, as well as increase serum level of **digoxin**, benzodiazepines and statins.

▶ *erythromycin ethylsuccinate* (B)(G) 400 mg qid x 7-10 days
Pediatric: 30-50 mg/kg/day in 4 divided doses x 7-10 days; may double dose with severe infection; max 100 mg/kg/day; *see page 574 for dose by weight*

EryPed *Oral susp:* 200 mg/5 ml (100, 200 ml) (fruit); 400 mg/5 ml (60, 100, 200 ml) (banana); *Oral drops:* 200, 400 mg/5 ml (50 ml) (fruit); *Chew tab:* 200 mg wafer (fruit)
E.E.S. *Oral susp:* 200, 400 mg/5 ml (100 ml) (fruit)
E.E.S. Granules *Oral susp:* 200 mg/5 ml (100 ml) (cherry)
E.E.S. 400 Tablets *Tab:* 400 mg

Comment: *erythromycin* may increase INR with concomitant **warfarin**, as well as increase serum level of **digoxin**, benzodiazepines and statins.

▶ *linezolid* (C)(G) 600 mg q 12 hours x 10-14 days
Pediatric: <5 years: 10 mg/kg q 8 hours x 10-14 days; 5-11 years: 10 mg/kg q 12 hours x 10-14 days; >11years: same as adult

Zyvox *Tab:* 400, 600 mg; *Oral susp:* 100 mg/5 ml (150 ml) (orange) (phenylalanine)

Comment: *linezolid* is indicated to treat susceptible vancomycin-resistant *E. faecium* infections of skin and skin structures, including diabetic foot without osteomyelitis.

▶ *loracarbef* (B) 200 mg bid x 10 days
Pediatric: 15 mg/kg/day in 2 divided doses x 10 days; *see page 581 for dose by weight*

Lorabid *Pulvule:* 200, 400 mg; *Oral susp:* 100 mg/5 ml (50, 100 ml); 200 mg/5 ml (50, 75, 100 ml) (strawberry bubble gum)

▶ *moxifloxacin* (C)(G) 400 mg once daily x 5 days
Pediatric: <18 years: recommended

Avelox *Tab:* 400 mg; *IV soln:* 400 mg/250 mg (latex-free, presservative-free)

Comment: *moxifloxacin* is contraindicated <18 years of age and during pregnancy and lactation. Risk of tendonitis or tendon rupture, especially 60 years-of-age and older.

▶ *oritavancin* (C) administer 1,200 mg as a single dose by IV infusion over 3 hours
Pediatric: <18 years: not established

Orbactiv *Vial:* 400 mg pwdr for reconstitution, single-use (10/carton) (mannitol; preservative-free)

Comment: Orbactiv is indicated for the treatment of adults with acute bacterial skin and skin structures infection (ABSSSI).

▶ *penicillin V potassium* (B) 250-500 mg q 6 hours x 5-7 days
Pediatric: >12 years: same as adult; *see page 583 for dose by weight*

Pen-Vee K *Tab:* 250, 500 mg; *Oral soln:* 125 mg/5 ml (100, 200 ml); 250 mg/5 ml (100, 150, 200 ml)

▶ *tedizolid phosphate* (C) administer 200 mg once daily x 6 days, via PO or IV infusion over 1 hour
Pediatric: <18 years: not established

Sivextro *Tab:* 200 mg (6/blister pck)

Comment: Sivextro is indicated for the treatment of adults with acute bacterial skin and skin structures infection (ABSSSI).

▶ *tigecycline* (D)(G) 100 mg as a single dose; then 50 mg q 12 hours x 5-14 days; with se-
vere hepatic impairment (Child Pugh C), 100 mg as a single dose; then 25 mg q 12 hours
Pediatric: <18 years: not recommended
  Tygacil *Vial:* 50 mg pwdr for reconstitution and IV infusion (preservative-free)

CERUMEN IMPACTION

OTIC ANALGESIC

▶ *antipyrine/benzocaine/zinc acetate dihydrate* otic (C) fill ear canal with solution;
then moisten cotton plug with solution and insert into meatus; may repeat every
1-2 hours prn
Pediatric: same as adult
  Otozin *Otic soln:* antipyr 5.4%/benz 1%/zinc1% per ml (10 ml w. dropper)

CERUMINOLYTICS

▶ *triethanolamine* (NE)(OTC)(G) fill ear canal and insert cotton plug for 15-30 minutes before irrigating with warm water
  Cerumenex *Soln:* 10% (6, 12 ml)
▶ *carbamide peroxide* (NE)(OTC)(G) instill 5-10 drops in ear canal; keep drops in ear
several minutes; then irrigate with warm water; repeat bid for up to 4 days
  Debrox *Soln:* 15, 30 ml squeeze bottle w. applicator

CHANCROID

ANTI-INFECTIVES

▶ *azithromycin* (B)(G) 500 mg x 1 dose on day 1, then 250 mg daily on days 2-5 <u>or</u>
500 mg daily x 3 days <u>or</u> **Zmax** 2 g in a single dose
Pediatric: 12 mg/kg/day x 5 days; max 500 mg/day; *see page 559 for dose by
weight*
  Zithromax *Tab:* 250, 500, 600 mg; *Oral susp:* 100 mg/5 ml (15 ml);
  200 mg 5 ml (15, 22.5, 30 ml) (cherry); *Pkt:* 1 g for reconstitution
  (cherry-banana)
  Zithromax Tri-pak *Tab:* 3 x 500 mg tabs/pck
  Zithromax Z-pak *Tab:* 6 x 250 mg tabs/pck
  Zmax *Oral susp:* 2 g ext-rel for reconstitution (cherry-banana) (148 mg Na⁺)
▶ *ceftriaxone* (B)(G) 250 mg IM in a single dose
Pediatric: <45 kg: 125 mg IM in a single dose; ≥45 kg: same as adult
  Rocephin *Vial:* 250, 500 mg; 1, 2 g
▶ *ciprofloxacin* (C) 500 mg bid x 3 days
Pediatric: <18 years: not recommended
  Cipro *Tab:* 250, 500, 750 mg; *Oral susp:* 250, 500 mg/5 ml (100 ml) (strawberry)
  Cipro XR *Tab:* 500, 1000 mg ext-rel
  ProQuin XR *Tab:* 500 mg ext-rel

Comment: *ciprofloxacin* is contraindicated <18 years-of-age, and during pregnancy
and lactation. Risk of tendonitis or tendon rupture, especially 60 years-of-age and
older.

▷ *erythromycin base* (B)(G) 500 mg qid x 7 days
    Pediatric: 30-50 mg/kg/day divided bid-qid; max 100 mg/kg/day
        Ery-Tab *Tab:* 250, 333, 500 mg ent-coat
        PCE *Tab:* 333, 500 mg
    Comment: *erythromycin* may increase INR with concomitant *warfarin*, as well as increase serum level of *digoxin*, benzodiazepines and statins.
▷ *erythromycin ethylsuccinate* (B)(G) 400 mg qid x 7 days
    Pediatric: 30-50 mg/kg/day in 4 divided doses x 7 days; may double dose with severe infection; max 100 mg/kg/day; *see page 574 for dose by weight*
        EryPed *Oral susp:* 200 mg/5 ml (100, 200 ml) (fruit); 400 mg/5 ml (60, 100, 200 ml) (banana); *Oral drops:* 200, 400 mg/5 ml (50 ml) (fruit); *Chew tab:* 200 mg wafer (fruit)
        E.E.S. *Oral susp:* 200, 400 mg/5 ml (100 ml) (fruit)
        E.E.S. Granules *Oral susp:* 200 mg/5 ml (100, 200 ml) (cherry)
        E.E.S. 400 Tablets *Tab:* 400 mg
    Comment: *erythromycin* may increase INR with concomitant *warfarin*, as well as increase serum level of *digoxin*, benzodiazepines and statins.

◐ CHICKENPOX (VARICELLA)

PROPHYLAXIS

▷ *Varicella virus* vaccine, live, attenuated (C)
        Varivax 0.5 ml SC; repeat 4-8 weeks later
        Pediatric: <12 months: not recommended; 12 months-12 years: 1 dose of 0.5 ml SC; repeat 4-6 weeks later
        Vial: 1350 PFU/0.5 ml single-dose w. diluent (preservative-free)
    Comment: Administer **Varivax** SC in the deltoid in adults and children.

TREATMENT

Antipyretics *see Fever page* 143

ORAL ANTIPRURITICS

▷ *diphenhydramine* (B)(OTC)(G) 25-50 mg q 6-8 hours; max 100 mg/day
    Pediatric: <2 years: not recommended; 2-6 years: 6.25 mg q 4-6 hours; max 37.5 mg/day; >6-12 years: 12.5-25 mg q 4-6 hours; max 150 mg/day; >12 years: same as adult
        Benadryl (OTC) *Chew tab:* 12.5 mg (grape; phenylalanine); *Liq:* 12.5 mg/5 ml (4, 8 oz); *Cap:* 25 mg; *Tab:* 25 mg; *dye-free soft gel:* 25 mg; *Dye-free liq:* 12.5 mg/5 ml (4, 8 oz)
▷ *hydroxyzine* (C)(G) 50-100 mg qid; max 600 mg/day
    Pediatric: <6 years: 50 mg/day divided qid; ≥6 years: 50-100 mg/day divided qid
        AtaraxR *Tab:* 10, 25, 50, 100 mg; *Syr:* 10 mg/5 ml (alcohol 0.5%)
        VistarilR *Cap:* 25, 50, 100 mg; *Oral susp:* 25 mg/5 ml (4 oz) (lemon)

ANTIVIRALS

▷ *acyclovir* (B)(G) 800 mg qid x 5 days
    Pediatric: <2 years: not recommended; ≥2 years, <40 kg: 20 mg/kg qid x 5 days; ≥2 years, >40 kg: 800 mg qid x 5 days; *see page 552 for dose by weight*

Zovirax *Cap:* 200 mg; *Tab:* 400, 800 mg
Zovirax Oral Suspension *Oral susp:* 200 mg/5 ml (banana)

 CHLAMYDIA TRACHOMATIS

Comment: The following treatment regimens for *C. trachomatis* are published in the **2015 CDC Sexually Transmitted Diseases Treatment Guidelines**. Treatment regimens are presented by generic drug name first, followed by information about brands and dose forms. Treat all sexual contacts. Patients who are HIV-positive should receive the same treatment as those who are HIV-negative. Sexual abuse must be considered a cause of chlamydial infection in preadolescent children, although perinatally transmitted *C. trachomatis* infections of the nasopharynx, urogenital tract, and rectum may persist for >1 year.

RECOMMENDED REGIMENS: ADOLESCENT AND ADULT, NON-PREGNANT
Regimen 1

▷ *azithromycin* 1 g in a single dose

Regimen 2

▷ *doxycycline* 100 mg bid x 7 days

ALTERNATIVE REGIMENS: ADOLESCENT AND ADULT, NON-PREGNANT
Regimen 1

▷ *erythromycin base* 500 mg qid x 7 days

Regimen 2

▷ *erythromycin ethylsuccinate* 800 mg qid x 7 days

Regimen 3

▷ *levofloxacin* 500 mg once daily x 7 days

Regimen 4

▷ *ofloxacin* 300 mg bid x 7 days

RECOMMENDED REGIMENS: PREGNANCY
Regimen 1

▷ *azithromycin* 1 g in a single dose

Regimen 2

▷ *amoxicillin* 500 mg tid x 7 days

ALTERNATE REGIMENS: PREGNANCY

Regimen 1

▷ *erythromycin base* 500 mg qid x 7 days

Regimen 2

▷ *erythromycin base* 250 mg qid x 14 days

Regimen 3

▷ *erythromycin ethylsuccinate* 800 mg qid x 7 days

Regimen 4

▷ *erythromycin ethylsuccinate* 400 mg qid x 14 days

ALTERNATE REGIMENS: CHILDREN (>8 YEARS)

Regimen 1

▷ *azithromycin* 1 g in a single dose

Regimen 2

▷ *doxycycline* 100 mg bid x 7 days

ALTERNATE REGIMEN: CHILDREN (>45 KG; <8 YEARS)

Regimen 1

▷ *azithromycin* 1 g in a single dose

ALTERNATE REGIMENS: INFANTS

Regimen 1

▷ *erythromycin base* 50 mg/kg/day in divided doses qid x 14 days

Regimen 2

▷ *erythromycin ethylsuccinate* 50 mg/kg/day divided qid x 14 days

DRUG BRANDS AND DOSE FORMS

▷ *azithromycin* (B)(G) 500 mg x 1 dose on day 1, then 250 mg daily on days 2-5 or 500 mg daily x 3 days or **Zmax** 2 g in a single dose
  Pediatric: 12 mg/kg/day x 5 days; max 500 mg/day; *see page 559 for dose by weight*
    Zithromax *Tab:* 250, 500, 600 mg; *Oral susp:* 100 mg/5 ml (15 ml); 200 mg/5 ml (15, 22.5, 30 ml) (cherry); *Pkt:* 1 g for reconstitution (cherry-banana)
    Zithromax Tri-pak *Tab:* 3 x 500 mg tabs/pck
    Zithromax Z-pak *Tab:* 6 x 250 mg tabs/pck
    Zmax *Oral susp:* 2 g ext-rel for reconstitution (cherry-banana) (148 mg Na⁺)
▷ *doxycycline* (D)(G)
    Actilate *Tab:* 75, 150**mg
    Adoxa *Tab:* 50, 75, 100, 150 mg ent-coat

Doryx *Tab:* 50, 75, 100, 150, 200 mg del-rel
Monodox *Cap:* 50, 75, 100 mg
Oracea *Cap:* 40 mg del-rel
Vibramycin *Tab:* 100 mg; *Cap:* 50, 100 mg; *Syr:* 50 mg/5 ml (raspberry-apple) (sulfites); *Oral susp:* 25 mg/5 ml (raspberry)
Vibra-Tab *Tab:* 100 mg film-coat

Comment: *doxycycline* is contraindicated <8 years-of-age, in pregnancy, and lactation (discolors developing tooth enamel). A side effect may be photo-sensitivity (photophobia). Do not give with antacids, calcium supplements, milk or other dairy, or within two hours of taking another drug.

▷ *erythromycin base* (B)(G)
Ery-Tab *Tab:* 250, 333, 500 mg ent-coat
PCE *Tab:* 333, 500 mg

Comment: *erythromycin* may increase INR with concomitant *warfarin*, as well as increase serum level of *digoxin*, benzodiazepines and statins.

▷ *erythromycin ethylsuccinate* (B)(G)
EryPed *Oral susp:* 200 mg/5 ml (100, 200 ml) (fruit); 400 mg/5 ml (60, 100, 200 ml) (banana); *Oral drops:* 200, 400 mg/5 ml (50 ml) (fruit); *Chew tab:* 200 mg wafer (fruit)
E.E.S. *Oral susp:* 200, 400 mg/5 ml (100 ml) (fruit)
E.E.S. Granules *Oral susp:* 200 mg/5 ml (100, 200 ml) (cherry)
E.E.S. 400 Tablets *Tab:* 400 mg

Comment: *erythromycin* may increase INR with concomitant *warfarin*, as well as increase serum level of *digoxin*, benzodiazepines and statins.

▷ *levofloxacin* (C)
Levaquin *Tab:* 250, 500, 750 mg

Comment: *levofloxacin* is contraindicated <18 years-of-age, and during pregnancy and lactation. Risk of tendonitis or tendon rupture, especially 60 years-of-age and older.

▷ *ofloxacin* (C)(G)
Floxin *Tab:* 200, 300, 400 mg

Comment: *ofloxacin* is contraindicated <18 years-of-age, and during pregnancy and lactation. Risk of tendonitis or tendon rupture, especially 60 years-of-age and older.

CHOLELITHIASIS

▷ *ursodiol* (B) 8-10 mg/kg/day in 2-3 divided doses
Pediatric: not recommended
Actigall *Cap:* 300 mg

Comment: **Actigall** is indicated for the dissolution of radiolucent, noncalciferous, gallstones <20 mm in diameter and for prevention of gallstones during rapid weight loss.

CHOLERA (*VIBRIO CHOLERAE*)

Comment: June 10, 2016, the FDA approved the first vaccine for the prevention of cholera caused by serogroup O1 (the most predominant cause of cholera globally [WHO]) in adults age 18-64 years traveling to cholera-affected areas. https://www.drugs.com/newdrugs/fda-approves-vaxchora-cholera-vaccine-live-oral-prevent-cholera-travelers-4396.html. Vaxchora (R) is the only FDA approved vaccine for the prevention of cholera. The bacterium Vibrio cholerae is acquired by ingesting contaminated water or food and causes nausea, vomiting, and watery diarrhea that may be mild to severe. Profuse fluid loss may cause life-threatening dehydration if antibiotics and fluid replacement are not initiated promptly.

VACCINE PROPHYLAXIS

▷ *Vibrio cholerae* vaccine

> **Vaxchora** reconstitute the buffer component in 100 ml purified bottled water; then add the active component (lyophilized V. cholerae CVD 103-HgR); total dose after reconstitution is 100 ml; instruct the patient to avoid eating or drinking fluids for 60 minutes before and after ingestion of the dose

Comment: **Vaxchora** is a live, attenuated vaccine that is taken as a single oral dose at least 10 days before travel to a cholera-affected area and at least 10 days before starting antimalarial prophylaxis. Diminished immune response when taken concomitantly with *chloroquine*. Avoid concomitant administration with systemic antibiotics since these agents may be active against the vaccine strain. Do not administer to patients who have received an oral or parental antibiotic within 14 days prior to vaccination. **Vaxchora** may be shed in the stool of recipients for at least 7 days. There is potential for transmission of the vaccine strain to non-vaccinated and immunocompromised close contacts. The Centers for Disease Control and Prevention and several health professional organizations state that vaccines given to a nursing mother do not affect the safety of breastfeeding for mothers or infants and that breastfeeding is not a contraindication to cholera vaccine. **Vaxchora** is not absorbed systemically, and maternal use is not expected to result in fetal exposure to the drug. The **Vaxchora** pregnancy exposure registry for reporting adverse events is 800-533-5899. There are 0 disease interactions, but at least 165 drug-drug interactions with **Vaxchora** (see mfr pkg insert).

TREATMENT

Comment: The first line treatment for *V. cholerae* is oral rehydration therapy (ORT) and intravenous fluid replacement as indicated. Antibiotic therapy may shorten the duration and severity of symptoms, but is optional in other than severe cases. Although *doxycycline* is contraindicated in pregnancy and in children under 7 years-of-age, the benefits may outweigh the risks (WHO, CDC, UNICEF). Although *ciprofloxacin* is contraindicated in children under 18 years-of-age, the benefits may outweigh the risks (WHO, CDC, UNICEF). Cholera is not transmitted from person to person, but rather the fecal-oral route. Therefore, chemoprophylaxis is not usually required with strict hand hygiene and sanitation measures, and avoidance of contaminated food and water. Drugs and dosages for chemoprophylaxis are the same as for treatment.

ADULTS 15 YEARS AND OLDER, NON-PREGNANT WOMEN

Regimen 1

▷ *doxycycline* (D)(G) 300 mg in a single dose

> **Actilate** *Tab:* 75, 150**mg
> **Adoxa** *Tab:* 50, 75, 100, 150 mg ent-coat
> **Doryx** *Tab:* 50, 75, 100, 150, 200 mg del-rel
> **Monodox** *Cap:* 50, 75, 100 mg

Oracea *Cap:* 40 mg del-rel
Vibramycin *Tab:* 100 mg; *Cap:* 50, 100 mg; *Syr:* 50 mg/ml (raspberry-apple)
(sulfites); *Oral susp:* 25 mg/5 ml (raspberry)
Vibra-Tab *Tab:* 100 mg film-coat

Regimen 2

▷ *azithromycin* (B) 1000 mg in a single dose
Zithromax *Tab:* 250, 500, 600 mg
Zmax *Oral susp:* 2 g ext-rel for reconstitution (cherry-banana) (148 mg Na$^+$)
or
▷ *ciprofloxacin* (C)(G) 1000 mg in a single dose
Cipro *Tab:* 250, 500, 750 mg;
Cipro XR *Tab:* 500, 1000 mg ext-rel
ProQuin XR *Tab:* 500 mg ext-rel

PREGNANT WOMEN, 15 YEARS AND OLDER

▷ *azithromycin* (B) 1000 mg in a single dose
Zithromax *Tab:* 250, 500, 600 mg
Zmax *Oral susp:* 2 g ext-rel for reconstitution (cherry-banana) (148 mg Na$^+$)
or
▷ *erythromycin* (B)(G) 500 mg q 6 hours x 3 days
E.E.S. 400 Tablets *Tab:* 400 mg
Ery-Tab *Tab:* 250, 333, 500 mg ent-coat
PCE *Tab:* 333, 500 mg

CHILDREN 3-15 YEARS WHO CAN SWALLOW TABLETS

Regimen 1

▷ *erythromycin* (B)(G) 12.5 mg/kg q 6 hours x 3 days
E.E.S. 400 Tablets *Tab:* 400 mg
Ery-Tab *Tab:* 250, 333, 500 mg ent-coat
PCE *Tab:* 333, 500 mg
or
▷ *azithromycin* (B) 20 mg/kg in a single dose; max 1 g
Zithromax *Tab:* 250, 500, 600 mg
Zmax *Oral susp:* 2 g ext-rel for reconstitution (cherry-banana) (148 mg Na$^+$)

Regimen 2

▷ *ciprofloxacin* (D)(G) 20 mg/kg in a single dose
Cipro *Tab:* 250, 500, 750 mg;
Cipro XR *Tab:* 500, 1000 mg ext-rel
ProQuin XR *Tab:* 500 mg ext-rel
or
▷ *doxycycline* (D)(G) 2-4 mg/kg in a single dose
Actilate *Tab:* 75, 150**mg
Adoxa *Tab:* 50, 75, 100, 150 mg ent-coat
Doryx *Tab:* 50, 75, 100, 150, 200 mg del-rel
Monodox *Cap:* 50, 75, 100 mg
Oracea *Cap:* 40 mg del-rel

Vibramycin *Tab:* 100 mg; *Cap:* 50, 100 mg; *Syr:* 50 mg/ml (raspberry-apple) (sulfites); *Oral susp:* 25 mg/5 ml (raspberry)
Vibra-Tab *Tab:* 100 mg film-coat

CHILDREN UNDER 3 YEARS

Regimen 1

▷ *erythromycin ethylsuccinate* (B)(G) 12.5 mg/kg q 6 hours x 3 days; use suspension
    E.E.S. *Oral susp:* 200, 400 mg/5 ml (100 ml) (fruit)
    E.E.S. Granules *Oral susp:* 200 mg/5 ml (100, 200 ml) (cherry, fruit); *Chew tab:* 200 mg wafer (fruit)
    EryPed *Oral susp:* 200 mg/5 ml (100, 200 ml) (fruit); 400 mg/5 ml (60, 100, 200 ml) (banana); *Oral drops:* 200, 400 mg/5 ml (50 ml) (fruit); *Chew tab:* 200 mg wafer (fruit)
        or
▷ *azithromycin* (B) 20 mg/kg in a single dose; max 1 g; use suspension
    Zithromax *Tab:* 250, 500, 600 mg; *Oral susp:* 100 mg/5 ml (15 ml); 200 mg/5 ml (15, 22.5, 30 ml) (cherry)
    Zmax *Oral susp:* 2 g ext-rel for reconstitution (cherry-banana) (148 mg Na$^+$)

Regimen 2

▷ *ciprofloxacin* (C)(G) 20 mg/kg in a single dose; use suspension
    Cipro *Oral susp:* 250, 500 mg/5 ml (100 ml) (strawberry)
        or
▷ *doxycycline* (D)(G) 2-4 mg/kg in a single dose; use suspension or syrup
    Vibramycin *Tab:* 100 mg; *Cap:* 50, 100 mg; *Syr:* 50 mg/5 ml (raspberry-apple) (sulfites); *Oral susp:* 25 mg/5 ml (raspberry)

◯ COLIC: INFANTILE

▷ *hyoscyamine* (C)(G)
    Levsin Drops
        Pediatric: 3-4 kg: 4 drops q 4 hours prn; max 24 drops/day; 5 kg: 5 drops q 4 hours prn; max 30 drops/day; 7 kg: 6 drops q 4 hours prn; max 36 drops/day; 10 kg: 8 drops q 4 hours prn; max 40 drops/day; *Oral drops:* 0.125 mg/ml (15 ml) (orange) (alcohol 5%)
▷ *simethicone* (C) 0.3 ml qid pc and HS
    Mylicon Drops (OTC) *Oral drops:* 40 mg/0.6 ml (30 ml)

◯ COMMON COLD (VIRAL UPPER RESPIRATORY INFECTION [URI])

Oral Drugs for Allergy, Cough, and Cold *see page* 535
Oral Decongestants *see page* 535

Oral Expectorants *see page* 535
Oral Antitussives *see page* 535
Oral Antipyretic-Analgesics *see Fever page* 143

NASAL SALINE DROPS/SPRAYS

Comment: Homemade saline nose drops: 1/4 tsp salt added to 8 oz boiled water, then cool water.
▷ *saline* nasal spray (NE)(G)
Afrin Saline Mist w. Eucalyptol and Menthol (OTC) 2-6 sprays in each nostril prn
Pediatric: 1 month-2 years: 1-2 sprays in each nostril prn; >2-12 years: 1-4 sprays in each nostril prn; >12 years: same as adult
Squeeze bottle: 45 ml
Afrin Moisturizing Saline Mist (OTC) 2-6 sprays in each nostril prn
Pediatric: 1 month-2 years: 1-2 sprays in each nostril prn; 2-12 years: 1-4 sprays in each nostril prn; >12 years: same as adult
Squeeze bottle: 45 ml
Ocean Mist (OTC) 2-6 sprays in each nostril prn
Pediatric: 1 month-2 years: 1-2 sprays in each nostril prn; >2-12 years: 1-4 sprays in each nostril prn; >12 years: same as adult
Squeeze bottle: saline 0.65% (45 ml) (alcohol-free)
Pediamist (OTC) 2-6 sprays in each nostril prn
Pediatric: 1 month-2 years: 1-2 sprays in each nostril prn; >2-12 years: 1-4 sprays in each nostril prn; >12 years: same as adult
Squeeze bottle: saline 0.5% (15 ml) (alcohol-free)

NASAL SYMPATHOMIMETICS

▷ *oxymetazoline* (C)(OTC) 2-3 drops <u>or</u> sprays in each nostril q 10-12 hours prn; max 2 doses/day; max duration 5 days
Pediatric: <6 years: not recommended; ≥6 years: same as adult
4-hour formulation: 2-3 drops <u>or</u> sprays q 4 hours prn; max duration 5 days
Pediatric: not recommended
Afrin 12-Hour Extra Moisturizing Nasal Spray
Afrin 12-Hour Nasal spray Pump Mist
Afrin 12-Hour Original Nasal spray
Afrin 12-Hour Original Nose Drops
Afrin 12-Hour Severe Congestion Nasal Spray
Afrin 12-Hour Sinus Nasal Spray
Nasal spray: 0.05% (45 ml); *Nasal drops:* 0.05% (45 ml)
Afrin 4-Hour Nasal Spray
Neo-Synephrine 12 Hour Nasal Spray
Neo-Synephrine 12 Hour Extra Moisturizing Nasal Spray
Nasal spray: 0.05% (15 ml)
▷ *phenylephrine* (C)
Afrin Allergy Nasal Spray (OTC) 2-3 sprays in each nostril q 4 hours prn; max duration 5 days
Pediatric: <12 years: not recommended; ≥12 years: same as adult

Nasal spray: 0.5% (15 ml)
Afrin Nasal Decongestant Childrens Pump Mist (OTC)
  Pediatric: <6 years: not recommended; ≥6 years: 2-3 sprays in each nostril q 4 hours prn; max duration 5 days
  Nasal spray: 0.25% (15 ml)
Neo-Synephrine Extra Strength (OTC) 2-3 sprays <u>or</u> drops in each nostril q 4 hours prn; max duration 5 days
  Pediatric: <12 years: not recommended; ≥12 years: same as adult
  Nasal spray: 0.1% (15 ml); *Nasal drops:* 0.1% (15 ml)
Neo-Synephrine Mild Formula (OTC) 2-3 sprays <u>or</u> drops in each nostril q 4 hours prn; max duration 5 days
  Pediatric: <6 years: not recommended; ≥6 years: same as adult
  Nasal spray: 0.25% (15 ml)
Neo-Synephrine Regular Strength (OTC) 2-3 sprays <u>or</u> drops in each nostril q 4 hours prn; max duration 5 days
  Pediatric: <12 years: not recommended; ≥12 years: same as adult
  Nasal spray: 0.5% (15 ml); *Nasal drops:* 0.5% (15 ml)
▷ *tetrahydrozoline* (C)
  Tyzine 2-4 drops <u>or</u> 3-4 sprays in each nostril q 3-8 hours prn; max duration 5 days
  Pediatric: <6 years: not recommended; ≥6 years: same as adult
  Nasal spray: 0.1% (15 ml); *Nasal drops:* 0.1% (30 ml)
  Tyzine Pediatric Nasal Drops 2-3 sprays <u>or</u> drops in each nostril q 3-6 hours prn
  Nasal drops: 0.05% (15 ml)

CONJUNCTIVITIS: ALLERGIC

Oral Prescription Drugs for the Management of Allergy, Cough, and Cold Symptoms
page 535

OPHTHALMIC CORTICOSTEROIDS

Comment: Concomitant contact lens wear is contraindicated during therapy. Ophthalmic steroids are contraindicated with ocular, fungal, mycobacterial, viral (except herpes zoster), and untreated bacterial infection. Ophthalmic steroids may mask <u>or</u> exacerbate infection, and may increase intraocular pressure, optic nerve damage, cataract formation, <u>or</u> corneal perforation. Limit ophthalmic steroid use to 2-3 days if possible; usual max 2 weeks. With prolonged or frequent use, there is risk of corneal and scleral thinning and cataract formation.
▷ *dexamethasone* (C) initially 1-2 drops hourly during the day and q 2 hours at night; then prolong dosing interval to 4-6 hours as condition improves
  Pediatric: not recommended
  Maxidex *Ophth susp:* 0.1% (5, 15 ml) (benzalkonium chloride)
▷ *dexamethasone phosphate* (C) initially 1-2 drops hourly during the day and q 2 hours at night; then 1 drop q 4-8 hours <u>or</u> more as condition improves
  Pediatric: not recommended
  Decadron *Ophth soln:* 0.1% (5 ml) (sulfites)

▷ *fluorometholone* (C) 1 drop bid-qid **or** 1/2 inch of ointment once daily-tid; may increase dose frequency during initial 24-48 hours
  Pediatric: <2 years: not recommended; ≥2 years: same as adult
    FML *Ophth susp:* 0.1% (5, 10, 15 ml) (benzalkonium chloride)
    FML Forte *Ophth susp:* 0.25% (5, 10, 15 ml) (benzalkonium chloride)
    FML S.O.P. Ointment *Ophth oint:* 0.1% (3.5 g)
▷ *fluorometholone acetate* (C) initially 2 drops q 2 hours during the first 24-48 hours; then 1-2 drops qid as condition improves
  Pediatric: not recommended
    Flarex *Ophth susp:* 0.1% (2.5, 5 10 ml) (benzalkonium chloride)
▷ *loteprednol etabonate* (C)
  Pediatric: not recommended
    Alrex 1 drop qid
      Ophth susp: 0.2% (5, 10 ml) (benzalkonium chloride)
    Lotemax 1-2 drops qid
      Ophth susp: 0.5% (5, 10, 15 ml) (benzalkonium chloride)
▷ *medrysone* (C) 1 drop up to q 4 hours
  Pediatric: not recommended
    HMS *Ophth susp:* 1% (5, 10 ml) (benzalkonium chloride)
▷ *rimexolone* (C) initially 1-2 drops hourly while awake x 1 week; then 1 drop q 2 hours while awake x 1 week; then taper as condition improves
  Pediatric: not recommended
    Vexol *Ophth susp:* 0.1% (5, 10 ml) (benzalkonium chloride)
▷ *prednisolone acetate* (C)
  Pediatric: not recommended
    Econopred 2 drops qid
      Ophth susp: 0.125% (5, 10 ml)
    Econopred Plus 2 drops qid
      Ophth susp: 1% (5, 10 ml)
    Pred Forte initially 2 drops hourly x 24-48 hours; then 1-2 drops bid-qid
      Ophth susp: 1% (1, 5, 10, 15 ml) (benzalkonium chloride, sulfites)
    Pred Mild initially 2 drops hourly x 24-48 hours; then 1-2 drops bid-qid
      Ophth susp: 0.12% (5, 10 ml) (benzalkonium chloride)
▷ *prednisolone sodium phosphate* (C) initially 1-2 drops hourly during the day and q 2 hours at night; then 1 drop q 4 hours; then 1 drop tid-qid as condition improves
  Pediatric: not recommended
    Inflamase Forte *Ophth soln:* 1% (5, 10, 15 ml) (benzalkonium chloride)
    Inflamase Mild *Ophth soln:* 1/8% (5, 10 ml) (benzalkonium chloride)

OPHTHALMIC H1 ANTAGONISTS (ANTIHISTAMINES)

Comment: May insert contact lens 10 minutes after administration of ophthalmic antihistamine.
▷ *emedastine* (C) 1 drop qid prn
  Pediatric: <3 years: not recommended; ≥3 years: same as adult
    Emadine *Ophth soln:* 0.05% (5 ml) (benzalkonium chloride)
▷ *levocabastine* (C) 1 drop qid prn
  Pediatric: not recommended
    Livostin *Ophth susp:* 0.05% (2.5, 5, 10 ml) (benzalkonium chloride)

OPHTHALMIC MAST CELL STABILIZERS

Comment: Concomitant contact lens wear is contraindicated during treatment.
▷ *cromolyn sodium* (B) 1-2 drops 4-6 x/day at regular intervals
    Pediatric: <4 years: not recommended; ≥4 years: same as adult
        Crolom *Ophth soln:* 4% (10 ml) (benzalkonium chloride)
▷ *lodoxamide tromethamine* (B) 1-2 drops qid up to 3 months
    Pediatric: <2 years: not recommended; ≥2 years: same as adult
        Alomide *Ophth soln:* 1% (10 ml) (benzalkonium chloride)
▷ *nedocromil* (B) 1-2 drops bid
    Pediatric: <3 years: not recommended; ≥3 years: same as adult
        Alocril *Ophth soln:* 2% (5 ml) (benzalkonium chloride)
▷ *pemirolast potassium* (C) 1-2 drops qid
    Pediatric: <3 years: not recommended; ≥3 years: same as adult
        Alamast *Ophth soln:* 0.1% (10 ml) (lauralkonium chloride)

OPHTHALMIC ANTIHISTAMINE/MAST CELL STABILIZER COMBINATIONS

▷ *alcaftadine* (B) 1 drop each eye daily
    Pediatric: <2 years: not recommended; ≥2 years: same as adult
        Lastacaft *Ophth soln:* 0.25% (6 ml) (benzalkonium chloride)
    Comment: May insert contact lens 10 minutes after ophthalmic administration.
▷ *azelastine* (C) 1 drop each eye bid
    Pediatric: <3 years: not recommended; ≥3 years: same as adult
        Optivar *Ophth soln:* 0.05% (6 ml) (benzalkonium chloride)
    Comment: May insert contact lens 10 minutes after ophthalmic administration.
▷ *bepotastine besilate* (C) 1 drop each eye bid
    Pediatric: <2 years: not recommended; ≥2 years: same as adult
        Bepreve *Ophth soln:* 1.5% (10 ml) (benzalkonium chloride)
    Comment: May insert contact lens 10 minutes after ophthalmic administration.
▷ *epinastine* (C)(G) 1 drop each eye bid
    Pediatric: <3 years: not recommended; ≥3 years: same as adult
        Elestat *Ophth soln:* 0.05% (5 ml) (benzalkonium chloride)
▷ *ketotifen fumarate* (C) 1 drop each eye q 8-12 hours
    Pediatric: <3 years: not recommended; ≥3 years: same as adult
        Alaway (OTC) *Ophth soln:* 0.025% (10 ml) (benzalkonium chloride)
        Claritin Eye (OTC) *Ophth soln:* 0.025% (5 ml) (benzalkonium chloride)
        Refresh Eye Itch Relief (OTC) *Ophth soln:* 0.025% (5 ml) (benzalkonium chloride)
        Zaditor (OTC) *Ophth soln:* 0.025% (5 ml)(benzalkonium chloride)
        Zyrtec Itchy Eye (OTC) *Ophth soln:* 0.025% (5 ml) (benzalkonium chloride)
▷ *olopatadine* (C) 1 drop each eye bid
    Pediatric: <3 years: not recommended; ≥3 years: same as adult
        Pataday (G) *Ophth soln:* 0.2% (2.5 ml) (benzalkonium chloride)
        Patanol *Ophth soln:* 0.1% (5 ml) (benzalkonium chloride)
        Pazeo *Ophth soln:* 0.7% (2.5 ml) (benzalkonium chloride)
    Comment: May insert contact lens 10 minutes after administration.

OPHTHALMIC VASOCONSTRICTORS

Comment: Concomitant contact lens wear is contraindicated during treatment.

▷ *naphazoline* (C) 1-2 drops each eye qid prn
  Pediatric: not recommended
    Vasocon-A *Ophth soln:* 0.1% (15 ml) (benzalkonium chloride)
▷ *oxymetazoline* (NE)(OTC) 1-2 drops each eye qid prn
  Pediatric: <6 years: not recommended; ≥6 years: same as adult
    Visine L-R *Ophth soln:* 0.025% (15, 30 ml)
▷ *tetrahydrozoline* (NE)(OTC)(G) 1-2 drops each eye qid prn
  Pediatric: <6 years: not recommended; ≥6 years: same as adult
    Visine *Ophth soln:* 0.05% (15, 22.5, 30 ml)

OPHTHALMIC VASOCONSTRICTOR/MOISTURIZER COMBINATION

Comment: Concomitant contact lens wear is contraindicated during treatment.
▷ *tetrahydrozoline/polyethylene glycol 400/povidone/dextran 70* (NE)(OTC) 1-2
  drops each eye qid prn
  Pediatric: <6 years: not recommended; ≥6 years: same as adult
    Advanced Relief Visine *Ophth soln:* tetra 0.025%/*poly* 1%/*pov* 1%/*dex* 0.1% (15,
    30 ml)

OPHTHALMIC VASOCONSTRICTOR/ASTRINGENT COMBINATION

Comment: Concomitant contact lens wear is contraindicated during treatment.
▷ *tetrahydrozoline/zinc sulfate* (NE)(OTC) 1-2 drops each eye qid prn
  Pediatric: <6 years: not recommended; ≥6 years: same as adult
    Visine AC *Ophth soln:* tetra 0.025%/*zinc* 0.05% (15, 30 ml)

OPHTHALMIC VASOCONSTRICTOR/ANTI-HISTAMINE COMBINATIONS

Comment: Concomitant contact lens wear is contraindicated during treatment.
▷ *naphazoline/pheniramine* (C) 1-2 drops each eye qid
  Pediatric: <6 years: not recommended; ≥6 years: same as adult
    Naphcon-A (OTC) *Ophth soln:* naph 0.025%/*phen* 0.3% (15 ml) (benzalkonium
    chloride)

OPHTHALMIC NSAIDs

Comment: Concomitant contact lens wear is contraindicated during treatment.
▷ *diclofenac* (B) 1 drop affected eye(s) qid
  Pediatric: not recommended
    Voltaren Ophthalmic Solution *Ophth soln:* 0.1% (2.5, 5 ml)
▷ *ketorolac tromethamine* (C) 1 drop affected eye(s) qid; max x 4 days
  Pediatric: <3 years: not recommended; ≥3 years: same as adult
    Acular *Ophth soln:* 0.5% (3, 5, 10 ml) (benzalkonium chloride)
    Acular LS *Ophth soln:* 0.4% (5 ml) (benzalkonium chloride)
    Acular PF *Ophth soln:* 0.5% (0.4 ml; 12 single-use vials/carton) (preserva-
    tive-free)
▷ *nepafenac* (C) 1 drop affected eye(s) tid
  Pediatric: <10 years: not recommended; ≥10 years: same as adult
    Nevanac Ophthalmic Suspension *Ophth susp:* 0.1% (3 ml) (benzalkonium
    chloride)

CONJUNCTIVITIS/BLEPHAROCONJUNCTIVITIS: BACTERIAL

OPHTHALMIC ANTI-INFECTIVES

▶ *azithromycin* ophthalmic solution **(B)(G)** 1 drop to affected eye(s) bid x 2 days; then 1 drop once daily for the next 5 days
Pediatric: <1 year: not recommended; ≥1 year: same as adult
   AzaSite Ophthalmic Solution *Ophth susp:* 1% (2.5 ml) (benzalkonium chloride)

▶ *bacitracin* ophthalmic ointment **(C)(G)** apply 1/2 inch ribbon to the lower conjunctival sac of affected eye(s) 1-3 x daily x 7 days
Pediatric: same as adult
   Bacitracin Ophthalmic Ointment *Ophth oint:* 500 units/g (3.5 g)

▶ *besifloxacin* ophthalmic solution **(C)** 1 drop to affected eye(s) tid x 7 days
Pediatric: <1 year: not recommended; ≥1 year: same as adult
   Besivance Ophthalmic Solution *Ophth susp:* 0.6% (5 ml) (benzalkonium chloride)

▶ *ciprofloxacin* ophthalmic ointment **(C)** apply 1/2 inch ribbon to the lower conjunctival sac of affected eye(s) tid x 2 days; then bid x 5 days
Pediatric: <2 years: not recommended; ≥2 years: same as adult
   Ciloxan Ophthalmic Ointment *Ophth oint:* 0.3% (3.5 g)

▶ *ciprofloxacin* ophthalmic solution **(C)** 1-2 drops to affected eye(s) q 2 hours while awake x 2 days; then, q 4 hours while awake x 5 days
Pediatric: <1 years: not recommended; ≥1 year: same as adult
   Ciloxan Ophthalmic Solution *Ophth soln:* 0.3% (2.5, 5, 10 ml) (benzalkonium chloride)

▶ *erythromycin* ophthalmic ointment **(B)** apply 1/2 inch ribbon to the lower conjunctival sac of affected eye(s) up to 6 x/day
Pediatric: same as adult
   Ilotycin Ophthalmic Ointment *Ophth oint:* 5 mg/g (1/8 oz)

▶ *gatifloxacin* ophthalmic solution **(C)**
Pediatric: <1 years: not recommended; ≥1 year: same as adult
   Zymar Ophthalmic Solution initially 1 drop to affected eye(s) q 2 hours while awake up to 8 times/day for 2 days; then 1 drop qid while awake x 5 more days
      Ophth soln: 0.3% (5 ml) (benzalkonium chloride)
   Zymaxid Ophthalmic Solution (G) initially 1 drop to affected eye(s) q 2 hours while awake up to 8 times/day on day 1; then 1 drop bid-qid while awake on days 2-7
      Ophth soln: 0.5% (2.5 ml) (benzalkonium chloride)

▶ *gentamicin sulfate* ophthalmic ointment **(C)(G)** apply 1/2 inch ribbon to the lower conjunctival sac of affected eye(s) bid-tid
Pediatric: same as adult
   Garamycin Ophthalmic Ointment *Ophth oint:* 3 mg/g (3.5 g) (preservative-free formulation available)
   Genoptic Ophthalmic Ointment *Ophth oint:* 3 mg/g (3.5 g)
   Gentacidin Ophthalmic Ointment *Ophth oint:* 3 mg/g (3.5 g)

▶ *gentamicin sulfate* ophthalmic solution **(C)(G)** 1-2 drops to affected eye(s) q 4 hours x 7-14 days; max 2 drops q 1 h
Pediatric: same as adult
   Garamycin Ophthalmic Solution *Ophth soln:* 0.3% (5 ml) (benzalkonium chloride)
   Genoptic Ophthalmic Solution *Ophth soln:* 0.3% (3, 5 ml)

▷ *levofloxacin* ophthalmic solution **(C)** 1-2 drops to affected eye(s) q 2 hours while awake on days 1 and 2 (max 8 times/day); then 1-2 drops q 4 hours while awake on days 3-7; max 4 x/day
Pediatric: <1 years: not recommended; ≥1 years: same as adult
   Quixin Ophthalmic Solution *Ophth soln:* 0.5% (2.5, 5 ml) (benzalkonium chloride)

▷ *moxifloxacin* ophthalmic solution **(C)** 1 drop to affected eye(s) tid x 7 days
Pediatric: <1 years: not recommended; ≥1 year: same as adult
   Moxeza Ophthalmic Solution (G) *Ophth soln:* 0.5% (3 ml)
   Vigamox Ophthalmic Solution *Ophth soln:* 0.5% (3 ml)

▷ *ofloxacin* ophthalmic solution **(C)** 1-2 drops to affected eye(s) q 2-4 hours x 2 days; then qid x 5 days
Pediatric: <1 years: not recommended; ≥1 year: same as adult
   Ocuflox Ophthalmic Solution *Ophth soln:* 0.3% (5, 10 ml) (benzalkonium chloride)

▷ *sulfacetamide* ophthalmic solution and ointment **(C)**
   Bleph-10 Ophthalmic Solution 1-2 drops to affected eye(s) q 2-3 hours x 7-10 days
      Pediatric: <2 months: not recommended; ≥2 months: 1-2 drops q 2-3 hours during the day x 7-10 days
      Ophth soln: 10% (2.5, 5, 15 ml) (benzalkonium chloride)
   Bleph-10 Ophthalmic Ointment apply 1/2 inch ribbon to the lower conjunctival sac of affected eye(s) q 3-4 hours and HS x 7-10 days
      Pediatric: <2 years: not recommended; ≥2 years: same as adult
      Ophth oint: 10% (3.5 g) (phenylmercuric acetate)
   Cetamide Ophthalmic Solution initially 1-2 drops to affected eye(s) q 2-3 hours; then increase dosing interval as condition improves
      Pediatric: <2 years: not recommended; ≥2 years: same as adult
      Ophth soln: 15% (5, 15 ml)
   Isopto Cetamide Ophthalmic Ointment initially 1/2 inch ribbon in lower conjunctival sac of affected eye(s) q 3-4 hours; then increase dosing interval as condition improves
      Pediatric: <2 years: not recommended; ≥2 years: same as adult
      Ophth oint: 10% (3.5 g)
   Isopto Cetamide Ophthalmic Solution initially 1-2 drops to affected eye(s) q 2-3 hours; then increase dosing interval as condition improves
      Pediatric: <2 years: not recommended; ≥2 years: same as adult
      Ophth soln: 15% (5, 15 ml)

▷ *tobramycin* **(B)**
   Tobrex Ophthalmic Solution 1-2 drops to affected eye(s) q 4 hours
      Pediatric: same as adult
      Ophth soln: 0.3% (5 ml) (benzalkonium chloride)
   Tobrex Ophthalmic Ointment apply 1/2 inch ribbon to the lower conjunctival sac of affected eye(s) bid-tid
      Pediatric: same as adult
      Ophth oint: 0.3% (3.5 g) (chlorobutanol)

OPHTHALMIC ANTI-INFECTIVE COMBINATIONS

▷ *polymyxin B sulfate/bacitracin* ophthalmic ointment **(C)** apply 1/2 inch ribbon to the lower conjunctival sac of affected eye(s) q 3-4 hours x 7-10 days
Pediatric: same as adult

Polysporin Ophthalmic Ointment *Ophth oint: poly b* 10,000 U/*bac* 500 U (3.75 g)

▷ *polymyxin B sulfate/bacitracin zinc/neomycin sulfate* ophthalmic ointment (C) apply 1/2 inch ribbon to the lower conjunctival sac of affected eye(s) q 3-4 hours x 7-10 days
Pediatric: same as adult
Neosporin Ophthalmic Ointment *Ophth oint: poly b* 10,000 U/*bac* 400 U/*neo* 3.5 mg/g (3.75 g)

▷ *polymyxin B sulfate/gramicidin/neomycin* ophthalmic solution (C) 1-2 drops to affected eye(s) q 1 hour x 2-3 doses; then 1-2 drops bid-qid x 7-10 days
Pediatric: not recommended
Neosporin Ophthalmic Solution *Ophth soln: poly b* 10,000 U/*gram* 0.025 mg/*neo* 1.7 mg/g (10 ml)

▷ *trimethoprim/polymyxin B sulfate* ophthalmic solution (C) 1 drop to affected eye(s) q 3 hours x 7-10 days; max 6 doses/day
Pediatric: <2 years: not recommended; ≥2 years: same as adult
Polytrim *Ophth soln: trim* 1 mg/*poly b* 10,000 U/ml (10 ml) (benzalkonium chloride)

OPHTHALMIC ANTI-INFECTIVE/STEROID COMBINATIONS

Comment: Ophthalmic corticosteroids are contraindicated after removal of a corneal foreign body, epithelial herpes simplex keratitis, *varicella*, other viral infections of the cornea or conjunctiva, fungal ocular infections, and mycobacterial ocular infections. Limit ophthalmic steroid use to 2-3 days if possible; usual max 2 weeks. With prolonged or frequent use, there is risk of corneal and scleral thinning and cataract formation.

▷ *gentamicin sulfate/prednisolone acetate* ophthalmic suspension (C)
Pediatric: not recommended
Pred-G Ophthalmic Suspension 1 drop to affected eye(s) bid-qid; max 20 ml/ therapeutic course
Ophth susp: gent 0.3%/*pred* 1%/ml (2, 5, 10 ml) (benzalkonium chloride)
Pred-G Ophthalmic Ointment apply 1/2 inch ribbon to the lower conjunctival sac of affected eye(s) once daily-tid; max 8 g/therapeutic course
Ophth oint: gent 0.3%/*pred* 0.6%/g (3.5 g)

▷ *neomycin sulfate/polymyxin B sulfate/dexamethasone* ophthalmic suspension (C)
Pediatric: not recommended
Maxitrol Ophthalmic Suspension 1-2 drops to affected eye(s) q 1 hour (severe infection) or qid (mild to moderate infection)
Ophth susp: neo 0.35%/*poly b* 10,000 U/*dexa* 1%/ml (5 ml) (benzalkonium chloride)
Maxitrol Ophthalmic Ointment apply 1/2 inch ribbon to the lower conjunctival sac of affected eye(s) q 1 hour (severe infection) or qid (mild to moderate infection)
Ophth oint: neo 0.35%/*poly b* 10,000 U/*dexa* 0.1%/g (3.5 g)

▷ *neomycin sulfate/polymyxin B sulfate/prednisolone acetate ophthalmic suspension* (C)
Pediatric: not recommended
Poly-Pred Ophthalmic Suspension 1-2 drops to affected eye(s) q 3-4 hours; more often as necessary; max 20 ml/therapeutic course.
Ophth susp: neo 0.35%/*poly b* 10,000 U/*pred* 0.5%/ml (10 ml)

▷ *polymyxin B sulfate/neomycin sulfate/hydrocortisone* ophthalmic suspension (C)
Pediatric: not recommended

Cortisporin Ophthalmic Suspension 1-2 drops to affected eye(s) tid-qid; more often if necessary; max 20 ml/therapeutic course
Ophth susp: poly b 10,000 U/*neo* 0.35%/*hydro* 1%/ml (7.5 ml) (thimerosal)

▶ *polymyxin B sulfate/neomycin sulfate/bacitracin zinc/hydrocortisone* ophthalmic ointment **(C)**
Pediatric: not recommended

Cortisporin Ophthalmic Ointment apply 1/2 inch ribbon to the lower conjunctival sac of affected eye(s) tid-qid; more often if necessary; max 8 g/therapeutic course
Ophth oint: poly b 10,000 U/*neo* 0.35%/*bac* 400 U/*hydro* 1%/g (3.5 g)

▶ *sulfacetamide sodium/fluorometholone* suspension **(C)** 1 drop to affected eye(s) qid; max 20 ml/therapeutic course
Pediatric: not recommended

FML-S *Ophth susp: sulfa* 10%/*fluoro* 0.1%/ml (5, 10, 15 ml) (benzalkonium chloride)

▶ *sulfacetamide sodium/prednisolone acetate* ophthalmic suspension and ointment **(C)**
Pediatric: <6 years: not recommended; ≥6 years: same as adult

Blephamide Liquifilm 2 drops to affected eye(s) qid and HS
Ophth susp: sulfa 10%/*pred* 0.2%/ml (5, 10 ml) (benzalkonium chloride)
Blephamide S.O.P. Ophthalmic Ointment apply 1/2 inch ribbon to the lower conjunctival sac of affected eye(s) tid-qid
Ophth oint: sulfa 10%/*pred* 0.2%/g (3.5 g) (benzalkonium chloride)

▶ *sulfacetamide sodium/prednisolone sodium phosphate* ophthalmic solution **(C)** 2 drops to affected eye(s) q 4 hours
Pediatric: <6 years: not recommended; ≥6 years: same as adult

Vasocidin Ophthalmic Solution *Ophth soln: sulfa* 10%/*pred* 0.25%/ml (5, 10 ml)

▶ *tobramycin/dexamethasone* ophthalmic solution and ointment **(C)**

TobraDex Ophthalmic Solution 1-2 drops to affected eye(s) q 2-6 hours x 24-48 hours; then 4-6 hours; reduce frequency of dose as condition improves; max 20 ml per therapeutic course
Pediatric: >2 years: not recommended; >2 years: 1-2 drops q 4-6 hours; may start with 1-2 drops q 2 hours first 1-2 days
Ophth susp: tobra 0.3%/*dexa* 0.1%/ml (2.5, 5 ml) (benzalkonium chloride)
TobraDex Ophthalmic Ointment apply 1/2 inch ribbon to the lower conjunctival sac of affected eye(s) tid-qid; may use at HS in conjunction with daytime drops; max 8 g/therapeutic course
Pediatric: <2 years: not recommended; >2 years: apply 1/2 inch ribbon to lower conjunctival sac tid-qid
Ophth oint: tobra 0.3%/*dexa* 0.1%/g (3.5 g) (chlorobutanol chloride)
TobraDex ST 1-2 drops to affected eye(s) q 2-6 hours x 24-48 hours; then 4-6 hours; reduce frequency of dose as condition improves; max 20 ml per therapeutic course
Pediatric: not recommended
Ophth susp: tobra 0.3%/*dexa* 0.05%/ml (2.5, 5, 10 ml) (benzalkonium chloride)

▶ *tobramycin/loteprednol etabonate* ophthalmic suspension **(C)**
Pediatric: not recommended

Zylet 1-2 drops to affected eye(s) q 1-2 hours first 24-48 hours; reduce frequency of dose to q 4-6 hours as condition improves; max 20 ml per therapeutic course
Ophth susp: tobra 0.3%/*lote etab* 0.5%/ml (2.5, 5, 10 ml) (benzalkonium chloride)

CONJUNCTIVITIS: CHLAMYDIAL

Comment: A chlamydial etiology should be considered for all infants aged ≤30 days that have conjunctivitis, especially if the mother has a history of chlamydia infection. Topical antibiotic therapy alone is inadequate for treatment for ophthalmia neonatorum caused by chlamydia and is unnecessary when systemic treatment is administered.

ANTI-INFECTIVES

▷ *amoxicillin* (B)(G) 500 mg tid x 7 days
Pediatric: <40 kg (88 lb): 20-40 mg/kg/day in 3 divided doses x 7 days >40 kg: same as adult; *see page 554 for dose by weight*
   Amoxil *Cap:* 250, 500 mg; *Tab:* 875*mg; *Chew tab:* 125, 200, 250, 400 mg (cherry-banana-peppermint) (phenylalanine); *Oral susp:* 125, 250 mg/5 ml (80, 100, 150 ml) (strawberry); 200, 400 mg/5 ml (50, 75, 100 ml) (bubble gum); *Oral drops:* 50 mg/ml (30 ml) (bubble gum)

RECOMMENDED 1ST LINE REGIMEN

▷ *erythromycin base* (B)(G) 250 mg qid x 14 days *or* 500 mg qid x 7 days
Pediatric: <45 kg: 50 mg/kg/day in 4 divided doses x 14 days; ≥45 kg: same as adult
   Ery-Tab *Tab:* 250, 333, 500 mg ent-coat
   PCE *Tab:* 333, 500 mg
Comment: *erythromycin* may increase INR with concomitant *warfarin*, as well as increase serum level of *digoxin*, benzodiazepines and statins.
▷ *erythromycin ethylsuccinate* (B)(G) 400 mg qid x 14 days *or* 800 mg qid x 7 days
Pediatric: 50 mg/kg/day in 4 divided doses x 7 days; max 100 mg/kg/day; *see page 574 for dose by weight*
   EryPed *Oral susp:* 200 mg/5 ml (100, 200 ml) (fruit); 400 mg/5 ml (60, 100, 200 ml) (banana); *Oral drops:* 200, 400 mg/5 ml (50 ml) (fruit); *Chew tab:* 200 mg wafer (fruit)
   E.E.S. *Oral susp:* 200, 400 mg/5 ml (100 ml) (fruit)
   E.E.S. Granules *Oral susp:* 200 mg/5 ml (100, 200 ml) (cherry)
   E.E.S. 400 Tablets *Tab:* 400 mg
Comment: *erythromycin* may increase INR with concomitant *warfarin*, as well as increase serum level of *digoxin*, benzodiazepines and statins.

ALTERNATE REGIMEN

▷ *azithromycin* (B) 500 mg x 1 dose on day 1; then 250 mg once daily on days; 2-5 *or* 500 mg daily x 3 days *or* 2 g in a single dose
Pediatric: 20 mg/kg in a single dose once daily x 3 days
   Zithromax *Tab:* 250, 500, 600 mg; *Oral susp:* 100 mg/5 ml (15 ml); 200 mg/5 ml (15, 22.5, 30 ml) (cherry); *Pkt:* 1 g for reconstitution (cherry-banana)
   Zithromax Tri-pak *Tab:* 3 x 500 mg tabs/pck
   Zithromax Z-pak *Tab:* 6 x 250 mg tabs/pck
   Zmax *Oral susp:* 2 g ext-rel for reconstitution (cherry-banana) (148 mg Na⁺)

◉ CONJUNCTIVITIS: FUNGAL

▷ *natamycin* ophthalmic suspension (C) 1 drop q 1-2 hours x 3-4 days; then 1 drop every 6 hours; treat for 14-21 days; withdraw dose gradually at 4- to -7-day intervals
Pediatric: <1 year: not recommended; ≥1 year: same as adult
   Natacyn Ophthalmic Suspension *Ophth susp:* 0.5% (15 ml) (benzalkonium chloride)

◉ CONJUNCTIVITIS: GONOCOCCAL

RECOMMENDED REGIMENS

Regimen 1

▷ *ceftriaxone* (B)(G) 250 mg IM x 1 dose
Pediatric: <45 kg: 50 mg/kg IM x 1 dose; max 125 mg IM
   Rocephin *Vial:* 250, 500 mg; 1, 2 g

Regimen 2

▷ *erythromycin base* (B)(G) 250 mg qid x 10-14 days
Pediatric: <45 kg: 50 mg/kg/day in 4 divided doses x 10-14 days; ≥45 kg: same as adult
   Ery-Tab *Tab:* 250, 333, 500 mg ent-coat
   PCE *Tab:* 333, 500 mg
   Comment: *erythromycin* may increase INR with concomitant *warfarin*, as well as increase serum level of *digoxin*, benzodiazepines and statins.
▷ *erythromycin ethylsuccinate* (B)(G) 400 mg qid x 14 days or 800 mg qid x 7 days
Pediatric: 50 mg/kg/day in 4 divided doses x 7 days; max 100 mg/kg/day; *see page 574 for dose by weight*
   EryPed *Oral susp:* 200 mg/5 ml (100, 200 ml) (fruit); 400 mg/5 ml (60, 100, 200 ml) (banana); *Oral drops:* 200, 400 mg/5 ml (50 ml) (fruit); *Chew tab:* 200 mg wafer (fruit)
   E.E.S. *Oral susp:* 200, 400 mg/5 ml (100 ml) (fruit)
   E.E.S. Granules *Oral susp:* 200 mg/5 ml (100, 200 ml) (cherry)
   E.E.S. 400 Tablets *Tab:* 400 mg
   Comment: *erythromycin* may increase INR with concomitant *warfarin*, as well as increase serum level of *digoxin*, benzodiazepines and statins.

ALTERNATE REGIMEN

▷ *azithromycin* (B) 500 mg x 1 dose on day 1; then 250 mg once daily on days; 2-5 or 500 mg daily x 3 days or 2 g in a single dose
Pediatric: not recommended for bronchitis in children
   Zithromax *Tab:* 250, 500, 600 mg; *Oral susp:* 100 mg/5 ml (15 ml); 200 mg/5 ml (15, 22.5, 30 ml) (cherry); *Pkt:* 1 g for reconstitution (cherry-banana)
   Zithromax Tri-pak *Tab:* 3 x 500 mg tabs/pck
   Zithromax Z-pak *Tab:* 6 x 250 mg tabs/pck
   Zmax *Oral susp:* 2 g ext-rel for reconstitution (cherry-banana) (148 mg Na⁺)

CONJUNCTIVITIS: VIRAL

Comment: For prevention of secondary bacterial infection, see agents listed under bacterial conjunctivitis. Ophthalmic corticosteroids are contraindicated with herpes simplex, keratitis, *Varicella*, and other viral infections of the cornea.

▶ *trifluridine* ophthalmic suspension **(C)** 1 drop q 2 hours while awake; max 9 drops/day; after re-epithelialization, 1 drop q 4 h x 7 days (at least 5 drops/day); max 21 days of therapy

Pediatric: <6 years: not recommended; ≥6 years: same as adult

Viroptic Ophthalmic Solution *Ophth soln:* 1% (7.5 ml) (thimerosal)

CONSTIPATION

CHRONIC IDIOPATHIC CONSTIPATION (CIC)

▶ *lubiprostone (chloride channel activator [GI motility enhancer])* **(C)** 1 cap bid with food

Pediatric: not recommended

Amitiza *Cap:* 24 mcg

▶ *linaclotide (guanylate cyclase-c agonist)* **(C)** 290 mcg once daily; take on an empty stomach at least 30 minutes before the first meal of the day; swallow whole

Pediatric: <6 years: not recommended; 6-17 years: avoid

Linzess *Cap:* 145, 290 mcg

BULK-FORMING AGENTS

▶ *calcium polycarbophil* **(C)**

FiberCon (OTC) 2 tabs once daily to qid

Pediatric: <6 years: not recommended; 6-12 years: 1 tab daily to qid

Cplt: 625 mg

Konsyl Fiber Tablets (OTC) *Tab:* 625 mg

▶ *methylcellulose*

Citrucel 1 heaping tbsp in 8 oz cold water tid

Pediatric: <6 years: not recommended; 6-12 years: 1/2 adult dose

Oral pwdr: 16, 24, 30 oz and single-dose pkts (orange)

Citrucel Sugar-Free 1 heaping tblsp in 8 oz cold water tid

Pediatric: <6 years: not recommended; 6-12 years: 1/2 adult dose

Oral pwdr: 16, 24, 30 oz and single-dose pkts (orange) (sugar-free, phenylalanine)

▶ *psyllium husk* **(B)**

Pediatric: <6 years: not recommended; 6-12 years: 1/2 adult dose in 8 oz liquid tid

Metamucil (OTC) wafer or cap or 1 pkt or 1 rounded tsp (1 rounded tblsp for sugar-containing form) in 8 oz liquid tid

Cap: psyllium husk 5.2 g (100, 150/carton); *Wafer: psyllium husk* 3.4 g/rounded tsp (24/carton) (apple crisp, cinnamon spice); *Plain and flavored pwdr:* 3.4 g/rounded tsp (15, 20, 24, 29, 30, 36, 44, 48 oz); *Efferv sugar-free flav pkts:* 3.4 g/pkt (30/pkt) (phenylalanine)

▶ *psyllium* hydrophilic mucilloid **(B)** 2 rounded tsp in 8 oz water qid

Pediatric: <6 years: not recommended; 6-12 years: 1 rounded tsp in 8 oz liquid tid

Konsyl (OTC) *Pwdr:* 6 g/rounded tsp (10.6, 15.9 oz); *Pwdr pkt:* 6 g/rounded tsp (30/carton)

Konsyl-D (OTC) *Pwdr:* 3.4 g/rounded tsp (11.5, 17.59 oz); *Pwdr pkt:* 3.4 g/rounded tsp (30/carton)
Konsyl Easy Mix Formula (OTC) *Pwdr:* 3.4 g/rounded tsp (8 oz) (sugar-free, low sodium)
Konsyl Orange (OTC) *Pwdr:* 3.4 g/rounded tsp (19 oz); *Pwdr pkt:* 3.4 g/rounded tsp (30/carton)
Konsyl Orange SF (OTC) *Pwdr:* 3.5 g/rounded tsp (15 oz) (phenylalanine); *Pwdr pkt:* 3.5 g/rounded tsp (30/carton) (phenylalanine)

STOOL SOFTENERS

▷ **docusate sodium** (OTC) 50-200 mg/day
  Pediatric: <3 years: 10-40 mg/day; 3-6 years: 20-60 mg/day; >6 years: 40-120 mg/day
    Cap: 50, 100 mg; *Liq:* 10 mg/ml (30 ml w. dropper); *Syr:* 20 mg/5 ml (8 oz) (alcohol ≤1%)
  Dialose 1 tab q HS
    Pediatric: <6 years: not recommended; ≥6 years: same as adult
    Tab: 100 mg
  Surfak (OTC) 240 mg/day
    Pediatric: not recommended
    Cap: 240 mg

OSMOTIC LAXATIVES

▷ **lactulose** (B)(G) take 10-20 g dissolved in 4 oz water once daily prn; max 40 g/day
  Pediatric: not recommended
    Kristalose *Crystals for oral soln:* 10, 20 g single-dose pkts (30/carton)
▷ **magnesium citrate** (B)(G) 1 full bottle (120-300 ml) once daily prn
  Pediatric: <2 years: not recommended; 2-6 years: 4-12 ml once daily prn; ≥6-12 years: 50-100 ml once daily prn
    Citrate of Magnesia (OTC) *Oral soln:* 300 ml
▷ **magnesium hydroxide** (B) 30-60 ml/day in a single or divided doses prn
  Pediatric: 2-5 years: 5-15 ml/day in a single or divided doses; 6-11 years: 15-30 ml/day in a single or divided doses; ≥12 years: same as adult
    Milk of Magnesia *Liq:* 390 mg/5 ml (10, 15, 20, 30, 100, 120, 180, 360, 720 ml)
▷ **polyethylene glycol (PEG)** (C)(OTC)(G) 1 tblsp (17 g) dissolved in 4-8 oz water per day for up to max 7 days; may need 2-4 days for results
  Pediatric: ≤17: not recommended
    GlycoLax Powder for Oral Solution *Oral pwdr:* 7, 14, 30, and 45 dose bottles w. 17 g dosing cup (gluten-free, sugar-free); 17 g single-dose pkts (20/carton)
    MiraLAX Powder for Oral Solution *Oral pwdr:* 7, 14, 30, and 45 dose bottles w. 17 g dosing cup (gluten-free, sugar-free)
    Polyethylene Glycol 3350 Powder for Oral Solution (G) *Oral pwdr:* 3350 g w. dosing cup; 17 g/scoop
Comment: *PEG* is an osmotic indicated for occasional constipation without affecting glucose and electrolyte levels. Contraindicated with suspected or known bowel obstruction.

STIMULANTS

▷ **bisacodyl** (B) 2-3 tabs or 1 suppository bid prn
    Dulcolax, Gentlax *Tab:* 5 mg; *Rectal supp:* 10 mg

Pediatric: <12 years: 1/2 suppository once daily prn; 6-12 years: 1 tablet or 1/2 suppository once daily prn; >12 years: same as adult

Senokot (OTC) initially 2-4 tabs or 1 level tsp at HS prn; max 4 tabs or 2 tsp bid
Pediatric: <2 years: not recommended; 2-6 years: 1/4 tab or 1/2 tsp once daily prn; max 1 tab or 1/2 tsp bid; 6-12 years: 1 tab or 1/2 tsp once daily prn; max 2 tabs or 1 tsp once daily
Tab: 8.6*mg; *Granules:* 15 mg/tsp (2, 6, 12 oz) (cocoa)

Senokot Syrup (OTC) initially 10-15 ml at HS prn; max 15 ml bid
Pediatric: use Childrens Syrup
Syr: 8.8 mg/5 ml (2, 8 oz) (chocolate) (alcohol-free)

Senokot Childrens Syrup (OTC)
Pediatric: <2 years: not recommended; 2-6 years: 2.5-3.75 ml once daily prn; max 3.75 ml bid prn; ≥6-12 years: 5-7.5 ml once daily prn; max 7.5 ml bid
Syr: 8.8 mg/5 ml (2.5 oz) (chocolate) (alcohol-free)

Senokot Xtra (OTC) 1 tab at HS prn; max 2 tabs bid
Pediatric: <2 years: not recommended; 2-6 years: use Childrens Syrup; 6-12 years: 1/2 tab once daily at HS; max 1 tab bid
Tab: 17*mg

BULK FORMING AGENT/STIMULANT COMBINATIONS

▷ *psyllium/senna* (B)
Perdiem (OTC) 1-2 rounded tsp swallowed with 8 oz cool liquid daily bid
Pediatric: <7 years: not recommended; 7-11 years: 1 rounded tsp swallowed with 8 oz cool liquid once daily-bid; ≥12 years: same as adult
Canister: 8.8, 14 oz; *Individual pkt:* 6 g (6/pck)

SennaPrompt (OTC) initially 2-5 caps bid
Pediatric: not recommended
Cap: psyl 500 mg/*senna* 9 mg

STOOL SOFTENER/STIMULANT COMBINATIONS

▷ *docusate/casanthranol* (C)
Doxidan (OTC) 1-3 caps/day; max 1 week
Pediatric: <2 years: not recommended; ≥2 years: 1 cap/day
Cap: doc 60 mg/*cas* 30 mg

Peri-Colace (OTC) 1-2 caps or 15-30 ml q HS; max 2 caps or 30 ml bid or 3 caps q HS
Pediatric: 5-15 ml q HS
Cap: doc 100 mg/*cas* 30 mg; *Syr: doc* 60 mg/*cas* 30 mg per 15 ml (8, 16 oz)

▷ *docusate/senna* concentrate (C)
Senokot S (OTC) 2 tabs q HS; max 4 tabs bid
Pediatric: <2 years: not recommended; 2-6 years: 1/2 tab daily; max 1 tab bid; >6-12 years: 1 tab daily; max 2 tabs bid
Tab: doc 50 mg/*senna* 8.6 mg

ENEMAS AND OTHER AGENTS

▷ *sodium biphosphate/sodium phosphate* enema (C)(OTC)
Fleets Adult 59-118 ml rectally
Pediatric: <2 years: not recommended; ≥2-12 years: 59 ml rectally

Enema: Na biphos 19 g/Na phos 7 g (59, 118 ml w. applicator)
Fleets Pediatric 59 ml
Pediatric: rectally
Enema: na biphos 19 g/*na phos* 7 g (59 ml w. applicator)
▷ *glycerin* suppositories (C)(OTC)
Pediatric: <6 years: 1 pediatric suppository; ≥6 years: 1 adult suppository

CORNEAL EDEMA

▷ *sodium chloride* (NE)(G)
Pediatric: same as adult
Various (OTC) 1-2 drops or 1 inch ribbon q 3-4 hours prn; reduce frequency as edema subsides
Ophth soln: 2, 5% (15, 30 ml); *Ophth oint:* 5% (3.5 g)

CORNEAL ULCERATION

ANTIBACTERIAL OPHTHALMIC SOLUTION/OINTMENT

see *Conjunctivitis/Blepharoconjunctivitis: Bacterial page* 89

COSTOCHONDRITIS (CHEST WALL SYNDROME)

Acetaminophen for IV Infusion *see Pain page* 306
Oral Prescription NSAIDs *see page* 501
Other Oral Analgesics *see Pain page* 308
Topical/Transdermal NSAIDs *see Pain page* 307
Parenteral Corticosteroids *see page* 511
Oral Corticosteroids *see page* 509
Topical Analgesic and Anesthetic Agents *see page* 499

CRAMPS: ABDOMINAL, INTESTINAL

ANTISPASMODIC/ANTICHOLINERGIC COMBINATIONS

▷ *dicyclomine* (B)(G) initially 20 mg bid-qid; may increase to 40 mg qid PO; usual IM dose 80 mg/day divided qid; do not use IM route for more than 1-2 days
Pediatric: not recommended
Bentyl *Tab:* 20 mg; *Cap:* 10 mg; *Syr:* 10 mg/5 ml (16 oz); *Vial:* 10 mg/ml (10 ml); *Amp:* 10 mg/ml (2 ml)
▷ *methscopolamine bromide* (B) 1 tab q 6 hours prn
Pediatric: not recommended
Pamine *Tab:* 2.5 mg
Pamine Forte *Tab:* 5 mg

ANTICHOLINERGICS

▷ *hyoscyamine* (C)(G)

Anaspaz 1-2 tabs q 4 hours prn; max 12 tabs/day
Pediatric: <2 years: not recommended; 2-12 years: 0.0625-0.125 mg q 4 hours prn; max 0.75 mg/day; ≥12 years: same as adult
Tab: 0.125*mg

Levbid 1-2 tabs q 12 hours prn; max 4 tabs/day
Pediatric: <12 years: not recommended; ≥12 years: same as adult
Tab: 0.375*mg ext-rel

Levsin 1-2 tabs q 4 hours prn; max 12 tabs/day
Pediatric: <6 years: not recommended; ≥6-12 years: 1 tab q 4 hours prn
Tab: 0.125*mg

Levsinex SL 1-2 tabs q 4 hours SL or PO; max 12 tabs/day
Pediatric: 2-12 years: 1 tab SL or PO q 4 hours; max 6 tabs/day
Tab: 0.125 mg sublingual

Levsinex Timecaps 1-2 caps q 12 hours; may adjust to 1 cap q 8 hours
Pediatric: 2-12 years: 1 cap q 12 hours; max 2 caps/day
Cap: 0.375 mg time-rel

NuLev dissolve 1-2 tabs on tongue, with or without water, q 4 hours prn; max 12 tabs/day
Pediatric: <2 years: not recommended; 2-12 years: dissolve 1 tab on tongue, with or without water, q 4 hours prn; max 6 tabs/day; >12 years: same as adult
ODT: 0.125 mg (mint) (phenylalanine)

▷ *simethicone* (C)(G) 0.3 ml qid pc and HS

Mylicon Drops (OTC) *Oral drops:* 40 mg/0.6 ml (30 ml)

▷ *phenobarbital/hyoscyamine/atropine/scopolamine* (C)(IV)(G)

Donnatal 1-2 tabs ac and HS
Pediatric: not recommended
Tab: pheno 16.2 mg/*hyo* 0.1037 mg/*atro* 0.0194 mg/*scop* 0.0065 mg

Donnatal Elixir 1-2 tsp ac and HS
Pediatric: 20 lb: 1 ml q 4 hours or 1.5 ml q 6 hours; 30 lb: 1.5 ml q 4 hours or 2 ml q 6 hours; 50 lb: 1/2 tsp q 4 hours or 3/4 tsp q 6 hours; 75 lb: 3/4 tsp q 4 hours or 1 tsp q 6 hours; 100 lb: 1 tsp q 4 hours or 1 tsp q 6 hours
Elix: pheno 16.2 mg/*hyo* 0.1037 mg/*atro* 0.0194 mg/*scop*
0.0065 mg per 5 ml (4, 16 oz)

Donnatal Extentabs 1 tab q 12 hours
Pediatric: not recommended
Tab: pheno 48.6 mg/*hyo* 0.3111 mg/*atro* 0.0582 mg/*scop*
0.0195 mg ext-rel

ANTICHOLINERGIC/SEDATIVE COMBINATION

▷ *chlordiazepoxide/clidinium* (D)(IV) 1-2 caps ac and HS; max 8 caps/day
Pediatric: not recommended
Librax *Cap: chlor* 5 mg/*clid* 2.5 mg

CROHN'S DISEASE

Comment: Standard treatment regimen for active disease (flare) is: antibiotic, antispasmodic, and bowel rest; progress to clear liquids; then progress to high-fiber diet.

Parenteral Corticosteroids *see page* 511
Oral Corticosteroids *see page* 509
▷ *azathioprine* (D)(G)
    Imuran *Tab:* 50*mg; *Injectable:* 100 mg
    Comment: **Imuran** is usually administered on a daily basis. The initial
    dose should be approximately 1.0 mg/kg (50 to 100 mg) as a single dose or
    divided bid. Dose may be increased beginning at 6-8 weeks, and thereafter
    at 4-week intervals, if there are no serious toxicities and if initial response is
    unsatisfactory. Dose increments should be 0.5 mg/kg/day, up to max 2.5 mg/kg
    per day. Therapeutic response usually occurs after 6-8 weeks of treatment. An
    adequate trial should be a minimum of 12 weeks. Patients not improved after
    12 weeks can be considered refractory. **Imuran** may be continued long-term
    in patients with clinical response, but patients should be monitored carefully,
    and gradual dosage reduction should be attempted to reduce risk of toxicities.
    Maintenance therapy should be at the lowest effective dose, and the dose given
    can be lowered decrementally with changes of 0.5 mg/kg or approximately 25
    mg daily every 4 weeks while other therapy is kept constant. The optimum
    duration of maintenance **Imuran** has not been determined. **Imuran** can be
    discontinued abruptly, but delayed effects are possible.
▷ *infliximab (tumor necrosis factor-alpha blocker)* (B) administer 5 mg/kg/dose by IV
infusion over at least 2 h; *Fistulizing disease:* initial dose; repeat dose at 2 weeks and
6 weeks (total 3 doses); then repeat dose every 8 weeks; *Maintenance:* usually 5 mg/
kg/dose every 8 weeks; may increase to 10 mg/kg/dose
Pediatric: not recommended
    Remicade *Vial:* 100 mg pwdr for IV infusion single-use (preservative-free)
▷ *mesalamine* (B)
    Asacol 800 mg tid x 6 weeks; maintenance 1.6 g/day in divided doses; swallow
    whole, do not crush or chew
        Pediatric: not recommended
        Tab: 400 mg del-rel
    Comment: 2 **Asacol** 400 mg tabs are not bioequivalent to 1 **Asacol HD** 800 mg tab.
    Asacol HD 1600 mg tid x 6 weeks; swallow whole, do not crush or chew
        Pediatric: not recommended
        Tab: 800 mg del-rel
    Comment: 1 **Asacol HD** 800 mg tab is not bioequivalent to 2 **Asacol** 400 mg
    tabs
    Canasa 1 g qid for up to 8 weeks
        Rectal supp: 1 g del-rel (30, 42/pck)
    Delzicol *Treatment:* 800 mg tid x 6 weeks; maintenance 1.6 g/day in 2-4 divided
    doses daily; swallow whole; do not crush or chew
        Pediatric: <5 years: not established; > years: same as adult
        Cap: 400 mg del-rel
    Comment: 2 **Delzicol** 400 mg caps are not bioequivalent to 1 *mesalamine*
    800 mg del-rel tab
    Lialda 2.4-4.8 g daily in a single dose for up to 8 weeks; swallow whole, do not
    crush or chew
        Pediatric: <18 years: not recommended
        Tab: 1.2 g del-rel
    Pentasa 1 g qid for up to 8 weeks; swallow whole, do not crush or chew
        Pediatric: not recommended

Cap: 250 mg cont-rel

Rowasa Enema 4 g rectally by enema q HS; retain for 8 hours x 3-6 weeks
Enema: 4 g/60 ml (7, 14, 28/pck; kit, 7, 14, 28/pck w. wipes)

Rowasa Suppository 1 suppository rectally bid x 3-6 weeks; retain for 1-3 hours or longer
Rectal supp: 500 mg

Sulfite-Free Rowasa Rectal Suspension 4 g rectally by enema q HS; retain for 8 hours x 3-6 weeks
Enema: 4 g/60 ml (7, 14, 28/pck; kit, 7, 14, 28/pck w. wipes)

➤ *olsalazine* (C)

Dipentum 1 g/day in 2 divided doses; max 2 g/day
Cap: 250 mg

Comment: Indicated in persons who cannot tolerate *sulfasalazine*.

➤ *sulfasalazine* (B)(G)

Azulfidine initially 1-2 g/day; increase to 3-4 g/day in divided doses pc until clinical symptoms controlled; maintenance 2 g/day; max 4 g/day
Tab: 500*mg
Pediatric: <2 years: not recommended; 2-16 years: initially 40-60 mg/kg/day in 3-6 divided doses; max 2 g/day

Azulfidine EN initially 500 mg in the PM x 7 days; then 500 mg bid x 7 days; then 500 mg in the AM and 1 g in the PM x 7 days; then 1 g bid; max 4 g/day
Pediatric: not recommended
Tab: 500 mg ent-coat

Comment: sulfasalazine

➤ *vedolizumab* (B) administer by IV infusion over 30 minutes; 300 mg at weeks 0, 2, 6; then once every 8 weeks
Pediatric: not established

Entyvio
Vial: 300 mg (20 ml) single dose, pwdr for IV infusion after reconstitution (preservative-free)

➤ *budesonide micronized* (C) (G)
Pediatric: not recommended

Entocort EC *Treatment* 9 mg once daily in the AM for up to 8 weeks; may repeat an 8-week course; *Maintenance of remission*: 6 mg once daily for up to 3 months
Cap: 3 mg ent-coat ext-rel granules

Comment: Taper other systemic steroids when transferring to **Entocort EC**. When corticosteroids are used chronically, systemic effects such as hypercorticism and adrenal suppression may occur. Corticosteroids can reduce the response of the hypothalamus-pituitary-adrenal (HPA) axis to stress. In situations where patients are subject to surgery or other stress situations, supplementation with a systemic corticosteroid is recommended. General precautions concerning corticosteroids should be followed.

ORAL ANTI-INFECTIVES

➤ *metronidazole* (not for use in 1st; B in 2nd, 3rd)(G) 500 mg tid or 750 mg bid; max 8 weeks
Pediatric: 35-50 mg/kg/day in 3 divided doses x 10 days
Flagyl *Tab:* 250*, 500*mg
Flagyl 375 *Cap:* 375 mg

Flagyl ER *Tab:* 750 mg ext-rel
Comment: Alcohol is contraindicated during treatment with oral ***metronidazole***
and for 72 hours after therapy due to a possible ***disulfiram***-like reaction (nausea,
vomiting, flushing, headache).

TUMOR NECROSIS FACTOR (TNF) BLOCKER

➤ ***adalimumab*** **(B)** 40 mg SC once every other week; may increase to once weekly without MTX; administer in abdomen <u>or</u> thigh; rotate sites
Pediatric: <2 years, <10 kg: not recommended; 10-<15 kg: 10 mg every other week;
15-<30 kg: 20 mg every other week; ≥30 kg: 40 mg every other week; 2-17 years,
supervise first dose
    Humira *Prefilled syringe:* 20 mg/0.4 ml; 40 mg/0.8 ml single-dose (2/pck; 2, 6/
starter pck) (preservative-free)
Comment: May use with methotrexate (MTX), DMARDS, corticosteroids, salicylates,
NSAIDs, <u>or</u> analgesics.
➤ ***certolzumab*** **(B)** 400 mg SC (2 x 200 mg inj at two different sites on day 1); then,
400 mg SC at weeks 2 and 4; maintenance 400 mg SC every 4 weeks; administer in
abdomen <u>or</u> thigh; rotate sites
Pediatric: not recommended
    Cimzia *Vial:* 200 mg (2/pck); *Prefilled syringe:* 200 mg/ml single-dose (2/pck; 2,
6/starter pck) (preservative-free)
➤ ***infliximab*** **(B)** administer by IV infusion over 2 hours; 5 mg/kg weeks 0, 2, 6; then
once every 8 weeks
Pediatric: <6 years: not recommended; ≥6 years: same as adult
    Remicade
        Vial: 100 mg pwdr for reconstitution for IV infusion (preservative-free)
➤ ***vedolizumab*** **(B)** administer by IV infusion over 30 minutes; 300 mg at weeks 0, 2, 6;
then 300 mg once every 8 weeks
Pediatric: not established
    Entyvio
        Vial: 300 mg (20 ml) single dose, pwdr for IV infusion after reconstitution
(preservative-free)

INTEGRIN RECEPTOR ANTAGONIST (IMMUNOMODULATOR)

➤ ***natalzumab*** **(C)** administer by IV infusion over 1 hour; monitor during and for 1
hour postinfusion; 300 mg every 4 weeks; discontinue after 12 weeks if no therapeutic response, <u>or</u> if unable to taper off chronic concomitant steroids within 6 months;
may continue aminosalicylates
Pediatric: not established
    Tysarbi
        Vial: 300 mg single-dose, soln after dilution for IV infusion
(preservative-free)

CRYPTOSPORIDIUM PARVUM

➤ ***nitazoxanide*** **(B)** 500 mg by mouth q 12 hours x 3 days
Pediatric: 12-47 months: 5 ml q 12 hours x 3 days; 4-11 years: 10 ml q 12 hours x 3
days; ≥12 years: same as adult

Alinia *Oral susp:* 100 mg/5 ml (60 ml)
Comment: **Alinia** is an antiprotozoal for the treatment of diarrhea due to *G. lamblia* <u>or</u> *C. parvum*.

CYSTIC FIBROSIS

▷ *acetylcysteine* (B)(G) administer via face mask, mouth piece, tracheostomy T-piece, mist tent, <u>or</u> croupette; routine tracheostomy care, 1 to 2 ml of a 10% to 20% solution may be administered by direct instillation into the tracheostomy every 1 to 4 hours
Pediatric: same as adult

Mucomyst *Vial:* 10, 20% (4, 10, 30 ml) soln for inhalation
Comment: **Mucomyst** is a mucolytic. For inhalation, the 10% concentration may be used undiluted; the 20% concentration should be diluted with sterile water <u>or</u> normal saline (either for injection <u>or</u> inhalation).

▷ *lumacaftor/ivacaftor* (B) 2 tabs q 12 hours; reduce dose with moderate to severe hepatic impairment
Pediatric: <12 years: not established

Orkambi *Tab:* luma 200 mg/iva 125 mg film-coat

DEEP VEIN THROMBOSIS (DVT)

Anticoagulation Therapy see page 527

DEHYDRATION

ORAL REHYDRATION AND ELECTROLYTE REPLACEMENT THERAPY

▷ *oral electrolyte replacement* (NE)(OTC)(G)

KaoLectrolyte 1 pkt dissolved in 8 oz water q 3-4 hours
Pediatric: not indicated <2 years *Pkt: sod* 12 mEq/*pot* 5 mEq/*chlor* 10 mEq/*citrate* 7 mEq/*dextrose* 5 g/*calories* 22 per 6.2 g

Pedialyte
Pediatric: <2 years: as desired and as tolerated; >2 years: 1-2 liters/day
Oral soln: dextrose 20 g/*fructose* 5 g/*sodium* 25 mEq/*potassium* 20 mEq/*chloride* 35 mEq/*citrate* 30 mEq/*calories* 100 per liter (8 oz, 1 L)

Pedialyte Freezer Pops
Pediatric: as desired and as tolerated
Pops: dextrose 1.6 g/*sodium* 2.8 mEq/*potassium* 1.25 mEq/*chloride* 2.2 mEq/*citrate* 1.88 mEq/*calories* 6.25 per 62.5 ml (2.1 fl oz) pop

DEMENTIA

Comment: Underlying cause should be explored, accurately diagnosed, and addressed. All antipsychotic agents are associated with increased risk of mortality in elderly patients with dementia-related psychosis (Black Box Warning.) APA recommends that non-emergency antipsychotic medication should only be used for the treatment of agitation or psychosis in patients with dementia when symptoms are severe, are dangerous <u>and/or</u> cause significant distress to the patient. APA recommends that before nonemergency treatment with an antipsychotic is initiated in patients with dementia, the potential risks and benefits are discussed with the patient and the patient's surrogate decision maker with input from family or others involved with the patient.

Alzheimer's Disease *see page* 11
Antidepressants *see* **Depression** *page* 105
Hypnotics/Sedatives *see* **Insomnia** *page* 242

ANTIPSYCHOTICS

▷ *haloperidol* **(C)(G)** 0.5-1 mg q HS
 Haldol *Tab*: 0.5, 1, 2, 5, 10, 20 mg
▷ *mesoridazine* **(C)** initially 25 mg tid; max 300 mg/day
 Serentil *Tab*: 10, 25, 50, 100 mg; *Conc*: 25 mg/ml (118 ml)
▷ *olanzapine* **(C)** initially 2.5-10 mg daily; increase to 10 mg/day within a few days; then by 5 mg/day at weekly intervals; max 20 mg/day
 Zyprexa *Tab*: 2.5, 5, 7.5, 10 mg
 Zyprexa Zydis *ODT*: 5, 10, 15, 20 mg (phenylalanine)
▷ *quetiapine fumarate* **(C)**
 SeroQUEL initially 25 mg bid, titrate q 2nd <u>or</u> 3rd day in increments of 25-50 mg bid-tid; usual maintenance 400-600 mg/day in 2-3 divided doses
  Tab: 25, 50, 100, 200, 300, 400 mg
 SeroQUEL XR administer once daily in the PM; *Day 1*: 50 mg; *Day 2*: 100 mg; *Day 3*: 200 mg; *Day 4*: 300 mg; usual range 400-600 mg/day
  Tab: 50, 150, 200, 300, 400 mg ext-rel
▷ *risperidone* **(C)** 0.5 mg bid x 1 day; adjust in increments of 0.5 mg bid; usual range 0.5-5 mg/day
 Risperdal *Tab*: 1, 2, 3, 4 mg; *Oral soln*: 1 mg/ml (100 ml)
 Risperdal M-Tab *Tab*: 0.5, 1, 2 mg
▷ *thioridazine* **(C)(G)** 10-25 mg bid
 Mellaril *Tab*: 10, 15, 25, 50, 100, 150, 200 mg; *Oral susp*: 25 mg/5 ml, 100 mg/5 ml; *Oral conc*: 30 mg/ml, 100 mg/ml (4 oz)

⬤ DENTAL ABSCESS

▷ *amoxicillin/clavulanate* **(B)(G)** 500 mg tid <u>or</u> 875 mg bid x 10 days
 Augmentin *Tab*: 250, 500, 875 mg; *Chew tab*: 125, 250 mg (lemon-lime); 200, 400 mg (cherry-banana) (phenylalanine); *Oral susp*: 125 mg/5 ml (banana), 250 mg/5 ml (75, 100, 150 ml) (orange); 200, 400 mg/5 ml (50, 75, 100 ml) (orange) (phenylalanine)
  Pediatric: 40-45 mg/kg/day divided tid x 10 days <u>or</u> 90 mg/kg/day divided bid x 10 days *see page* 556 *for dose by weight*
 Augmentin ES-600 *Oral susp*: 600 mg/5 ml (50, 75, 100, 125, 150, 200 ml) (strawberry cream) (phenylalanine)
  Pediatric: <3 months: not recommended; ≥3 months, <40 kg: 90 mg/kg/day in 2 divided doses; ≥40 kg: not recommended
 Augmentin XR 2 tabs q 12 hours x 7-10 days
  Pediatric: <16 years: use other forms; ≥16 years: same as adult
  Tab: 1000*mg ext-rel

➤ *clindamycin* (B) (administer with fluoroquinolone in adults and TMP-SMX in children) 300 mg qid x 10 days
  Pediatric: 8-16 mg/kg/day in 3-4 divided doses x 10 days
    Cleocin (G) *Cap:* 75 (tartrazine), 150 (tartrazine), 300 mg
    Cleocin Pediatric Granules (G) *Oral susp:* 75 mg/5 ml (100 ml) (cherry)
➤ *erythromycin base* (B)(G) 500 mg q 6 hours x 10 days
  Pediatric: 30-40 mg/kg/day in 4 divided doses x 10 days
    Ery-Tab *Tab:* 250, 333, 500 mg ent-coat
    PCE *Tab:* 333, 500 mg
  Comment: *erythromycin* may increase INR with concomitant *warfarin*, as well as increase serum level of *digoxin*, benzodiazepines and statins.
➤ *erythromycin ethylsuccinate* (B)(G) 400 mg qid x 7 days
  Pediatric: 30-50 mg/kg/day in 4 divided doses x 7 days; may double dose with severe infection; max 100 mg/kg/day; *see page 574 for dose by weight*
    EryPed *Oral susp:* 200 mg/5 ml (100, 200 ml) (fruit); 400 mg/5 ml (60, 100, 200 ml) (banana); *Oral drops:* 200, 400 mg/5 ml (50 ml) (fruit); *Chew tab:* 200 mg wafer (fruit)
    E.E.S. *Oral susp:* 200, 400 mg/5 ml (100 ml) (fruit)
    E.E.S. Granules *Oral susp:* 200 mg/5 ml (100, 200 ml) (cherry)
    E.E.S. 400 Tablets *Tab:* 400 mg
  Comment: *erythromycin* may increase INR with concomitant *warfarin*, as well as increase serum level of *digoxin*, benzodiazepines and statins.
➤ *penicillin V potassium* (B) 250-500 mg q 6 hours x 5-7 days
  Pediatric: 25-50 mg/kg/day divided q 6 hours x 5-7 days; >12 years: same as adult; *see page 583 for dose by weight*
    Pen-Vee K *Tab:* 250, 500 mg; *Oral soln:* 125 mg/5 ml (100, 200 ml); 250 mg/5 ml (100, 150, 200 ml)

◯ DENTURE IRRITATION

DEBRIDING AGENT/CLEANSER

➤ *carbamide peroxide 10%* (NE)(OTC) apply 10 drops to affected area; swish x 2-3 minutes, then spit; do not rinse; repeat treatment qid
  Pediatric: with adult supervision only
    Gly-Oxide *Liq:* 10% (15, 60 ml, squeeze bottle w. applicator)

◯ DEPRESSION, MAJOR DEPRESSIVE DISORDER (MDD)

Comment: Abrupt withdrawal or interruption of treatment with an antidepressant medication is sometimes associated with an antidepressant discontinuation syndrome which may be mediated by gradually tapering the drug over a period of two weeks or longer, depending on the dose strength and length of treatment. Common symptoms of antidepressant withdrawal include flu-like symptoms, insomnia, nausea, imbalance, sensory disturbances, and hyperarousal. These medications include SSRIs, TCAs, MAOIs, and atypical agents such as *venlafaxine* (Effexor), *mirtazapine* (Remeron), trazodone (Desyrel), and duloxetine (Cymbalta). Common symptoms of the serotonin discontinuation syndrome include flu-like symptoms (nausea, vomiting, diarrhea, headaches, sweating), sleep disturbances (insomnia, nightmares, constant sleepiness), mood disturbances (dysphoria, anxiety, agitation), cognitive disturbances (mental confusion, hyperarousal), sensory and movement disturbances (imbalance, tremors, vertigo, dizziness, electric-shock-like sensations in the brain, often described by sufferers as "brain zaps."

SELECTIVE SEROTONIN REUPTAKE INHIBITORS (SSRIs)

Comment: Co-administration of SSRIs with TCAs requires extreme caution. Concomitant use of MAOIs and SSRIs is absolutely contraindicated. Avoid St. John's wort and other serotonergic agents. A potentially fatal adverse event is *serotonin syndrome*, caused by serotonin excess. Milder symptoms require HCP intervention to avert severe symptoms which can be rapidly fatal without urgent/emergent medical care. Symptoms include restlessness, agitation, confusion, tachycardia, hypertension, dilated pupils, muscle twitching, muscle rigidity, loss of muscle coordination, diaphoresis, diarrhea, headache, shivering, piloerection, hyperpyrexia, cardiac arrhythmias, seizures, loss of consciousness, coma, death. Common symptoms of the *serotonin discontinuation syndrome* include flu-like symptoms (nausea, vomiting, diarrhea, headaches, sweating), sleep disturbances (insomnia, nightmares, constant sleepiness), mood disturbances (dysphoria, anxiety, agitation), cognitive disturbances (mental confusion, hyperarousal, hallucinations), sensory and movement disturbances (imbalance, tremors, vertigo, dizziness, electric-shock-like sensations in the brain, often described by sufferers as "brain zaps."

▷ *citalopram* (C)(G) initially 20 mg daily; may increase after one week to 40 mg; max 40 mg
  Pediatric: not recommended
      Celexa *Tab:* 10, 20, 40mg; *Oral soln:* 10 mg/5 ml (120 ml) (pepper mint) (sugar-free, alcohol-free, parabens)
▷ *escitalopram* (C)(G) initially 10 mg daily; may increase to 20 mg daily after 1 week; elderly or hepatic impairment, 10 mg once daily
  Pediatric: <12 years: not recommended; 12-17 years: initially 10 mg daily; may increase to 20 mg daily after 3 weeks
      Lexapro *Tab:* 5, 10*, 20*mg
      Lexapro Oral Solution *Oral soln:* 1 mg/ml (240 ml) (peppermint) (parabens)
▷ *fluoxetine* (C)(G)
      Prozac initially 20 mg daily; may increase after 1 week; doses >20 mg/day should be divided into AM and noon doses; max 80 mg/day
          Pediatric: <8 years: not recommended; 8-17 years: initially 10 mg/day; may increase after 1 week to 20 mg/day; range 20-60 mg/day; range for lower weight children, 20-30 mg/day
          Cap: 10, 20, 40 mg; *Tab:* 30*, 60*mg; *Oral soln:* 20 mg/5 ml (4 oz) (mint)
      Prozac Weekly following daily fluoxetine therapy at 20 mg/day for 13 weeks, may initiate **Prozac Weekly** 7 days after the last 20 mg fluoxetine dose
          Pediatric: not recommended
          Cap: 90 mg ent-coat del-rel pellets
▷ *levomilnacipran* (C) swallow whole; initially 20 mg once daily for 2 days; then increase to 40 mg once daily; may increase dose in 40 mg increments at intervals of ≥2 days; max 120 mg once daily; *CrCl 30-59 mL/min:* max 80 mg once daily; *CrCl 15-29 mL/min:* max 40 mg once daily

Fetzima
> *Pediatric:* not recommended
> *Cap:* 20, 40, 80, 120 mg ext-rel

▷ *paroxetine maleate* (D)(G)
> *Pediatric:* not recommended
>> **Paxil** initially 20 mg daily in AM; may increase by 10 mg/day at weekly intervals
>> as needed; max 60 mg/day
>>> *Tab:* 10*, 20*, 30, 40 mg
>> **Paxil CR** initially 25 mg daily in AM; may increase by 12.5 mg at weekly intervals
>> as needed; max 62.5 mg/day
>>> *Tab:* 12.5, 25, 37.5 mg cont-rel ent-coat
>> **Paxil Suspension** initially 20 mg daily in AM; may increase by 10 mg/day at
>> weekly intervals as needed; max 60 mg/day
>>> *Oral susp:* 10 mg/5 ml (250 ml) (orange)

▷ *sertraline* (C)(G) initially 50 mg daily; increase at 1 week intervals if needed; max 200
mg daily; dilute oral concentrate immediately prior to administration in 4 oz water,
ginger ale, lemon/lime soda, lemonade, <u>or</u> orange juice
> *Pediatric:* <6 years: not recommended; 6-12 years: initially 25 mg daily; max 200
> mg/day; 13-17 years: initially 50 mg daily; max 200 mg/day
>> **Zoloft** *Tab:* 25*, 50*, 100*mg; *Oral conc:* 20 mg per ml (60 ml) (alcohol 12%)

SEROTONIN AND NOREPINEPHRINE REUPTAKE INHIBITORS (SNRIs)

▷ *desvenlafaxine* (C)(G) swallow whole; initially 50 mg once daily; max 120 mg/day
> *Pediatric:* not recommended
>> **Pristiq** *Tab:* 50, 100 mg ext-rel

▷ *duloxetine* (C)(G) swallow whole; initially 30 mg once daily x 1 week; then, increase
to 60 mg once daily; max 120 mg/day
> *Pediatric:* not recommended
>> **Cymbalta** *Cap:* 20, 30, 40, 60 mg del-rel

▷ *venlafaxine* (C)(G)
>> **Effexor** initially 75 mg/day in 2-3 divided doses; may increase at 4 day intervals
>> in 75 mg increments to 150 mg/day; max 225 mg/day
>>> *Pediatric:* <18 years: not recommended
>>> *Tab:* 37.5, 75, 150, 225 mg
>> **Effexor XR** initially 75 mg q AM; may start at 37.5 mg daily x 4-7 days, then
>> increase by increments of up to 75 mg/day at intervals of at least 4 days; usual
>> max 375 mg/day
>>> *Pediatric:* not recommended
>>> *Tab/Cap:* 37.5, 75, 150 mg ext-rel

▷ *vortioxetine* (C) initially 10 mg once daily; max 30 mg/day
> *Pediatric:* <18 years: not restablished
>> **Brintellix** *Tab:* 5, 10, 15, 20 mg

SELECTIVE SEROTONIN REUPTAKE INHIBITOR (SSRI)/5-HT-14 RECEPTOR PARTIAL AGONIST COMBINATION

▷ *vilazodone* (C) take with food; initially 10 mg once daily x 7 days; then, 20 mg once
daily x 7 days; then, 40 mg once daily
> *Pediatric:* <18 years: not restablished
>> **Viibryd** *Tab:* 10, 20, 40 mg

THIENOBENZODIAZEPINE/SSRI COMBINATION

▶ *olanzapine/fluoxetine* (C) initially one 6/25 cap in the PM; titrate; max one 18/75 cap once daily in the PM
  Pediatric: <10 years: not established; <10 years: same as adult
    Symbyax
      Cap: **Symbyax 3/25:** *olan* 3 mg/*fluo* 25 mg
            Symbyax 6/25: *olan* 6 mg/*fluo* 25 mg
            Symbyax 6/50: *olan* 6 mg/*fluo* 50 mg
            Symbyax 12/25: *olan* 12 mg/*fluo* 25 mg
            Symbyax 12/50: *olan* 12 mg/*fluo* 50 mg
    Comment: **Symbyax** is a thienobenzodiazepine-SSRI indicated for the treatment of depressive episodes associated with bipolar depression disorder and treatment resistant depression (TRD).

TRICYCLIC ANTIDEPRESSANTS (TCAs)

Comment: Co-administration of TCAs with SSRIs requires extreme caution.
▶ *amitriptyline* (C)(G) initially 75 mg/day in divided doses or 50-100 mg in a single dose at HS; max 300 mg/day
  Pediatric: not recommended
    Tab: 10, 25, 50, 75, 100, 150 mg
▶ *amoxapine* (C) initially 50 mg bid-tid; after 1 week may increase to 100 mg bid-tid; usual effective dose 200-300 mg/day; if total dose exceeds 300 mg/day, give in divided doses (max 400 mg/day); may give as a single bedtime dose (max 300 mg q HS)
  Pediatric: not recommended
    Tab: 25, 50, 100, 150 mg
▶ *desipramine* (C)(G) 100-200 mg/day in single or divided doses; max 300 mg/day
  Pediatric: not recommended
    Norpramin *Tab:* 10, 25, 50, 75, 100, 150 mg
▶ *doxepin* (C)(G) 75 mg/day; max 150 mg/day
  Pediatric: not recommended
    Cap: 10, 25, 50, 75, 100, 150 mg; *Oral conc:* 10 mg/ml (4 oz w. dropper)
▶ *imipramine* (C)(G)
  Pediatric: not recommended
    Tofranil initially 75 mg daily (max 200 mg); adolescents initially 30-40 mg daily (max 100 mg/day); if maintenance dose exceeds 75 mg daily, may switch to **Tofranil PM** for divided or bedtime dose
      Tab: 10, 25, 50 mg
    Tofranil PM initially 75 mg daily 1 hour before HS; max 200 mg
      Cap: 75, 100, 125, 150 mg
    Tofranil Injection 50 mg IM; lower dose for adolescents; switch to oral form as soon as possible
      Amp: 25 mg/2 ml (2 ml)
▶ *nortriptyline* (D)(G) initially 25 mg tid-qid; max 150 mg/day
  Pediatric: not recommended
    Pamelor *Cap:* 10, 25, 50, 75 mg; *Oral soln:* 10 mg/5 ml (16 oz)
▶ *protriptyline* (C) initially 5 mg tid; usual dose 15-40 mg/day in 3-4 divided doses; max 60 mg/day
  Pediatric: <12 years: not recommended

      Vivactyl *Tab:* 5, 10 mg
▷ *trimipramine* (C) initially 75 mg/day in divided doses; max 200 mg/day
    Pediatric: not recommended
      Surmontil *Cap:* 25, 50, 100 mg

AMINOKETONES

▷ *bupropion HBr* (C)(G)
    Pediatric: not established
      Aplenzin initially 100 mg bid for at least 3 days; may increase to 375 or 400 mg/day after several weeks; then after at least 3 more days, 450 mg in 4 divided doses; max 450 mg/day, 174 mg/single-dose
      Tab: 174, 348, 522 mg
      Forfivo XL do not use for initial treatment; use immediate-release bupropion forms for initial titration; switch to **Forfivo XL** 450 mg once daily when total dose/day reaches 450 mg; may switch to **Forfivo XL** when total dose/day reaches 300 mg for 2 weeks and patient needs 450 mg/day to reach therapeutic target; swallow whole, do not crush or chew
      Tab: 450 mg ext-rel
▷ *bupropion HCl* (C)(G)
    Pediatric: <18 years: not recommended
      Wellbutrin initially 100 mg bid for at least 3 days; may increase to 375 or 400 mg/day after several weeks; then after at least 3 more days, 450 mg in 4 divided doses; max 450 mg/day, 150 mg/single-dose
      Tab: 75, 100 mg
      Wellbutrin SR initially 150 mg in AM for at least 3 days; increase to 150 mg bid if well tolerated; usual dose 300 mg/day; max 400 mg/day
      Tab: 100, 150 mg sust-rel
      Wellbutrin XL initially 150 mg in AM for at least 3 days; increase to 150 mg bid if well tolerated; usual dose 300 mg/day; max 450 mg/day
      Tab: 150, 300 mg sust-rel

MONOAMINE OXIDASE INHIBITORS (MAOIs)

Comment: Many drug and food interactions with this class of drugs, use cautiously. Should be reserved for refractory depression that has not responded to other classes of antidepressants. Concomitant use of MAOIs and SSRIs is an absolute contraindication. See mfr pkg insert for drug and food interactions.
▷ *isocarcatronazid* (C)(G) initially 10 mg bid; increase by 10 mg every 2-4 days up to 40 mg/day; may increase by 20 mg/week to max 60 mg/day divided bid-qid
    Marplan
      Pediatric: <16 years: not recommended; ≥16 years: same as adult
      Tab: 10 mg
▷ *phenelzine* (C)(G) initially 15 mg tid; max 90 mg/day
    Nardil
      Pediatric: <16 years: not recommended; ≥16 years: same as adult
      Tab: 15 mg
▷ *selegiline* (C) initially 10 mg tid; max 60 mg/day
      Emsam *Transdermal patch:* 6 mg/24 h, 9 mg/24 h, 12 mg/24 h
      Comment: With the **Emsam** transdermal patch 6 mg/24 h dose, the dietary restrictions commonly required when using nonselective MAOIs are not necessary.

▶ *tranylcypromine* (C) initially 10 mg tid; may increase in 10 mg/day every 1-3 weeks; max 60 mg/day
    Parnate *Tab:* 10 mg

TETRACYCLICS

▶ *maprotiline* (B)(G) initially 75 mg/day for 2 weeks then change gradually as needed in 25 mg increments; max 225 mg/day
Pediatric: <18 years: not recommended
    Ludiomil *Tab:* 25, 50, 75 mg
▶ *mirtazapine* (C) initially 15 mg q HS; increase at intervals of 1-2 weeks; usual range 15-45 mg/day; max 45 mg/day
Pediatric: not recommended
    Remeron *Tab:* 15*, 30*, 45*mg
    Remeron SolTab *ODT:* 15, 30, 45 mg (orange) (phenylalanine)
▶ *chlordiazepoxide/amitriptyline* (C)(IV)
Pediatric: not recommended
    Limbitrol 3-4 tabs in divided doses
        Tab: chlor 5 mg/*amit* 12.5 mg
    Limbitrol DS 3-4 tabs in divided doses; max 6 tabs/day
        Tab: chlor 10 mg/*amit* 25 mg
▶ *trazodone* (C)(G) initially 150 mg/day in divided doses with food; increase by 50 mg/day q 3-4 days; max 400 mg/day in divided doses
Pediatric: <18 years: not recommended
    Oleptro *Tab:* 50, 100*, 150*, 200, 250, 300 mg

ATYPICAL ANTIPSYCHOTICS

▶ *aripiprazole* (C)(G) initially 15 mg daily; may increase to max 30 mg/day
Pediatric: <10 years: not recommended; 10-17 years: initially 2 mg/day for 2 days; then, increase to 5 mg/day for 2 days; then, increase to target dose of 10 mg/day; may increase by 5 mg/day at 1 week intervals as needed to max 30 mg/day
    Abilify *Tab:* 2, 5, 10, 15, 20, 30 mg
    Abilify Discmelt *Tab:* 15 mg orally disintegrating (vanilla) (phenylalanine)
    Abilify Maintena *Vial:* 300, 400 mg ext-rel pwdr for IM injection after reconstitution; 300, 400 mg single-dose prefilled dual-chamber syringes w. supplies
    Comment: **Abilify** is indicated for acute and maintenance treatment of manic or mixed episodes in bipolar I disorder, as monotherapy or as an adjunct to *lithium* or *valproate*, as adjunct to antidepressants for major depressive disorder (MDD), and for irritability associated with autistic disorder.
▶ *brexpiprazole* (C) initially 0.5 or 1 mg once daily; titrate weekly up to target 2 mg/day; max 3 mg/day; *Moderate-severe hepatic impairment, renal impairment,* or *ESRD,* max 2 mg/day
Pediatric: not established
    Rexulti *Tab:* 0.25, 0.5, 1, 2, 3, 4 mg

◯ DERMATITIS: ATOPIC (ECZEMA)

Oral Antihistamines: *see* **Oral Drugs for Allergy, Cough, and Cold** *see page* 535
Parenteral Corticosteroids *see page* 511

Oral Corticosteroids *see page* 509

TOPICAL STEROIDS

(For other topical steroids, *see* **Topical Corticosteroids** *page* 506)
Comment: Topical steroids should be applied sparingly and for the shortest time necessary. Do not use in the diaper area. Do not use an occlusive dressing. Systemic absorption of topical corticosteroids can induce reversible hypothalamic-pituitary-adrenal (HPA) axis suppression with the potential for clinical corticosteroids insufficiency.

▶ *desonide* 0.05% topical gel **(C)** apply sparingly bid-tid; max 4 weeks
  Pediatric: <3 months: not recommended; ≥3 months: same as adult
    Desonate *Gel:* 0.05% (60 g) (89% purified water; fragrance-free, surfactant-free, alcohol-free)

PHOSPHODIESTERASE 4 INHIBITOR

▶ *crisaborole* 2% **(C)** apply sparingly bid; max 4 weeks
  Pediatric: <2 years: not recommended; ≥2 years: same as adult
    Eucrisa *Oint:* 2% (60 g)

MOISTURIZING AGENTS

Aquaphor Healing Ointment (OTC) *Oint:* 1.75, 3.5, 14 oz (alcohol)
Eucerin Daily Sun Defense (OTC) *Lotn:* 6 oz (fragrance-free)
Comment: Eucerin Daily Sun Defense is a moisturizer with SPF-15 sunscreen.
Eucerin Facial Lotion (OTC) *Lotn:* 4 oz
Eucerin Light Lotion (OTC) *Lotn:* 8 oz
Eucerin Lotion (OTC) *Lotn:* 8, 16 oz
Eucerin Original Creme (OTC) *Crm:* 2, 4, 16 oz (alcohol)
Eucerin Plus Creme (OTC) *Crm:* 4 oz
Eucerin Plus Lotion (OTC) *Lotn:* 6, 12 oz
Eucerin Protective Lotion (OTC) *Lotn:* 4 oz (alcohol)
Comment: Eucerin Protective Lotion is a moisturizer with SPF-25 sunscreen.
Lac-Hydrin Cream (OTC) *Crm:* 280, 385 g
Lac-Hydrin Lotion (OTC) *Lotn:* 25, 400 g
Lubriderm Dry Skin Scented (OTC) *Lotn:* 6, 10, 16, 32 oz
Lubriderm Dry Skin Unscented (OTC) *Lotn:* 3.3, 6, 10, 16 oz (fragrance-free)
Lubriderm Sensitive Skin Lotion (OTC) *Lotn:* 3.3, 6, 10, 16 oz (lanolin-free)
Lubriderm Dry Skin (OTC) *Lotn (scented):* 2.5, 6, 10, 16 oz;
    Lotn (fragrance-free): 1, 2.5, 6, 10, 16 oz
Lubriderm Bath 1-2 capfuls in bath or rub onto wet skin as needed, then rinse
    Oil: 8 oz
Moisturel apply as needed
    Crm: 4, 16 oz; *Lotn:* 8, 12 oz; *Clnsr:* 8.75 oz

OATMEAL COLLOIDS

Aveeno (OTC) add to bath as needed
    Regular: 1.5 oz (8/pck); *Moisturizing:* 0.75 oz (8/pck)
Aveeno Oil (OTC) add to bath as needed
    Oil: 8 oz

Aveeno Moisturizing (OTC) apply as needed
Lotn: 2.5, 8, 12 oz; *Crm:* 4 oz
Aveeno Cleansing Bar (OTC) *Bar:* 3 oz
Aveeno Gentle Skin Cleanser (OTC) *Liq clnsr:* 6 oz

TOPICAL OIL

▷ *fluocinolone acetamide* 0.01% topical oil (C)
Pediatric: <6 years: not recommended; ≥6 years: apply sparingly bid for up to 4 weeks
Derma-Smoothe/FS Topical Oil apply sparingly tid
Topical oil: 0.01% (4 oz) (peanut oil)

TOPICAL ANALGESICS

▷ *capsaicin* cream (B)(G) apply tid-qid prn
Pediatric: <2 years: not recommended; ≥2 years: apply sparingly tid-qid prn
Axsain *Crm:* 0.075% (1, 2 oz)
Capsin (OTC) *Lotn:* 0.025, 0,075% (59 ml)
Capzasin-P (OTC) *Crm:* 0.025% (1.5 oz); *Lotn:* 0.025% (2 oz)
Capzasin-HP (OTC) *Crm:* 0.075% (1.5 oz); *Lotn:* 0.075% (2 oz)
Dolorac *Crm:* 0.025% (28 g)
Double Cap (OTC) *Crm:* 0.05% (2 oz)
R-Gel *Gel:* 0.025% (15, 30 g)
Zostrix (OTC) *Crm:* 0.025% (0.7, 1.5, 3 oz)
Zostrix HP (OTC) *Emol crm:* 0.075% (1, 2 oz)
Comment: Provides some relief by 1-2 weeks; optimal benefit may take 4-6 weeks.
Avoid contact with mucous membranes.
▷ *doxepin* (B) cream apply to affected area qid at intervals of at least 3-4 hours;
max 8 days
Pediatric: not recommended
Prudoxin *Crm:* 5% (45 g)
Zonalon *Crm:* 5% (30, 45 g)
▷ *pimecrolimus* 1% cream (C) apply to affected area bid; do not occlude
Pediatric: <2 years: not recommended; ≥2 years: same as adult
Elidel *Crm:* 1% (30, 60, 100 g)
Comment: *pimecrolimus* is indicated for short-term and intermittent long-term
use. Discontinue use when resolution occurs. Contraindicated if the patient is
immunosuppressed. Change to the 0.1% preparation or if secondary bacterial
infection is present.
▷ *tacrolimus* (C) apply to affected area bid; do not occlude or apply to wet skin; continue for 1 week after clearing
Pediatric: <2 years: not recommended; 2-15 years: use 0.03% strength; apply to
affected area bid; continue for 1 week after clearing; >15 years: same as adult
Protopic *Oint:* 0.03, 0.1% (30, 60, 100 g)

TOPICAL ANESTHETIC

▷ *lidocaine* (B) apply to affected area bid-tid prn
Pediatric: reduce dosage commensurate with age, body weight, and physical condition
Lidoderm *Crm:* 3% (85 g)

DERMATITIS: CONTACT

PROPHYLAXIS

▷ *bentoquatam* (NE) apply as a wet film to exposed skin at least 15 minutes prior to possible contact; reapply at least q 4 hours; remove with soap and water
Pediatric: <6 years: not recommended; ≥6 years: same as adult
IvyBlock (OTC) *Soln:* 120 ml
Comment: Provides protection against genus rhus (poison ivy, oak, and sumac).

TREATMENT

Oatmeal Colloids

Aveeno (OTC) add to bath as needed
Regular: 1.5 oz (8/pck); *Moisturizing:* 0.75 oz (8/pck)
Aveeno Oil (OTC) add to bath as needed
Oil: 8 oz
Aveeno Moisturizing (OTC) apply as needed
Lotn: 2.5, 8, 12 oz; *Crm:* 4 oz
Aveeno Cleansing Bar (OTC) *Bar:* 3 oz
Aveeno Gentle Skin Cleanser (OTC) *Liq clnsr:* 6 oz
Oral Drugs for Allergy, Cough, and Cold *see page 535*
Topical Corticosteroids *see page 506*
Parenteral Corticosteroids *see page 511*
Oral Corticosteroids *see page 509*

DERMATITIS: SEBORRHEIC

ANTIFUNGAL SHAMPOOS AND TOPICAL AGENTS

▷ *chloroxine* shampoo (C) massage onto wet scalp; wait 3 minutes, rinse, repeat, and rinse thoroughly; use twice weekly
Pediatric: not recommended
Capitrol Shampoo *Shampoo:* 2% (4 oz)
▷ *ciclopirox* (B) apply gel once daily or apply cream or lotion twice daily, x 4 weeks or shampoo twice weekly; massage shampoo onto wet scalp; wait 3 minutes, rinse, repeat, and rinse thoroughly; shampoo twice weekly
Loprox Cream
Pediatric: <10 years: not recommended; ≥10 years: same as adult
Crm: 0.77% (15, 30, 90 g)
Loprox Gel
Pediatric: <16 years: not recommended; ≥16 years: same as adult
Gel: 0.77% (30, 45 g)
Loprox Lotion
Pediatric: <10 years: not recommended; ≥10 years: same as adult
Lotn: 0.77% (30, 60 ml)
Loprox Shampoo *Shampoo:* 1% (120 ml)
▷ *coal tar* (C)(G)
Pediatric: same as adult
Scytera (OTC) apply once daily-qid; use lowest effective dose

Foam: 2%

T/Gel Shampoo Extra Strength (OTC) use every other day; max 4 x/week; massage into wet scalp for 5 minutes; rinse; repeat *Shampoo:* 1%

T/Gel Shampoo Original Formula (OTC) use every other day; max 7 x/week; massage into wet scalp for 5 minutes; rinse; repeat
  Shampoo: 0.5%

T/Gel Shampoo Stubborn Itch Control (OTC) use every other day; max 7 x/week; massage into wet scalp for 5 minutes; rinse; repeat
  Shampoo: 0.5%

▷ *fluocinolone acetamide* (C)

Derma-Smoothe/FS Shampoo apply up to 1 oz to scalp daily, lather, and leave on x 5 minutes, then rinse twice
  Pediatric: not recommended
  Shampoo: 0.01% (4 oz)

Derma-Smoothe/FS Topical Oil *fluocinolone acetamide* 0.01% topical oil (C) apply sparingly tid; for scalp psoriasis wet <u>or</u> dampen hair <u>or</u> scalp, then apply a thin film, massage well, cover with a shower cap and leave on for at least 4 hours <u>or</u> overnight, then wash hair with regular shampoo and rinse
  Pediatric: <6 years: not recommended; ≥6 years: apply sparingly bid for up to 4 weeks
  Topical oil: 0.01% (4 oz) (peanut oil)

▷ *ketoconazole* (C) apply cream or gel once daily x 4 week <u>or</u> apply up to 1 oz shampoo to scalp daily, lather, leave on x 5 minutes, then rinse twice
Pediatric: not recommended

Nizoral Cream *Crm:* 2% (15, 30, 60 g)

Nizoral Shampoo *Shampoo:* 2% (4 oz)

Xolegel *Gel:* 2% (45 g)

Xolegel Duo *Kit:* **Xolegel** *Gel:* 2% (45 g) + **Xolex** *Shampoo:* 2% (4 oz)

▷ *selenium sulfide* (C) massage cream into scalp twice weekly x 2 weeks <u>or</u> massage into wet scalp, wait 2-3 minutes, rinse; repeat twice weekly x 2 weeks; may continue treatment with lotion of shampoo 1-2 x weekly as needed
Pediatric: not recommended

Exsel Shampoo *Shampoo:* 2.5% (4 oz)

Selsun Rx *Lotn:* 2.5% (4 oz)

Selsun Shampoo *Shampoo:* 1% (120, 210, 240, 330 ml); 2.5% (120 ml)

▷ *sodium sulfacetamide/sulfur* (C)

Clinia Emollient Cream apply daily tid
  Emol crm: sod sulfa 10%/*sulfur* 5% (10 oz)

Clinia Foaming Wash wash 1-2 x/daily
  Wash: sod sulfa 10%/*sulfur* 5% (6, 12 oz)

Rosula Gel apply daily tid
  Gel: sod sulfa 10%/*sulfur* 5% (45 ml)

Rosula Lotion apply daily tid
  Lotn: sod sulfa 10%/*sulfur* 5% (45 ml) (alcohol-free)

Rosula Wash wash bid
  Clnsr: sod sulfa 10%/*sulfur* 5% (335 ml)

TOPICAL STEROID

▷ *betamethasone valerate* 0.12% foam (C)(G) apply twice daily in AM and PM; invert can and dispense a small amount of foam onto a clean saucer <u>or</u> other cool surface

(do not apply directly to hand) and massage a small amount into affected area until foam disappears
Pediatric: not recommended
> **Luxiq** *Foam:* 100 g
Other Topical Corticosteroids *see page* 506

◯ DIABETIC PERIPHERAL NEUROPATHY

NUTRITIONAL SUPPLEMENT

➤ *L-methylfolate calcium (as metafolin)/pyridoxyl 5-phosphate/methyl-cobalamin* (NE) 1 cap twice daily or 2 caps once daily
Pediatric: not recommended
> **Metanx** *Cap: meta* 3 mg/*pyr* 35 mg/*methyl* 2 mg
> **Comment: Metanx** is indicated as adjunct treatment for patients with endothelial cell dysfunction, who have loss of protective sensation and neuropathic pain associated with diabetic peripheral neuropathy.
Acetaminophen for IV Infusion *see Pain page* 306

ORAL ANALGESICS

➤ *acetaminophen* (B)(G) *see Fever page* 143
➤ *aspirin* (D)(G) *see Fever page* 144
> **Comment:** *aspirin*-containing medications are contraindicated with history of allergic-type reaction to *aspirin*, children and adolescents with *Varicella* or other viral illness, and 3rd trimester pregnancy.
➤ *tramadol* (C)(IV)(G)
> **Rybix ODT** initially 100 mg once daily; may increase by 100 mg every 5 days; max 300 mg/day; *CrCl <30 mL/min* or *severe hepatic impairment*: not recommended; *Cirrhosis:* max 50 mg q 12 hours
>> *Pediatric:* <17 years: not recommended
>> *ODT:* 50 mg (mint) (phenylalanine)
> **Ryzolt** initially 100 mg once daily; may increase by 100 mg every 5 days; max 300 mg/day; *CrCl <30 mL/min* or *severe hepatic impairment*: not recommended
>> *Pediatric:* <16 years: not recommended; ≥16 years: same as adult
>> *Tab:* 100, 200, 300 mg ext-rel
> **Ultram** 50-100 mg q 4-6 hours prn; max 400 mg/day; *CrCl <30 mL/min*, max 100 mg q 12 hours; cirrhosis, max 50 mg q 12 hours
>> *Pediatric:* <16 years: not recommended
>> *Tab:* 50*mg
> **Ultram ER** initially 100 mg once daily; may increase by 100 mg every 5 days; max 300 mg/day; *CrCl <30 mL/min* or *severe hepatic impairment*: not recommended
>> *Pediatric:* <18 years: not recommended
>> *Tab:* 100, 200, 300 mg ext-rel
➤ *tramadol/acetaminophen* (C)(IV)(G) 2 tabs q 4-6 hours; max 8 tabs/day x 5 days; *CrCl <30 mL/min:* max 2 tabs q 12 hours; max 4 tabs/day x 5 days
Pediatric: <16 years: not recommended
> **Ultracet** *Tab: tram* 37.5/*acet* 325 mg
Other Oral Analgesics *see Pain page* 306

TOPICAL ANALGESICS

▷ *capsaicin* cream **(B)(G)** apply tid-qid after lesions have healed
  Pediatric: <2 years: not recommended; ≥2 years: same as adult
    Axsain *Crm:* 0.075% (1, 2 oz)
    Capsin *Lotn:* 0.025, 0.075% (59 ml)
    Capsaicin-P (OTC) *Crm:* 0.025% (1.5 oz); *Lotn:* 0.025% (2 oz)
    Capsaicin-HP (OTC) *Crm:* 0.075% (1.5 oz); *Lotn:* 0.075% (2 oz); *Crm:* 0.025% (45, 90 g)
    Dolorac *Crm:* 0.025% (28 g)
    Double Cap (OTC) *Crm:* 0.05% (2 oz)
    R-Gel *Gel:* 0.025% (15, 30 g)
    Zostrix (OTC) *Crm:* 0.025% (0.7, 1.5, 3 oz)
    Zostrix HP *Emol crm:* 0.075% (1, 2 oz)
▷ *capsaicin* 8% patch **(B)** apply up to 4 patches for one 60-minute application to clean dry skin; may prep area with topical anesthetic; wear nonlatex gloves; patches may be cut to size/shape; treatment may be repeated every 3 months
  Pediatric: <18 years: not recommended
    Qutenza *Patch:* 8% 1640 mcg/cm (179 mg) (1 or 2 patches w. 1-50 g tube cleansing gel/carton)
▷ *lidocaine* 5% patch **(B)(G)** apply up to 3 patches at one time for up to 12 hours/24-hour period (12 hours on/12 hours off); patches may be cut into smaller sizes before removal of the release liner; do not re-use
  Pediatric: not recommended
    Lidoderm *Patch:* 5% 10x14 cm (30 patches/carton)

ANTICONVULSANTS

Gamma Aminobutyric Acid Analog

▷ *gabapentin* **(C)**
  Pediatric: <3 years: not recommended; 3-12 years: initially 10-15 mg/kg/day in 3 divided doses; max 12 hours between doses; titrate over 3 days; 3-4 years: titrate to 40 mg/kg/day; 5-12 years: titrate to 25-35 mg/kg/day; max 50 mg/kg/day
    Gralise (C) initially 300 mg on Day 1; then 600 mg on Day 2; then 900 mg on Days 3-6; then 1200 mg on Days 7-10; then 1500 mg on Days 11-14; titrate up to 1800 mg on Day 15; take entire dose once daily with the evening meal; do not crush, split, or chew
      Tab: 300, 600 mg
    Neurontin (G) *Tab:* 600*, 800* mg; *Cap:* 100, 300, 400 mg; *Oral soln:* 250 mg/5 ml (480 ml) (strawberry-anise)
▷ *gabapentin enacarbil* **(C)** 600 mg once daily at about 5:00 PM; if dose not taken at recommended time, next dose should be taken the following day; swallow whole; take with food; *CrCl 30-59 mL/min:* 600 mg on Day 1, Day 3, and every day thereafter; *CrCl <30 mL/min:* or on hemodialysis: not recommended
  Pediatric: not recommended
    Horizant *Tab:* 300, 600 mg ext-rel
Comment: Avoid abrupt cessation of *gabapentin* and *gabapentin enacarbil*. To discontinue, withdraw gradually over 1 week or longer.
▷ *pregabalin (GABA analog)* **(C)(V)** initially 50 mg tid; may titrate to 100 mg tid within one week; max 600 mg divided tid; discontinue over 1 week
  Pediatric: <18 years: not recommended

Lyrica *Cap:* 25, 50, 75, 100, 150, 200, 225, 300 mg; *Oral soln:* 20 mg/ml

TRICYCLIC ANTIDEPRESSANTS (TCAs)

Comment: Co-administration of TCAs with SSRIs requires extreme caution.
▷ *amitriptyline* (C)(G) titrate to achieve pain relief; max 300 mg/day
   Pediatric: not recommended
    Tab: 10, 25, 50, 75, 100, 150 mg
▷ *amoxapine* (C) titrate to achieve pain relief; if total dose exceeds 300 mg/day, give
in divided doses; max 400 mg/day
   Pediatric: not recommended
    Tab: 25, 50, 100, 150 mg
▷ *desipramine* (C)(G) titrate to achieve pain relief; max 300 mg/day
   Pediatric: not recommended
    Norpramin *Tab:* 10, 25, 50, 75, 100, 150 mg
▷ *doxepin* (C)(G) titrate to achieve pain relief; max 150 mg/day
   Pediatric: not recommended
    Cap: 10, 25, 50, 75, 100, 150 mg; *Oral conc:* 10 mg/ml (4 oz w. dropper)
▷ *imipramine* (C)(G)
   Pediatric: not recommended
    Tofranil titrate to achieve pain relief; max 200 mg/day; adolescents max 100 mg/
    day; if maintenance dose exceeds 75 mg/day, may switch to **Tofranil PM** at bedtime
      Tab: 10, 25, 50 mg
    Tofranil PM titrate to achieve pain relief; initially 75 mg at HS; max 200 mg at HS
      Cap: 75, 100, 125, 150 mg
    Tofranil Injection 50 mg IM; lower dose for adolescents; switch to oral form as
    soon as possible
      Amp: 25 mg/2 ml (2 ml)
▷ *nortriptyline* (D)(G) titrate to achieve pain relief; initially 10-25 mg tid-qid; max
150 mg/day; lower doses for elderly and adolescents
   Pediatric: not recommended
    Pamelor titrate to achieve pain relief; max 150 mg/day
      Cap: 10, 25, 50, 75 mg; *Oral soln:* 10 mg/5 ml (16 oz)
▷ *protriptyline* (C) titrate to achieve pain relief; initially 5 mg tid; max 60 mg/day
   Pediatric: <12 years: not recommended
    Vivactyl *Tab:* 5, 10 mg
▷ *trimipramine* (C) titrate to achieve pain relief; max 200 mg/day
   Pediatric: not recommended
    Surmontil *Cap:* 25, 50, 100 mg

 DIAPER RASH

Topical Corticosteroids *see page 506*
Comment: Low to intermediate potency topical corticosteroids are indicated if
inflammation is present.

PROTECTIVE BARRIERS

▷ *aloe/vitamin E/zinc oxide* (NE) ointment apply at each diaper change after thoroughly cleansing skin
   Balmex *Oint:* 2, 4 oz tube; 16 oz jar

▷ *vitamin A&D* **(NE) (G)** ointment apply at each diaper change after thoroughly cleansing skin
  A&D Ointment *Oint:* 1.5, 4 oz
▷ *zinc oxide* **(NE)(G)** cream and ointment apply at each diaper change after thoroughly cleansing the skin
  A&D Ointment with Zinc Oxide *Oint:* 10% (1.5, 4 oz)
  Desitin *Oint:* 40% (1, 2, 4, 9 oz)
  Desitin Cream *Crm:* 10% (2, 4 oz)

TOPICAL ANTIFUNGALS

Comment: Use if caused by *Candida albicans.*
▷ *butenafine* **(B)(G)** apply bid x 1 week or once daily x 4 weeks
  Pediatric: <12 years: not recommended
  Lotrimin Ultra (C)(OTC) *Crm:* 1% (12, 24 g)
  Mentax *Crm:* 1% (15, 30 g)
  Comment: *butenafine* is a benzylamine, not an azole. Fungicidal activity continues for at least 5 weeks after last application.
▷ *clotrimazole* **(B)** apply to affected area bid x 7 days
  Pediatric: same as adult
  Lotrimin (OTC) *Crm:* 1% (15, 30, 45 g)
  Lotrimin AF (OTC) *Crm:* 1% (12 g); *Lotn:* 1% (10 ml); *Soln:* 1% (10 ml)
▷ *econazole* **(C)** apply bid x 7 days
  Spectazole *Crm:* 1% (15, 30, 85 g)
▷ *ketoconazole* **(C)(G)**
  Nizoral Cream *Crm:* 2% (15, 30, 60 g)
▷ *miconazole* 2% **(C)(G)** apply bid x 7 days
  Pediatric: same as adult
  Lotrimin AF Spray Liquid (OTC) *Spray liq:* 2% (113 g) (alcohol 17%)
  Lotrimin AF Spray Powder (OTC) *Spray pwdr:* 2% (90 g) (alcohol 10%)
  Monistat-Derm *Crm:* 2% (1, 3 oz); *Spray liq:* 2% (3.5 oz); *Spray pwdr:* 2% (3 oz)
▷ *nystatin* **(C)(G)** apply bid x 7 days
  Mycostatin *Crm:* 100,000 U/g (15, 30 g)

COMBINATION AGENT

▷ *clotrimazole/betamethasone* **(C)(G)** cream apply bid x 7 days
  Lotrisone *Crm:* 15, 45 g

 DIARRHEA: ACUTE

▷ *attapulgite* **(C)**
  Donnagel (OTC) 30 ml after each loose stool; max 7 doses/day x 2 days
  Pediatric: <3 years: not recommended; 3-6 years: 7.5 ml; >6-12 years: 15 ml; >12 years: same as adult
  Liq: 600 mg/15 ml (120, 240 ml)

Donnagel Chewable Tab (OTC) 2 tabs after each loose stool; max 14 tabs/day
   Pediatric: <3 years: not recommended; 3-6 years: 1/2 tab after each loose stool; max 7 doses/day; >6-12 years: 1 tab after each loose stool; max 7 tabs/day
   Chew tab: 600 mg

Kaopectate (OTC) 30 ml after each loose stool; max 7 doses/day x 2 days
   Pediatric: <3 years: not recommended; 3-6 years: 7.5 ml after each loose stool; >6-12 years: 15 ml after each loose stool; >12 years: same as adult
   Liq: 600 mg/15 ml (120, 240 ml)

▷ *bismuth subsalicylate* (C; D in 3rd)(G)
   Pepto-Bismol (OTC) 2 tabs or 30 ml q 30-60 minutes as needed; max 8 doses/day
   Pediatric: <3 years (14-18 lb): 2.5 ml q 4 hours; max 6 doses/day; <3 years (18-28 lb): 5 ml q 4 hours; max 6 doses/day; 3-6 years: 1/3 tab or 5 ml q 30-60 minutes; max 8 doses/day; >6-9 years: 2/3 tab or 10 ml q 30-60 minutes; max 8 doses/day; >9-12 years: 1 tab or 15 ml q 30-60 minutes; max 8 doses/day
   Chew tab: 262 mg; *Liq:* 262 mg/15 ml (4, 8, 12, 16 oz)

   Pepto-Bismol Maximum Strength (OTC) 30 ml q 60 minutes; max 4 doses/day
   Pediatric: <3 years: not recommended; 3-6 years: 5 ml q 60 minutes; max 4 doses/day; >6-9 years: 10 ml q 60 minutes; max 4 doses/day; >9-12 years: 15 ml q 60 minutes; max 4 doses/day
   Liq: 525 mg/15 ml (4, 8, 12, 16 oz)

Comment: *aspirin*-containing medications are contraindicated with history of allergic-type reaction to ***aspirin***, children and adolescents with *Varicella* or other viral illness, and 3rd trimester pregnancy.

▷ *calcium polycarbophil* (C)
   Pediatric: <6 years: not recommended; 6-12 years: 1 tab daily qid; >12 years: same as adult
   Fibercon (OTC) 2 tabs daily qid
   Cplt: 625 mg

▷ *crofelemer* (C) 2 tabs once daily; swallow whole with or without food; do not crush or chew
   Pediatric: not established
   Mytesi
   Tab: 125 mg del-rel

Comment: *crofelemer* is indicated for the symptomatic relief of non-infectious diarrhea in adult patients with HIV/AIDS on antiretroviral therapy.

▷ *difenoxin/atropine* (C)
   Pediatric: <2 years: not recommended; ≥2 years: same as adult
   Motofen 2 tabs, then 1 tab after each loose stool or 1 tab q 3-4 hours as needed; max 8 tab/day x 2 days
   Tab: dif 1 mg/atro 0.025 mg

▷ *diphenoxylate/atropine* (C)(V)(G)
   Pediatric: <2 years: not recommended; 2-12 years: initially 0.3-0.4 mg/kg/day in 4 divided doses; >12 years: same as adult
   Lomotil 2 tabs or 10 ml qid until diarrhea is controlled
   Tab: diphen 2.5 mg/atrop 0.025 mg; *Liq:* diphen 2.5 mg/atrop 0.025 mg per 5 ml (2 oz)

▷ *loperamide* (B)(OTC)(G)
   Imodium 4 mg initially, then 2 mg after each loose stool; max 16 mg/day x 2 days

Pediatric: <5 years: not recommended; ≥5 years: same as adult
Cap: 2 mg

Imodium A-D 4 mg initially, then 2 mg after each loose stool; usual max 8 mg/day x 2 days

Pediatric: <2 years: not recommended; 2-5 years (24-47 lb): 1 mg up to tid x 2 days; 6-8 years (48-59 lb): 2 mg initially, then 1 mg after each loose stool; max 4 mg/day x 2 days; 9-11 years (60-95 lb): 2 mg initially, then 1 mg after each loose stool; max 6 mg/day x 2 days

Cplt: 2 mg; *Liq:* 1 mg/5 ml (2, 4 oz) (cherry-mint) (alcohol 0.5%)

▷ *loperamide/simethicone* (B)(OTC)(G)

Imodium Advanced 2 tabs chewed after loose stool, then 1 after the next loose stool; max 4 tabs/day

Pediatric: 6-8 years: chew 1 tab after loose stool, then chew 1/2 tab after next loose stool; 9-11 years: chew 1 tab after loose stool, then chew 1/2 tab after next loose stool; max 3 tabs/day; ≥12 years: same as adult

Chew tab: loper 2 mg/*simeth* 125 mg (vanilla-mint)

ORAL REHYDRATION AND ELECTROLYTE REPLACEMENT THERAPY

▷ *oral electrolyte replacement* (NE)(OTC)

CeraLyte 50 dissolve in 8 oz water

Pediatric: <4 years: not indicated; ≥4 years, same as adult

Pkt: sodium 50 mEq/*potassium* 20 mEq/*chloride* 40 mEq/*citrate* 30 mEq/*rice syrup solids* 40 g/*calories* 190 per liter (mixed berry) (gluten-free)

CeraLyte 70 dissolved in 8 oz water

Pediatric: <4 years: not indicated; ≥4 years: same as adult

Pkt: sodium 70 mEq/*potassium* 20 mEq/*chloride* 60 mEq/*citrate* 30 mEq/*rice syrup solids* 40 g/*calories* 165 per liter (natural or lemon) (gluten-free)

KaoLectrolyte 1 pkt dissolved in 8 oz water q 3-4 hours

Pediatric: <2 years: not indicated; ≥2 years: same as adult

Pkt: sod 12 mEq/*pot* 5 mEq/*chlor* 10 mEq/*citrate* 7 mEq/*dextrose* 5 g/calories 22 per 6.2 g

Pedialyte

Pediatric: <2 years: as desired and as tolerated; ≥2 years: 1-2 L/day

Oral soln: dextrose 20 g/*fructose* 5 g/*sodium* 25 mEq/*potassium* 20 mEq/*chloride* 35 mEq/*citrate* 30 mEq/*calories* 100 per liter (8 oz, 1 L)

Pedialyte Freezer Pops

Pediatric: as desired and as tolerated

Pops: dextrose 1.6 g/*sodium* 2.8 mEq/*potassium* 1.25 mEq/*chloride* 2.2 mEq/*citrate* 1.88 mEq/*calories* 6.25 per 6.25 ml pop (8 oz, 1 L)

◯ DIARRHEA: CHRONIC

▷ *cholestyramine* (C)

Questran Powder for Oral Suspension initially 1 pkt or scoop daily; usual maintenance 2-4 pkts or scoops daily in 2 doses; max 6 pkts or scoops daily

Oral pwdr: 9 g pkts; 9 g equal 4 g *anhydrous cholestyramine resin* (60/pck); *Bulk can:* 378 g w. scoop

Questran Light initially 1 pkt <u>or</u> scoop daily; usual maintenance 2-4 pkts <u>or</u>
scoops daily in 2 doses
> *Light:* 5 g pkts; 5 g equals 4 g *anhydrous cholestyramine resin* (60/pck); *Bulk*
> *can:* 210 g w. scoop

Comment: Use *cholestyramine* only if diarrhea is due to bile salt malabsorption.
▷ *crofelemer* (C) 2 tabs once daily; swallow whole with <u>or</u> without food; do not crush
<u>or</u> chew
Pediatric: not established
> **Mytesi**
> > *Tab:* 125 mg del-rel

Comment: *crofelemer* is indicated for the symptomatic relief of non-infectious
diarrhea in adult patients with HIV/AIDS on antiretroviral therapy.
▷ *difenoxin/atropine* (C)
Pediatric: <2 years: not recommended; ≥2 years: same as adult
> **Motofen** 2 tabs, then 1 tab after each loose stool <u>or</u> 1 tab q 3-4 hours prn; max 8
> tab/day x 2 days
> > *Tab:* dif 1 mg/atrop 0.025 mg
▷ *diphenoxylate/atropine* (B)(V)(G)
Pediatric: <2 years: not recommended; 2-12 years: initially 0.3-0.4 mg/kg/day in 4
divided doses; >12 years: same as adult
> **Lomotil** 5-20 mg/day in divided doses
> > *Tab:* diphen 2.5 mg/atrop 0.025 mg; *Liq:* diphen 2.5 mg/atrop 0.025 mg per
> > 5 ml (2 oz w. dropper)
▷ *attapulgite* (C)(G)
> **Donnagel** (OTC) 30 ml after each loose stool; max 7 doses/day
> > *Pediatric:* <2 years: not recommended; 2-6 years: 7.5 ml after each loose
> > stool; >6 years: same as adult
> > *Liq:* 600 mg/15 ml (120, 240 ml)
> **Donnagel Chewable Tab** 2 tabs after each loose stool; max 14 tabs/day
> > *Pediatric:* <3 years: not recommended; 3-6 years: 1/2 tab after each stool;
> > max 7 doses/day; >6-12 years: 1 tab after each loose stool; max 7 tabs/day;
> > >12 years: same as adult
▷ *loperamide* (B)(OTC)(G)
> **Imodium** (OTC) 4-16 mg/day in divided doses
> > *Pediatric:* <5 years: not recommended; ≥5 years: same as adult
> > *Cap:* 2 mg
> **Imodium A-D** (OTC) 4-16 mg/day in divided doses
> > *Pediatric:* <2 years: not recommended; 2-5 years (24-47 lb): 1 mg up to
> > tid x 2 days; 6-8 years (48-59 lb): 2 mg initially, then 1 mg after after each
> > loose stool; max 4 mg/day x 2 days; 9-11 years (60-95 lb): 2 mg initially,
> > then 1 mg after each loose stool; max 6 mg/day x 2 days; ≥12 years: same
> > as adult
> > *Cplt:* 2 mg; *Liq:* 1 mg/5 ml (2, 4 oz)
▷ *loperamide/simethicone* (B)(OTC)(G)
> **Imodium Advanced** 2 tabs chewed after loose stool, then 1 after the next loose
> stool; max 4 tabs/day
> > *Pediatric:* 6-8 years: chew 1 tab after loose stool, then chew 1/2 tab after next
> > loose stool; 9-11 years: chew 1 tab after loose stool, then chew 1/2 tab after
> > next loose stool; max 3 tabs/day
> > *Chew tab:* loper 2 mg/simeth 125 mg

⬤ DIARRHEA: TRAVELERS

➤ *ciprofloxacin* (C) 500 mg bid x 3 days
   Pediatric: <18 years: not recommended
      Cipro (G) *Tab:* 250, 500, 750 mg; *Oral susp:* 250, 500 mg/5 ml (100 ml) (strawberry)
      Cipro XR *Tab:* 500, 1000 mg ext-rel
      ProQuin XR *Tab:* 500 mg ext-rel
   Comment: *ciprofloxacin* is contraindicated <18 years-of-age, and during pregnancy and lactation. Risk of tendonitis or tendon rupture, especially 60 years-of-age and older.
➤ *rifaximin* (C) 200 mg tid x 3 days; discontinue if diarrhea worsens or persists more than 24 hours; not for use if diarrhea is accompanied by fever or blood in the stool or if causative organism other than *E. coli* is suspected.
   Pediatric: <12 years: not recommended; ≥12 years: same as adult
      Xifaxan *Tab:* 200 mg
➤ *trimethoprim/sulfamethoxazole* (C)(G) bid x 10 days
   Pediatric: <2 months: not recommended; >2 months: 40 mg/kg/day of *sulfamethoxazole* in 2 divided doses x 10 days; *see page 587 for dose by weight*
      Bactrim, Septra 2 tabs bid x 10 days
         Tab: trim 80 mg/*sulfa* 400 mg*
      Bactrim DS, Septra DS 1 tab bid x 10 days
         Tab: trim 160 mg/*sulfa* 800 mg*
      Bactrim Pediatric Suspension, Septra Pediatric Suspension
         Oral susp: trim 40 mg/*sulfa* 200 mg per 5 ml (100 ml) (cherry) (alcohol 0.3%)
   Comment: *trimethoprim/sulfamethoxazole* is not recommended in pregnancy or lactation. *CrCl 15-30 mL/min:* reduce dose by 1/2; *CrCl <15 mL/min:* not recommended

⬤ DIGITALIS TOXICITY

Comment: The digitalis therapeutic index is narrow, 0.8-1.2 ng/mL. Whether acute or chronic toxicity, the patient should be treated in the emergency department and/ or admitted to in-patient service for continued monitoring and care. Signs and symptoms of digitalis toxicity include: loss of appetite, nausea, vomiting, abdominal pain, diarrhea, visiual disturbances (diplopia, blurred, or yellow vision, yellow-green halos around lights and other visual images, spots, blind spots), decreased urine output, generalized edema, orthopnea, confusion, delerium, decreased consciousness, potentially lethal cardiac arrhythmias (ranging from ventricular tachycardia (VT) and ventricular fibrillation (VF) to sino-atrial heart block AVB). Treatment measures include repeated doses of charcoal via NG tube administered after gastric lavage for acute ingestion (methods to induce vomiting are usually discouraged because vomiting can worsen bradyarrhythmias), digitalis binders. Monitoring includes: serial ECGs, serum digitalis level, chemistries, potassium (hyperkalemia), magnesium (hypomagnesemia), BUN and creatinine.

DIGOXIN BINDER

➤ *digoxin (immune fab [ovine])* (B)
      Digibind contents of one vial of **Digibind** neutralizes 0.5 mg digoxin; dose based on amount of *digoxin* or *digitoxin* to be neutralized; see mfr pkg insert

Pediatric: see mfr pkg insert
Vial: 38 mg
Digifab dose is based on amount of digoxin <u>or</u> digitoxin to be neutralized (see mfr pkg insert for dosage; contents of 1 vial neutralizes 0.5 mg digoxin.
Pediatric: see mfr pkg insert
Vial: 40 mg for IV injection after reconstitution (preservative-free)

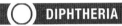

DIPHTHERIA

Prophylaxis see *Childhood Immunizations* page 478

POSTEXPOSURE PROPHYLAXIS FOR NON-IMMUNIZED PERSONS

▷ *erythromycin base* **(B)(G)** 500 mg qid x 14 days
Pediatric: <45 kg: 50 mg/kg/day in 4 divided doses x 14 days; ≥45 kg: same as adult
Ery-Tab *Tab:* 250, 333, 500 mg ent-coat
PCE *Tab:* 333, 500 mg
Comment: *erythromycin* may increase INR with concomitant *warfarin*, as well as increase serum level of *digoxin*, benzodiazepines and statins.

▷ *erythromycin ethylsuccinate* **(B)(G)** 400 mg qid x 14 days
Pediatric: 30-50 mg/kg/day in 4 divided doses x 14 days; may double dose with severe infection; max 100 mg/kg/day; *see page 574 for dose by weight*
EryPed *Oral susp:* 200 mg/5 ml (100, 200 ml) (fruit); 400 mg/5 ml (60, 100, 200 ml) (banana); *Oral drops:* 200, 400 mg/5 ml (50 ml) (fruit); *Chew tab:* 200 mg wafer (fruit)
E.E.S. *Oral susp:* 200, 400 mg/5 ml (100 ml) (fruit)
E.E.S. Granules *Oral susp:* 200 mg/5 ml (100, 200 ml) (cherry)
E.E.S. 400 Tablets *Tab:* 400 mg
Comment: *erythromycin* may increase INR with concomitant *warfarin*, as well as increase serum level of *digoxin*, benzodiazepines and statins.

▷ *Immunization Series*
see *Childhood Immunizations* page 478

POSTEXPOSURE PROPHYLAXIS FOR IMMUNIZED PERSONS

▷ *Diphtheria* immunization booster

DIVERTICULITIS

▷ *amoxicillin* **(B)(G)** 500 mg q 8 hours <u>or</u> 875 mg q 12 hours x 7 days
Amoxil *Cap:* 250, 500 mg; *Tab:* 875*mg; *Chew tab:* 125, 200, 250, 400 mg (cherry-banana-peppermint) (phenylalanine); *Oral susp:* 125, 250 mg/5 ml (80, 100, 150 ml) (strawberry); 200, 400 mg/5 ml (50, 75, 100 ml) (bubble gum); *Oral drops:* 50 mg/ml (30 ml) (bubble gum)
Moxatag *Tab:* 775 mg ext-rel

Trimox *Tab:* 125, 250 mg; *Cap:* 250, 500 mg; *Oral susp:* 125, 250 mg/5 ml (80, 100, 150 ml) (raspberry-strawberry)

▷ *amoxicillin/clavulanate* **(B)(G)** 500 mg tid <u>or</u> 875 mg bid x 10 days

Augmentin *Tab:* 250, 500, 875 mg; *Chew tab:* 125, 250 mg (lemon-lime); 200, 400 mg (cherry-banana) (phenylalanine); *Oral susp:* 125 mg/5 ml (banana), 250 mg/5 ml (75, 100, 150 ml) (orange); 200, 400 mg/5 ml (50, 75, 100 ml) (orange) (phenylalanine)

Pediatric: 40-45 mg/kg/day divided tid x 10 days <u>or</u> 90 mg/kg/day divided bid x 10 days *see pages 556-557 for dose by weight*

Augmentin ES-600 *Oral susp:* 600 mg/5 ml (50, 75, 100, 125, 150, 200 ml) (strawberry cream) (phenylalanine) every 12 hours

Pediatric: <3 months: not recommended; ≥3 months, <40 kg: 90 mg/kg/day in 2 divided doses; ≥40 kg: not recommended

Augmentin XR 2 tabs q 12 hours x 7-10 days

Pediatric: <16 years: use other forms; ≥16 years: same as adult

Tab: 1000*mg ext-rel

▷ *ciprofloxacin* **(C)** 500 mg bid x 7 days

Cipro (G) *Tab:* 250, 500, 750 mg; *Oral susp:* 250, 500 mg/5 ml (100 ml) (strawberry)

Cipro XR *Tab:* 500, 1000 mg ext-rel

ProQuin XR *Tab:* 500 mg ext-rel

Comment: *ciprofloxacin* is contraindicated <18 years-of-age, and during pregnancy and lactation. Risk of tendonitis or tendon rupture, especially 60 years-of-age and older.

▷ *metronidazole* **(not for use in 1st; B in 2nd, 3rd)(G)** 250-500 mg q 8 hours <u>or</u> 750 mg q 12 hours x 7 days

Flagyl *Tab:* 250*, 500*mg

Flagyl 375 *Cap:* 375 mg

Flagyl ER *Tab:* 750 mg ext-rel

Comment: Alcohol is contraindicated during treatment with oral *metronidazole* and for 72 hours after therapy due to a possible *disulfiram*-like reaction (nausea, vomiting, flushing, headache).

▷ *trimethoprim/sulfamethoxazole* **(D)(G)** bid x 7 days

Bactrim, Septra 2 tabs bid x 7 days

Tab: trim 80 mg/*sulfa* 400 mg*

Bactrim DS, Septra DS 1 tab bid x 7 days

Tab: trim 160 mg/*sulfa* 800 mg*

Bactrim Pediatric Suspension, Septra Pediatric Suspension 20 ml bid x 7 days

Oral susp: trim 40 mg/sulfa 200 mg per 5 ml (100 ml) (cherry) (alcohol 0.3%)

Comment: *trimethoprim/sulfamethoxazole* is not recommended in pregnancy <u>or</u> lactation. *CrCl 15-30 mL/min:* reduce dose by 1/2; *CrCl <15 mL/min:* not recommended

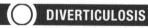

DIVERTICULOSIS

BULK-PRODUCING AGENTS

*see **Constipation** page 95*

◯ DRY EYE SYNDROME

OPHTHALMIC IMMUNOMODULATOR/ANTI-INFLAMMATORY

▷ *cyclosporine* (C) 1 drop q 12 hours
    Pediatric: <16 years: not recommended
        Restasis *Ophth emul:* 0.05% (0.4 ml) (preservative-free)
Comment: Ophthalmic Immunomodulators are contraindicated with active ocular
infection. Allow at least 15 minutes between doses of artificial tears. May re-insert
contact lenses 15 minutes after treatment.

OCULAR LUBRICANTS

Comment: Remove contact lens prior to using an ocular lubricant.
▷ *dextran 70/hypromellose* (NE) 1-2 drops prn
    Pediatric: same as adult
        Bion Tears (OTC) *Ophth soln:* single-use containers (28/pck) (preservative-free)
▷ *hydroxypropyl cellulose* (NE) **apply** 1/2 inch ribbon or 1 insert in each inferior cul-
de-sac 1-2 times/day prn
    Pediatric: same as adult
        Lacrisert *Ophth inserts:* 5 mg (60/pck) (preservative-free)
        Hypotears Ophthalmic Ointment (OTC) *Ophth oint:* 1% (3.5 g)
        (preservative-free)
Comment: Place insert in the inferior cul-de-sac of the eye, beneath the base of the tarsus,
not in apposition to the cornea nor beneath the eyelid at the level of the tarsal plate.
▷ *hydroxypropyl methylcellulose* (NE) 1-2 drops prn
    Pediatric: same as adult
        GenTeal Mild, GenTeal Moderate (OTC) *Ophth soln:* (15 ml) (perborate)
        GenTeal Severe (OTC) *Ophth soln:* (15 ml) (carbopol 980, perborate)
▷ *petrolatum/mineral oil* (NE) apply 1/2 inch ribbon prn
    Pediatric: same as adult
        Hypotears Ophthalmic Ointment (OTC) *Ophth oint:* 1% (3.5 g) (benzalkonium
        chloride, alcohol 1%)
        Hypotears PF Ophthalmic Ointment (OTC) *Ophth oint:* 1% (3.5 g) (preserva-
        tive-free, alcohol 1%)
        Lacri-Lube (OTC) *Ophth oint:* 1% (3.5, 7 g)
        Lacri-Lube NP (OTC) *Ophth oint:* 1% (0.7 g, 24/pck) (preservative-free)
▷ *petrolatum/lanolin/mineral oil* (NE) apply 1/4 inch ribbon prn
    Pediatric: same as adult
        Duratears Naturale (OTC) *Ophth oint:* 3.5 g (preservative-free)
▷ *polyethylene glycol/glycerin/hydroxypropyl methylcellulose* (NE) 1-2 drops prn
    Pediatric: same as adult
        Visine Tears (OTC) *Ophth soln:* 1% (15, 30 ml)
▷ *polyethylene glycol* 400 0.4%/*propylene glycol* 0.3% (NE) 1-2 drops prn
    Pediatric: same as adult
        Systane (OTC) *Ophth soln:* (15, 30, 40 ml) (polyquaternium-1, zinc chloride);
        Vial: 0.01 oz (28) (preservative-free)
        Systane Ultra (OTC) *Ophth soln:* (10, 20 ml) (aminomethylpropanol, polyqua-
        ternium-1, sorbitol (zinc chloride); *Vial:* 0.01 oz (24) (preservative-free)
▷ *polyvinyl alcohol* (NE) 1-2 drops prn
    Pediatric: same as adult

Hypotears (OTC) *Ophth soln:* 1% (15, 30 ml)
Hypotears PF (OTC) 1-2 drops q 3-4 hours prn
Ophth soln: 1% (0.02 oz single-use containers, 30/pck) (preservative-free)
 propylene glycol 0.6% (NE) 1-2 drops prn
Pediatric: same as adult
Systane Balance (OTC) *Ophth soln:* (10 ml) (polyquaternium-1)

DYSHIDROSIS

Topical Corticosteroids *see page* 506
Comment: Intermediate to high potency ophthalmic steroid treatment is indicated for dyshidrosis.

DYSFUNCTIONAL UTERINE BLEEDING (DUB)

 medroxyprogesterone acetate (X) 10 mg daily x 10-13 days
Provera *Tab:* 2.5, 5, 10 mg
▷ *Oral contraceptives* (X) with 35 mcg estrogen equivalent
see Combined Oral Contraceptives *page* 486
Oral Prescription NSAIDs *see page* 501
Other Oral Analgesics *see Pain page* 308

DYSLIPIDEMIA (HYPERCHOLESTEROLEMIA, HYPERLIPIDEMIA, MIXED DYSLIPIDEMIA)

OMEGA 3-FATTY ACID ETHYL ESTERS

Comment: *Vascepa, Lovaza,* and *Epanova* are indicated for the treatment of TG ≥500 mg/dL.
▷ *icosapent ethyl (omega 3-fatty acid ethyl ester of EPA)* (C) 2 caps bid with food; max 4 g/day; swallow whole, do not crush <u>or</u> chew
Pediatric: <18 years: not recommended
Vascepa sgc: 0.5, 1 g (α-tocopherol 4 mg/cap)
▷ *omega 3-fatty acid ethyl esters* (C)(G) 2 g bid <u>or</u> 4 g once daily; swallow whole, do not crush <u>or</u> chew
Pediatric: <18 years: not recommended
Lovaza *Soft gelcap:* 1 g (α-tocopherol 4 mg/cap) *omega 3-carcartonyl acids* (C) take 2-4 gel caps (2-4 g) daily without regard to meals
Epanova *Gelcap:* 1 g

MICROSOMAL TRIGLYCERIDE-TRANSFER PROTEIN (MTP) INHIBITOR

▷ *lomitapide mesylate* (X) 10 mg daily
Pediatric: not established
Juxtapid *Cap:* 5, 10, 20 mg
Comment: Juxtapid is an adjunct to low-fat diet and other lipid-lowering treatments, including LDL apheresis where available, to reduce LDL-C, total cholesterol, apoB, and non-HDL-C in patients with homozygous familial hypercholesterolemia (HoFH); not for patients with hypercholesterolemia who do not have HoFH.

OLIGONUCLEOTIDE INHIBITOR OF APO B-100 SYNTHESIS

▷ *mipomersen* (B) administer 200 mg SC once weekly, on the same day, in the upper arm, abdomen, or thigh; administer 1st injection under appropriate professional supervision
Pediatric: not established
    Kynamro *Vial/Prefilled syringe:* 200 mg mg/ml soln for SC inj single-use vial (preservative-free)
    Comment: **Kynamro** is an adjunct to low-fat diet and other lipid-lowering treatments, to reduce LDL-C, apo-B, total cholesterol (TC), non-HDL-C in patients with homozygous familial hypercholesterolemia (HoFH).

CHOLESTEROL ABSORPTION INHIBITOR

▷ *ezetimibe* (C)(G) 10 mg daily
Pediatric: <10 years: not recommended; ≥10 years: same as adult
    Zetia *Tab:* 10 mg
    Comment: *ezetimibe* is contraindicated with concomitant statins in liver disease, persistent elevations in serum transaminase, pregnancy, and nursing mothers. Concomitant fibrates are not recommended. Potentiated by *fenofibrate*, *gemfibrozil*, and possibly *cyclosporine*. Separate dosing of bile acid sequestrants is required; take *ezetimibe* at least 2 hours before or 4 hours after.

PROPROTEIN CONVERTASE SUBTILISIN KEXIN TYPE 9 (PCSK9) INHIBITOR

Comment: PCSK9 inhibitors are an adjunct to maximally tolerated statin therapy in persons who require additional lowering of LDL-C.
▷ *alirocumab* (NE)
Pediatric: not established
    Praluent administer SC in the upper outer arm, abdomen, or thigh; initially 75 mg SC once every 2 weeks; measure LDL 4-8 weeks after initiation or titration; if inadequate response, may increase to 150 mg SC every 2 weeks
        Soln for SC inj: 75, 150 mg/ml single-use prefilled syringe (preservative-free)
        Comment: Although **Praluent**, does not have an assigned pregnancy category, it is contraindicated in the 2nd and 3rd trimester of pregnancy.
▷ *evolocumab* (NE)
Pediatric: HeFH, primary hyperlipidemia: not established; HoFH: <13 years: not established; >13 years: same as adult
    Repatha administer SC in the upper outer arm, elbow, or thigh; measure LDL 4-8 weeks after initiation; *HeFH or primary hyperlipidemia:* 140 mg SC once every 2 weeks or 420 mg once monthly; *HoFH:* 420 mg once monthly
        Soln for SC inj: single-use prefilled syringe; 140 mg/syringe; single-use prefilled SureClick autoinjector (140 mg/syringe preservative-free)
        Comment: To administer 420 mg of **Repatha**, administer 150 mg SC x 3 within 30 minutes. Although **Repatha**, does not have an assigned pregnancy category, it is contraindicated in pregnancy.

HMG-COA REDUCTASE INHIBITORS (STATINS)

Comment: The statins decrease total cholesterol, LDL-C, TG, and apo-B, and increase HDL-C. Before initiating and at 4-6 weeks, 3 months, and 6 months of therapy, check fasting lipid profile and LFTs. Side effects include myopathy and increased liver enzymes. Relative contraindications include concomitant use of cyclosporine, a macrolide antibiotic, various oral antifungal agents, and CYP-450 inhibitors. An absolute contraindication is active or chronic liver disease.

➤ *atorvastatin* (X)(G) initially 10 mg daily; usual range 10-80 mg/day
    Pediatric: <10 years: not recommended; ≥10 years (female post-menarche): same as adult
        Lipitor *Tab:* 10, 20, 40, 80 mg

➤ *fluvastatin* (X)(G) initially 20-40 mg q HS; usual range 20-80 mg/day
    Pediatric: <18 years: not recommended
        Lescol *Cap:* 20, 40 mg
        Lescol XL *Tab:* 80 mg ext-rel

➤ *lovastatin* (X)
    Mevacor initially 20 mg daily at evening meal; may increase at 4-week intervals; max 80 mg/day in single or divided doses; if concomitant fibrates, niacin, or CrCl <30 mL/min, usual max 20 mg/day
        Pediatric: <10 years: not recommended; 10-17 years: initially 10-20 mg daily at evening meal; may increase at 4-week intervals; max 40 mg daily
        Tab: 10, 20, 40 mg
    Altoprev initially 20 mg daily at evening meal; may increase at 4-week intervals; max 60 mg/day; if concomitant fibrates, or *niacin* >1 g/day, usual max 40 mg/day; if concomitant cyclosporine, *amiodarone*, or *verapamil*, or CrCl <30 mL/min, usual max 20 mg/day
        Pediatric: <20 years: not recommended
        Tab: 10, 20, 40, 60 mg ext-rel

➤ *pitavastatin* (X) initially 2 mg q HS; may increase to 4 mg after 4 weeks; max 4 mg/day; if concomitant *erythromycin* or CrCl <60 ml/min; 1 mg/day with usual max 2 mg/day; if concomitant rifampin, max 2 mg once daily
    Pediatric: not established
        Livalo *Tab:* 1, 2, 4 mg

➤ *pravastatin* (X) initially 10-20 mg q HS; usual range 10-40 mg/day; may start at 40 mg/day
    Pediatric: <8 years: not recommended; 8-13 years: 20 mg daily; 14-18 years: 40 mg daily
        Pravachol *Tab:* 10, 20, 40, 80 mg

➤ *rosuvastatin* (X)(G) initially 10-20 mg q HS; usual range 5-40 mg/day; adjust at 4-week intervals
    Pediatric: <10 years: not recommended; 10-17 years: 5-20 mg/day; max 20 mg/day
        Crestor *Tab:* 5, 10, 20, 40 mg

➤ *simvastatin* (X) initially 20 mg q PM; usual range 5-80 mg/day; adjust at 4-week intervals
    Pediatric: <10 years: not recommended; ≥10 years (female postmenarche): same as adult
        Zocor *Tab:* 5, 10, 20, 40, 80 mg

CHOLESTEROL ABSORPTION INHIBITOR/HMG-COA REDUCTASE INHIBITOR COMBINATION

➤ *ezetimibe/simvastatin* (X)(G) Take once daily in the PM; may start at 10/40; swallow whole
    Pediatric: <17 years: not recommended
    Tab: **Vytorin 10/10** *ezet* 10 mg/*simva* 10 mg
        Vytorin 10/20 *ezet* 10 mg/*simva* 20 mg
        Vytorin 10/40 *ezet* 10 mg/*simva* 40 mg
        Vytorin 10/80 *ezet* 10 mg/*simva* 80 mg

ISOBUTYRIC ACID DERIVATIVES AND FIBRATE

Comment: These agents decrease total cholesterol, LDL-C, and TG; increase HDL-C. They are indicated when the primary problem is very high TG level. Side effects include epigastric discomfort, dyspepsia, abdominal pain, cholelithiasis, myopathy, and neutropenia. Before initiating, and at 4-6 weeks, 3 months, and 6 months of therapy, check fasting CBC, lipid profile, LFT, and serum creatinine. Absolute contraindications include severe renal disease and severe hepatic disease.

ISOBUTYRIC ACID DERIVATIVES

▷ *gemfibrozil* (C)(G) 600 mg bid 30 minutes before AM and PM meal
   Pediatric: not recommended
     Lopid *Tab:* 600*mg

FIBRATES (FIBRIC ACID DERIVATIVES)

▷ *fenofibrate* (C)(G) take with meals; adjust at 4- to 8-week intervals; discontinue if inadequate response after 2 months; lowest dose <u>or</u> contraindicated with renal impairment and the elderly
   Pediatric: not recommended
     Antara 43-130 mg daily; max 130 mg/day
        Cap: 43, 87, 130 mg
     Fenoglide 40-120 mg daily; max 120 mg/day
        Tab: 40, 120 mg
     FibriCor 30-105 mg daily; max 105 mg/day
        Tab: 30, 105 mg
     TriCor 48-145 mg daily; max 145 mg/day
        Tab: 48, 145 mg
     TriLipix 45-135 mg daily; max 135 mg/day
        Cap: 45, 135 mg del-rel
     Lipofen 50-150 mg daily; max 150 mg/day
        Cap: 50, 150 mg
     Lofibra 67-200 mg daily; max 200 mg/day
        Tab: 67, 134, 200 mg

NICOTINIC ACID DERIVATIVES

Comment: Nicotinic acid derivatives decrease total cholesterol, LDL-C, and TG; increase HDL-C. Before initiating and at 4-6 weeks, 3 months, and 6 months of therapy, check fasting lipid profile, LFT, glucose, and uric acid. Side effects include hyperglycemia, upper GI distress, hyperuricemia, hepatotoxicity, and significant transient skin flushing. Take with food and take *aspirin* 325 mg 30 minutes before dose to decrease flushing. Relative contraindications include diabetes, hyperuricemia (gout), and PUD and absolute contraindications include severe gout and chronic liver disease.
▷ *niacin* (C)
     Niaspan (G) 375 mg daily for 1st week, then 500 mg daily for 2nd week, then 750 mg daily for 3rd week, then 1 g daily for weeks 4-7; may increase by 500 mg q 4 weeks; usual range 1-2 g/day; max 2 g/day
        Pediatric: <21 years: not recommended
        Tab: 500, 750, 1000 mg ext-rel
     Slo-Niacin one 250 <u>or</u> 500 mg tab q AM <u>or</u> HS <u>or</u> one-half 750 mg tab q AM <u>or</u> HS

Pediatric: not recommended
Tab: 250, 500, 750 mg cont-rel

BILE ACID SEQUESTRANTS

Comment: Bile acid sequestrants decrease total cholesterol, LDL-C, and increase HDL-C, but have no effect on triglycerides. A relative contraindication is TG ≥200 mg/dL and an absolute contraindication is TG ≥400 mg/dL. Before initiating and at 4-6 weeks, 3 months, and 6 months of therapy, check fasting lipid profile. Side effects include sandy taste in mouth, abdominal gas, abdominal cramping, and constipation. These agents decrease the absorption of many other drugs.

▷ *cholestyramine* (C)
  Pediatric: see mfr pkg insert
    Questran Powder for Oral Suspension initially 1 pkt or scoop daily; usual maintenance 2-4 pkts or scoops daily in 2 divided doses; max 6 pkts or scoops daily
      Pwdr: 9 g pkts; 9 g equals 4 g anhydrous *cholestyramine* resin for reconstitution (60/pck); *Bulk can:* 378 g w. scoop
    Questran Light initially 1 pkt or scoop daily; usual maintenance 2-4 pkts or scoops daily in 2 doses
      Light: 5 g pkts; 5 g equals 4 g anhydrous *cholestyramine* resin (60/pck): *Bulk can:* 210 g w. scoop
▷ *colesevelam* (B)
    Monotherapy: 3 tabs bid or 6 tabs once daily or one 1.875 g pkt bid or one 3.75 g pkt once daily
      Pediatric: not recommended
    WelChol *Tab:* 625 mg; *Pwdr for oral susp:* 1.875 g pwdr pkts (60/carton); 3.75 g pwdr pkts (30/carton) (citrus) (phenylalanine)
    Comment: **WelChol** is indicated as adjunctive therapy to improve glycemic control in adults with type 2 diabetes. It can be added to *metformin*, sulfonylureas, or insulin alone or in combination with other antidiabetic agents
▷ *colestipol* (C)
  Pediatric: not recommended
    Colestid tabs: 2-16 g daily in a single or divided doses; granules: 5-30 g daily in a single or divided dose
      Tabs: 1 g (120); *Granules:* unflavored: 5 g pkt (30, 90/carton); unflavored bulk: 300, 500 g w. scoop; orange-flavored: 7.5 g pkt (60/carton) (aspartame); orange-flavored bulk: 450 g w. scoop (aspartame) flavored: 7.5 g pkt; flavored bulk: 450 g w. scoop
    Colestid Tab initially 2 g bid; increase by 2 g bid at 1-2-month intervals; usual maintenance 2-16 g/day
      Tab: 1 g
  Comment: *colestipol* lowers LDL and total cholesterol.

ANTILIPID COMBINATIONS

Nicotinic Acid Derivative/HMG-CoA Reductase Inhibitors

▷ *niacin/lovastatin* (X)
  Pediatric: <18 years: not recommended
    Advicor swallow whole at bedtime with a low-fat snack; may pretreat with aspirin; start at lowest niacin dose; may titrate niacin by no more than 500 mg/day every 4 weeks; max 2000/40 daily

Tab: **Advicor 500/20** *nia* 500 mg ext-rel/*lova* 20 mg
Advicor 750/20 *nia* 750 mg ext-rel/*lova* 20 mg
Advicor 1000/20 *nia* 1000 mg ext-rel/*lova* 20 mg
Advicor 1000/40 *nia* 1000 mg ext-rel/*lova* 40 mg

▷ *niacin/simvastatin* (X)
Pediatric: <18 years: not recommended
Simcor swallow whole at bedtime with a low-fat snack; may pretreat with *aspirin*; start at lowest *niacin* dose; may titrate *niacin* by no more than 500 mg/day every 4 weeks; max 2000/40 daily
Tab: **Simcor 500/20** *nia* 500 mg ext-rel/*simva* 20 mg
Simcor 750/20 *nia* 750 mg ext-rel/*simva* 20 mg
Simcor 1000/20 *nia* 1000 mg ext-rel/*simva* 20 mg
Simcor 500/40 *nia* 500 mg ext-rel/*simva* 40 mg
Simcor 1000/40 *nia* 1000 mg ext-rel/*simva* 40 mg

ANTIHYPERTENSIVE/ANTILIPID COMBINATIONS

Calcium Channel Blocker/HMG-CoA Reductase Inhibitor (Statin) Combinations

▷ *amlodipine/atorvastatin* (X)(G)
Caduet select according to blood pressure and lipid values; titrate amlodipine over 7-14 days; titrate atorvastatin according to monitored lipid values; max amlodipine 10 mg/day and max atorvastatin 80 mg/day; refer to contraindications and precautions for CCB and statin therapy
Pediatric: <10 years: not recommended; ≥10 years (female, post-menarche): same as adult
Tab: **Caduet 5/10** *amlo* 5 mg/*ator* 10 mg
Caduet 5/20 *amlo* 5 mg/*ator* 20 mg
Caduet 5/40 *amlo* 5 mg/*ator* 40 mg
Caduet 5/80 *amlo* 5 mg/*ator* 80 mg
Caduet 10/10 *amlo* 10 mg/*ator* 10 mg
Caduet 10/20 *amlo* 10 mg/*ator* 20 mg
Caduet 10/40 *amlo* 10 mg/*ator* 40 mg
Caduet 10/80 *amlo* 10 mg/*ator* 80 mg

 DYSMENORRHEA: PRIMARY

Acetaminophen for IV Infusion *see Pain page* 306
Oral Prescription NSAIDs *see page* 501
Other Oral Analgesics *see Pain page* 308

BENZENEACETIC ACID DERIVATIVE

▷ *diclofenac* (C) 50-100 mg once; then 50 tid
Pediatric: <14 years: not recommended; ≥14 years: same as adult
Cataflam *Tab:* 50 mg
Voltaren *Tab:* 25, 50, 75 mg ent-coat
Voltaren-XR *Tab:* 100 mg ext-rel
Comment: *diclofenac* is contraindicated with *aspirin* allergy and late (≥30 weeks) pregnancy.

FENAMATE

▷ *mefenamic acid* (C) 500 mg once; then 250 mg q 6 hours for up to 2-3 days; take with food
Pediatric: <14 years: not recommended
    Ponstel *Cap:* 250 mg
Comment: Avoid *aspirin* with a fenamate.

COX-2 INHIBITORS

Comment: Cox-2 inhibitors are contraindicated with history of asthma, urticaria, and allergic-type reactions to *aspirin*, other NSAIDs, and sulfonamides, 3rd trimester of pregnancy, and coronary artery bypass graft (CABG) surgery.
▷ *celecoxib* (C)(G) 400 mg x 1 dose; then 200 mg more on 1st day if needed; then 400 mg daily-bid; max 800 mg/day
Pediatric: <18 years: not recommended
    Celebrex *Cap:* 50, 100, 200, 400 mg
▷ *meloxicam* (C)(G) initially 7.5 mg once daily; max 15 mg once daily
Pediatric: <2 years: not recommended; ≥2 years: 0.125 mg/kg; max 7.5 mg once daily
    Mobic *Tab:* 7.5, 15 mg; *Oral susp:* 7.5 mg/5 ml (100 ml) (raspberry)
    Vivlodex *Cap:* 5, 10 mg
Combined Oral Contraceptives *see page 486*

DYSPAREUNIA, POSTMENOPAUSAL/ PAINFUL INTERCOURSE

Comment: Vulvar and vaginal atrophy due to menopause can cause painful intercourse.
Oral Hormonal and Transdermal Therapy *see Menopause page 264*

NONHORMONAL THERAPY

▷ *ospemifene*
    Osphena *Tab:* 60 mg

VAGINAL PREPARATIONS (WITHOUT UTERUS)

Comment: Vaginal preparations provide relief from vaginal and urinary symptoms only (i.e., atrophic vaginitis, dyspareunia, dysuria, and urinary frequency).
▷ *estradiol* (X)(G)
    Vagifem *Tabs* insert one 10 mcg or 25 mcg vaginal tablet once daily x 2 weeks; then twice weekly x 2 weeks (e.g., tues/fri); consider the addition of a progestin
        Vag tab: 10, 25 mcg (8, 18/blister pck with applicator)
    Yuvafem Vaginal Tablet insert one 10 mcg or 25 mcg vaginal tablet once daily x 2 weeks; then twice weekly x 2 weeks (e.g., tues/fri); consider the addition of a progestin
        Vag tab: 10, 25 mcg (8, 18/blister pck with applicator)
▷ *prasterone (dehydroepiandrosterone [DHEA])* (X) 1 tab intravaginally daily
    Intrarosa Tabs *Vag tab:* 10, 25 mcg (8, 18/blister pck with applicator)
    Comment: *prosterone* is an active endogenous steroid converted into active androgens and/or estrogens.
        Vag tab: 6.5 mg (7 tabs, 4 blister packs)

EDEMA

THIAZIDE DIURETICS

▷ *chlorthalidone* (B)(G) initially 30-60 mg daily or 60 mg on alternate days; max 90-120 mg/day
   Thalitone *Tab:* 15 mg
▷ *chlorothiazide* (B)(G) 0.5-1 g/day in a single or divided doses; max 2 g/day
   Pediatric: <6 months: up to 15 mg/lb/day in 2 divided doses; ≥6 months: 10 mg/lb/day in 2 divided doses; max 375 mg/day
   Diuril *Tab:* 250*, 500*mg; *Oral susp:* 250 mg/5 ml (237 ml)
▷ *hydrochlorothiazide* (B)(G)
   Pediatric: not recommended
      Esidrix 25-200 mg daily
         Tab: 25, 50, 100 mg
      Microzide 12.5 mg daily; usual max 50 mg/day
         Cap: 12.5 mg
▷ *hydroflumethiazide* (B) 50-200 mg/day in a single or 2 divided doses
   Pediatric: not recommended
      Saluron *Tab:* 50 mg
▷ *methyclothiazide/deserpidine* (B) initially 2.5 mg daily; max 5 mg daily
   Pediatric: not recommended
      Enduronyl *Tab: methy* 5 mg/*deser* 0.25 mg*
      Enduronyl Forte *Tab: methy* 5 mg/*deser* 0.5 mg*
▷ *polythiazide* (C) 1-4 mg daily
   Pediatric: not recommended
      Renese *Tab:* 1, 2, 4 mg

POTASSIUM-SPARING DIURETICS

▷ *amiloride* (B)(G) initially 5 mg; may increase to 10 mg; max 20 mg
   Pediatric: not recommended
      Tab: 5 mg
▷ *spironolactone* (D)(G) initially 25-200 mg in a single or divided doses; titrate at 2-week intervals
   Pediatric: not recommended
      Aldactone *Tab:* 25, 50*, 100*mg
▷ *triamterene* (B) 100 mg bid; max 300 mg
   Pediatric: not recommended
      Dyrenium *Cap:* 50, 100 mg

LOOP DIURETICS

▷ *bumetanide* (C)(G) 0.5-2 mg daily; *Tab:* 5 mg; may repeat at 4-5 hour intervals; max 10 mg/day
   Pediatric: <18 years: not recommended
      Tab: 1* mg
   Comment: *bumetanide* is contraindicated with sulfa drug allergy.
▷ *ethacrynic acid* (B)(G) initially 50-100 mg once daily-bid; max 400 mg/day
   Pediatric: Infants: not recommended; ≥1 month: initially 25 mg/day; then adjust dose in 25 mg increments

    Edecrin *Tab:* 25, 50 mg
▷ *ethacrynate sodium* **(B)(G)** for IV injection
    Sodium Edecrin *Vial:* 50 mg single-dose
    Comment: Sodium Edecrin is more potent than more commonly used loop and thiazide diuretics.
▷ *furosemide* **(C)(G)** initially 20-80 mg as a single dose
    Pediatric: not recommended
        Lasix *Tab:* 20, 40*, 80 mg; *Oral soln:* 10 mg/ml (2, 4 oz w. dropper)
    Comment: *furosemide* is contraindicated with sulfa drug allergy.
▷ *torsemide* **(B)** 5 mg daily; may increase to 10 mg daily
    Pediatric: not recommended
        Demadex *Tab:* 5*, 10*, 20*, 100*mg

OTHER DIURETICS

▷ *indapamide* **(B)** initially 1.25 mg daily; may titrate every 4 weeks if needed; max 5 mg/day
    Pediatric: not recommended
        Lozol *Tab:* 1.25, 2.5 mg
    Comment: *indapamide* is contraindicated with sulfa drug allergy.
▷ *metolazone* **(B)**
    Pediatric: not recommended
        Mykrox initially 0.5 mg q AM; max 1 mg/day
            Tab: 0.5 mg
        Zaroxolyn 2.5-5 mg once daily
            Tab: 2.5, 5, 10 mg
    Comment: *metolazone* is contraindicated with sulfa drug allergy.

DIURETIC COMBINATIONS

▷ *amiloride/hydrochlorothiazide* **(B)(G)** initially 1 tab daily; may increase to 2 tabs/day in a single <u>or</u> divided doses
    Pediatric: not recommended
        Moduretic *Tab: amil* 5 mg/*hydro* 50 mg*
▷ *spironolactone/hydrochlorothiazide* **(D)(G)** usual maintenance is 100 mg each of spironolactone and hydrochlorothiazide daily, in a single dose or in divided doses; range 25-200 mg of each component daily depending on the response to the initial titration
    Pediatric: not recommended
        Aldactazide 25
            Tab: spiro 25 mg/*hydro* 25 mg
        Aldactazide 50
            Tab: spiro 50 mg/*hydro* 50 mg
▷ *triamterene/hydrochlorothiazide* **(C)(G)**
    Pediatric: not recommended
        Dyazide 1-2 caps once daily
            Cap: triam 37.5 mg/*hydro* 25 mg
        Maxzide 1 tab once daily
            Tab: triam 75 mg/*hydro* 50 mg*
        Maxzide-25 1-2 tabs once daily
            Tab: triam 37.5 mg/*hydro* 25 mg*

⭕ EMPHYSEMA

Inhaled Corticosteroids *see Asthma page* 34
Parenteral Corticosteroids *see page* 511
Oral Corticosteroids *see page* 509
Inhaled Beta Agonists (Bronchodilators) *see Asthma page* 31
Oral Beta-Agonists (Bronchodilators) *see Asthma page* 35

LONG-ACTING INHALED BETA AGONIST (LABA)

▷ *indacaterol* (C)
> **Arcapta Neohaler** inhale contents of one 75 mcg cap once daily
> *Neohaler Device/Cap:* 75 mcg (5 blister cards, 6 caps/card)
> Comment: Remove cap from blister cap immediately before use. For oral
> inhalation with neohaler device only. **Arcapta Neohaler** is indicated for the long-
> term maintenance treatment of bronchoconstriction in persons with COPD. It is
> not indicated for treating asthma, for primary treatment of acute symptoms, <u>or</u>
> for acute deterioration of COPD.

▷ *olodaterol* (C)
> *Pediatric:* not established
> **Striverdi Respimat** 12 mcg q 12 hours
> *Inhal soln:* 2.5 mcg/cartridge (metered actuation) (40 g, 60 metered actuations)
> (benzalkonium chloride)

CORTICOSTEROID/INHALED LONG-ACTING BETA-AGONIST (LABA)

▷ *fluticasone furoate/vilanterol* (C) 1 inhalation 100/25 <u>or</u> 200/25 once daily at the
same time each day
> *Pediatric:* <17 years: not established
> **Breo Ellipta 100/25** *Inhal pwdr: flu* 100 mcg/*vil* 25 mcg dry pwdr per inhal
> (30 doses)
> **Breo Ellipta 200/25** *Inhal pwdr: flu* 200 mcg/*vil* 25 mcg dry pwdr per inhal
> (30 doses)
> Comment: **Breo Ellipta** is contraindicated with severe hypersensitivity to milk
> proteins.

INHALED ANTICHOLINERGICS (ANTIMUSCARINICS)

▷ *ipratropium* (B)(G)
> **Atrovent** 2 inhalations qid; max 12 inhalations/day
> *Inhaler:* 14 g (200 inh)
> **Atrovent Inhaled Solution** 500 mcg by nebulizer tid to qid
> *Inhal soln:* 0.02%; 500 mcg (2.5 ml)

INHALED LONG-ACTING ANTICHOLINERGICS (ANTIMUSCARINICS)

Comment: Inhales LAA's are indicated for prophylaxis and chronic treatment, only.
Not for primary (rescue) treatment of acute attack. Avoid getting powder in eyes.
Caution with narrow-angle glaucoma, BPH, bladder neck obstruction, and pregnancy.
Contraindicated with allergy to atropine <u>or</u> its derivatives (e.g., *ipratropium*). Avoid
other anticholinergic agents.

▷ *aclidinium bromide* (C) 1 inhalation twice daily using inhaler
  Pediatric: not recommended
    Tudorza Pressair *Inhal device:* 400 mcg/actuation (60 doses per inhalation device)

INHALED LONG-ACTING ANTICHOLINERGICS

▷ *glycopyrrolate* (C) inhale the contents of 1 capsule 2 x/day at the same times of day, AM and PM, using the neohaler; do not swallow caps
  Pediatric: not established
    Seebri Neohaler *Inhal cap:* 15.6 mcg (60/blister pck) dry pwdr for inhalation w. 1 Neohaler device (lactose)

▷ *tiotropium (as bromide monohydrate)* (C) 2 inhalations once daily using inhalation device; do not swallow caps
  Pediatric: <12 years: not recommended; ≥12 years: same as adult
    Spiriva HandiHaler *Inhal device:* 18 mcg/cap pwdr for inhalation (5, 30, 90 caps w. inhalation device)
    Spiriva Respimat *Inhal device:* 1.25, 2.5 mcg/actuation cartridge w. inhalation device (4 g, 60 metered actuations) (benzylkonian chloride)
  Comment: *tiotropium is f*or prophylaxis and chronic treatment, only. Not for primary (rescue) treatment of acute attack. Avoid getting powder in eyes. Caution with narrow-angle glaucoma, BPH, bladder neck obstruction, and pregnancy. Contraindicated with allergy to *atropine* or its derivatives (e.g., *ipratropium*).

▷ *umeclidinium* (C) one inhalation once daily at the same time each day
  Pediatric: not established
    Incruse Ellipta *Inhal pwdr:* 62.5 mcg/inhalation (30 doses) (lactose)
  Comment: **Incruse Ellipta** is contraindicated with allergy to atropine or its derivatives.

INHALED BRONCHODILATOR/ANTICHOLINERGIC COMBINATION

▷ *ipratropium/albuterol* (C)
    Combivent MDI 2 inhalations qid; max 12 inhalations/day
      Inhaler: 14.7 g (200 inh)

INHALED ANTICHOLINERGIC/LONG-ACTING BETA AGONIST (LABA) COMBINATIONS

▷ *indacaterol/glycopyrrolate* (C)
    Utibron Neohaler inhale the contents of 1 capsule 2 x/day at the same times of day, AM and PM, using the neohaler; do not swallow caps
      Inhal cap: indac 27.5 mcg/*glycop* 15.6 mcg per cap (60/blister pck) dry pwdr for inhalation w. 1 Neohaler device (lactose)

▷ *ipratropium/albuterol* (C) 1 inhalation qid; max 6 inhalations/day
    Combivent Respimat *Inhal soln: ipra* 20 mcg/*alb* 100 mcg per inhal (4 g, 120 inhal)
    Comment: When the labeled number of metered actuations (120) has been dispensed from the **Combivent Respimat** inhaler, the locking mechanism engages and no more actuations can be dispensed. **Combivent Respimat** is contraindicted with atropine allergy.

▷ *tiotropium/olodaterol* (C) 2 inhalations once daily at the same time each day; max 2 inhalations/day
    Stiolto Respimat *Inhal soln: tio* 2.5 mcg/*olo* 2.5 mcg per actuation (4 g, 60 inh) (benzalkonium chloride)
    Comment: **Stiolto Respimat** is not for treating asthma, for relief of acute bronchospasm, or acutely deteriorating COPD.

▷ *umeclidinium/vilanterol* (C) 1 inhalation once daily at the same time each day
    Anoro Ellipta *Inhal soln:* ume 62.5 mcg/*vila* 25 mcg per inhal (30 doses)
    Comment: **Anoro Ellipta** is contraindicated with severe hypersensitivity to milk proteins.

METHYLXANTHINES

see Asthma page 28

METHYLXANTHINE/EXPECTORANT COMBINATION

▷ *dyphylline/guaifenesin* (C)
    Pediatric: not recommended
    Lufyllin GG 1 tab qid
        Tab: dyph 200 mg/*guaif* 200 mg
    Lufyllin GG Elixir 30 ml qid
        Elix: dyph 100 mg/*guaif* 100 mg per 15 ml (16 oz)

OTHER METHYLXANTHINE COMBINATION

▷ *theophylline/potassium iodide/ephedrine/phenobarbital* (X)(II) 1 tab tid-qid prn; add an additional dose q HS as needed
    Pediatric: <6 years: not recommended; ≥6-12 years: 1/2 tab tid
    Quadrinal *Tab:* theo 130 mg/*pot iod* 320 mg/*ephed* 24 mg/*phenol 24 mg*

⦿ ENCOPRESIS

INITIAL BOWEL EVACUATION

▷ *mineral oil* (C) 1 oz x 1 day
▷ *bisacodyl* (B)
    Pediatric: <12 years: 1/2 suppository daily pen
    Dulcolax *Rectal supp:* 10 mg
▷ *glycerin* suppository
    Pediatric: <6 years: 1 pediatric suppository; ≥6 years: 1 adult suppository

MAINTENANCE

▷ *mineral oil* (C) 5-15 ml once daily
▷ *multivitamin* (A) 1 daily
    Comment: Mineral oil can inhibit absorption of fat-soluble vitamins.

⦿ ENDOMETRIOSIS

Acetaminophen for IV Infusion *see Pain page* 306
Oral Prescription NSAIDs *see page* 501
Other Oral Analgesics *see Pain page* 308
Contraceptives *see page* 486
▷ *medroxyprogesterone* (X) 30 mg daily
    Provera *Tab:* 2.5, 5, 10 mg
▷ *medroxyprogesterone acetate* injectable (X) 100-400 mg IM monthly
    Depo-Provera Injectable: 300 mg/ml (2.5, 10 ml)

▷ *norethindrone acetate* (X) initially 5 mg daily x 2 weeks; then increase by 2.5 mg/day every 2 weeks up to 15 mg/day maintenance dose; then continue for 6 to 9 months unless breakthrough bleeding is intolerable

    Aygestin *Tab:* 5*mg

GONADOTROPIN-RELEASING HORMONE ANALOGS

▷ *goserelin (GnRH analogue)* implant (X) implant SC into upper abdominal wall; 1 SC implant q 28 days for up to 6 months; re-treatment not recommended

    Pediatric: <18 years: not recommended

    Zoladex SC implant in syringe: 3.6 mg

▷ *leuprolide acetate (GnRH analogue)* (X)

    Pediatric: <18 years: not recommended

    Lupron Depot 3.75 mg 3.75 mg SC monthly for up to 6 months; may repeat one 6-month cycle

        Syringe: 3.75 mg (single-dose depo susp for SC injection)

    Lupron Depot-3 Month 22.5 mg SC q 3 months (84 days); max 2 injections

        Syringe: 22.5 mg (single-dose depo susp for IM injection)

Comment: Do not split doses.

▷ *nafarelin acetate* (X) 1 spray (200 mcg) into one nostril q AM, then 1 spray (200 mcg) into the other nostril q PM x 6 months; if no response after 2 months, may increase to 2 sprays (400 mcg) bid

    Synarel *Nasal spray:* 2 mg/ml (10 ml)

Comment: Start on 3rd <u>or</u> 4th day of menstrual period <u>or</u> after a negative pregnancy test.

OTHER AGENTS

▷ *danazol* (X) initially 400 mg bid; gradual downward titration of dosage may be considered dependent upon patient response; mild cases may respond to 100-200 mg bid

    Danocrine *Cap:* 50, 100, 200 mg

◯ ENURESIS: PRIMARY, NOCTURNAL

VASOPRESSIN

▷ *desmopressin acetate* (B)

    DDAVP usual dosage 0.1-1.2 mg/day in 2-3 divided doses; 0.2 mg q HS prn for nocturnal enuresis

    Pediatric: <6 years: not recommended

    Tab: 0.1*, 0.2*mg

    DDAVP Rhinal Tube

    Pediatric: <6 years: not recommended; ≥6 years: 10 mcg <u>or</u> 0.1 ml of soln each nostril (20 mcg total dose) q HS prn; max 40 mcg total dose

    Nasal spray: 10 mcg/actuation (5 ml, 50 sprays); *Rhinal tube:* 0.1 mg/ml (2.5 ml)

TRICYCLIC ANTIDEPRESSANT(TCA)

▷ *imipramine* (C)(G)

    Pediatric: <6 years: not recommended; 6-12 years: 25 mg 1 hour before bedtime; after 1 week, may increase to 50 mg; max 50 mg; >12 years: 25 mg 1 hour before bedtime; after 1 week, may increase to 50 mg; max 75 mg; *Early night bedwetters:* administer 25 mg in the afternoon and repeat at bedtime; max 2.5 mg/kg/day

Comment: If drug response favorable, consider gradual tapering and attempting drug-free periods.

> **Tofranil** initially 75 mg daily (max 200 mg); if maintenance dose exceeds 75 mg daily, may switch to **Tofranil PM** for divided <u>or</u> bedtime dose
> > *Tab:* 10, 25, 50 mg
>
> **Tofranil PM** initially 75 mg 1 hour before HS; max 200 mg
> > *Cap:* 75, 100, 125, 150 mg

 EPICONDYLITIS

Acetaminophen for IV Infusion *see **Pain** page* 306
Oral Prescription NSAIDs *see page* 501
Other Oral Analgesics *see **Pain** page* 308
Topical/Transdermal NSAIDs *see **Pain** page* 307
Parenteral Corticosteroids *see page* 511
Oral Corticosteroids *see page* 509
Topical Analgesic and Anesthetic Agents *see page* 499

 EPIDIDYMITIS

Comment: The following treatment regimens for epididymitis are published in the **2015 CDC Transmitted Diseases Treatment Guidelines**. Treatment regimens are presented by generic drug name first, followed by information about brands and dose forms. Empiric treatment requires concomitant treatment of chlamydia. Treat all sexual contacts. Patients who are HIV-positive should receive the same treatment as those who are HIV-negative.

RECOMMENDED REGIMEN

Regimen 1

▷ *ceftriaxone* (B)(G) 250 mg IM in a single dose
   plus
▷ *doxycycline* (D)(G) 100 mg bid x 10 days

RECOMMENDED REGIMENS: LIKELY CAUSED BY ENTERIC ORGANISMS

Regimen 1

▷ *levofloxacin* (C) 500 mg daily x 10 days

Regimen 2

▷ *ofloxacin* (C)(G) 300 mg bid x 10 day

DRUG BRANDS AND DOSE FORMS

▷ *ceftriaxone* (B)(G)
      Rocephin *Vial:* 250, 500 mg; 1, 2 g
▷ *doxycycline* (D)(G)
      Actilate *Tab:* 75, 150**mg
      Adoxa *Tab:* 50, 75, 100, 150 mg ent-coat
      Doryx *Tab:* 50, 75, 100, 150, 200 mg del-rel
      Monodox *Cap:* 50, 75, 100 mg

Oracea *Cap:* 40 mg del-rel
Vibramycin *Tab:* 100 mg; *Cap:* 50, 100 mg; *Syr:* 50 mg/5 ml (raspberry-apple) (sulfites); *Oral susp:* 25 mg/5 ml (raspberry)
Vibra-Tab *Tab:* 100 mg film-coat

Comment: *doxycycline* is contraindicated <8 years-of-age, in pregnancy, and lactation (discolors developing tooth enamel). A side effect may be photo-sensitivity (photophobia). Do not give with antacids, calcium supplements, milk or other dairy, or within two hours of taking another drug.

▷ *levofloxacin* (C)
Levaquin *Tab:* 250, 500, 750 mg; *Oral soln:* 25 mg/ml (480 ml) (benzyl alcohol)
Comment: *levofloxacin* is contraindicated <18 years-of-age, and during pregnancy and lactation. Risk of tendonitis or tendon rupture, especially 60 years-of-age and older.

▷ *ofloxacin* (C)(G)
Floxin *Tab:* 200, 300, 400 mg
Comment: *ofloxacin* is contraindicated <18 years-of-age, and during pregnancy and lactation. Risk of tendonitis or tendon rupture, especially 60 years-of-age and older.

 ERECTILE DYSFUNCTION (ED)

Comment: Due to a degree of cardiac risk with sexual activity, consider cardiovascular status of patient before instituting therapeutic measures for erectile dysfunction.

PHOSPHODIESTERASE TYPE 5 (PDE5) INHIBITORS, CGMP-SPECIFIC

Comment: Oral PDE5 inhibitors (**Cialis**, **Levitra**, **Staxyn**, **Viagra**) are contraindicated in patients taking nitrates. Caution with history of recent MI, stroke, life-threatening arrhythmia, hypotension, hypertension, cardiac failure, unstable angina, retinitis pigmentosa, CYP3A4 inhibitors (e.g., *cimetidine*, the azoles, *erythromycin*, grapefruit juice), protease inhibitors (e.g., *ritonavir*), CYP3A4 inducers (e.g., *rifampin*, *carbamazepine*, *phenytoin*, *phenobarbital*), alcohol, antihypertensive agents. Side effects include headache, flushing, nasal congestion, rhinitis, dyspepsia, and diarrhea. Use with caution in patients with anatomical deformation of the penis (e.g., angulation, cavernosal fibrosis, or Peyronie's disease) or in patients who have conditions, which may predispose them to priapism (e.g., sickle cell anemia, multiple myeloma, or leukemia). In the event of an erection that persists longer than 4 hours, the patient should seek immediate medical assistance. If priapism (painful erection greater than 6 hours in duration) is not treated immediately, penile tissue damage and permanent loss of potency could result.

▷ *avanafil* (B) initially 100 mg taken 30 min prior to sexual activity; may decrease to 50 mg or increase to 200 mg based on response; max one administration/day
Stendra *Tab:* 50, 100, 200 mg

▷ *sildenafil citrate* (B)(G) one dose about 1 hour (range 30 min-4 hrs) before sexual activity; usual initial dose 50 mg; may decrease to 25 mg or increase to max 100 mg/ dose based on response; max one administration/day
Viagra *Tab:* 25, 50, 100 mg

▷ *tadalafil* (B) initially 10 mg prior to sexual activity up to once daily; may decrease to 5 mg or increase to 20 mg based on response; max one administration/day; effect may last 36 hours
Cialis *Tab:* 2.5, 5, 10, 20 mg

▷ *vardenafil* (B) initially 10 mg taken 60 min prior to sexual activity; may decrease to 5 mg or increase to 20 mg based on response; max one administration/day

Levitra *Tab:* 2.5, 5, 10, 20 mg film-coat
Comment: **Levitra** is not interchangeable with **Staxyn**.

▷ *vardenafil (as HCl)* **(B)(G)** dissolve 1 tab on tongue 60 min prior to sexual activity, max once daily
Staxyn *Tab:* 10 mg orally disintegrating (peppermint) (phenylalanine)
Comment: **Staxyn** is not interchangeable with **Levitra**.

▷ *alprostadil* **(X)** *urethral suppository* initially 125 or 250 mcg inserted in the urethra after urination; adjust dose in stepwise manner on separate occasions; max two administrations/day
Muse *Urethral supp:* 125, 250, 500, 1000 mcg
Comment: Contraindicated with urethral stricture, balanitis, severe hypospadias and curvature, urethritis, predisposition to venous thrombosis, hyperviscosity syndrome. Extreme caution with anticoagulant therapy (e.g., warfarin, heparin). Potential for hypotension and/or syncope.

▷ *alprostadil* **(X)** *injection* inject over 5-10 seconds into the dorsal lateral aspect of the proximal third of the penis; avoid visible veins; rotate injection sites and sides; if no initial response, may give next higher dose within 1 hour; if partial response, give next higher dose after 24 hours; max 60 mcg and 3 self-injections/week; allow at least 24 hours between doses; reduce dose if erection lasts >1 hour.
Caverject *Vial:* 5, 10, 20, 40 mcg/vial (pwdr for reconstitution w. diluent)
Caverject Impulse *Cartridge:* 10, 20 mcg (2 cartridge starter and refill pcks)
Edex *Vial:* 5, 10, 20, 40 mcg (6/pck); *Syringe:* 5, 10, 20, 40 mcg (4/pck); *Cartridge:* 10, 20, 40 mcg (2 cartridge starter and refill pcks)
Comment: Determine dose of injectable prostaglandins in the office. Contraindicated with predisposition to priapism, penile angulation, cavernosal fibrosis, Peyronies disease, penile implant. Extreme caution with anticoagulant therapy (e.g., *warfarin*, *heparin*).

 ERYSIPELAS

Comment: Erysipelas is most commonly due to GABHS (Group A beta-hemolytic Strept).

TREATMENT OF CHOICE

▷ *penicillin V potassium* **(B)** 250-500 mg q 6 hours x 10 days
Pediatric: 25-50 mg/kg/day divided q 6 hours x 10 days; *see page 583 for dose by weight*
Pen-Vee K *Tab:* 250, 500 mg; *Oral soln:* 125 mg/5 ml (100, 200 ml); 250 mg/5 ml (100, 150, 200 ml)

TREATMENT IF PENICILLIN ALLERGIC

▷ *erythromycin base* **(B)(G)** 250 mg q 6 hours x 10 days
Pediatric: 30-40 mg/kg/day divided q 6 hours x 10 days; >40 kg: same as adult
Ery-Tab *Tab:* 250, 333, 500 mg ent-coat
PCE *Tab:* 333, 500 mg
Comment: *erythromycin* may increase INR with concomitant *warfarin*, as well as increase serum level of *digoxin*, benzodiazepines and statins.

▷ *erythromycin ethylsuccinate* **(B)(G)** 400 mg qid x 7 days
Pediatric: 30-50 mg/kg/day in 4 divided doses x 7 days; may double dose with severe infection; max 100 mg/kg/day; *see page 574 for dose by weight*

EryPed *Oral susp:* 200 mg/5 ml (100, 200 ml) (fruit); 400 mg/5 ml (60, 100, 200 ml) (banana); *Oral drops:* 200, 400 mg/5 ml (50 ml) (fruit); *Chew tab:* 200 mg wafer (fruit)
E.E.S. *Oral susp:* 200, 400 mg/5 ml (100 ml) (fruit)
E.E.S. Granules *Oral susp:* 200 mg/5 ml (100, 200 ml) (cherry)
E.E.S. 400 Tablets *Tab:* 400 mg
Comment: *erythromycin* may increase INR with concomitant *warfarin*, as well as increase serum level of *digoxin*, benzodiazepines and statins.

⊙ ESOPHAGITIS, EROSIVE

Antacids *see GERD page* 151
H₂ Antagonists *see GERD page* 153
Proton Pump Inhibitors *see GERD page* 154
▷ *sucralfate* (B)(G) *Active ulcer:* 1 g qid; *Maintenance:* 1 g bid
    Carafate *Tab:* 1*g; *Oral susp:* 1 g/10 ml (14 oz)

⊙ EYE PAIN

Acetaminophen for IV Infusion *see Pain page* 306

OPHTHALMIC NSAIDs

Comment: Concomitant contact lens wear is contraindicated during therapy. Etiology of eye pain must be known prior to use of these agents
▷ *diclofenac* (B) 1 drop affected eye qid
    Pediatric: not recommended
    Voltaren Ophthalmic Solution *Ophth soln:* 0.1% (2.5, 5 ml)
▷ *ketorolac tromethamine* (C) 1 drop affected eye qid for up to 4 days
    Pediatric: <3 years: not recommended; ≥3 years: same as adult
    Acular *Ophth soln:* 0.5% (3, 5, 10 ml; benzalkonium chloride)
    Acular LS *Ophth soln:* 0.4% (5 ml; benzalkonium chloride)
    Acular PF *Ophth soln:* 0.5% (0.4 ml; 12 single-use vials/carton)
    (preservative-free)
▷ *nepafenac* (C) 1 drop affected eye tid
    Pediatric: <10 years: not recommended; ≥10 years: same as adult
    Nevanac Ophthalmic Suspension *Ophth susp:* 0.1% (3 ml) (benzalkonium chloride)

OPHTHALMIC STEROIDS

Comment: Contraindications: ocular fungal, viral, or mycobacterial infections. Effectiveness of treatment should be assessed after 2 days. The corticosteroid should be tapered and treatment concluded within 14 days if possible due to risk of corneal and/or scleral thinning with prolonged use.
▷ *difluprednate* (C) 1 drop affected eye qid; *Post-op Pain:* beginning 24 hours after surgery, 1 drop affected eye qid; continue for 2 weeks post-op; then bid x 1 week; then taper until resolved
    Pediatric: not recommended
    Durezol Ophthalmic Solution *Ophth emul:* 0.05% (5 ml)

▷ *etabonate* (C) 1 drop affected eye qid
  Pediatric: not recommended
    Alrex Ophthalmic Solution *Ophth emul:* 0.2% (5 ml) (benzylkonium chloride)

⬤ FACIAL HAIR, EXCESSIVE/UNWANTED

TOPICAL HAIR GROWTH RETARDANT

▷ *eflornithine* 13.9% cream (C) apply a thin layer to affected areas of face and under the chin bid at least 8 hours apart; rub in thoroughly; do not wash treated area for at least 4 hours following application
  Pediatric: not recommended
    Vaniqa *Crm:* 13.9% (30, 60 g)
    Comment: After **Vaniqa** dries, may apply cosmetics or sunscreen. Hair removal techniques may be continued as needed.

⬤ FECAL ODOR

▷ *bismuth subgallate powder* (B)(OTC) 1-2 tabs tid with meals
    Devron *Chew tab:* 200 mg; *Cap:* 200 mg
    Comment: **Devron** is an internal (oral) deodorant for control of odors from ileostomy or colostomy drainage or fecal incontinence.

⬤ FEVER (PYREXIA)

ACETAMINOPHEN FOR IV INFUSION

▷ *acetaminophen* injectable (B)(G) administer by IV infusion over 15 minutes; 1000 mg q 6 hours prn or 650 mg q 4 hours prn; max 4,000 mg/day
  Pediatric: <2 years: not recommended; 2-13 years <50 kg: 15 mg/kg q 6 hours prn or 12.5 mg/kg q 4 hours prn; max 750 mg single-dose; max 75 mg/kg per day
    Ofirmev *Vial:* 10 mg/ml (100 ml) (preservative-free)
    Comment: The **Ofirmev** vial is intended for single-use. If any portion is withdrawn from the vial, use within 6 hours. Discard the unused portion. For pediatric patients, withdraw the intended dose and administer via syringe pump. Do not ad-mix **Ofirmev** with any other drugs. **Ofirmev** is physically incompatable with diazepam and chlorpromazine hydrochloride.
▷ *acetaminophen* (B)(G)
    Children's Tylenol (OTC) 10-20 mg/kg q 4-6 hours prn
      Oral susp: 80 mg/tsp
        4-11 months (12-17 lb): 1/2 tsp q 4 hours prn; 12-23 months (18-23 lb): 3/4 tsp q 4 hours prn; 2-3 years (24-35 lb): 1 tsp q 4 hours prn; 4-5 years (36-47 lb): 1 tsp q 4 hours prn; 6-8 years (48-59 lb): 2 tsp q 4 hours prn; 9-10 years (60-71 lb): 2 tsp q 4 hours prn; 11 years (72-95 lb): 3 tsp q 4 hours prn; All: max 5 doses/day
      Elix: 160 mg/5 ml (2, 4 oz)

Chew tab: 80 mg

 2-3 years (24-35 lb): 2 tabs q 4 hours prn; 4-5 years (36-47 lb): 3 tabs q 4 hours prn; 6-8 years (48-59 lb): 4 tabs q 4 hours prn; 9-10 years (60-71 lb): 5 tabs q 4 hours prn; 11 years (72-95 lb): 6 tabs q 4 hours prn; All: max 5 doses/day

Junior Strength:

 6-8 years: 2 tabs q 4 hours prn; 9-10 years: 2 tabs q 4 hours prn; 11 years: 3 tabs q 4 hours prn; 12 years: 4 tabs q 4 hours prn; All: max 5 doses/day

Chew tab: 160 mg

Junior cplt: 160 mg

Infant's Drops and Suspension: 80 mg/0.8 ml (1/2, 1 oz)

 <3 months: 0.4 ml q 4 hours prn; 4-11 months: 0.8 ml q 4 hours prn; 12-23 months: 1.2 ml q 4 hours prn; 2-3 years (24-35 lb): 1.6 ml q 4 hours prn; 4-5 years (36-47 lb): 2.4 ml q 4 hours prn; All: max 5 doses/day

Extra Strength Tylenol (OTC) 1 g q 4-6 hours prn; max 4 g/day

 Pediatric: not recommended

 Tab/Cplt/Gel tab/Gel cap: 500 mg; *Liq:* 500 mg/15 ml (8 oz)

FeverAll Extra Strength Tylenol (OTC)

 Pediatric: <3 months: not recommended; 3-36 months: 80 mg q 4 hours prn; 3-6 years: 120 mg q 4 hours prn; ≥6 years: 325 mg q 4 hours prn; *Rectal supp:* 80, 120, 325 mg (6/carton)

Maximum Strength Tylenol Sore Throat (OTC) 500-1000 mg q 4-6 hours prn

 Pediatric: not recommended

 Liq: 1000 mg/30 ml (8 oz)

Tylenol (OTC) 650 mg q 4-6 hours; max 4 g/day

 Pediatric: <6 years: not recommended; 6-11 years: 325 mg q 4-6 hours prn; max 1.625 g/day; ≥12 years: same as adult

▷ *aspirin* (D)(G)

Bayer (OTC) 325-650 mg q 4 hours prn; max: 5 doses/day

 Pediatric: not recommended

 Tab/Cplt: 325 mg ext-rel

Extra Strength Bayer (OTC) 500 mg-1 g q 4-6 hours prn; max 4 g/day

 Pediatric: not recommended

 Cplt: 500 mg

Extended-Release Bayer 8 Hour (OTC) 650-1300 mg q 8 hours prn

 Pediatric: not recommended

 Cplt: 650 mg ext-rel

Comment: *aspirin*-containing medications are contraindicated with history of allergic-type reaction to *aspirin*, children and adolescents with *Varicella* or other viral illness, and 3rd trimester pregnancy.

▷ *aspirin/caffeine* (D)(G)

Anacin (OTC) 800 mg q 4 hours prn; max 4 g/day

 Pediatric: <6 years: not recommended; 6-12 years: 400 mg q 4 hours prn; max 2 g/day; ≥12 years: same as adult

 Tab/Cplt: 400 mg

Anacin Maximum Strength (OTC) 1 g tid-qid

 Pediatric: not recommended

 Tab: 500 mg

Comment: *aspirin*-containing medications are contraindicated with history of allergic-type reaction to aspirin, children and adolescents with *Varicella* or other viral illness, and 3rd trimester pregnancy.

▷ *aspirin/antacid* (D)(G)

Extra Strength Bayer Plus (OTC) 500 mg-1 g q 4-6 hours prn; usual max 4 g/day
Pediatric: not recommended
Cplt: 500 mg *aspirin* with *calcium carbonate*

Bufferin (OTC) 650 mg q 4 hours; max 3.9 mg/day
Pediatric: not recommended
Tab: 325 mg *aspirin* with *calcium carbonate*, *magnesium carbonate*, and *magnesium oxide*

Comment: *aspirin*-containing medications are contraindicated with history of allergic-type reaction to **aspirin**, children and adolescents with *Varicella* or other viral illness, and 3rd trimester pregnancy.

▷ *ibuprofen* (B; not for use in 3rd)(G)

Comment: *ibuprofen* is contraindicated in children <6 months-of-age.

Children's Advil (OTC), ElixSure IB (OTC), Motrin (OTC), PediaCare (OTC), PediaProfen (OTC)
Pediatric: 5-10 mg/kg q 6-8 hours; max 40 mg/kg/day; <24 lb (<2 years): individualize; 24-35 lb (2-3 years): 5 ml q 6-8 hours prn; 36-47 lb (4-5 years): 7.5 ml q 6-8 hours prn; 48-59 lb (6-8 years): 10 ml or 2 tabs q 6-8 hours prn; 60-71 lb (9-10 years): 12.5 ml or 2 tabs q 6-8 hours prn; 72-95 lb (11 years): 15 ml or 3 tabs q 6-8 hours prn
Oral susp: 100 mg/5 ml (2, 4 oz) (berry); *Junior tabs:* 100 mg

Children's Motrin Drops (OTC), PediaCare Drops (OTC)
Pediatric: <24 lb (<2 years): individualize; 24-35 lb (2-3 years): 2.5 ml q 6-8 hours prn; *Oral drops:* 50 mg/1.25 ml (15 ml; berry)

Children's Motrin Chewables and Caplets (OTC)
Pediatric: 48-59 lb (6-8 years): 200 mg q 6-8 hours prn; 60-71 lb (9-10 years): 250 mg q 6-8 hours prn; 72-95 lb (11 years): 300 mg q 6-8 hours prn; ≥12 years: same as adult
Chew tab: 100*mg (citrus; phenylalanine)
Cplt: 100 mg

Motrin (OTC) 400 mg q 6 hours prn
Pediatric: <6 months: not recommended; >6 months, fever <102.5: 5 mg/kg q 6-8 hours prn; >6 months, fever >102.5: 10 mg/kg q 6-8 hours prn
All: max 40 mg/kg/day
Tab: 400 mg; *Cplt:* 100*mg; *Chew tab:* 50*, 100*mg (citrus; phenylalanine); *Oral susp:* 100 mg/5 ml (4, 16 oz) (berry); *Oral drops:* 40 mg/ml (15 ml) (berry)

Advil (OTC), Motrin IB (OTC), Nuprin (OTC) 200-400 mg q 4-6 hours; max 1.2 g/day
Pediatric: not recommended
Tab/Cplt/Gel cap: 200 mg

▷ *naproxen* (B)(G)
Pediatric: <2 years: not recommended; ≥2 years: 2.5-5 mg/kg bid-tid; max: 15 mg/kg/day

Aleve (OTC) 400 mg x 1 dose; then 200 mg q 8-12 hours prn; max 10 days
Tab/Cplt/Gel cap: 200 mg

Anaprox 550 mg x 1 dose; then 550 mg q 12 hours <u>or</u> 275 mg q 6-8 hours prn; max 1.375 g first day and 1.1 g/day thereafter
   Tab: 275 mg
Anaprox DS 1 tab bid
   Tab: 550 mg
EC-Naprosyn 375 <u>or</u> 500 mg bid prn; may increase dose up to max 1500 mg/day as tolerated
   Tab: 375, 500 mg del-rel
Naprelan 1 g daily <u>or</u> 1.5 g daily for limited time; max 1 g/day thereafter
   Tab: 375, 500 mg
Naprosyn initially 500 mg, then 500 mg q 12 hours <u>or</u> 250 mg q 6-8 hours prn; max 1.25 g first day and 1 g/day thereafter
   Tab: 250, 375, 500 mg; *Oral susp:* 125 mg/5 ml (473 ml) (pineapple-orange)

FIBROCYSTIC BREAST DISEASE

Contraceptives *see page* 486
➤ *spironolactone* (D)(G) 10 mg bid premenstrually
   Aldactone *Tab:* 25, 50*, 100*mg
➤ *vitamin E* (A) 400-600 IU daily
➤ *vitamin B6* (A) 50-100 mg daily
➤ *danazol* (X) 50-200 mg bid x 2-6 months
   Danocrine *Cap:* 50, 100, 200 mg
Comment: Start on 3rd <u>or</u> 4th day of menstrual period <u>or</u> after a negative pregnancy test.

FIBROMYALGIA

Acetaminophen for IV Infusion *see Pain page* 306
Oral Prescription NSAIDs *see page* 501
Other Oral Analgesics *see Pain page* 308
Topical/Transdermal NSAIDs *see Pain page* 307
Parenteral Corticosteroids *see page* 511
Oral Corticosteroids *see page* 509
Topical Analgesic and Anesthetic Agents *see page* 499

SEROTONIN AND NOREPINEPHRINE REUPTAKE INHIBITORS (SNRIs)

➤ *duloxetine* (C)(G) swallow whole; initially 30 mg once daily x 1 week; then increase to 60 mg once daily; max 120 mg/day
Pediatric: not recommended
   Cymbalta
      Cap: 20, 30, 60 mg ent-coat pellets
➤ *milnacipran* (C)(G) *Day 1:* 12.5 mg once; *Days 2-3:* 12.5 mg bid; *Days 4-7:* 25 mg bid; max 100 mg bid
Pediatric: <17 years: not recommended
   Savella
      Tab: 12.5, 25, 50, 100 mg

GAMMA-AMINOBUTYRIC ACID ANALOG

▷ *gabapentin* (C)
Pediatric: not applicable
▷ *Gralise* initially 300 mg on Day 1; then 600 mg on Day 2; then 900 mg on Days 3-6; then 1200 mg on Days 7-10; then 1500 mg on Days 11-14; titrate up to 1800 mg on Day 15; take entire dose once daily with the evening meal; do not crush, split, or chew
Tab: 300, 600 mg
    Neurontin (G) 100 mg daily x 1 day; then 100 mg bid x 1 day; then 100 mg tid continuously or 300 mg bid; max 900 mg tid
        Tab: 600*, 800* mg; *Cap:* 100, 300, 400 mg; *Oral soln:* 250 mg/5 ml (480 ml) (strawberry-anise)
▷ *gabapentin enacarbil* (C) 600 mg once daily at about 5:00 PM; if dose not taken at recommended time, next dose should be taken the following day; swallow whole; take with food; *CrCl 30-59 mL/min:* 600 mg on Day 1, Day 3, and every day thereafter; *CrCl <30 mL/min:* or on hemodialysis: not recommended
Pediatric: not recommended
    Horizant *Tab:* 300, 600 mg ext-rel
Comment: Avoid abrupt cessation of *gabapentin* and *gabapentin* enacarbil. To discontinue, withdraw gradually over 1 week or longer.

α₂-DELTA LIGAND

▷ *pregabalin (GABA analog)* (C)(V) initially 50 mg tid; may titrate to 100 mg tid within one week; max 600 mg divided tid; discontinue over one week
Pediatric: <18 years: not recommended
    Lyrica *Cap:* 25, 50, 75, 100, 150, 200, 225, 300 mg; *Oral soln:* 20 mg/ml

OTHER AGENTS

▷ *amitriptyline* (C)(G) 20 mg q HS; may increase gradually to max 50 mg q HS
Pediatric: not recommended
Tab: 10, 25, 50, 75, 100, 150 mg
▷ *cyclobenzaprine* (B)(G) 10 mg tid; usual range 20-40 mg/day in divided doses; max 60 mg/day x 2-3 weeks or 15 mg ext-rel once daily; max 30 mg ext-rel/day x 2-3 weeks
Pediatric: <15 years: not recommended
    Amrix *Cap:* 15, 30 mg ext-rel
    Fexmid *Tab:* 7.5 mg
    Flexeril *Tab:* 5, 10 mg
▷ *eszopiclone* (C)(IV)(G) (pyrrolopyrazine) 1-3 mg; max 3 mg/day x 1 month; do not take if unable to sleep for at least 8 hours before required to be active again; delayed effect if taken with a meal
Pediatric: <18 years: not recommended
    Lunesta *Tab:* 1, 2, 3 mg
▷ *flurazepam* (X)(IV)(G) 15 mg q HS; may increase to 30 mg q HS
    Dalmane *Cap:* 15, 30 mg
▷ *trazodone* (C)(G) 50 mg q HS
    Desyrel *Tab:* 50, 100, 150, 300 mg
▷ *triazolam* (X)(IV)(G) 0.125 mg q HS, may increase gradually to 0.5 mg
    Halcion *Tab:* 0.125, 0.25*mg

➤ *zaleplon* (C)(IV) (imidazopyridine) 5-10 mg at HS <u>or</u> after going to bed if unable to sleep; do not take if unable to sleep for at least 4 hours before required to be active again; max 20 mg/day x 1 month; delayed effect if taken with a meal
Pediatric: not recommended
    Sonata *Cap:* 5, 10 mg (tartrazine)
    Comment: **Sonata** is indicated for the treatment of insomnia when a middle-of-the-night awakening is followed by difficulty returning to sleep.
➤ *zolpidem* oral solution spray (C)(IV) (imidazopyridine hypnotic) 2 actuations (10 mg) immediately before bedtime; *Elderly, debilitated,* <u>or</u> *hepatic impairment:* 2 actuations (5 mg); max 2 actuations (10 mg)
Pediatric: not recommended
    ZolpiMist *Oral soln spray:* 5 mg/actuation (60 metered actuations) (cherry)
    Comment: The lowest dose of *zolpidem* in all forms is recommended for women as drug elimination is slower than in men.
➤ *zolpidem* tabs (B)(IV)(G) (pyrazolopyrimidine hypnotic) 5-10 mg <u>or</u> 6.25-12.5 extrel q HS prn; max 12.5 mg/day x 1 month; do not take if unable to sleep for at least 8 hours before required to be active again; delayed effect if taken with a meal
Pediatric: ≤18 years: not recommended
    Ambien *Tab:* 5, 10 mg
    Ambien CR *Tab:* 6.25, 12.5 mg ext-rel
    Comment: The lowest dose of *zolpidem* in all forms is recommended for women as drug elimination is slower than in men.
➤ *zolpidem* sublingual tabs (C)(IV) (imidazopyridine hypnotic) dissolve 1 tab under the tongue; allow to disintegrate completely before swallowing; take only once per night and only if at least 4 hours of bedtime remain before planned time for awakening
    Edluar *SL Tab:* 5, 10 mg
    Intermezzo *SL Tab:* 1.75, 3.5 mg
    Comment: **Intermezzo** is indicated for the treatment of insomnia when a middle-of-the-night awakening is followed by difficulty returning to sleep. The lowest dose of *zolpidem* in all forms is recommended for women as drug elimination is slower than in men.

FIFTH DISEASE (ERYTHEMA INFECTIOSUM)

Antipyretics *see Fever page* 143

FLATULENCE

➤ *simethicone* (C)(G)
    Gas-X (OTC) 2-4 tabs pc and HS prn
        Tab: 40, 80, 125 mg; *Cap:* 125 mg
    Mylicon (OTC) 2-4 tabs pc and HS prn
        Tab: 40, 80, 125 mg; *Cap:* 125 mg
    Phazyme-95 1-2 tabs with each meal and HS prn
        Tab: 95 mg
    Phazyme Infant Oral Drops
        Pediatric: <2 years: 0.3 ml qid pc and HS prn; 2-12 years: 0.6 ml qid pc and HS prn; >12 years: 1.2 ml qid pc and HS prn;

Oral drops: 40 mg/0.6 ml (15, 30 ml w. calibrated dropper) (orange) (alcohol-free)
Maximum Strength Phazyme 1-2 caps with each meal and HS prn
Cap: 125 mg

 ## FLUORIDATION, WATER, <0.6 PPM

▷ *fluoride* (NE)(G)
    Luride
    Pediatric: Water fluoridation 0.3-0.6 ppm: <3 years: use drops; 3-6 years: 0.25 mg
    daily; 7-16 years: 0.5 mg daily; *Water fluoridation <0.3 ppm:* <3 years: use drops;
    6 months-3 years: 0.25 mg daily; 4-6 years: 0.5 mg daily; 7-16 years: 1 mg daily
    Chew tab: 0.25, 0.5, 1 mg (sugar-free)
    Luride Drops
    Pediatric: Water fluoridation 0.3-0.6 ppm: 6 months-3 years: 0.25 ml once
    daily; 4-6 years: 0.5 ml once daily; 7-16 years: 1 ml once daily; *Water fluori-*
    dation <0.3 ppm: 6 months-3 years: 0.5 ml once daily; 4-6 years: 1 ml once
    daily; 7-16 years: 2 ml daily
    Oral drops: 0.5 mg/ml (50 ml) (sugar-free)

COMBINATION AGENTS

▷ *fluoride/vitamin a/vitamin d/vitamin c* (NE)(G)
Pediatric: Water fluoridation 0.3-0.6 ppm: <3 years: not recommended; 3-6 years:
0.25 mg fluoride/day; 7-16 years: 0.5 mg fluoride/day; *Water fluoridation <0.3 ppm:*
<6 months: not recommended; 6 months-3 years: 0.25 mg fluoride/day; 4-6 years:
0.5 mg fluoride/day; 7-16 years: 1 mg fluoride/day
    Tri-Vi-Flor Drops
    Oral drops: fluoride 0.25 mg/*vit a* 1500 u/*vit d* 400 u/*vit c* 35 mg per ml (50 ml)
    Oral drops: fluoride 0.5 mg/*vit a* 1500 u/*vit d* 400 u/*vit c* 35 mg per ml (50 ml)
▷ *fluoride/vitamin a/vitamin d/vitamin c/iron* (NE)
Pediatric: Water fluoridation 0.3-0.6 ppm: <3 years: not recommended; 3-6 years:
0.25 mg fluoride/day; 7-16 years: 0.5 mg fluoride/day; *Water fluoridation <0.3 ppm:*
<6 months: not recommended; 6 months-3 years: 0.25 mg fluoride/day; 4-6 years:
0.5 mg fluoride/day; 7-16 years: 1 mg fluoride/day
    Tri-Vi-Flor w. Iron Drops
    Oral drops: fluoride 0.25 mg/*vit a* 1500 u/*vit d* 400 u/*vit c* 35 mg/*iron* 10 mg
    per ml (50 ml)

FOLLICULITIS BARBAE

TOPICAL AGENTS

▷ *benzoyl peroxide* (B) 5% apply once daily after shaving
    Pediatric: same as adult
    see *Acne Vulgaris for benzoyl peroxide preparations* page 4
▷ *clindamycin* topical (B) apply bid
    Pediatric: same as adult
    Cleocin T *Pad:* 1% (60/pck; alcohol 50%); *Lotn:* 1% (60 ml); *Gel:* 1% (30, 60 g);
    Soln w. applicator: 1% (30, 60 ml) (alcohol 50%)

    Clindagel *Gel:* 1% (42, 77 g)
    Clindets *Pad:* 1% (60/pck)
    Evoclin *Foam:* 1% (50, 100 g) (alcohol)
▷ *clindamycin/benzoyl peroxide* topical **(C)**
  Pediatric: <12 years: not recommended; ≥12 years: same as adult
    Acanya (G) apply once daily-bid
     Gel: clin 1.2%/*benz* 2.5% (50 g)
    BenzaClin apply bid
     Gel: clin 1%/*benz* 5% (25, 50 g)
    Duac apply daily in the evening
     Gel: clin 1%/*benz* 5% (45 g)
    Onexton Gel apply once daily
     Gel: clin 1.2%/*benz* 3.75% (50 g pump) (alcohol-free) (preservative-free)
▷ *dapsone* topical **(C)** apply bid
  Pediatric: <12 years: not recommended; ≥12 years: same as adult
    Aczone *Gel:* 5% (30 g)
▷ *hydrocortisone* 1% **(C)(OTC)(G)** apply q HS
  Pediatric: same as adult
  see **Topical Corticosteroids** *page* 506
▷ *tazarotene* **(X)** apply daily at HS
  Pediatric: not recommended
    Avage Cream *Crm:* 0.1% (30 g)
    Tazorac Cream *Crm:* 0.05, 0.1% (15, 30, 60 g)
    Tazorac Gel *Gel:* 0.05, 0.1% (30, 100 g)
▷ *tretinoin* **(C)** apply q HS
  Pediatric: <12 years: not recommended
    Avita *Crm/Gel:* 0.025% (20, 45 g)
    Renova *Crm:* 0.02% (40 g); 0.05% (40, 60 g)
    Retin-A Cream *Crm:* 0.025, 0.05, 0.1% (20, 45 g)
    Retin-A Gel *Gel:* 0.01, 0.025% (15, 45 g) (alcohol 90%)
    Retin-A Liquid *Liq:* 0.05% (28 ml) (alcohol 55%)
    Retin-A Micro *Microspheres:* 0.04, 0.1% (20, 45 g)

◯ FOREIGN BODY: ESOPHAGUS

▷ *glucagon* **(B)** 0.02 mg/kg IV or IM with serial x-rays; max 1 mg
  Glucagon (rDNA origin or beef/pork derived)
   Vial: 1 mg/ml w. diluent
Comment: *glucagon* facilitates passage of foreign body from esophagus into stomach.

◯ FOREIGN BODY: EYE

▷ *proparacaine* **(NE)** 1-2 drops to anesthetize surface of eye; then flush with normal saline
  Ophthaine *Ophth soln:* 0.5% (15 ml)
Comment: *proparacaine* facilitates the search, location, and removal of foreign body and examination of the cornea.

◯ GASTRITIS

Antacids *see GERD* page 151
H₂ Antagonists *see GERD* page 153

◯ GASTROESOPHAGEAL REFLUX DISEASE (GERD)

Comment: Precipitators of gastric reflux include narcotics, benzodiazepines, calcium antagonists, alcohol, nicotine, chocolate, and peppermint.

ANTACIDS

Comment: Antacids with *aluminum hydroxide* may potentiate constipation. Antacids with *magnesium hydroxide* may potentiate diarrhea.
▷ *aluminum hydroxide* (C)
ALTernaGEL (OTC) 5-10 ml between meals and HS prn; max 90 ml/day
Pediatric: not recommended
Liq: 500 mg/5 ml (5, 12 oz)
Amphojel (OTC) 10 ml 5-6 times/day between meals and HS prn; max 60 ml/day
Pediatric: not recommended
Oral susp: 320 mg/5 ml (12 oz)
Amphojel Tab (OTC) 600 mg 5-6 times/day between meals and HS prn; max 3.6 g/day
Pediatric: not recommended
Tab: 300, 600 mg
▷ *aluminum hydroxide/magnesium hydroxide* (C)(OTC)(G)
Maalox 10-20 ml qid and HS prn
Pediatric: not recommended
Oral susp: alum 225 mg/*mag* 200 mg per 5 ml (5, 12, 26 oz) (mint, lemon, cherry)
Maalox Therapeutic Concentrate 10-20 ml qid pc and HS prn
Pediatric: not recommended
Oral susp: alum 600 mg/*mag* 300 mg per 5 ml (12 oz) (mint)
▷ *aluminum hydroxide/magnesium hydroxide/simethicone* (C)(OTC)(G)
Maalox Plus 10-20 ml qid pc and HS prn
Pediatric: not recommended
Tab: alum 200 mg/*mag* 200 mg/*sim* 25 mg
Extra Strength Maalox Plus 10-20 ml qid pc and HS prn
Pediatric: not recommended
Tab: alum 350 mg/*mag* 350 mg/*sim* 30 mg
Oral susp: alum 500 mg/*mag* 450 mg/*sim* 40 mg per 5 ml (5, 12, 26 oz)
Extra Strength Maalox Plus Tab 1-3 tabs qid pc and HS prn
Pediatric: not recommended
Tab: alum 350 mg/*mag* 350 mg/*sim* 30 mg
Mylanta 10-20 ml between meals and HS prn
Pediatric: not recommended
Liq: alum 200 mg/*mag* 200 mg/*sim* 20 mg per 5 ml (5, 12, 24 oz)
Mylanta Double Strength 10-20 ml between meals and HS prn
Pediatric: not recommended
Liq: alum 700 mg/*mag* 400 mg/*sim* 40 mg per 5 ml (5, 12, 24 oz)

▷ *aluminum hydroxide/magnesium carbonate* (C)(OTC)(G)

    Maalox HRF 10-20 ml qid pc and HS prn

        Pediatric: not recommended

        Oral susp: alum 280 mg/*mag* 350 mg per 10 ml (10 oz)

▷ *aluminum hydroxide/magnesium trisilicate* (C)(G)

    Gaviscon chew 2-4 tabs qid pc and HS prn

        Pediatric: not recommended

        Tab: alum 80 mg/*mag* 20 mg

    Gaviscon Liquid 15-30 ml qid pc and HS prn

        Pediatric: not recommended

        Liq: alum 95 mg/*mag* 359 mg per 15 ml (6, 12 oz)

    Gaviscon Extra Strength 2-4 tabs qid pc and HS prn

        Pediatric: not recommended

        Tab: alum 160 mg/*mag* 105 mg

    Gaviscon Extra Strength Liquid 10-20 ml qid prn

        Pediatric: not recommended

        Liq: alum 508 mg/*mag* 475 mg per 10 ml (12 oz)

▷ *aluminum hydroxide/magnesium hydroxide/simethicone* (C)(OTC)(G)

    Maalox Maximum Strength 10-20 ml qid prn; max 60 ml/day

        Pediatric: not recommended

        Oral susp: alum 500 mg/*mag* 450 mg/*sim* 40 mg per 5 ml (5, 12, 26 oz) (mint, cherry)

▷ *calcium carbonate* (C)(OTC)(G)

    Children's Mylanta Tab

        Pediatric: <2 years: not recommended; 2-5 years (24-47 lb): 1 tab as needed up to tid; 6-11 years (48-95 lb): 2 tabs as needed up to tid

        Tab: 400 mg

    Children's Mylanta

        Pediatric: <2 years: not recommended; 2-5 years (24-47 lb): 1 tab as needed up to tid; 6-11 years (48-95 lb): 2 tabs as needed up to tid

        Liq: 400 mg/5 ml (4 oz)

    Maalox Tab chew 2-4 tabs prn; max 12 tabs/day

        Pediatric: not recommended

        Chew tab: 600 mg (wild berry, lemon, wintergreen) (phenylalanine)

    Maalox Maximum Strength Tab 1-2 tabs prn; max 8 tabs/day

        Pediatric: not recommended

        Tab: 1 g (wild berry, lemon, wintergreen; phenylalanine)

    Rolaids Extra Strength 1-2 tabs dissolved in mouth o͟r chewed q 1 hour prn; max 8 tabs/day

        Tab: 1000 mg

    Tums 1-2 tabs dissolved in mouth o͟r chewed q 1 hour prn; max 16 tabs/day

        Tab: 500 mg

    Tums E-X 1-2 tabs dissolved in mouth o͟r chewed q 1 hour prn; max 16 tabs/day

        Tab: 750 mg

▷ *calcium carbonate/magnesium hydroxide* (C)

    Mylanta Tab 2-4 tabs between meals and HS prn

        Pediatric: not recommended

        Tab: calib 350 mg/*mag* 150 mg

    Mylanta DS Tab 2-4 tabs between meals and HS prn

        Pediatric: not recommended

    Tab: calib 700 mg/*mag* 300 mg
    Rolaids Sodium-Free 1-2 tabs dissolved in mouth <u>or</u> chewed q 1 hour as needed
        Tab: calib 317 mg/*mag* 64 mg
▷ *calcium carbonate/magnesium carbonate* (C)
    Mylanta Gel Caps (OTC) 2-4 caps prn
        Gel cap: calib 550 mg/*mag* 125 mg
▷ *dihydroxyaluminum* (NE)
    Rolaids (OTC) 1-2 tabs dissolved in mouth <u>or</u> chewed q 1 hour prn; max 24 tabs/day
        Tab: 334 mg

H2 ANTAGONISTS

▷ *cimetidine* (B)(OTC)(G) 800 mg bid <u>or</u> 400 mg qid; max 12 weeks
  Pediatric: <16 years: not recommended; ≥16 years: same as adult
    Tagamet 800 mg bid or 400 mg qid; max 12 weeks
        Tab: 200, 300, 400*, 800*mg
    Tagamet HB *Prophylaxis:* 1 tab ac; *Treatment:* 1 tab bid
        Tab: 200 mg
    Tagamet HB Oral Suspension *Prophylaxis:* 1-3 tsp ac; *Treatment:* 1 tsp bid
        Oral susp: 200 mg/20 ml (12 oz)
    Tagamet Liquid *Liq:* 300 mg/5 ml (mint-peach) (alcohol 2.8%)
▷ *famotidine* (B)(OTC)(G)
  Pediatric: 0.5 mg/kg/day q HS prn <u>or</u> in 2 divided doses; max 40 mg/day
    Maximum Strength Pepcid AC 1 tab ac
        Tab: 20 mg
    Pepcid 20-40 mg bid; max 6 weeks
        Tab: 20 mg; *Tab:* 40 mg; *Oral susp:* 40 mg/5 ml (50 ml)
    Pepcid AC 1 tab ac; max 2 doses/day
        Tab/Rapid dissolving tab: 10 mg
    Pepcid Complete (OTC) 1 tab ac; max 2 doses/day
        Tab: fam 10 mg/*CaCO2* 800 mg/*mg hydroxide* 165 mg
    Pepcid RPD *Tab:* 20, 40 mg rapid dissolv
▷ *nizatidine* (B)(OTC)(G) 150 mg bid <u>or</u> 300 mg once daily
  Pediatric: not recommended
    Axid *Cap:* 150, 300 mg; *Oral soln:* 15 mg/ml (480 ml) (bubble gum)
▷ *ranitidine* (B)(OTC)(G)
  Pediatric: <1 month: not recommended; 1 month to 16 years: 2-4 mg/kg/day in 2 divided doses; max 300 mg/day; *Duodenal/Gastric Ulcer:* 2-4 mg/kg/day divided bid; max 300 mg/day; *Erosive Esophagitis:* 5-10 mg/kg/day divided bid; max 300 mg/day; 20 lb, 9 kg: 0.6 ml; 30 lb, 13.6 kg: 0.9 ml; 40 lb, 18.2 kg: 1.2 ml; 50 lb, 22.7 kg: 1.5 ml; 60 lb, 27.3 kg: 1.8 ml; 70 lb, 31.8 kg: 2.1 ml
    Zantac 150 mg bid <u>or</u> 300 mg q HS
        Tab: 150, 300 mg
    Zantac 75 1 tab ac
        Tab: 75 mg
    Zantac EFFERdose dissolve 25 mg tab in 5 ml water and dissolve 150 mg tab in 6-8 oz water
        Efferdose: 25, 150 mg effervescent
    Zantac Syrup *Syr:* 15 mg/ml (peppermint) (alcohol 7.5%)

▷ *ranitidine bismuth citrate* (C) 400 mg bid
  Pediatric: not recommended
    Tritec *Tab:* 400 mg

PROTON PUMP INHIBITORS

▷ *dexlansoprazole* (B)(G) 30-60 mg daily for up to 4 weeks
  Pediatric: <18 years: not recommended
    Dexilant *Cap:* 30, 60 mg ent-coat del-rel granules; may open and sprinkle on
    applesauce; do not crush or chew granules
    Dexilant SoluTab *Tab:* 30 mg del-rel orally disint
▷ *esomeprazole* (B)(OTC)(G) 20-40 mg once daily; max 8 weeks; take 1 hour before
  food; swallow whole or mix granules with food or juice and take immediately; do not
  crush or chew granules
  Pediatric: <1 month: not established; 1 month-<1 year, 3-5 kg: 2.5 mg; 5-7.5 kg: 5
  mg; >7.5-12 kg: 10 mg; 1-11 years, <20 kg: 10 mg; ≥20 kg: 10-20 mg; 12-17 years:
  20 mg; max 8 weeks
    Nexium *Cap:* 20, 40 mg ent-coat del-rel pellets
    Nexium for Oral Suspension *Oral susp:* 10, 20, 40 mg ent-coat del-rel granules/
    pkt; mix in 2 tblsp water and drink immediately; 30 pkt/carton
▷ *lansoprazole* (B)(OTC)(G) 15-30 mg daily for up to 8 weeks; may repeat course; take
  before eating
  Pediatric: <1 year: not recommended; 1-11 years, <30 kg: 15 mg once daily;
  >11 years: same as adult
    Prevacid *Cap:* 15, 30 mg ent-coat del-rel granules; swallow whole or mix gran-
    ules with food or juice and take immediately; do not crush or chew granules;
    follow with water
    Prevacid for Oral Suspension *Oral susp:* 15, 30 mg ent-coat del-rel granules/
    pkt; mix in 2 tblsp water and drink immediately; 30 pkt/carton (strawberry)
    Prevacid SoluTab *ODT:* 15, 30 mg (strawberry) (phenylalanine)
    Prevacid 24HR 15 mg ent-coat del-rel granules; swallow whole or mix granules
    with food or juice and take immediately; do not crush or chew granules; follow
    with water
▷ *omeprazole* (C)(OTC)(G) 20-40 mg daily for 14 days; may repeat course in 4 months;
  take before eating; swallow whole or mix granules with applesauce and take immediately; do not crush or chew granules; follow with water
  Pediatric: <1 year: not recommended; 5-<10 kg: 5 mg daily; 10-<20 kg: 10 mg daily;
  ≥20 kg: same as adult
    Prilosec *Cap:* 10, 20, 40 mg ent-coat del-rel granules
      Pediatric: <1 year: not recommended; 5-<10 kg: 5 mg daily; 10-<20 kg: 10
      mg daily; ≥20 kg: same as adult
    Prilosec OTC *Tab:* 20 mg del-rel (regular, wildberry)
      Pediatric: <18 years: not recommended
▷ *pantoprazole* (B) 40 mg daily
  Pediatric: not recommended
    Protonix (G)
      Tab: 40 mg ent-coat del-rel
    Protonix for Oral Suspension *Oral susp:* 40 mg ent-coat del-rel granules/pkt;
    mix in 1 tsp apple juice for 5 seconds or sprinkle on 1 tsp apple sauce, and
    swallow immediately; do not mix in water or any other liquid or food; take
    approximately 30 minutes prior to a meal; 30 pkt/carton

▷ *rabeprazole* **(B)(OTC)(G)** *Tab:* 20 mg daily after breakfast; do not crush or chew;
Cap: open cap and sprinkle contents on a small amount of soft food or liquid
Pediatric: <1 year: not recommended; 1-11 years, <15 kg: 5 mg once daily for up to
12 weeks; ≥12 years, ≥15 kg: same as adult
  AcipHex *Tab:* 20 mg ent-coat del-rel
  AcipHex Sprinkle *Cap:* 5, 10 mg del-rel

PROTON PUMP INHIBITORS/SODIUM BICARBONATE COMBINATION

▷ *omeprazole/na bicarbonate* **(B)(G)** 20 mg daily; do not crush or chew; max 8 weeks
Pediatric: <18 years: not recommended
  Zegerid *Cap: omep* 20 mg/*na bicarb* 1100 mg; *omep* 40 mg/*na bicarb* 1100 mg
  Zegerid OTC (OTC) *Cap: omep* 20 mg/*na bicarb* 1100 mg
  Zegerid for Oral Suspension *Pwdr for oral susp: omep* 20 mg/*na bicarb* 1680
  mg; *omep* 40 mg/*na bicarb* 1680 mg (30 pkt/carton)

PROMOTILITY AGENT

▷ *metoclopramide* **(B)(G)** 10-15 mg qid 30 minutes ac and HS prn; up to 20 mg prior
to provoking situation; max 12 weeks per therapeutic course
Pediatric: <18 years: not recommended
  Metozolv ODT *ODT:* 5, 10 mg (mint)
  Reglan *Tab:* 5*, 10 mg; *Syr:* 5 mg/5 ml
  Reglan ODT *ODT:* 5, 10 mg (orange)
Comment: *metoclopropamide* is contraindicated when stimulation of GI
motility may be dangerous. Observe for tardive dyskinesia and Parkinsonism.
Avoid concomitant drugs which may cause an extrapyramidal reaction (e.g.,
phenothiazines, *haloperidol*).

◯ GIARDIASIS (*GIARDIA LAMBLIA*)

▷ *metronidazole* **(not for use in 1st; B in 2nd, 3rd)(G)** 250 mg tid x 5-10 days
Pediatric: 35-50 mg/kg/day in 3 divided doses x 10 days
  Flagyl *Tab:* 250*, 500*mg
  Flagyl 375 *Cap:* 375 mg
  Flagyl ER *Tab:* 750 mg ext-rel
Comment: Alcohol is contraindicated during treatment with oral *metronidazole*
and for 72 hours after therapy due to a possible *disulfiram*-like reaction (nausea,
vomiting, flushing, headache).
▷ *tinidazole* **(not for use in 1st; B in 2nd, 3rd)** 2 g in a single dose; take with food
Pediatric: <3 years: not recommended; ≥3 years: 50 mg/kg daily in a single dose;
take with food; max 2 g
  Tindamax *Tab:* 250*, 500*mg
Comment: Alcohol is contraindicated during treatment with oral *tinidazole* and for
72 hours after therapy due to a possible *disulfiram*-like reaction (nausea, vomiting,
flushing, headache).
▷ *nitazoxanide* **(B)** 500 mg q 12 hours x 3 days; take with food
Pediatric: <1 year: not recommended; 1-3 years; 100 mg q 12 hours x 3 days; 4-11
years: 200 mg q 12 hours x 3 days; ≥12 years: same as adult
  Alinia *Tab:* 500 mg; *Oral susp:* 100 mg/5 ml (60 ml)

Comment: **Alinia** is an antiprotozoal for the treatment of diarrhea due to *G. lamblia* or *C. parvum*.

◯ GINGIVITIS/PERIODONTITIS

ANTI-INFECTIVE ORAL RINSES

Comment: Oral treatments should be preceded by brushing and flossing the teeth. Avoid foods and liquids for 2-3 hours after a treatment.

▷ *chlorhexidine gluconate* **(B)(G)** swish 15 ml undiluted for 30 seconds bid; do not swallow; do not rinse mouth after treatment.
  Peridex, PerioGard *Oral soln:* 0.12% (480 ml)

◯ GLAUCOMA: OPEN ANGLE

Comment: Other ophthalmic medications should not be administered within 5-10 minutes of administering an ophthalmic antiglaucoma medication. Contact lenses should be removed prior to instillation of antiglaucoma medications and may be replaced 15 minutes later. Interactions with ophthalmic anti-glaucoma agents include MAOIs, CNS depressants, beta-blockers, tricyclic antidepressants, and hypoglycemics.

OPHTHALMIC ALPHA-2-AGONISTS

Comment: Ophthalmic alpha-2-agonists are contraindicated with concomitant MAOI use. Cautious use with CNS depressants, beta-blockers (ocular and systemic), antihypertensives, cardiac glycosides, and tricyclic antidepressants.

▷ *apraclonidine* ophthalmic solution **(C)** 1-2 drops affected eye tid
  Pediatric: not recommended
    Iopidine *Ophth soln:* 0.5% (5 ml) (benzalkonium chloride)
▷ *brimonidine tartrate* ophthalmic solution **(B)** 1 drop affected eye q 8 hours
  Pediatric: <2 years: not recommended; ≥2 years: 1 drop affected eye q 8 hours
    Alphagan P *Ophth soln:* 0.1, 0.15% (5, 10, 15 ml) (purite)

OPHTHALMIC CARBONIC ANHYDRASE INHIBITORS

Comment: Ophthalmic carbonic anhydrase inhibitors are contraindicated in patients with sulfa allergy.

▷ *brinzolamide* ophthalmic suspension **(C)** 1 drop affected eye tid
  Pediatric: not recommended
    Azopt *Ophth susp:* 1% (2.5, 5, 10, 15 ml) (benzalkonium chloride)
▷ *dorzolamide* ophthalmic solution **(C)(G)** 1 drop affected eye tid
  Pediatric: same as adult
    Trusopt *Ophth soln:* 2% (10 ml) (benzalkonium chloride)

OPHTHALMIC ALPHA-2 ADRENERGIC RECEPTOR AGONIST/CARBONIC ANHYDRASE INHIBITOR

▷ *brimonidine/brinzolamide* **(C)** 1 drop affected eye tid
  Pediatric: not recommended
    Simbrinza *Ophth soln: brim* 1% mg/*brinz* 0.2% per ml (10 ml)

OPHTHALMIC CHOLINERGICS (MIOTICS)

▷ *carbachol/hydroxypropyl methylcellulose* ophthalmic solution (C) 2 drops affected eye tid
  Pediatric: not recommended
  Isopto Carbachol *Ophth soln: carb* 0.75% or 2.25%/*hydroxy* 1% (15 ml); *carb* 1.5% or 3%/*hydroxy* 1% (15, 30 ml) (benzalkonium chloride)
▷ *pilocarpine* (C)(G)
  Pediatric: not recommended
  Isopto Carpine 2 drops affected eye tid-qid
    Ophth soln: 1, 2, 4% (15 ml) (benzalkonium chloride)
  Ocusert Pilo change ophthalmic insert once weekly
    Ophth inserts: 20 mcg/hr (8/pck)
  Pilocar Ophthalmic Solution 1-2 drops affected eye 1-6 times/day
    Ophth soln: 0.5, 1, 2, 3, 4, 6, 8% (15 ml)
  Pilopine HS apply 1/2 inch ribbon in lower conjunctival sac q HS
    Opth gel: 4% (4 g)

OPHTHALMIC CHOLINESTERASE INHIBITORS

▷ *demecarium bromide* ophthalmic solution (X) 1-2 drops affected eye q 12-48 hours
  Pediatric: not recommended
  Humorsol Ocumeter *Ophth soln:* 0.125, 0.25% (5 ml)
▷ *echothiophate iodide* ophthalmic solution (C) initially 1 drop of 0.03% affected eye bid; then increase strength as needed
  Pediatric: not recommended
  Phospholine Iodide *Ophth soln:* 0.03, 0.06, 0.125, 0.25% (5 ml)

OPHTHALMIC CARDIOSELECTIVE BETA-BLOCKERS

Comment: Ophthalmic beta-blockers are generally contraindicated in severe COPD, history of or current bronchial asthma, sinus bradycardia, 2nd or 3rd degree AV block.
▷ *betaxolol* ophthalmic solution (C)(G) 1-2 drops affected eye bid
  Pediatric: not recommended
  Betoptic *Ophth soln:* 0.5% (5, 10, 15 ml) (benzalkonium chloride)
  Betoptic S *Ophth soln:* 0.25% (2.5, 5, 10, 15 ml) (benzalkonium chloride)

OPHTHALMIC BETA-BLOCKERS (NONCARDIOSELECTIVE)

Comment: Ophthalmic beta-blockers are generally contraindicated in severe COPD, history of or current bronchial asthma, sinus bradycardia, 2nd or 3rd degree AV block.
▷ *carteolol* ophthalmic solution (C)(G) 1 drop affected eye bid
  Pediatric: not recommended
  Ocupress *Ophth soln:* 1% (5, 10, 15 ml) (benzalkonium chloride)
▷ *levobunolol* ophthalmic solution (C) 1-2 drops affected eye bid
  Pediatric: not recommended
  Betagan *Ophth soln:* 0.5% (5, 10, 15 ml) (benzalkonium chloride)
▷ *metipranolol* ophthalmic solution (C)(G) 1 drop affected eye bid
  Pediatric: not recommended
  OptiPranolol *Ophth soln:* 0.3% (5, 10 ml) (benzalkonium chloride)
▷ *timolol* ophthalmic solution and gel (C)(G)
  Pediatric: not recommended

Betimol 1 drop affected eye bid
Ophth soln: 0.25, 0.5% (5, 10, 15 ml) (benzalkonium chloride)
Istalol 1 drop affected eye daily
Ophth soln: 0.5% (2.5, 5 ml) (preservative-free)
Timoptic 1 drop affected eye bid
Ophth soln: 0.25, 0.5% (5, 10, 15 ml) (benzalkonium chloride)
Timoptic Ocudose 1 drop bid
Ophth soln: 0.25, 0.5% (0.2 ml/dose, 60 dose) (preservative-free)
Timoptic-XE 1 drop affected eye bid
Ophth gel: 0.25, 0.5% (2.5, 5 ml) (preservative-free)

OPHTHALMIC ALPHA-2 AGONIST/BETA-BLOCKER (NONCARDIOSELECTIVE) COMBINATION

Comment: Generally contraindicated in severe COPD, history of <u>or</u> current bronchial asthma, sinus bradycardia, 2nd <u>or</u> 3rd degree AV block.
▷ *brimonidine tartrate/timolol* ophthalmic solution **(C)** 1 drop affected eye bid
Pediatric: <2 years: not recommended; ≥2 years: same as adult
Combigan *Ophth soln: brimo* 0.2%/*timo* 0.5% (5, 10, 15 ml) (benzalkonium chloride)

OPHTHALMIC PROSTAMIDE ANALOGUES

▷ *bimatropost* ophthalmic solution **(C)(G)** 1 drop q affected eye HS
Pediatric: <16 years: not recommended; ≥16 years: same as adult
Lumigan *Ophth soln:* 0.01, 0.03% (2.5, 5, 7.5 ml) (benzalkonium chloride)
▷ *latanoprost* ophthalmic solution **(C)** 1 drop affected eye q HS
Pediatric: not recommended
Xalatan *Ophth soln:* 0.005% (2.5 ml) (benzalkonium chloride)
▷ *tafluprost* ophthalmic solution **(C)** 1 drop affected eye q HS
Pediatric: not recommended
Zioptan *Ophth soln:* 0.0015% (0.3 ml single-use, 30-60/carton) (preservative-free)
▷ *travoprost* ophthalmic solution **(C)(G)** 1 drop affected eye q HS
Pediatric: <16 years: not recommended; ≥16 years: same as adult
Travatan *Ophth soln:* 0.004% (2.5, 5 ml) (benzalkonium chloride)
Travatan Z *Ophth soln:* 0.004% (2.5, 5 ml) (boric acid, propylene glycol, sorbitol, zinc chloride)

OPHTHALMIC SYMPATHOMIMETICS

Comment: Contraindicated in narrow-angle glaucoma. Use with caution in cardiovascular disease, hypertension, hyperthyroidism, diabetes, and asthma.
▷ *dipivefrin* ophthalmic solution **(B)** 1 drop affected eye q 12 hours
Propine *Ophth soln:* 0.1% (5, 10, 15 ml) (benzalkonium chloride)

OPHTHALMIC CARBONIC ANHYDRASE INHIBITOR/NONCARDIOSELECTIVE OPHTHALMIC CARBONIC ANHYDRASE INHIBITOR/BETA-BLOCKER

▷ *dorzolamide/timolol* ophthalmic solution **(C)** 1 drop affected eye bid
Pediatric: not recommended
Cosopt *Ophth soln: dorz* 2%/*tim* 0.5% (10 ml) (benzalkonium chloride)
Cosopt PF *Ophth soln: dorz* 2%/*tim* 0.5% (10 ml) (preservative-free)

OPHTHALMIC SYNTHETIC DOCOSANOID

▷ *unoprostone isopropyl* ophthalmic solution (C) 1 drop affected eye bid
    Pediatric: not recommended
        Rescula *Ophth soln:* 0.15% (5 ml) (benzalkonium chloride)

ORAL CARBONIC ANHYDRASE INHIBITORS

▷ *acetazolamide* (C) 250-1000 mg/day in divided doses <u>or</u> 500 mg bid sust-rel tabs;
  max 1 g/day
    Pediatric: not recommended
        Diamox *Tab:* 125*, 250*mg
        Diamox Sequels *Tab:* 500 mg sust-rel
▷ *methazolamide* (C)(G) 50-100 mg bid-tid times daily
    Pediatric: not recommended
        Neptazane *Tab:* 25, 50 mg
Comment: Administer ophthalmic osmotic and miotic agents concomitantly.

GONORRHEA (*NEISSERIA GONORRHOEAE*)

Comment: The following treatment regimens for *N. gonorrhoeae* are published in
the **2015 CDC Transmitted Diseases Treatment Guidelines**. Treatment regimens are
presented by generic drug name first, followed by information about brands and dose
forms. Empiric treatment requires concomitant treatment of chlamydia. Treat all sexual
contacts. Patients who are HIV-positive should receive the same treatment as those who
are HIV-negative. Sexual abuse must be considered a cause of gonococcal infection in
preadolescent children.

RECOMMENDED REGIMENS: ADULT; UNCOMPLICATED INFECTIONS OF THE CERVIX, URETHRA, AND RECTUM

Regimen 1

▷ *ceftriaxone* 250 mg IM in a single dose
    <u>plus</u>
▷ *azithromycin* 1 g in a single dose

Regimen 2

▷ *ceftriaxone* 250 mg IM in a single dose
    <u>plus</u>
▷ *doxycycline* 100 mg bid x 7 days

RECOMMENDED REGIMENS: ADULT; UNCOMPLICATED INFECTIONS OF THE PHARYNX

Regimen 1

▷ *ceftriaxone* 250 mg IM in a single dose
    <u>plus</u>
▷ *azithromycin* 1 g in a single dose

Regimen 2

▷ *ceftriaxone* 250 mg IM in a single dose
    plus
▷ *doxycycline* 100 mg bid x 7 days

RECOMMENDED REGIMENS: CHILDREN >45 KG, >8 YEARS; UNCOMPLICATED INFECTIONS OF THE CERVIX, URETHRA, AND RECTUM

Regimen 1

▷ *ceftriaxone* 250 mg IM in a single dose
    plus
▷ *azithromycin* 1 g in a single dose

RECOMMENDED REGIMEN: CHILDREN >45 KG

Regimen 1

▷ *ceftriaxone* 250 mg IM in a single dose

RECOMMENDED REGIMEN: CHILDREN >45 KG WHO HAVE GONOCOCCAL BACTEREMIA <u>OR</u> ARTHRITIS

Regimen 1

▷ *ceftriaxone* 50 mg/kg IM <u>or</u> IV in a single dose daily x 7 days

RECOMMENDED REGIMENS: CHILDREN <45 KG, <8 YEARS; UNCOMPLICATED GONOCOCCAL VULVOVAGINITIS, CERVICITIS, URETHRITIS, PHARYNGITIS, <u>OR</u> PROCTITIS

Regimen 1

▷ *ceftriaxone* 250 mg IM in a single dose

RECOMMENDED REGIMEN: CHILDREN <45 KG, <8 YEARS WHO HAVE GONOCOCCAL BACTEREMIA <u>OR</u> ARTHRITIS

Regimen 1

▷ *ceftriaxone* 50 mg/kg (max dose 1 g) IM <u>or</u> IV in a single dose daily x 7 days

DRUG BRANDS AND DOSE FORMS

▷ *azithromycin* (B)
    Zithromax *Tab:* 250, 500, 600 mg; *Oral susp:* 100 mg/5 ml (15 ml); 200 mg/5 ml
    (15, 22.5, 30 ml) (cherry); *Pkt:* 1 g for reconstitution (cherry-banana)
    Zithromax Tri-pak *Tab:* 3 x 500 mg tabs/pck
    Zithromax Z-pak *Tab:* 6 x 250 mg tabs/pck
    Zmax *Oral susp:* 2 g ext-rel for reconstitution (cherry-banana) (148 mg Na$^+$)
▷ *ceftriaxone* (B)(G)
    Rocephin *Vial:* 250, 500 mg; 1, 2 g
▷ *doxycycline* (D)(G)
    Actilate *Tab:* 75, 150** mg

Adoxa *Tab:* 50, 75, 100, 150 mg ent-coat
Doryx *Tab:* 50, 75, 100, 150, 200 mg del-rel
Monodox *Cap:* 50, 75, 100 mg
Oracea *Cap:* 40 mg del-rel
Vibramycin *Tab:* 100 mg; *Cap:* 50, 100 mg; *Syr:* 50 mg/5 ml (raspberry-apple) (sulfites); *Oral susp:* 25 mg/5 ml (raspberry)
Vibra-Tab *Tab:* 100 mg film-coat

ALTERNATIVE THERAPY

▶ *azithromycin* (B) 2 g x 1 dose
  Pediatric: not recommended for treatment of gonorrhea in children
    Zithromax *Tab:* 250, 500, 600 mg; *Oral susp:* 100 mg/5 ml (15 ml); 200 mg/5 ml (15, 22.5, 30 ml) (cherry); *Pkt:* 1 g for reconstitution (cherry-banana)
    Zithromax Tri-pak *Tab:* 3 x 500 mg tabs/pck
    Zithromax Z-pak *Tab:* 6 x 250 mg tabs/pck
    Zmax *Oral susp:* 2 g ext-rel for reconstitution (cherry-banana) (148 mg Na$^+$)
▶ *cefotaxime* 500 mg IM x 1 dose
    Claforan *Vial:* 500 mg; 1, 2 g
▶ *cefotetan* 1 g IM x 1 dose
  Pediatric: not recommended
    Cefotan *Vial:* 1, 2 g
▶ *cefoxitin* (B) 2 g IM x 1 dose
  Pediatric: <3 months: not recommended
    Mefoxin *Vial:* 1, 2 g
      <u>plus</u>
▶ *probenecid* (B)(G)
    Benemid 1 g 30 minutes before *cefoxitin*
      Pediatric: <2 years: not recommended; 2-14 years: 25 mg/kg 30 minutes before *cefoxitin*; >14 years: same as adult
      Tab: 500*mg; *Cap:* 500 mg
▶ *cefpodoxime proxetil* (B) 200 mg x 1 dose
  Pediatric: <2 months: not recommended; 2 months-12 years: 10 mg/kg/day (max 400 mg/dose) <u>or</u> 5 mg/kg/day bid (max 200 mg/dose)
    Vantin *Tab:* 100, 200 mg; *Oral susp:* 50, 100 mg/5 ml (50, 75, 100 mg) (lemon creme)
▶ *ceftizoxime* (B) 1 g IM x 1 dose
  Pediatric: <6 months: not recommended
    Cefizox *Vial:* 500 mg; 1, 2, 10 g
▶ *cefuroxime axetil* (B)(G) 1000 mg x 1 dose
  Pediatric: 30 mg/kg/day in 2 divided doses x 10 days
    Ceftin *Tab:* 250, 500 mg; *Oral susp:* 125, 250 mg/5 ml (50, 100 ml) (tutti-frutti)
▶ *demeclocycline* (X) 600 mg initially, followed by 300 mg q 12 hours x 4 days (total 3 g)
  Pediatric: <8 years: not recommended
    Declomycin *Tab:* 300 mg
Comment: *demeclocycline* is contraindicated <8 years-of-age, in pregnancy, and lactation (discolors developing tooth enamel). A side effect may be photosensitivity (photophobia). Do not give with antacids, calcium supplements, milk or other dairy, or within two hours of taking another drug.
▶ *enoxacin* (C) 400 mg x 1 dose
  Pediatric: <18 years: not recommended

Penetrex *Tab:* 200, 400 mg
▷ *imipramine* (C) 400 mg x 1 dose
   Pediatric: <18 years: not recommended
   Maxaquin *Tab:* 400 mg
▷ *norfloxacin* (C) 800 mg x 1 dose
   Pediatric: <18 years: not recommended
   Noroxin *Tab:* 400 mg
▷ *spectinomycin* (B) 2 g IM x 1 dose
   Pediatric: 40 mg/kg IM x 1 dose
   Trobicin *Vial:* 2 g

 GOUT

Pseudogout *see Pseudogout page* 364
Acetaminophen for IV Infusion *see page* 306
Oral Prescription NSAIDs *see page* 501
Other Oral Analgesics *see Pain page* 308
Topical/Transdermal NSAIDs *see Pain page* 307
Parenteral Corticosteroids *see page* 511
Oral Corticosteroids *see page* 509

PEGYLATED URIC ACID SPECIFIC ENZYME

▷ *pegloticase* (C) premedicate with antihistamine and corticosteroid; 8 mg once every
   2 weeks; administer IV infusion after dilution over at least 2 hours; observe at least
   1 hour post-infusion
   Pediatric: <18 years: not recommended
   Krystexxa *Vial:* 8 mg/ml (1 ml) single-use pwdr for IV infusion after dilution
   Comment: Slow rate, or stop and restart at lower rate, if infusion reaction
   occurs (e.g., **Krystexxa** is contraindicated with G6PD deficiency; screen patients
   of African or Mediterranean descent). **Krystexxa** is not for the treatment of
   asymptomatic hyperuricemia.

PROPHYLAXIS

▷ *allopurinol* (C)(G) initially 100 mg daily; increase by 100 mg weekly; max 800 mg/
   day and 300 mg/dose; usual range for mild symptoms 200-300 mg/day; for severe
   symptoms 400-600 mg/day; take with food
   Pediatric: not recommended
   Zyloprim *Tab:* 100*, 300*mg
   Comment: Do not take concurrent with *colchicine*.
▷ *colchicine* (C)(G) 0.6-1.2 mg at first sign of attack; then 0.6 mg every hour or 1.2 mg every
   2 hours until pain relief; then consider 0.6 mg/day or every other day for maintenance
   Pediatric: not recommended
   Colcrys *Tab:* 0.6 mg
   Mitigare *Cap:* 0.6 mg
   Comment: Do not take concurrent with *allopurinol*.
▷ *febuxostat* (C) initially 40 mg daily; after 2 weeks, may increase to 80 mg daily.
   Pediatric: <18 years: not recommended
   Uloric *Tab:* 40, 80 mg

Comment: Gout flare prophylaxis with *colchicine* or NSAID is recommended on initiation of *febuxostat* and up to 6 months.

URICOSURIC AGENT

▷ *probenecid* (C)(G) 250 mg bid x 1 week; maintenance 500 mg bid
   Pediatric: not recommended
   Tab: 500*mg; *Cap:* 500 mg
   Comment: Avoid concomitant use of *probenecid* and salicylates.

URICOSURIC/ANTI-INFLAMMATORY COMBINATIONS

▷ *probenecid/colchicine* (NE)(G) 1 tab once daily x 1 week; then, 1 tab bid thereafter
   Pediatric: not recommended
   Tab: prob 500 mg/*colch* 0.5 mg
   Comment: *probenecid/colchicine* is contraindicated in the treatment of acute gout attack, patients with blood dyscrasias, and patients with uric acid kidney stones. Concomitant salicylates antagonize the uricosuric effects.
▷ *sulfinpyrazone* (C) initially 200-400 mg bid; may gradually increase to 800 mg bid
   Anturane *Cap:* 100, 200 mg
Comment: Goal is serum uric acid <6.5 mg/dL.

XANTHINE OXIDASE INHIBITOR

▷ *febuxostat* (C) 40 mg once daily x 2 weeks; if serum uric acid is not <6 mg/dL, may increase to 80 mg once daily
   Pediatric: <18 years: not established
   Uloric *Tab:* 40, 80 mg

SELECTIVE URIC ACID REABSORPTION INHIBITOR (SURI)

▷ *lesinurad* (C) 200 mg once daily in combination with a xanthine oxidase inhibitor (XOI)
   Pediatric: <18 years: not established
   Zurampic *Tab:* 200 mg
   Comment: **Zurampic** inhibits URATI, a urate transporter, which is responsible for the majority of renal absorption of uric acid and (OAT) 4, organic anion transporter, a uric acid transporter involved in diuretic-induced hyperuricemia. Do not use as monotherapy. Use in combination with an XOI, such as *allopurinol* or *febuxostat*, (to reduce the production of uric acid). Do not initiate if CrCl <45 mL/min, ESRD, dialysis, or kidney transplant.

◉ GOUTY ARTHRITIS

Acetaminophen for IV Infusion *see Pain page* 306
Oral Prescription NSAIDs *see Pain page* 501
Other Oral Analgesics *see Pain page* 308
Topical/Transdermal NSAIDs *see Pain page* 307
Parenteral Corticosteroids *see page* 511
Oral Corticosteroids *see page* 509
Topical Analgesic and Anesthetic Agents *see page* 499

TOPICAL ANALGESICS

▷ *capsaicin* (B)(G) apply tid-qid prn to intact skin
    Pediatric: <2 years: not recommended; ≥2 years: same as adult
        Axsain *Crm:* 0.075% (1, 2 oz)
        Capsin *Lotn:* 0.025, 0.075% (59 ml)
        Capzasin-P (OTC) *Crm:* 0.025% (1.5 oz); *Lotn:* 0.025% (2 oz)
        Dolorac *Crm:* 0.025% (28 g)
        Double Cap (OTC) *Crm:* 0.05% (2 oz)
        R-Gel *Gel:* 0.025% (15, 30 g)
        Zostrix (OTC) *Crm:* 0.025% (0.7, 1.5, 3 oz)
        Zostrix HP (OTC) *Emol crm:* 0.075% (1, 2 oz)
Comment: Provides some relief by 1-2 weeks; optimal benefit may take 4-6 weeks.

ORAL SALICYLATE

▷ *indomethacin* (C) initially 25 mg bid-tid; increase as needed at weekly intervals by
    25-50 mg/day; max 200 mg/day
    Pediatric: <14 years: usually not recommended; >2 years, if risk warranted: 1-2 mg/
    kg/day in divided doses; max 3-4 mg/kg/day (or 150-200 mg/day, whichever is
    less); <14 years, ER cap not recommended
    Cap: 25, 50 mg; *Susp:* 25 mg/5 ml (pineapple-coconut, mint; alcohol 1%); *Supp:*
    50 mg; *ER Cap:* 75 mg ext-rel
    Comment: *indomethacin* is indicated only for acute painful flares. Administer with
    food and/or antacids. Use lowest effective dose for shortest duration.

NSAID PLUS PPI

▷ *esomeprazole/naproxen* (C; not for use in 3rd)(G) 1 tab bid; use lowest effective dose
    for the shortest duration; swallow whole; take at least 30 minutes before a meal
    Pediatric: <18 years: not recommended
        Vimovo *Tab:* nap 375 mg/*eso* 20 mg ext-rel; *nap* 500 mg/*eso* 20 mg ext-rel

COX-2 INHIBITORS

Comment: Cox-2 inhibitors are contraindicated with history of asthma, urticaria, and
allergic-type reactions to *aspirin*, other NSAIDs, and sulfonamides, 3rd trimester of
pregnancy, and coronary artery bypass graft (CABG) surgery.
▷ *celecoxib* (C)(G) 100-400 mg bid; max 800 mg/day
    Pediatric: <18 years: not recommended
        Celebrex *Cap:* 50, 100, 200, 400 mg
▷ *meloxicam* (C)(G) initially 7.5 mg once daily; max 15 mg once daily
    Pediatric: <2 years: not recommended; ≥2 years: 0.125 mg/kg; max 7.5 mg once
    daily
        Mobic *Tab:* 7.5, 15 mg; *Oral susp:* 7.5 mg/5 ml (100 ml) (raspberry)
        Vivlodex *Cap:* 5, 10 mg

 GRANULOMA INGUINALE (DONOVANOSIS)

Comment: The following treatment regimens are published in the **2015 CDC Sexually
Transmitted Diseases Treatment Guidelines**. Treatment regimens are for adults only;

consult a specialist for treatment of patients less than 18 years-of-age. Treatment regimens are presented by generic drug name first, followed by information about brands and dose forms. Persons who have sexual contact with a patient who has had granuloma inguinale within the past 60 days before onset of the patient's symptoms should be examined and offered therapy. Patients who are HIV-positive should receive the same treatment as those who are HIV-negative; however, the addition of a parenteral aminoglycoside (e.g., *gentamicin*) can also be considered.

RECOMMENDED REGIMEN

▷ *doxycycline* 100 mg bid x at least 3 weeks and until all lesions have completely healed

ALTERNATE REGIMENS

▷ *azithromycin* 1 g once weekly for at least 3 weeks and until all lesions have completely healed
▷ *ciprofloxacin* 750 mg bid x at least 3 weeks and until all lesions have completely healed
▷ *erythromycin base* 500 mg qid x 14 days <u>or</u> *erythromycin ethylsuccinate* 400 mg qid x 14 days
▷ *trimethoprim/sulfamethoxazole* 1 double-strength (160/800) dose bid x at least 3 weeks and until all lesions have completely healed

DRUG BRANDS AND DOSE FORMS

▷ *azithromycin* (B)
  Zithromax *Tab:* 250, 500, 600 mg; *Oral susp:* 100 mg/5 ml (15 ml); 200 mg/5 ml (15, 22.5, 30 ml) (cherry); *Pkt:* 1 g for reconstitution (cherry-banana)
  Zithromax Tri-pak *Tab:* 3 x 500 mg tabs/pck
  Zithromax Z-pak *Tab:* 6 x 250 mg tabs/pck
  Zmax *Oral susp:* 2 g ext-rel for reconstitution (cherry-banana) (148 mg Na⁺)
▷ *ciprofloxacin* (C)
  Cipro (G) *Tab:* 250, 500, 750 mg; *Oral susp:* 250, 500 mg/5 ml (100 ml) (strawberry)
  Cipro XR *Tab:* 500, 1000 mg ext-rel
  ProQuin XR *Tab:* 500 mg ext-rel
  Comment: *ciprofloxacin* is contraindicated <18 years-of-age, and during pregnancy and lactation. Risk of tendonitis or tendon rupture, especially 60 years-of-age and older.
▷ *doxycycline* (D)(G)
  Actilate *Tab:* 75, 150**mg
  Adoxa *Tab:* 50, 75, 100, 150 mg ent-coat
  Doryx *Tab:* 50, 75, 100, 150, 200 mg del-rel
  Monodox *Cap:* 50, 75, 100 mg
  Oracea *Cap:* 40 mg del-rel
  Vibramycin *Tab:* 100 mg; *Cap:* 50, 100 mg; *Syr:* 50 mg/5 ml (raspberry-apple) (sulfites); *Oral susp:* 25 mg/5 ml (raspberry)
  Vibra-Tab *Tab:* 100 mg film-coat
  Comment: *doxycycline* is contraindicated <8 years-of-age, in pregnancy, and lactation (discolors developing tooth enamel). A side effect may be photo-sensitivity (photophobia). Do not give with antacids, calcium supplements, milk or other dairy, or within two hours of taking another drug.

▷ *erythromycin base* (B)(G)
    Ery-Tab *Tab:* 250, 333, 500 mg ent-coat
    PCE *Tab:* 333, 500 mg
    Comment: *erythromycin* may increase INR with concomitant *warfarin*, as well as increase serum level of *digoxin*, benzodiazepines and statins.
▷ *erythromycin ethylsuccinate* (B)(G)
    EryPed *Oral susp:* 200 mg/5 ml (100, 200 ml) (fruit); 400 mg/5 ml (60, 100, 200 ml) (banana); *Oral drops:* 200, 400 mg/5 ml (50 ml) (fruit); *Chew tab:* 200 mg wafer (fruit)
    E.E.S. *Oral susp:* 200, 400 mg/5 ml (100 ml) (fruit)
    E.E.S. Granules *Oral susp:* 200 mg/5 ml (100, 200 ml) (cherry)
    E.E.S. 400 Tablets *Tab:* 400 mg
    Comment: *erythromycin* may increase INR with concomitant *warfarin*, as well as increase serum level of *digoxin*, benzodiazepines and statins.
▷ *trimethoprim/sulfamethoxazole* (C)(G)
    Bactrim, Septra
      Tab: trim 80 mg/*sulfa* 400 mg*
    Bactrim DS, Septra DS
      Tab: trim 160 mg/*sulfa* 800 mg*
    Bactrim Pediatric Suspension, Septra Pediatric Suspension
      Oral susp: trim 40 mg/*sulfa* 200 mg per 5 ml (100 ml) (cherry) (alcohol 0.3%)
    Comment: *trimethoprim/sulfamethoxazole* is not recommended in pregnancy or lactation. *CrCl 15-30 mL/min:* reduce dose by 1/2; *CrCl <15 mL/min:* not recommended

⊘ GROWTH FAILURE

Comment: Administer growth hormones by SC injection into thigh, buttocks, or abdomen. Rotate sites with each dose. Contraindicated in children with fused epiphyses or evidence of neoplasia.
▷ *mecasermin* (recombinant human insulin-like growth factor-1 [rhIGF-1])
    Increlex (B) see mfr pkg insert
    Vial: 10 mg/ml (benzyl alcohol)
    Comment: **Increlex** is indicated for growth failure in children with severe primary IGF-1 deficiency (primary IGFD) or in those with growth hormone (GH) gene deletion who have developed neutralizing antibodies to GH.
▷ *somatropin* (rDNA origin)
    Genotropin (B) initially not more than 0.04 mg/kg/week divided into 6-7 doses; may increase at 4-8 week intervals; max 0.08 mg/kg/week divided into 6-7 doses
    Pediatric: usually 0.16-0.024 mg/kg/week divided into 6-7 doses
    Intra-Mix Device: 1.5 mg (1.3 mg/ml after reconstitution), 5.8 mg (5 mg/ml after reconstitution) (two-chamber cartridge w. diluent); *Pen or Intra-Mix Device:* 5.8 mg (5 mg/ml after reconstitution), 13.8 mg (512 mg/ml after reconstitution) (two-chamber cartridge w. diluent)
    Genotropin Miniquick (B) initially not more than 0.04 mg/kg/week divided into 6-7 doses; may increase at 4-8-week intervals; max 0.08 mg/kg/week divided into 6-7 doses

Pediatric: usually 0.16-0.024 mg/kg/week divided into 6-7 doses
MiniQuick: 0.2, 0.4, 0.6, 0.8, 1, 1.2, 1.4, 1.6, 1.8, 2 mg/0.25 ml (pwdr for SC injection after reconstitution) (2-chamber cartridge w. diluent)

Humatrope (C)
Pediatric: initially 0.18 mg/kg/week IM o̱r SC divided into equal doses given either on 3 alternate days o̱r 6 x/week; max 0.3 mg/kg/week
Vial: 5 mg w. 5 ml diluent

Norditropin (C)
Pediatric: 0.024-0.034 mg/kg 6 to 7 times/week SC
Vial: 4 mg (12 IU), 8 mg (24 IU); *Cartridge for inj:* 5, 10, 15 mg/1.5 ml; *Flex-Pro prefilled pen:* 5, 10, 15 mg/1.5 ml
NordiFlex prefilled pen: 5, 10, 15 mg/1.5 ml; 30 mg/3 ml

Nutropin (C)
Pediatric: 0.7 mg/kg/week SC in divided daily doses
Vial: 5, 10 mg/vial w. diluent

Nutropin AQ (C)
<35 years: initially not more than 0.006 mg/kg SC daily; may increase to max 0.025 mg/kg SC daily; ≥35 years: initially not more than 0.006 mg/kg SC daily; may increase to max 0.0125 mg/kg SC daily
Pediatric: Prepubertal: up to 0.043 mg/kg SC daily; *Pubertal:* up to 0.1 mg/kg SC daily; *Turner Syndrome:* up to 0.0375 mg/kg/week divided into equal doses 3-7 times/week
Vial: 5 mg/ml (2 ml)

Nutropin Depot (C) 1.5 mg/kg SC monthly on same day each month; max 22.5 mg/inj; divide injection if >22.5 mg
Pediatric: same as adult
Vial: 13.5, 18, 22.5 mg/vial (pwdr for injection after reconstitution; single-use w. diluent and needle)

Omnitrope (B) 0.16-0.24 mg/kg/week SC divided 3-7 times/week
Vial: 5.8 mg

Omnitrope Pen 5 (B) 0.16-0.24 mg/kg/week SC divided 3-7 times/week
Cartridge for inj: 5 mg/1.5 ml

Omnitrope Pen 10 (B) 0.16-0.24 mg/kg/week SC divided 3-7 times/week
Cartridge for inj: 10 mg/1.5 ml

Saizen (B) 0.18 mg/kg/week IM o̱r SC divided 3-7 times/week
Vial: 5 mg (pwdr for SC injection w. diluent)

Serostem (B) 0.1 mg/kg SC once daily at HS; max 6 mg
Vial: 5, 4, 6, 8.8 mg (pwdr for SC injection w. diluent) (benzyl alcohol)

 HEADACHE: MIGRAINE/CLUSTER

ERGOTAMINE AGENTS

Comment: Do not use an ergotamine-type drug within 24 hours of any triptan o̱r other 5-HT agonist.

▶ *dihydroxyergotamine mesylate* (X)
DHE 45 1 mg SC, IM, o̱r IV; may repeat at 1 hour intervals; max 3 mg/day SC o̱r IM/day; max 2 mg IV/day; max 6 mg/week

   Pediatric: not recommended
    Amp: 1 mg/ml (1 ml)
  Migranal 1 spray in each nostril; may repeat 15 minutes later; max 6 sprays/day
  and 8 sprays/week
   Pediatric: not recommended
   Nasal spray: 4 mg/ml; 0.5 mg/spray (caffeine)
▷ *ergotamine* (X)(G) 1 tab SL at onset of attack; then q 30 minutes as needed; max
 3 tabs/day and 5 tabs/week
 Tab: 2 mg
▷ *ergotamine/caffeine* (X)(G)
  Cafergot 2 tabs at onset of attack; then 1 tab every 1/2 hour if needed; max
  6 tabs/attack and 10 tabs/week
   Pediatric: not recommended
   Tab: ergot 1 mg/*caf* 100 mg
  Cafergot Suppository 1 suppository rectally at onset of headache; may repeat x
  1 after 1 hour; max 2/attack, 5/week
   Rectal supp: ergot 2 mg/*caf* 100 mg

5-HT RECEPTOR AGONISTS

Comment: Contraindications to 5-HT receptor agonists include cardiovascular
disease, ischemic heart disease, cerebral vascular syndromes, peripheral vascular
disease, uncontrolled hypertension, hemiplegic <u>or</u> basilar migraine. Do not use any
triptan within 24 hours of ergot-type drugs <u>or</u> other 5-HT1A agonists, <u>or</u> within 2
weeks of taking an MAOI.
▷ *almotriptan* (C)(G) 6.25 <u>or</u> 12.5 mg; may repeat once after 2 hours; max 2 doses/day
  Pediatric: <12 years: not recommended; ≥12 years: same as adult
  Axert *Tab:* 6.25 mg (6/card), 12.5 mg (12/card)
  Comment: *almotriptan* is indicated for patients 12-17 years-of-age with PMHx
  migraine headache lasting ≥4 hours untreated.
▷ *eletriptan* (C) 20 <u>or</u> 40 mg; may repeat once after 2 hours; max 80 mg/day
 Pediatric: <18 years: not recommended
  Relpax *Tab:* 20, 40 mg
▷ *frovatriptan* (C)(G) 2.5 mg with fluids; may repeat once after 2 hours; max 7.5 mg/day
 Pediatric: <18 years: not recommended
  Frova *Tab:* 2.5 mg
▷ *naratriptan* (C) 1 <u>or</u> 2.5 mg with fluids; may repeat once after 4 hours; max 5 mg/day
 Pediatric: <18 years: not recommended
  Amerge *Tab:* 1, 2.5 mg
▷ *rizatriptan* (C) initially 5 <u>or</u> 10 mg; may repeat in 2 hours if needed; max 30 mg/day
 Pediatric: <18 years: not recommended
  Maxalt *Tab:* 5, 10 mg
  Maxalt-MLT *ODT:* 5, 10 mg (peppermint) (phenylalanine)
▷ *sumatriptan* (C)(G)
 Pediatric: <18 years: not recommended
  Alsuma 6 mg SC to the upper arm <u>or</u> lateral thigh only; may repeat after 1 hour
  if needed; max 2 doses/day
   Prefilled syringe: 6 mg/0.5 ml (2/pck with auto injector)
  Imitrex Injectable 4-6 mg SC; may repeat after 1 hour if needed; max 2 doses/day
   Prefilled syringe: 4, 6 mg/0.5 ml (2/pck with <u>or</u> without autoinjector)

Imitrex Nasal Spray (G) 5-20 mg intranasally; may repeat once after 2 hours if needed; max 40 mg/day

Nasal spray: 5, 20 mg/spray (single-dose)

Imitrex Tab 25-200 mg x 1 dose; may be repeated at intervals of at least 2 hours if needed; max 200 mg/day

Tab: 25, 50, 100 mg rapid-rel

Imitrex STATdose Pen 6 mg/0.5 mg SC; may repeat once after 2 hours if needed; max 2 doses/day

Prefilled needle-free autoinjector delivery system: 6 mg/0.5 ml (6/pck)

Onzetra Xsail each disposable white nosepiece contains half a dose of medication (11 mg of sumatriptan). A full dose is 22 mg. Do not use more than 2 nosepieces per dose; attach the mouthpiece and one nasal piece; then press the white button on the delivery device to pierce the capsule in the nasal piece, then insert the nasal piece into one nostril and blow into the mouth piece to deliver the nasal powder in the contents of one capsule (11 mg); repeat in the opposite nostril for a total single 22 mg dose

Cap: 11 mg nasal pwdr; *Kit:* nosepieces (2), capsules (2), reusable breath powered delivery device (1)

Sumavel DosePro 6 mg SC to the upper arm <u>or</u> lateral thigh only; may repeat after 1 hour if needed; max 2 doses/day

Prefilled needle-free delivery system: 6 mg/0.5 ml (6/pck)

Zembrace SymTouch administer 3 mg SC at onset of headache; may repeat hourly; max 12 mg/24 hours

Pediatric: <18 years: not recommended

Autoinjector: 3 mg/0.5 ml (prefilled single-dose disposable autoinjector)

▷ *zolmitriptan* (C)(G) initially 2.5 mg; may repeat after 2 hours if needed; max 10 mg/day

Pediatric: <18 years: not recommended

Zomig *Tab:* 2.5*, 5 mg

Zomig Nasal Spray *Nasal spray:* 5 mg/spray (6 single dose/carton)

Zomig-ZMT *ODT:* 2.5 mg (6 tabs), 5*mg (3 tabs) (orange) (phenylalanine)

Comment: Do not use any ***triptan*** within 24 hours of ergotamine-type drugs <u>or</u> other 5-HT agonists, <u>or</u> within 2 weeks of taking an MAOI.

5-HT IB/ID RECEPTOR AGONIST/NSAID COMBINATION

▷ *sumatriptan/naproxen* (C; D in 3rd)

Pediatric: <18 years: not recommended

Treximet initially 1 tab; may repeat after 2 hours; max 2 doses/day

Tab: suma 85 mg/*naprox* 500 mg (9/blister card)

Comment: Do not use ***sumatriptan*** within 24 hours of ergot-type drugs <u>or</u> other 5-HT agonists, <u>or</u> within 2 weeks of taking an MAOI.

OTHER ANALGESICS

▷ *acetaminophen/aspirin/caffeine* (D)(G)

Comment: ***aspirin***-containing medications are contraindicated with history of allergic-type reaction to ***aspirin***, children and adolescents with *Varicella* <u>or</u> other viral illness, and 3rd trimester pregnancy.

> **Excedrin Migraine (OTC)** 2 tabs q 6 hours prn; max 8 tabs/day x 2 days
>> *Pediatric:* not recommended
>> *Tab:* acet 250 mg/*asp* 250 mg/*caf* 65 mg

▷ *diclofenac potassium powder for oral solution* (C; D ≥30 weeks)(G) empty the contents of one pkt into a cup containing 1-2 oz or 2-4 tbsp (30-60 ml) of water, mix well, and drink immediately; water only, no other liquids; take on an empty stomach; use the losest effective dose for the shortest duration of time; safety and effectiveness of a 2nd dose has not been established

Pediatric: <18 years: not established; ≥18 years: same as adult

> **Cambia** *Pwdr for oral soln:* 50 mg/pkt (3 pkts/set, conjoined with a perforated border

Comment: Cambia is not indicated for migraine prophylaxis. May not be bioequivalent with other *diclofenac* forms (e.g., *diclofenac sodium* ent-coat tabs, *diclofenac sodium* ext-rel tabs, *diclofenac potassium* immed-rel tabs) even of the mg strength is the same, therefore, it is not possible to convert dosing from any other diclofenac formulation to **Cambia. Cambia** is contraindicated in the setting of coronary artery bypass graft. Use of **Cambia** should not be considered with hepatic impairment, gastric/duodenal ulcer, starting at 30 weeks gestation (risk of premature closure of the ductus arteriosus in the fetus), concomitant NSAIDs, SSRIs, anticoagulants/antiplatelets, any risk factor for potential bleeding.

▷ *isometheptene mucate/dichloralphenazone/acetaminophen* (C)(IV)

> **Midrin** 2 caps initially; then 1 cap q 1 hour until relieved; max 5 caps/12 hours
>> *Pediatric:* not recommended
>> *Cap:* iso 65 mg/*dichlor* 100 mg/*acet* 325 mg

PROPHYLAXIS

▷ *topiramate* (D)(G) initially 25 mg daily in the PM and titrate up daily as tolerated; then 25 mg bid; then, 25 mg in the AM and 50 mg in the PM; then, 50 mg bid

Pediatric: <12 years: not recommended

> **Topamax** *Tab:* 25, 50, 100, 200 mg
> **Topamax Sprinkle Caps** *Cap:* 15, 25 mg

BETA-BLOCKERS

▷ *atenolol* (D)(G) initially 25 mg bid; max 150 mg/day in divided doses

Pediatric: not recommended

> **Tenormin** *Tab:* 25, 50, 100 mg

▷ *metoprolol succinate* (C)

Pediatric: not recommended

> **ToprolR-XL** initially 25-100 mg in a single dose daily; increase weekly if needed; max 400 mg/day
>> *Tab:* 25*, 50*, 100*, 200*mg ext-rel

▷ *metoprolol tartrate* (C)

Pediatric: not recommended

> **Lopressor (G)** initially 25-50 mg bid; increase weekly if needed; max 400 mg/day
>> *Tab:* 25, 37.5, 50, 75, 100 mg

▷ *nadolol* (C)(G) initially 20 mg daily; max 240 mg/day in divided doses

Pediatric: not recommended

> **Corgard** *Tab:* 20*, 40*, 80*, 120*, 160*mg

▷ *propranolol* (C)(G)

    Inderal initially 10 mg bid; usual range 160-320 mg/day in divided doses

        Pediatric: not recommended

        Tab: 10*, 20*, 40*, 60*, 80*mg

    Inderal LA initially 80 mg daily in a single dose; increase q 3-7 days; usual range 120-160 mg/day; max 320 mg/day in a single dose

        Pediatric: not recommended

        Cap: 60, 80, 120, 160 mg sust-rel

    InnoPran XL initially 80 mg q HS; max 120 mg/day

        Cap: 80, 120 mg ext-rel

▷ *timolol* (C)(G) initially 5 mg bid; max 60 mg/day in divided doses

  Pediatric: not recommended

    Blocadren *Tab:* 5, 10*, 20*mg

CALCIUM ANTAGONISTS

▷ *diltiazem* (C)(G)

    Cardizem initially 30 mg qid; may increase gradually every 1-2 days; max 360 mg/day in divided doses

        Pediatric: not recommended

        Tab: 30, 60, 90, 120 mg

    Cardizem CD initially 120-180 mg once daily; adjust at 1- to 2-week intervals; max 480 mg/day

        Pediatric: not recommended

        Cap: 120, 180, 240, 300, 360 mg ext-rel

    Cardizem LA initially 180-240 mg once daily; titrate at 2-week intervals; max 540 mg/day

        Pediatric: not recommended

        Tab: 120, 180, 240, 300, 360, 420 mg ext-rel

    Cardizem SR initially 60-120 mg bid; adjust at 2-week intervals; max 360 mg/day

        Pediatric: not recommended

        Cap: 60, 90, 120 mg sust-rel

▷ *nifedipine* (C)(G)

  Pediatric: not recommended

    Adalat initially 10 mg tid; usual range 10-20 mg tid; max 180 mg/day

        Cap: 10, 20 mg

    Procardia initially 10 mg tid; titrate over 7-14 days: max 30 mg/dose and 180 mg/day in divided doses

        Cap: 10, 20 mg

    Procardia XL initially 30-60 mg daily; titrate over 7-14 days; max 90 mg/day in divided doses

▷ *verapamil* (C)(G)

  Pediatric: not recommended

    Calan 80-120 mg tid; increase daily <u>or</u> weekly if needed

        Tab: 40, 80*, 120*mg

    Covera HS initially 180 mg q HS; titrate in steps to 240 mg; then to 360 mg; then to 480 mg if needed

        Tab: 180, 240 mg ext-rel

    Isoptin initially 80-120 mg tid

        Tab: 40, 80, 120 mg

Isoptin SR initially 120-180 mg in the AM; may increase to 240 mg in the AM; then, 180 mg q 12 hours <u>or</u> 240 mg in the AM and 120 mg in the PM; then, 240 mg q 12 hours
Tab: 120, 180*, 240*mg sust-rel

Tricyclic Antidepressants (TCAs)

Comment: Co-administration of TCAs with SSRIs requires extreme caution.
▷ *amitriptyline* (C)(G) 10-20 mg q HS
Pediatric: not recommended
Tab: 10, 25, 50, 75, 100, 150 mg
▷ *doxepin* (C)(G) 10-200 mg q HS
Pediatric: not recommended
Cap: 10, 25, 50, 75, 100, 150 mg; *Oral conc:* 10 mg/ml (4 oz w. dropper)
▷ *imipramine* (C)(G) 10-200 mg q HS
Tofranil 25-50 mg; max 200 mg/day; if maintenance dose exceeds 75 mg daily, may switch to **Tofranil PM**
Pediatric: <6 years: not recommended; 6-12 years: initially 25 mg; >12 years: 50 mg max 2.5 mg/kg/day
Tab: 10, 25, 50 mg
Tofranil PM initially 75 mg once daily 1 hour before HS; max 200 mg
Cap: 75, 100, 125, 150 mg
▷ *nortriptyline* (D)(G) 10-150 mg q HS
Pediatric: not recommended
Pamelor *Cap:* 10, 25, 50, 75 mg; *Oral soln:* 10 mg/5 ml (16 oz)

SSRI ANTIDEPRESSANTS

Comment: Co-administration of SSRIs with TCAs requires extreme caution. Concomitant use of MAOIs and SSRIs is absolutely contraindicated. Avoid other serotonergic drugs. A potentially fatal adverse event is Serotonin Syndrome, caused by serotonin excess. Milder symptoms require HCP intervention to avert severe symptoms which can be rapidly fatal without urgent/emergent medical care. Symptoms include restlessness, agitation, confusion, hallucinations, tachycardia, hypertension, dilated pupils, muscle twitching, muscle rigidity, loss of muscle coordination, diaphoresis, diarrhea, headache, shivering, piloerection, hyperpyrexia, cardiac arrhythmias, seizures, loss of consciousness, coma, death. Abrupt withdrawal or interruption of treatment with an antidepressant medication is sometimes associated with an Antidepressant Discontinuation Syndrome which may be mediated by gradually tapering the drug over a period of two weeks or longer, depending on the dose strength and length of treatment. Common symptoms of the Serotonin Discontinuation Syndrome include flu-like symptoms (nausea, vomiting, diarrhea, headaches, sweating), sleep disturbances (insomnia, nightmares, constant sleepiness), mood disturbances (dysphoria, anxiety, agitation), cognitive disturbances (mental confusion, hyperarousal), sensory and movement disturbances (imbalance, tremors, vertigo, dizziness, electric-shock-like sensations in the brain, often described by sufferers as "brain zaps."
▷ *fluoxetine* (C)(G)
Prozac initially 20 mg daily; may increase after 1 week; doses >20 mg/day may be divided into AM and noon doses; max 80 mg/day

Pediatric: <8 years: not recommended; 8-17 years: initially 10-20 mg/day; start lower weight children at 10 mg/day; if starting at 10 mg daily, may increase after 1 week to 20 mg once daily

Cap: 10, 20, 40 mg; *Tab:* 30*, 60*mg; *Oral soln:* 20 mg/5 ml (4 oz) (mint)

Prozac Weekly following daily fluoxetine therapy at 20 mg/day for 13 weeks, may initiate **Prozac Weekly** 7 days after the last 20 mg fluoxetine dose

Pediatric: not recommended

Cap: 90 mg ent-coat del-rel pellets

OTHER AGENTS

▷ *divalproex sodium* (D) *Delayed-release*: initially 250 mg bid; titrate weekly to usual max 500 mg bid; *Extended-release*: initially 500 mg once daily; may increase after one week to 1 g once daily

Pediatric: <10 years: not recommended; ≥10 years: same as adult

Depakene *Cap:* 250 mg del-rel; syr: 250 mg/5 ml (16 oz)

Depakote *Tab:* 125, 250, 500 mg del-rel

Depakote ER *Tab:* 250, 500 mg ext-rel

Depakote Sprinkle *Cap:* 125 mg del-rel

▷ *methysergide* (C) 4-8 mg daily in divided doses with food; max 8 mg/day; max 6 month treatment course; wean off over last 2-3 weeks of treatment course; separate treatment courses by 3-4 week drug-free interval

Sansert *Tab:* 2 mg

MAGNESIUM SUPPLEMENTS

▷ *magnesium* (B)

Slow-Mag 2 tabs daily

Tab: 64 mg (as chloride)/110 mg (as carbonate)

▷ *magnesium oxide* (B)

Mag-Ox 400 1-2 tabs daily

Tab: 400 mg

HEADACHE: TENSION (MUSCLE CONTRACTION HEADACHE)

Acetaminophen for IV Infusion *see Pain page* 306
Oral Prescription NSAIDs *see page* 501
Other Oral Analgesics *see Pain page* 308
Topical/Transdermal NSAIDs *see Pain page* 307
Parenteral Corticosteroids *see page* 511
Oral Corticosteroids *see page* 509
Topical Analgesic and Anesthetic Agents *see page* 499

TRICYCLIC ANTIDEPRESSANTS (TCAs)

Comment: Co-administration of TCAs with SSRIs requires extreme caution.

▷ *amitriptyline* (C)(G) 50-100 mg/day

Pediatric: not recommended

Tab: 10, 25, 50, 75, 100, 150 mg

▷ *desipramine* (C)(G) 50-100 mg bid
   Pediatric: not recommended
     Norpramin *Tab:* 10, 25, 50, 75, 100, 150 mg
▷ *imipramine* (C)(G)
   Pediatric: not recommended
     Tofranil initially 75 mg daily (max 200 mg); adolescents initially 30-40 mg daily
     (max 100 mg/day); if maintenance dose exceeds 75 mg daily, may switch to
     Tofranil PM for divided <u>or</u> bedtime dosing
       Tab: 10, 25, 50 mg
     Tofranil PM initially 75 mg once daily 1 hour before HS; max 200 mg
       Cap: 75, 100, 125, 150 mg
     Tofranil Injection 50 mg IM; lower dose for adolescents; switch to oral form as
     soon as possible
       Amp: 25 mg/2 ml (2 ml)
▷ *nortriptyline* (D)(G) 25-50 mg/day
   Pediatric: not recommended
     Pamelor *Cap:* 10, 25, 50, 75 mg; *Oral soln:* 10 mg/5 ml (16 oz)

ANALGESICS

▷ *butalbital/acetaminophen* (C)(G)
   Pediatric: <12 years: not recommended; ≥12 years: same as adult
     Phrenilin 1-2 tabs q 4 hours prn; max 6 tabs/day
       Tab: but 50 mg/acet 325 mg
     Phrenilin Forte 1 tab <u>or</u> cap q 4 hours prn; max 6 caps/day
       Cap/Tab: but 50 mg/acet 650 mg
▷ *butalbital/acetaminophen/caffeine* (C)(G)
   Pediatric: not recommended
     Fioricet 1-2 tabs q 4 hours prn; max 6/day
       Tab: but 50 mg/acet 325 mg/caf 40 mg
     Zebutal 1 cap q 4 hours prn; max 5/day
       Cap: but 50 mg/acet 500 mg/caf 40 mg
▷ *butalbital/acetaminophen/codeine/caffeine* (C)(III)(G)
   Pediatric: <12 years: not recommended
     Fioricet with Codeine 1-2 tabs at onset q 4 hours prn; max 6 tabs/day
       Tab: but 50 mg/acet 325 mg/cod 30 mg/caf 40 mg
▷ *butalbital/aspirin/caffeine* (C)(III)(G)
   Pediatric: <12 years: not recommended; ≥12 years: same as adult
     Fiorinal 1-2 tabs <u>or</u> caps q 4 hours prn; max 6 caps/tabs/day
       Tab/Cap: but 50 mg/asa 325 mg/caf 40 mg
▷ *butalbital/aspirin/codeine/caffeine* (C)(III)(G)
   Pediatric: <12 years: not recommended; ≥12 years: same as adult
     Fiorinal with Codeine 1-2 caps q 4 hours prn; max 6 caps/day
       Cap: but 50 mg/asp 325 mg/cod 30 mg/caf 40 mg
▷ *butorphanol tartrate* (C)(IV)(G) initially 1 spray (1 mg) in one nostril and may repeat after 60-90 minutes (*Elderly* 90-120 minutes) in opposite nostril if needed <u>or</u> 1
   spray in each nostril and may repeat q 3-4 hours prn
   Pediatric: <18 years: not recommended
     Butorphanol Nasal Spray *Nasal spray:* 1 mg/actuation (10 mg/ml, 2.5 ml)
     Stadol Nasal Spray *Nasal spray:* 10 mg/ml, 1 mg/actuation (10 mg/ml, 2.5 ml)

▷ *tramadol* (C)(IV)(G)

> **Rybix ODT** initially 100 mg once daily; may increase by 100 mg every 5 days; max 300 mg/day; *CrCl <30 mL/min* or *severe hepatic impairment*: not recommended; *Cirrhosis:* max 50 mg q 12 hours
>> *Pediatric:* <17 years: not recommended
>> *ODT:* 50 mg (mint) (phenylalanine)

> **Ryzolt**
>> *Pediatric:* <16 years: not recommended; ≥16 years: same as adult
>> *Tab:* 100, 200, 300 mg ext-rel

> **Ultram**
>> *Pediatric:* <16 years: not recommended; ≥16 years: same as adult
>> *Tab:* 50*mg

> **Ultram ER**
>> *Pediatric:* <18 years: not recommended
>> *Tab:* 100, 200, 300 mg ext-rel

▷ *tramadol/acetaminophen* (C)(IV)(G) 2 tabs q 4-6 hours prn; max 8 tabs/day; 5 days; *CrCl <30 mL/min:* max 2 tabs q 12 hours; max 4 tabs/day x 5 days; *Cirrhosis or other liver disease:* contraindicated

> *Pediatric:* <16 years: not recommended; ≥16 years: same as adult
>> **Ultracet** *Tab:* tram 37.5/acet 325 mg

Other Oral Analgesics *see* **Pain** *page* 308

MAGNESIUM SUPPLEMENTS

▷ *magnesium* (B)

> **Slow-Mag** 2 tabs daily
>> *Tab:* 64 mg (as chloride)/110 mg (as carbonate)

▷ *magnesium oxide* (B)

> **Mag-Ox 400** 1-2 tabs daily
>> *Tab:* 400 mg

HEART FAILURE (HF)

ACE INHIBITORS (ACEIs)

▷ *captopril* (C; D in 2nd, 3rd)(G) initially 25 mg tid; after 1-2 weeks may increase to 50 mg tid; max 450 mg/day

Pediatric: not recommended

> **Capoten** *Tab:* 12.5*, 25*, 50*, 100*mg

▷ *enalapril* (D) initially 5 mg daily; usual dosage range 10-40 mg/day; max 40 mg/day

Pediatric: not recommended

> **Epaned Oral Solution** *Oral soln:* 1mg/ml (150 ml) (mixed berry)
> **Vasotec** (G) *Tab:* 2.5*, 5*, 10, 20 mg

▷ *fosinopril* (C; D in 2nd, 3rd) initially 10 mg daily, usual maintenance 20-40 mg/day in a single or divided doses

Pediatric: <6 years, <50 kg: not recommended; 6-12 years, ≥50 kg: 5-10 mg daily; >12 years: same as adult

> **Monopril** *Tab:* 10*, 20, 40 mg

▷ *lisinopril* **(D)** initially 5 mg daily
    Prinivil initially 10 mg daily; usual range 20-40 mg/day
      Pediatric: not recommended
        Tab: 5*, 10*, 20*, 40 mg
    Qbrelis Oral Solution administer as a single dose once daily
      Pediatric: <6 years, GFR <30 mL/min: not recommended; ≥6 years, GFR >30
      mL/min: initially 0.07 mg/kg, max 5 mg; adjust according to BP up to a max
      0.61 mg/kg (40 mg) once daily
        Oral soln: 1 mg/ml (150 ml)
    Zestril initially 10 mg daily; usual range 20-40 mg/day
      Pediatric: not recommended
        Tab: 2.5, 5*, 10, 20, 30, 40 mg
▷ *quinapril* **(C; D in 2nd, 3rd)** initially 5 mg bid; increase weekly to 10-20 mg bid
  Pediatric: not recommended
    Accupril *Tab:* 5*, 10, 20, 40 mg
▷ *ramipril* **(C; D in 2nd, 3rd)** initially 2.5 mg bid; usual maintenance 5 mg bid
  Pediatric: not recommended
    Altace *Tab/Cap:* 1.25, 2.5, 5, 10 mg
▷ *trandolapril* **(C; D in 2nd, 3rd)** initially 1 mg daily; titrate to dose of 4 mg daily as
tolerated
  Pediatric: not recommended
    Mavik *Tab:* 1*, 2, 4 mg

BETA-BLOCKERS (CARDIOSELECTIVE)

▷ *carvedilol* **(C)**
    Coreg initially 3.125 mg bid; may increase at 1-2 week intervals to 12.5 mg bid;
    usual max 50 mg bid
      Pediatric: <18 years: not recommended
        Tab: 3.125, 6.25, 12.5, 25 mg
    Coreg CR initially 10 mg once daily x 2 weeks; may double dose at 2 week inter-
    vals; max 80 mg once daily; may open caps and sprinkle on food
      Pediatric: <18 years: not recommended
        Cap: 10, 20, 40, 80 mg cont-rel
▷ *metoprolol succinate* **(C)**
  Pediatric: not recommended
    Toprol-XL initially 12.5-25 mg in a single dose daily; increase weekly if needed;
    reduce if symptomatic bradycardia occurs; max 400 mg/day
      Tab: 25*, 50*, 100*, 200*mg ext-rel
▷ *metoprolol tartrate* **(C)**
  Pediatric: not recommended
    Lopressor (G) initially 25-50 mg bid; increase weekly if needed; max
    400 mg/day
      Tab: 25, 37.5, 50, 75, 100 mg

ANGIOTENSIN II RECEPTOR BLOCKERS (ARBs)

▷ *valsartan* **(C; D in 2nd, 3rd)** initially 40 mg bid; increase to 160 mg bid as tolerated
<u>or</u> 320 mg daily after 2-4 weeks; usual range 80-320 mg/day
  Pediatric: not recommended
    Diovan *Tab:* 40*, 80, 160, 320 mg

NEPRILYSIN INHIBITOR/ARB COMBINATION

➤ *sacubitril/valsartan* (D) initially 49/51 bid; double dose after 2-4 weeks; maintenance 97/103 bid; *GFR <30 mL/min* or *moderate hepatic impairment:* initially 24/26 bid; double dose every 2-4 weeks to target maintenance 97/103 bid
Pediatric: not established
    Entresto
      Tab: **Entresto 24/26:** *sacu* 24 mg/*val* 26 mg
             Entresto 49/51: *sacu* 49 mg/*val* 51 mg
             Entresto 97/103: *sacu* 97 mg/*val* 103 mg

ALDOSTERONE RECEPTOR BLOCKER

➤ *eplerenone* (B) initially 25 mg once daily; titrate within 4 weeks to 50 mg once daily; adjust dose based on serum K^+
Pediatric: not recommended
    Inspra *Tab:* 25, 50 mg
    Comment: Inspra is contraindicated with concomitant potent CYP3A4 inhibitors. Risk of hyperkalemia with concomitant ACEI or ARB. Monitor serum potassium at baseline, 1 week, and 1 month. Caution with serum *Cr >2 mg/dL* (male) or *>1.8 mg/dL* (female) and/or *CrCl <50 mL/min*, and DM with proteinuria.

THIAZIDE DIURETICS

Comment: Monitor hydration status, blood pressure, urine output, serum K^+.
➤ *chlorothiazide* (C)(G) 0.5-1 g/day in single or divided doses; max 2g/day
Pediatric: <6 months: up to 15 mg/lb/day in 2 divided doses; ≥6 months: 10 mg/lb/day in 2 divided doses
    Diuril *Tab:* 250*, 500*mg; *Oral susp:* 250 mg/5 ml (237 ml)
➤ *hydrochlorothiazide* (B)(G)
Pediatric: not recommended
    Esidrix 25-100 mg once daily
      Tab: 25, 50, 100 mg
    Microzide 12.5 mg daily; usual max 50 mg/day
      Cap: 12.5 mg
➤ *methyclothiazide/deserpidine* (B) initially 2.5 mg once daily; max 5 mg once daily
Pediatric: not recommended
    Enduronyl *Tab: methy* 5 mg/*deser* 0.25 mg*
    Enduronyl Forte *Tab: methy* 5 mg/*deser* 0.5 mg*
➤ *polythiazide* (C) 2-4 mg once daily
Pediatric: not recommended
    Renese *Tab:* 1, 2, 4 mg

POTASSIUM-SPARING DIURETICS

Comment: Monitor hydration status, blood pressure, urine output, serum K^+.
➤ *amiloride* (B) initially 5 mg once daily; may increase to 10 mg; max 20 mg
Pediatric: not recommended
    Midamor *Tab:* 5 mg
➤ *spironolactone* (D)(G) initially 50-100 mg in a single or divided doses; titrate at 2 week intervals

Pediatric: not established
> **Aldactone** *Tab:* 25, 50*, 100*mg

LOOP DIURETICS

Comment: Monitor hydration status, blood pressure, urine output, serum K+.
➤ *bumetanide* (C)(G) 0.5-2 mg as a single dose; may repeat at 4-5 hour intervals; max 10 mg/day
Pediatric: <18 years: not recommended
> **Bumex** *Tab:* 0.5*, 1*, 2*mg

Comment: *bumetanide* is contraindicated with sulfa drug allergy.
➤ *ethacrynic acid* (B)(G) initially 50-200 mg once daily
Pediatric: infants: not recommended; >1 month: initially 25 mg/day; then adjust dose in 25 mg increments
> **Edecrin** *Tab:* 25, 50 mg

➤ *ethacrynate sodium* (B)(G) for IV injection
> **Sodium Edecrin** *Vial:* 50 mg single-dose

Comment: **Sodium Edecrin** is more potent than more commonly used loop and thiazide diuretics.
➤ *furosemide* (C)(G) initially 40 mg bid
Pediatric: not recommended
> **Lasix** *Tab:* 20, 40*, 80 mg; *Oral soln:* 10 mg/ml (2, 4 oz w. dropper)

Comment: *furosemide* is contraindicated with sulfa drug allergy.
➤ *torsemide* (B) 5 mg once daily; may increase to 10 mg daily
Pediatric: not recommended
> **Demadex** *Tab:* 5*, 10*, 20*, 100*mg

OTHER DIURETICS

Comment: Monitor hydration status, blood pressure, urine output, serum K+.
➤ *indapamide* (B) initially 1.25 mg once daily; may titrate dosage upward every 4 weeks if needed; max 5 mg/day
> **Lozol** *Tab:* 1.25, 2.5 mg

Comment: *indapamide* is contraindicated with sulfa drug allergy.
➤ *metolazone* (B) 2.5-5 mg once daily
Pediatric: not recommended
> **Zaroxolyn** *Tab:* 2.5, 5, 10 mg

Comment: *metolazone* is contraindicated with sulfa drug allergy.

DIURETIC COMBINATIONS

Comment: Monitor hydration status, blood pressure, urine output, serum K+.
➤ *amiloride/hydrochlorothiazide* (B)(G) initially 1 tab once daily; may increase to 2 tabs/day in a single <u>or</u> divided doses
Pediatric: not recommended
> **Moduretic** *Tab:* amil 5 mg/hydro 50 mg*

➤ *spironolactone/hydrochlorothiazide* (D)(G)
Pediatric: not recommended
> **Aldactazide 25** usual maintenance 50-100 mg in a single <u>or</u> divided doses
> *Tab:* spiro 25 mg/hydro 25 mg
> **Aldactazide 50** usual maintenance 50-100 mg in a single <u>or</u> divided doses
> *Tab:* spiro 50 mg/hydro 50 mg

➤ *triamterene/hydrochlorothiazide* (C)(G)
    Pediatric: not recommended
        Dyazide 1-2 caps daily
            Cap: triam 37.5 mg/*hydro* 25 mg
        Maxzide 1 tab once daily
            Tab: triam 75 mg/*hydro* 50 mg*
        Maxzide-25 1-2 tabs once daily
            Tab: triam 37.5 mg/*hydro* 25 mg*

NITRATE/PERIPHERAL VASODILATOR COMBINATION

➤ *isosorbide dinitrate/hydralazine* (C) initially 1 tab tid; may reduce to 1/2 tab tid if not tolerated; titrate as tolerated after 3-5 days; max 2 tabs tid
    Pediatric: not recommended
        BiDil *Tab: isosor* 20 mg/*hydral* 37.5 mg
        Comment: **BiDil** is an adjunct to standard therapy in self-identified black persons to improve survival, to prolong time to hospitalization for heart failure, and to improve patient-reported functional status.

CARDIAC GLYCOSIDES

Comment: Therapeutic serum level of is 0.8-2 mcg/ml.
➤ *digoxin* (C)(G) 1-1.5 mg IM, IV, or PO in divided doses over 1-3 days as a loading dose; usual maintenance 0.125-0.5 mg/day
    Pediatric: Total oral pediatric digitalizing dose (in 24 hours): <2 years: 40-50 mcg/kg; 2-10 years: 30-40 mcg/kg; >10 years: 0.75-1.5 mg; *Daily oral pediatric maintenance dose (single-dose):* <2 years: 10-12 mcg/kg; 2-10 years: 8-10 mcg/kg; >10 years: 0.125–0.5 mg
    Comment: For more information on the use of digoxin in pediatric heart failure, see **Jain, S. & Vaidyanathan B.** Ann Pediatr Cardiol. 2009 Jul-Dec; 2(2): 149–152.
        Lanoxicaps
            Pediatric: <10 years: use elixir or parenteral form
            Cap: 0.05, 0.1, 0.2 mg soln-filled (alcohol)
        Lanoxin
            Pediatric: <10 years: use elixir or parenteral form
            Tab: 0.0625, 0.125*, 0.1875, 0.25*mg; *Elix:* 0.05 mg/ml (2 oz w. dropper) (lime) (alcohol 10%)
        Lanoxin Injection *Amp:* 0.25 mg/ml (2 ml)
        Lanoxin Injection Pediatric *Amp:* 0.1 mg/ml (1 ml)

OTHER

➤ *ivabradine* (D) initially 5 mg bid with food; assess after 2 weeks and adjust dose to achieve a resting heart rate 50-60 bpm; thereafter, adjust dose as needed based on resting heart rate and tolerability; max 7.5 mg bid; in patients with a history of conduction defects, or for whom bradycardia could lead to hemodynamic compromise, initiate at 2.5 mg bid before increasing the dose based on heart rate
    Pediatric: <18 years: not established
        Corlanor *Tab:* 5, 7.5 mg
        Comment: **Corlanor** is indicated to reduce the risk of hospitalization for worsening heart failure inpatients with stable, symptomatic, chronic heart failure with left ventricular ejection fraction (LVEF) ≤35%, who are in sinus

rhythm with resting heart rate ≤70 bpm and either are on maximally tolerated doses of beta-blockers or have a contraindication to beta-blocker use. **Corlanor** is contraindicated with acute decompensated heart failure, BP <90/50, sick sinus syndrome (SSS), sinoatrial block, and 3rd degree AV block (unless patient has a functioning demand pacemaker). **Corlanor** may cause fetal toxicity when administered pregnant women based on embryo-fetal toxicity and cardiac teratogenic to effects observed in animal studies. Therefore, females should be advised to use effective contraception when taking this drug.

 ## HELICOBACTER PYLORI (H. PYLORI) INFECTION

ERADICATION REGIMENS

Comment: There are many H2 receptor blocker-based and PPI-based treatment regimens suggested in the professional literature for the eradication of the *H. pylori* organism and subsequent ulcer healing. Generally, regimens range from 10-14 days for eradication and 2-6 more weeks of continued gastric acid suppression. A three- or four-antibiotic combination may increase treatment effectiveness and decrease the likelihood of resistant strain emergence. Empirical treatment is not recommended. Diagnosis should be confirmed before treatment is started. Antibiotic choices include *doxycycline, tetracycline, amoxicillin, amoxicillin/clavulanate, clarithromycin, clindamycin*, and *metronidazole*. Follow-up visits are recommended at 2 and 6 weeks to evaluate treatment outcomes.

➤ **Regimen 1: Helidac Therapy (D)** *bismuth subsalicylate* 525 mg qid + *tetracycline* 500 mg qid + *metronidazole* 250 mg qid x 14 days
Pediatric: not recommended
Pack: bismuth subsalicylate chew tab: 262.4 mg (112/pck); *tetracycline cap:* 500 mg (56/pck); *metronidazole Tab:* 250 mg (56/pck)

➤ **Regimen 2: PrevPac (D)(G)** *amoxicillin* 500 mg 2 caps bid + *lansoprazole* 30 mg bid + *clarithromycin* 500 mg bid x 14 days (one card per day)
Pediatric: not recommended
Kit: lansoprazole cap: 30 mg (2/card); *amoxicillin cap:* 500 mg (4/card); *clarithromycin tab:* 500 mg (2/card) (14 daily cards/carton)

➤ **Regimen 3: Pylera (D)** take 3 caps qid after meals and at bedtime x 10 days; take with 8 oz water plus *omeprazole* 20 mg bid, with breakfast and dinner, for 10 days
Pediatric: not recommended
Cap: bismuth subsalicylate 140 mg/*tetracycline* 125 mg/*metronidazole* 125 mg (120 caps)
Comment: *omeprazole* not included with Pylera.

➤ **Regimen 4: Omeclamox-Pak (C)** *omeprazole* 20 mg bid + *amoxicillin* 1000 bid + *clarithromycin* 500 mg bid x 10 days
Kit: omeprazole cap: 20 mg (2/pck); *amoxicillin cap:* 500 mg (4/pck); *clarithromycin tab:* 500 mg (2/pck) (10 pcks/carton)

➤ **Regimen 5: (C)** *omeprazole* 40 mg daily + *clarithromycin* 500 mg tid x 2 weeks; then continue *omeprazole* 10-40 mg daily x 6 more weeks

➤ **Regimen 6: (B)** *lansoprazole* 30 mg tid + *amoxicillin* 1 g tid x 10 days; then continue *lansoprazole* 15-30 mg daily x 6 more weeks

➤ **Regimen 7: (C)** *omeprazole* 40 mg daily + *amoxicillin* 1 g bid + *clarithromycin* 500 mg bid x 10 days; then continue *omeprazole* 10-40 mg daily x 6 more weeks

➤ **Regimen 8: (D)** *bismuth subsalicylate* 525 mg qid + *metronidazole* 250 mg qid + *tetracycline* 500 mg qid + H2 receptor agonist x 2 weeks; then continue H2 receptor agonist x 6 more weeks

▷ **Regimen 9:** (not for use in 1st; B in 2nd, 3rd) *bismuth subsalicylate* 525 mg qid + *metronidazole* 250 mg qid + *amoxicillin 500 mg qid + H2 receptor agonist x 2 weeks; then continue H2 receptor agonist x 6 more weeks* receptor agonist x 2 weeks; then continue H2 receptor agonist x 6 more weeks

▷ **Regimen 10:** (C) *ranitidine bismuth citrate* 400 mg bid + *clarithromycin* 500 mg bid x 2 weeks; then continue *ranitidine bismuth citrate* 400 mg bid x 2 more weeks

▷ **Regimen 11:** (D) *omeprazole* 20 mg or *lansoprazole* 30 mg q AM + *bismuth subsalicylate* 524 mg qid + *metronidazole* 500 mg tid + *tetracycline* 500 mg qid x 2 weeks; then continue *omeprazole* 20 mg or *lansoprazole* 30 mg q AM for 6 more weeks

◯ HEMORRHOIDS

▷ *dibucaine* (C)(OTC)(G) 1 applicatorful or suppository bid and after each stool; max 6/day
Pediatric: not recommended
  Nupercainal (OTC) *Rectal oint:* 1% (30, 60 g); *Rectal supp:* 1% (12, 14/pck)
▷ *hydrocortisone* (C)(OTC)(G)
Pediatric: not recommended
  Anusol-HC 1 suppository rectally bid-tid or 2 suppositories bid x 2 weeks
    Rectal supp: 25 mg (12, 24/pck)
  Anusol-HC Cream 2.5% apply bid-qid prn
    Rectal crm: 2.5% (30 g)
  Anusol HC-1 apply tid-qid prn; max 7 days
    Rectal crm: 1% (0.7 oz)
  Hydrocortisone Rectal Cream
    Rectal crm: 1, 2.5% (30 g)
  Nupercainal apply tid-qid prn
    Rectal crm: 1% (30 g)
  Proctocort 1 suppository rectally bid-tid prn or 2 suppositories bid
  x 2 weeks
    Rectal supp: 30 mg (12/pck)
  Proctocream HC 2.5% apply rectally bid-qid prn
    Rectal crm: 2.5% (30 g)
  Proctofoam HC 1% apply rectally tid-qid prn
    Rectal foam: 1% (14 applications/10 g)
▷ *hydrocortisone/pramoxine* (C) 1 applicatorful tid-qid and after each stool; max 2 weeks
Pediatric: not recommended
  Procort *Rectal crm: hydro* 1.85%/*pramox* 1.15% (30 g)
▷ *hydrocortisone/lidocaine* (B) apply bid-tid prn
Pediatric: not recommended
  AnaMantle HC, LidaMantle HC *Crm/Lotn: hydrocort* 5%/*lido* 3% (1 oz)
▷ *petrolatum/mineral oil/shark liver oil/phenylephrine* (C)(OTC)(G)
  Preparation H Ointment apply up to qid prn
    Rectal oint: 1, 2 oz
▷ *petrolatum/glycerin/shark liver oil/phenylephrine* (C)(OTC)(G)
  Preparation H Cream apply up to qid prn
    Rectal crm: 0.9, 1.8 oz
▷ *phenylephrine/cocoa butter/shark liver oil* (C)(OTC)(G)
  Preparation H Suppositories 1 suppository or 1 application of rectal ointment
  or cream, up to qid

> *Rectal supp:* phenyle 0.25%/*cocoa* 85.5%/*shark* 3% (12, 24, 45/pck); *Rectal oint:* phenyle 0.25%/*petro* 1.9%/*mineral oil* 14%/*shark liv* 3% (1, 2 oz); *Rectal crm:* phenyle 0.25%/*petro* 18%/*gly* 12%/*shark liv* 3% (0.9, 1.8 oz)

➤ *witch hazel* topical solution/gel **(NE)(OTC)**
> **Tucks** apply up to 6 x/day; leave on x 5-15 minutes
> > *Pad:* 12, 40, 100/pck; *Gel:* 19.8 g

➤ *lidocaine* 3% cream **(B)** apply bid-tid prn
> *Pediatric:* reduce dosage commensurate with age, body weight, and physical condition
> > **LidaMantle** *Crm:* 3% (1 oz)

Bulk-forming Agents, Stool Softeners, and Stimulant Laxatives *see* **Constipation** *page* 97

⬤ HEPATITIS A (HAV)

Comment: Administer a 2-dose series. Schedule first immunization at least 2 weeks before expected exposure. Booster dose recommended 6-12 months later. Under 1 year-of-age administer in the vastus lateralis; over 1 year-of-age administer in deltoid.

PROPHYLAXIS (HEPATITIS A)

➤ *hepatitis A vaccine, inactivated* **(C)**
> **Havrix** 1,440 El.U IM; repeat in 6-12 months
> > *Pediatric:* <2 years: not recommended; 2-18 years: 720 El.U IM; repeat in 6-12 months or 360 El.U IM; repeat in 1 month
> **Vaqta** 25 U (1 ml) IM; repeat in 6 months
> > *Pediatric:* <2 years: not recommended; 2-18 years: 0.5 ml IM; repeat in 6-18 months
> > *Vial:* 25 U/ml single-dose (preservative-free); *Prefilled syringe:* 25 U/ml, (0.5, 1 ml single-dose)

PROPHYLAXIS (HEPATITIS A AND B COMBINATION)

➤ *hepatitis A inactivated/hepatitis B surface antigen (recombinant vaccine)* (C)
> *Pediatric:* <18 years: not recommended
> **Twinrix** 1 ml IM in deltoid; repeat in 1 month and 6 months
> > *Vial (soln): hepatitis A* inactivated 720 IU/*hepatitis B* surface antigen (recombinant) 20 mcg/ml (1, 10 ml); *Prefilled syringe: hepatitis A* inactivated 720 IU/*hepatitis B* surface antigen (recombinant) 20 mcg/ml

⬤ HEPATITIS B (HBV)

PROPHYLAXIS (HEPATITIS B)

Comment: Administer IM; under 1 year-of-age, administer in vastus lateralis. Over 1 year-of-age, administer in the deltoid. Administer a 3-dose series; *First dose:* newborn (or now); *Second dose:* 1-2 months after first dose; *Third dose:* 6 months after first dose.

➤ *hepatitis B recombinant vaccine* (C)
> **Engerix-B Adult** 20 mcg (1 ml) IM; repeat in 1 and 6 months
> > *Pediatric:* infant-19 years: 10 mcg (1/2 ml) IM; repeat in 1 and 6 months
> > *Vial:* 20 mcg/ml single-dose (preservative-free, thimerosal); *Prefilled syringe:* 20 mcg/ml

Engerix-B Pediatric/Adolescent
> *Pediatric:* infant-19 years: 10 mcg IM; repeat in 1 and 6 months; *Vial:* 10 mcg/0.5 ml single-dose (preservative-free, thimerosal)
> *Prefilled syringe:* 10 mcg/0.5 ml

Recombivax HB Adult 10 mcg (1 ml) IM in deltoid; repeat in 1 and 6 months
> *Vial:* 10 mcg/ml single-dose; *Vial:* 10 mcg/3 ml multi-dose

Recombivax HB Pediatric/Adolescent 5 mcg (0.5 ml) IM; repeat in 1 and 6 months
> *Pediatric:* birth-19 years: 5 mcg (0.5 ml) IM; repeat in 1 and 6 months; >19 years: use adult formulation or 10 mcg (1 ml) pediatric/adolescent formulation
> *Vial:* 5 mcg/0.5 ml single-dose

PROPHYLAXIS (HEPATITIS A AND B COMBINATION)

Comment: Administer IM; under 1 year-of-age, administer in vastus lateralis. Over 1 year-of-age, administer in the deltoid. Administer a 3-dose series; *First dose:* newborn (or now); *Second dose:* 1-2 months after first dose; *Third dose:* 6 months after first dose.

▷ *hepatitis A inactivated/hepatitis B surface antigen (recombinant) vaccine* (C)
> *Pediatric:* <18 years: not recommended
> **Twinrix** 1 ml IM in deltoid; repeat in 1 months and 6 months
> > *Vial (soln): hepatitis A* inactivated 720 IU/*hepatitis B* surface antigen (recombinant) 20 mcg/ml (1, 10 ml); *Prefilled syringe: hepatitis A* inactivated 720 IU/*hepatitis B* surface antigen (recombinant) 20 mcg/ml

CHRONIC HBV INFECTION TREATMENT

Nucleoside Analogs (Reverse Transcriptase Inhibitors and HBV Polymerase Inhibitors)

Comment: Nucleoside analogs are indicated for chronic hepatitis infection with viral replication and either elevated ALT/AST or histologically active disease.

▷ *adefovir dipivoxil* (C)(G) 10 mg daily; *CrCl 20-49 mL/min:* 10 mg q 48 hours; *CrCl 10-19 mL/min:* 10 mg q 72 hours
> *Pediatric:* not recommended
> **Hepsera** *Tab:* 10 mg

▷ *entecavir* (C)(G) take on an empty stomach
> *Nucleoside naïve:* 0.5 mg daily; *Nucleoside naïve, CrCl 30-49 mL/min:* 0.25 mg daily; *Nucleoside naïve, CrCl 10-29 mL/min:* 0.15 mg daily; *Nucleoside naïve, CrCl <10 mL/min:* 0.05 mg daily; *lamivudine-refractory:* 1 mg daily; *lamivudine-refractory, renal impairment:* see mfr pkg insert
> > *Pediatric:* <16 years: not recommended
> **Baraclude** *Tab:* 0.5, 1 mg; *Oral Soln:* 0.05 mg/ml (orange; parabens)

▷ *lamivudine* (C)(G) 100 mg daily; *CrCl <5 mL/min:* 35 mg for 1st dose, then 10 mg once daily; *CrCl 5-14 mL/min:* 35 mg for 1st dose, then 15 mg once daily; *CrCl 15-29 mL/min:* 100 mg for 1st dose, then 25 mg once daily; *CrCl 30-49 mL/min:* 100 mg for 1st dose, then 50 mg once daily
> *Pediatric:* <2 years: not recommended; 2-17 years: 3 mg/kg (max 100 mg) once daily
> **Epivir-HBV** *Tab:* 100 mg
> **Epivir-HBV Oral Solution** *Oral Soln:* 5 mg/ml (240 ml) (strawberry-banana)

▷ *telbivudine* (C) 600 mg daily; *CrCl <40 mL/min:* 600 mg q 72 hours; *CrCl 30-49 mL/min:* 600 mg q 48 hours
> *Pediatric:* <16 years: not recommended
> **Tyzeka** *Tab:* 600 mg

➤ *tenofovir alafenamide (TAF)* **(C)** take with food; take 1 tab once daily with concomitant carbamazepine 2 tablets
Pediatric: <18 years: not established
> **Vemlidy** *Tab:* 25 mg
>
> Comment: No dosage adjustment of **Vemlidy** is required in patients with mild hepatic impairment (Child-Pugh A). The safety and efficacy of **Vemlidy** in patients with decompensated cirrhosis (Child-Pugh B or C) have not been established; therefore **Vemlidy** is not recommended in patients with decompensated (Child-Pugh B or C) hepatic impairment, Healthcare providers are encouraged to register patients by calling the Antiretroviral Pregnancy Registry (APR) at 1-800-258-4263.

Interferon Alpha

➤ *interferon alfa-2b* **(C)** 5 million IU SC or IM daily or 10 million IU SC or IM 3 times/week x 16 weeks; reduce dose by half or interrupt dose if WBCs, granulocyte count, or platelet count decreases
Pediatric: <1 year: not recommended; >1 year: 3 million IU/m^2 3 times/week x 1 week; then increase to 6 million IU/m^2 3 times/week to 16-24 weeks; max 10 million IU/dose; reduce dose by half or interrupt dose if WBCs, granulocyte count, or platelet count decreases
> **Intron A** *Vial (pwdr):* 5, 10, 18, 25, 50 million IU/vial (pwdr + diluent; single-dose) (benzoyl alcohol); *Vial (soln):* 3, 5, 10 million IU/vial (single-dose); *Multi-dose vials (soln):* 18, 25 million IU/vial soln; *Multi-dose pens (soln):* 3, 5, 10 million IU/0.2 ml (6 doses/pen)

◯ HEPATITIS C (HCV)

CHRONIC HCV INFECTION TREATMENT

Nucleoside Analogs (Reverse Transcriptase Inhibitors)

Comment: Nucleoside analogs are indicated for patients with compensated liver disease previously untreated with *alpha interferon* or who have relapsed after *alpha interferon* therapy. Primary toxicity is hemolytic anemia. Contraindicated in male partners of pregnant women; use 2 forms of contraception during therapy and for 6 months after discontinuation.

➤ *ribavirin* **(X)(G)** take with food in 2 divided doses; *Genotype 2, 3:* 800 mg/day x 24 weeks; *Genotype 1, 4, <75 kg:* 1 gm/day x 48 weeks; ≥75 km 1.2 gm/day x 48 weeks; *HIV co-infection:* 800 mg/day x 48 weeks; *CrCl 30-50 mL/min:* alternate 200 mg and 400 mg every other day; *CrCl <30 mL/min or hemodialysis:* reduce dose or discontinue if hematologic abnormalities occur
Pediatric: <5 years: not established; ≥5-<18 years: 23-33 kg: 400 mg/day; 34-46 kg: 600 mg/day; 47-59 kg: 800 mg/day; 60-75 kg: 1 gm/day; 1.2 gm/day; ≥75 kg: *Genotype 2, 3:* treat for 24 weeks; *Genotype 1, 4:* treat for 48 weeks; reduce dose or discontinue if hematologic abnormalities occur; ≥18 years: same as adult
> **Copegus** *Tab:* 200 mg
> **Rebetol** *Cap:* 200mg
> **Rebetol Oral Solution** *Oral soln:* 40 mg/ml (120 ml) (bubble gum)
> **Ribashere RibaPak 600 mg** *Tab:* 600 mg (14/pck)

Interferon Alpha

▷ *interferon alfacon-1* (C)
  Pediatric: <18 years: not recommended
    Infergen 9 mcg SC 3 times/week x 24 weeks, then 15 mcg SC 3 times/week x 6
    months; allow at least 48 hours between doses
      Vial (soln): 9, 15 mcg/vial soln (6-single dose/pck; preservative-free)
▷ *interferon alfa-2b* (C)
    Intron A *Vial (pwdr):* 5, 10, 18, 25, 50 million IU/vial (pwdr w. diluent; sin-
    gle-dose) (benzoyl alcohol); *Vial (soln):* 3, 5, 10 million IU/vial (single-dose);
    Multi-dose vials (soln): 18, 25 million IU/vial; *Multi-dose pens (soln):* 3, 5, 10
    million IU/0.2 ml (6 doses/pen)
▷ *peginterferon alfa-2a* (C) administer 180 mcg SC once weekly (on the same day of
  the week); treat for 48 weeks; consider discontinuing if adequate response after 12-
  24 weeks
  Pediatric: <18 years: not recommended
    PEGasys *Vial:* 180 mcg/ml (single-dose); *Monthly pck (vials):* 180 mcg/ml (1 ml,
    4/pck)
▷ *peginterferon alfa-2b* (C) administer SC once weekly (on the same day of the week);
  treat for 1 year; consider discontinuing if inadequate response after 24 weeks; 37-45
  kg: 40 mcg (100 mg/ml, 0.4 ml); 46-56 kg: 50 mcg (100 mg/ml, 0.5 ml); 57-72 kg: 64
  mcg (160 mg/ml, 0.4 ml); 73-88 kg: 80 mcg (160 mg/ml, 0.5 ml); 89-106 kg: 96 mcg
  (240 mg/ml, 0.4 ml); 107-136 kg: 120 mcg (240 mg/ml, 0.5 ml); 137-160 kg: 150 mcg
  (300 mg/ml, 0.5 ml)
  Pediatric: <18 years: not recommended
    PEG-Intron *Vial:* 50, 80, 120, 150 mcg/ml (single-dose)
    PEG-Intron Redipen *Pen:* 50, 80, 120, 150 mcg/ml (disposable pens)

HCV NS5A Inhibitor

▷ *daclatasvir* (X) 60 mg once daily for 12 weeks (with *sofosbuvir*); if *sofosbuvir* is discontinued, daclatasvir should also be discontinued; with concomitant CY3P inhibitors, reduce dose to 30 mg once daily; with concomitant CY3P inducers, increase
  dose to 90 mg once daily
    Daklinza *Tab:* 30, 60 mg
    Comment: **Daklinza** is indicated in combination with *sofosbuvir* with or
    without *ribavirin*, for the treatment of HCV genotypes 1 and 3, and in patients
    with co-morbid HIV-1 infection, advanced cirrhosis, or post-liver transplant
    recurrence of HCV.

HCV NS5A Inhibitor/HCV NS3/4A Protease Inhibitor Combinations

▷ *elbasvir/grazoprevir* (NE) 1 tab as a single dose once daily; see mfr pkg insert for
  length of treatment
  Pediatric: <18 years: not recommended
    Zepatier *Tab:* elba 50 mg/grazo 100/mg
    Comment: **Zepatier** is contraindicated with moderate or severe hepatic
    impairment, concomitant *azanavir*, *carbamazepine*, *cyclosporine*, *darunavir*,
    efavirenz, *lopinavir, phenatoin, rifampin, saquinavir*, St. John's wort, *tipranavir*.
    When co-administered with *ribavirin*, pregnancy category (X)

HCV NS5A Inhibitor/HCV NS3/4A Protease Inhibitor/ CYP3A Inhibitor Combinations

▷ *ombitasvir/paritaprevir/ritonavir* (B) take 2 tabs once daily in the AM x 12 weeks
Pediatric: <18 years: not established
> **Technivie** *Tab:* omvi 25 mg/pari 75 mg/rito 50 mg (4 x 7 daily dose pcks/carton)
> Comment: **Technivie** is indicated for use in chronic HCV genotype 4 without cirrhosis. **Technivie** is not for use with moderate hepatic impairment.

HCV NS3/4A Protease Inhibitor Combinations

▷ *boceprevir* (C) 800 mg 3 times/day; take with food (not low-fat); not for monotherapy; start after 4 weeks therapy with *peginterferon* and discontinue if HCV-RNA levels indicate futility *ribavirin*; *Without cirrhosis:* continue as indicated by HCV-RNA levels at weeks 8, 12, and 24; *With cirrhosis:* continue for 44 weeks; do not reduce dose
Pediatric: <18 years: not recommended
> **Victrelis** *Cap:* 200 mg
▷ *simeprevir* (C) 150 mg once daily; swallow whole; take with food, not for monotherapy; do not reduce dose or interrupt therapy; if discontinued, do not reinitiate; discontinue if HCV-RNA levels indicate futility; discontinue if *peginterferon, ribavirin,* or *sofobuvir* is permanently discontinued; *Treatment naïve, treatment relapses, with or without cirrhosis:* treat x 12 weeks (*simeprevir + peginterferon + ribavirin*) followed by additional 12 weeks *peginterferon + ribavirin* (total = 24 weeks). *Partial and non-responders, with or without cirrhosis:* treat x 12 weeks (*simeprevir + peginterferon + ribavirin*) followed by additional 36 weeks *peginterferon + ribavirin* (total = 48 weeks); *Treatment naïve or treatment experienced without cirrhosis:* treat x 12 weeks (*simeprevir + sofobuvir*); *Treatment naïve or treatment experienced with cirrhosis:* treat x 24 weeks (*simeprevir + sofobuvir*)
> **Olysio** *Cap:* 150 mg

HCV NS5A Inhibitor/HCV NS5B Polymerase Inhibitor Combinations

▷ *ledipasvir/sofosbuvir* (NE) *Treatment naïve, without cirrhosis, with pretreatment HCV RNA <6 million IU/ml:* 1 tab daily x 8 weeks; *Treatment naïve with or without cirrhosis or treatment-experienced without cirrhosis:* 1 tab daily x 12 weeks; *Treatment-experienced with cirrhosis:* 1 tab daily x 24 weeks; *In combination with ribavirin:* 1 tab daily x 12 weeks
Pediatric: <18 years: not established
> **Harvoni** *Tab:* ledi 90 mg/sofo 400 mg
> Comment: **Harvoni** is indicated for patients with advanced liver disease, genotytpe 1, 4, 5, or 6 infection: chronic HCV genotype 1- or 4-infected liver transplant recipients with or without cirrhosis or with compensated cirrhosis (Child-Pugh A), and for HCV genotype 1-infected patients with decompensated cirrhosis (Child-Pugh B/C), including those who have undergone liver transplantation. No adequate human data are available to establish whether or not **Harvoni** poses a risk to pregnancy outcomes; the background risk of major birth defects and miscarriage for the indicated population is unknown. If **Harvoni** is administered with *ribavirin*, the combination regimen is contraindicated (**X**) in pregnant women and in men whose female partners are pregnant. It is not known whether **Harvoni** and its metabolites are present in human breast milk, affect human milk production

<u>or</u> have effects on the breastfed infant. If **Harvoni** is administered with *ribavirin*, the nursing mother's information for *ribavirin* also applies to this combination regimen.

▷ *sofosbuvir/velpatasvir* (NE) *Without cirrhosis or compensated cirrhosis* (*Child-Pug A*): 1 tablet daily x 12 weeks; *Decompensated cirrhosis* (*Child Pugh B or C*): 1 tablet daily <u>plus</u> *ribavirin* (RBV)
Pediatric: <18 years: not established
    Epclusa *Tab: sofo* 400 mg/*velpa* 100 mg
    Comment: **Epclusa** is indicated for patients with chronic HCV with genotytpe 1, 2, 3, 4, 5, <u>or</u> 6 infection.

HCV NS5A Inhibitor/HCV NS3/4A Protease Inhibitor/CYP3A Inhibitor Combination

▷ *sofosbuvir/velpatasvir* (B) 1 tab daily
Pediatric: not established
    Viekira XR *Tab: dasa* 200 mg/*omvi* 8.33 mg/*pari* 50 mg/*rito* 33.33 mg ext-rel (4 weekly cartons, each containing 7 daily dose packs/carton)
    Comment: **Viekira XR** is indicated for HCV genotype 1 with mild liver dysfunction (Child-Pugh A). **Viekira XR** is contraindicated for moderate (Child-Pugh B) to severe (Child-Pugh C) liver dysfunction. No adjustment is recommended with mild, moderate, <u>or</u> severe renal dysfunction.

HCV NS5A Inhibitor/HCV NS3/4A Protease Inhibitor/CYP3A Inhibitor <u>PLUS</u> HCV NS5B Polymerase Inhibitor Combination

▷ *ombitasvir/paritaprevir/ritonavir* <u>plus</u> *dasabuvir* (B)
Pediatric: not established
    Viekira Pak *ombitasvir/paritaprevir/ritonavir* fixed-dose combination tablet: 2 tablets orally once a day (in the morning); *dasabuvir*: 250 mg orally twice a day (morning and evening)
    Tab: omvi 12.5 mg/*pari* 75 mg/*rito* 50 mg <u>plus</u> *Tab: dasa* 250 mg (28 day supply/pck)
    Comment: **Viekira Pak** is indicated for mild liver dysfunction (Child-Pugh A). **Viekira Pak** is contraindicated for moderate (Child-Pugh B) to severe (Child-Pugh C) liver dysfunction. No adjustment is recommended with mild, <u>or</u> severe renal dysfunction.

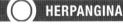

HERPANGINA

ANALGESICS

▷ *acetaminophen* (B) *see Fever page* 143
▷ *tramadol* (C)(IV)(G)
    Rybix ODT initially 100 mg once daily; may increase by 100 mg every 5 days; max 300 mg/day; *CrCl <30 mL/min* <u>or</u> *severe hepatic impairment:* not recommended; *Cirrhosis:* max 50 mg q 12 hours
    Pediatric: <17 years: not recommended
    ODT: 50 mg (mint) (phenylalanine)
    Ryzolt initially 100 mg once daily; may increase by 100 mg every 5 days; max 300 mg/day; *CrCl <40 mL/min* <u>or</u> *severe hepatic impairment:* not recommended
    Pediatric: <16 years: not recommended; ≥16 years: same as adult

  Tab: 100, 200, 300 mg ext-rel
 Ultram 50-100 mg q 4-6 hours prn; max 400 mg/day; *CrCl <40 mL/min:* max 100 mg q 12 hours; *Cirrhosis:* max 50 mg q 12 hours
  Pediatric: <16 years: not recommended; ≥16 years: same as adult
  Tab: 50*mg
 Ultram ER initially 100 mg once daily; may increase by 100 mg every 5 days; max 300 mg/day; *CrCl <40 mL/min* or *severe hepatic impairment:* not recommended
  Pediatric: <18 years: not recommended
  Tab: 100, 200, 300 mg ext-rel

▷ *tramadol/acetaminophen* **(C)(IV)(G)** 2 tabs q 4-6 hours; max 8 tabs/day; 5 days; *CrCl <40 mL/min:* max 2 tabs q 12 hours; max 4 tabs/day x 5 days
 Pediatric: <16 years: not recommended; ≥16 years: same as adult
  Ultracet *Tab:* tram 37.5/acet 325 mg

Other Oral Analgesics *see Pain page 308*

TOPICAL ANESTHETICS

▷ *lidocaine* viscous soln **(B)** 15 ml gargle or mouthwash; repeat after 3 hours; max 8 doses/day
 Pediatric: <4 years: apply 1.25 ml to affected area with cotton-tipped applicator; may repeat after 3 hours; max 8 doses/day
  Xylocaine 2% Viscous Solution *Viscous soln:* 2% (20, 100, 450 ml)
  Antipyretics *see Fever page 143*

◯ HERPES GENITALIS (HSV TYPE II)

Comment: The following treatment regimens are published in the **2015 CDC Sexually Transmitted Diseases Treatment Guidelines**. Treatment regimens are for adults only; consult a specialist for treatment of patients less than 18 years-of-age. Treatment regimens are presented in alphabetical order by generic drug name, followed by brands and dose forms.

RECOMMENDED REGIMENS: FIRST CLINICAL EPISODE

Regimen 1

▷ *acyclovir* 400 mg tid x 7-10 days or 200 mg 5 times/day x 10 days or until clinically resolved

Regimen 2

▷ *acyclovir* cream apply q 3 hours 6 x/day x 7 days

Regimen 3

▷ *famciclovir* 250 mg tid x 7-10 days or until clinically resolved

Regimen 4

▷ *valacyclovir* 1 g bid x 10 days or until clinically resolved

RECOMMENDED RECURRENT/EPISODIC REGIMENS

Comment: Initiate treatment of recurrent episodes within 1 day of onset of lesions.

Regimen 1
▷ *acyclovir* 200 mg 5 times/day x 5 days

Regimen 2
▷ *famciclovir* 125 mg bid x 5 days

Regimen 3
▷ *valacyclovir* 500 mg bid x 3-5 days <u>or</u> until clinically resolved

SUPPRESSION THERAPY REGIMENS
Regimen 1
▷ *acyclovir* 400 mg bid x 1 year

Regimen 2
▷ *famciclovir* 250 mg bid x 1 year

Regimen 3
▷ *valacyclovir* 500 mg daily x 1 year (for ≤9 recurrences/year) <u>or</u> 1 g daily x 1 year (for ≥10 recurrences/year)

DAILY SUPPRESSIVE REGIMENS FOR PERSONS WITH HIV
Regimen 1
▷ *acyclovir* 400-800 mg bid-tid

Regimen 2
▷ *famciclovir* 500 mg bid

Regimen 3
▷ *valacyclovir* 500 mg bid

RECURRENT/EPISODIC REGIMENS FOR PERSONS WITH HIV
Regimen 1
▷ *acyclovir* 400 mg tid x 5-10 days

Regimen 2
▷ *famciclovir* 500 mg bid x 5-10 days

Regimen 3
▷ *valacyclovir* 1 g bid x 5-10 days

DRUG BRANDS AND DOSE FORMS
▷ *acyclovir* (B)(G)

Zovirax *Cap:* 200 mg; *Tab:* 400, 800 mg
Zovirax Oral Suspension *Oral susp:* 200 mg/5 ml (banana)
Zovirax Cream *Crm:* 5% (3, 15 g); *Oint:* 5% (3, 15 g)
▷ *famciclovir* (B)
Famvir *Tab:* 125, 250, 500 mg
▷ *valacyclovir* (B)
Valtrex *Cplt:* 500, 1,000 mg

HERPES LABIALIS/HERPES FACIALIS (HERPES SIMPLEX VIRUS TYPE I, COLD SORE, FEVER BLISTER)

PRIMARY INFECTION

▷ *acyclovir* (B)(G) do not chew, crush, <u>or</u> swallow the buccal tab; apply within 1 hour of symptom onset and before appearance of lesion; apply a single buccal tab to the upper gum region on the affected side and hold in place for 30 seconds
Pediatric: not established
Sitavig *Buccal tab:* 50 mg
Pediatric: see page 552 for dose by weight
Comment: **Sitavig** is contraindicated with allergy to milk protein concentrate.
▷ *valacyclovir* (B) 2 g q 12 hours x 1 day
Valtrex *Cplt:* 500, 1,000 mg

SUPPRESSION THERAPY (FOR 6 <u>OR</u> MORE OUTBREAKS/YEAR)

▷ *acyclovir* (B)(G) 200 mg 2-5 x/day x 1 year
Pediatric: <2 years: not recommended; >2 years, <40 kg: 20 mg/kg 2-5 times/day x 1 year; >2 years, >40 kg: 200 mg 2-5 times/day x 1 year; *see page 552 for dose by weight*
Zovirax *Cap:* 200 mg; *Tab:* 400, 800 mg
Zovirax Oral Suspension *Oral susp:* 200 mg/5 ml (banana)

TOPICAL ANTIVIRAL THERAPY

▷ *acyclovir* (B)(G) apply q 3 hours 6 times/day x 7 days
Pediatric: <2 years: not recommended; ≥2 years: same as adult
Zovirax Cream *Crm:* 5% (3, 15 g); *Oint:* 5% (3, 15 g)
▷ *docosanol* (B) apply and gently rub in 5 times daily until healed
Pediatric: not recommended
Abreva (OTC) *Crm:* 10% (2 g)
▷ *penciclovir* (B) apply q 2 hours while awake x 4 days
Pediatric: not recommended
Denavir *Crm:* 1% (2 g)

TOPICAL ANTIVIRAL/CORTICOSTEROID THERAPY

▷ *acyclovir/hydrocortisone* (B)(G) cream apply to affected area 5 x/day x 5 days
Pediatric: <12 years: not recommended; ≥12 years: same as adult
Crm: 1% (2, 5 g)

◯ HERPES ZOSTER (SHINGLES)

ORAL ANTIVIRALS

▷ *famciclovir* (B) 500 mg tid x 7 days
  Pediatric: <18 years: not recommended
    Famvir *Tab:* 125, 250, 500 mg
▷ *valacyclovir* (B) 1 g tid x 7 days
  Pediatric: not recommended
    Valtrex *Cplt:* 500, 1,000 mg
▷ *acyclovir* (B)(G) 800 mg 5 x/day x 7-10 days
  Pediatric: <2 years: not recommended; ≥2 years, <40 kg: 20 mg/kg 5 x/day x 7-10
  days; >2 years, >40 kg: 800 mg 5 x/day x 7-10 days; *see page 552 for dose by weight*
    Zovirax *Cap:* 200 mg; *Tab:* 400, 800 mg
    Zovirax Oral Suspension *Oral susp:* 200 mg/5 ml (banana)

PROPHYLAXIS AGAINST SECONDARY INFECTION

▷ *silver sulfadiazine* (B) apply qid
  Pediatric: not recommended
    Silvadene *Crm:* 1% (20, 50, 85, 400, 1,000 g jar; 20 g tube)

ANALGESICS

▷ *acetaminophen* (B) *see Fever page 143*
▷ *aspirin* (D)(G) *see Fever page 144*
  Comment: *aspirin*-containing medications are contraindicated with history of allergic-type reaction to *aspirin*, children and adolescents with *varicella* or other viral
  illness, and 3rd trimester pregnancy.
▷ *tramadol* (C)(IV)(G)
    Rybix ODT initially 100 mg once daily; may increase by 100 mg every 5 days;
    max 300 mg/day; *CrCl <30 mL/min or severe hepatic impairment:* not recom-
    mended; *Cirrhosis:* max 50 mg q 12 hours
      Pediatric: <17 years: not recommended
      ODT: 50 mg (mint) (phenylalanine)
    Ryzolt initially 100 mg once daily; may increase by 100 mg every 5 days; max 300
    mg/day; *CrCl <30 mL/min or severe hepatic impairment,* not recommended
      Pediatric: <16 years: not recommended; ≥16 years: same as adult
      Tab: 100, 200, 300 mg ext-rel
    Ultram 50-100 mg q 4-6 hours prn; max 400 mg/day; *CrCl <40 mL/min:* max
    100 mg q 12 hours; *Cirrhosis:* max 50 mg q 12 hours
      Pediatric: <16 years: not recommended: ≥16 years: same as adult
      Tab: 50*mg
    Ultram ER initially 100 mg once daily; may increase by 100 mg every 5 days; max
    300 mg/day; *CrCl <30 mL/min or severe hepatic impairment:* not recommended
      Pediatric: <18 years: not recommended
      Tab: 100, 200, 300 mg ext-rel
▷ *tramadol/acetaminophen* (C)(IV)(G) 2 tabs q 4-6 hours; max 8 tabs/day x 5 days;
  CrCl <40 mL/min: max 2 tabs q 12 hours; max 4 tabs/day x 5 days
  Pediatric: <16 years: not recommended; ≥16 years: same as adult
    Ultracet *Tab:* tram 37.5/*acet* 325 mg

Other Oral Analgesics *see Pain page* 308
Postherpetic Neuralgia *see page* 351

SECONDARY INFECTION PROPHYLAXIS

▷ *silver sulfadiazine* (B) apply qid
  Pediatric: not recommended
    Silvadene *Crm:* 1% (20, 50, 85, 400, 1,000 g/jar; 20 g tube)

◯ HICCUPS: INTRACTABLE

▷ *chlorpromazine* (C) 25-50 mg tid-qid
  Pediatric: <6 months: not recommended; ≥6 months: 0.25 mg/lb orally q 4-6 hours
  prn <u>or</u> 0.5 mg/lb rectally q 6-8 hours prn
    Thorazine *Tab:* 10, 25, 50, 100, 200 mg; *Spansule:* 30, 75, 150 mg sust-rel; *Syr:*
    10 mg/5 ml (4 oz; orange custard); *Oral conc:* 30 mg/ml (4 oz); 100 mg/ml
    (2, 8 oz); *Supp:* 25, 100 mg

◯ HIDRADENITIS SUPPURATIVA

ORAL ANTI-INFECTIVES

▷ *doxycycline* (D)(G) 100 mg bid x 7-14 days
  Pediatric: <8 years: not recommended; ≥8 years, <100 lb: 2 mg/lb on first day in
  2 divided doses, followed by 1 mg/lb/day in 1-2 divided doses; ≥8 years, ≥100 lb:
  same as adult; *see page 572 for dose by weight*
    Actilate *Tab:* 75, 150** mg
    Adoxa *Tab:* 50, 75, 100, 150 mg ent-coat
    Doryx *Tab:* 50, 75, 100, 150, 200 mg del-rel
    Monodox *Cap:* 50, 75, 100 mg
    Oracea *Cap:* 40 mg del-rel
    Vibramycin *Tab:* 100 mg; *Cap:* 50, 100 mg; *Syr:* 50 mg/5 ml (raspberry-apple);
    (sulfites); *Oral susp:* 25 mg/5 ml (raspberry)
    Vibra-Tab *Tab:* 100 mg film-coat
  Comment: *doxycycline* is contraindicated <8 years-of-age, in pregnancy, and
  lactation (discolors developing tooth enamel). A side effect may be photo-
  sensitivity (photophobia). Do not give with antacids, calcium supplements, milk or
  other dairy, or within two hours of taking another drug.
▷ *erythromycin base* (B)(G) 1-1.5 g divided qid x 7-14 days
  Pediatric: <45 kg: 30-50 mg in 2-4 divided doses x 7-14 days; ≥45 kg: same as adult
    Ery-Tab *Tab:* 250, 333, 500 mg ent-coat
    PCE *Tab:* 333, 500 mg
  Comment: *erythromycin* may increase INR with concomitant *warfarin*, as well as
  increase serum level of *digoxin*, benzodiazepines and statins.
▷ *erythromycin ethylsuccinate* (B)(G) 1200-1600 mg divided qid x 7-14 days
  Pediatric: 30-50 mg/kg/day in 4 divided doses x 7 days; may double dose with
  severe infection; max 100 mg/kg/day; see page 574 for dose by weight
    EryPed *Oral susp:* 200 mg/5 ml (100, 200 ml) (fruit); 400 mg/5 ml (60, 100,
    200 ml) (banana); *Oral drops:* 200, 400 mg/5 ml (50 ml) (fruit); *Chew tab:* 200
    mg wafer (fruit)

E.E.S. *Oral susp:* 200, 400 mg/5 ml (100 ml) (fruit)
E.E.S. Granules *Oral susp:* 200 mg/5 ml (100, 200 ml) (cherry)
E.E.S. 400 Tablets *Tab:* 400 mg

Comment: *erythromycin* may increase INR with concomitant *warfarin*, as well as increase serum level of *digoxin*, benzodiazepines and statins.

▷ *minocycline* (D)(G) 100 mg bid x 7-14 days
Pediatric: <8 years: not recommended, ≥8 years: same as adult
Dynacin *Cap:* 50, 100 mg
Minocin *Cap:* 50, 75, 100 mg; *Oral susp:* 50 mg/5 ml (60 ml) (custard) (sulfites, alcohol 5%)

Comment: *minocycline* is contraindicated <8 years-of-age, in pregnancy, and lactation (discolors developing tooth enamel). A side effect may be photosensitivity (photophobia). Do not give with antacids, calcium supplements, milk or other dairy, or within two hours of taking another drug.

▷ *tetracycline* (D)(G) 250 mg qid <u>or</u> 500 mg tid x 7-14 days
Pediatric: <8 years: not recommended; ≥8 years, <100 lb: 25-50 mg/kg/day in 2-4 divided doses x 7-14 days; ≥8 years, ≥100 lb: same as adult; *see page 585 for dose by weight*
Achromycin V *Cap:* 250, 500 mg
Sumycin *Tab:* 250, 500 mg; *Cap:* 250, 500 mg; *Oral susp:* 125 mg/5 ml (100, 200 ml) (fruit, sulfites)

Comment: *tetracycline* is contraindicated <8 years-of-age, in pregnancy, and lactation (discolors developing tooth enamel). A side effect may be photosensitivity (photophobia). Do not give with antacids, calcium supplements, milk or other dairy, or within two hours of taking another drug.

TOPICAL ANTI-INFECTIVES

▷ *clindamycin* (B) topical apply bid x 7-14 days
Cleocin T *Pad:* 1% (60/pck; alcohol 50%); *Lotn:* 1% (60 ml); *Gel:* 1% (30, 60 g); *Soln w. applicator:* 1% (30, 60 ml; alcohol 50%)

HOOKWORM (UNCINARIASIS, CUTANEOUS LARVAE MIGRANS)

ANTHELMINTICS

▷ *albendazole* (C) 400 mg as a single dose; may repeat in 3 weeks
Pediatric: <2 years: 200 mg daily x 3 days; may repeat in 3 weeks; ≥2-12 years: 400 mg daily x 3 days; may repeat in 3 weeks
Albenza *Tab:* 200 mg

▷ *mebendazole* (C) chew, swallow, <u>or</u> mix with food; 100 mg bid x 3 days; may repeat in 3 weeks if needed; take with a meal
Pediatric: <2 years: not recommended; ≥2 years: same as adult
Emverm *Chew tab:* 100 mg
Vermox (G) *Chew tab:* 100 mg

▷ *pyrantel pamoate* (C) 11 mg/kg x 1 dose; max 1 g/dose
Pediatric: 25-37 lb: 1/2 tsp x 1 dose; 38-62 lb: 1 tsp x 1 dose; 63-87 lb: 1 tsp x 1 dose; 88-112 lb: 2 tsp x 1 dose; 113-137 lb: 2 tsp x 1 dose; 138-162 lb: 3 tsp x 1 dose; 163-187 lb: 3 tsp x 1 dose; >187 lb: 4 tsp x 1 dose

Pin-X (OTC) *Cap:* 180 mg; *Liq:* 50 mg/ml (30 ml); 144 mg/ml (30 ml); *Oral susp:* 50 mg/ml (30 ml)

⬤ HUMAN IMMUNODEFICIENCY VIRUS (HIV) EXPOSURE, ANTIRETROVIRAL PEP/nPEP

Antiretroviral drug brand names and dose forms (*see Anti-HIV Drugs page* 523)
Comment: Antiretroviral prophylactic treatment regimens for occupational HIV exposure (PEP) and nonoccupational exposure (nPEP) are referenced from the **2015 CDC Sexually Transmitted Diseases Treatment Guidelines, MMWR, and NIH** available at: www.cdc.gov/mmwr/preview/mmwrhtml/rr5402a1.htm and www .aidsinfo.nih.gov/guidelines/default_db2.asp?id=50.

In this section, the 2015 CDC-recommended highly active antiretroviral treatment (HAART) regimens are followed by a listing of the single and combination drugs with dosing regimens and dose forms. Appendix S is an alphabetical listing of the HIV drugs and dose forms. For more information on the management of HIV infection in adults and adolescents, see *Guidelines for the Use of Antiretroviral Agents in HIV-1-Infected Adults and Adolescents:* https://aidsinfo.nih.gov/contentfiles/lvguidelines/ adultandadolescentgl.pdf. For specific dosing information in the management of HIV infection in children, see *Guidelines for Use of Antiretroviral Agents in Pediatric HIV Infection:* https://www.aidsinfo.nih.gov/contentfiles/lvguidelines/pediatricguidelines. pdf. Providers should consult, and/refer HIV-infected patients to, a specialist and/or specialty community services for age-appropriate dosing regimens and other patient-specific needs.

Initiation of PEP/nPEP with ART as soon as possible increases the likelihood of prophylactic benefit. Treatment regimens must be initiated ≥72 hours following exposure. A 28-day course of ART is recommended for persons with *substantial risk for HIV exposure* (i.e., exposure of vagina, rectum, eye, mouth, or other mucous membrane, non-intact skin, or percutaneous contact with blood, semen, vaginal secretions, breast milk, or any body fluid that is visibly contaminated with blood, when the source is known to be infected with HIV). ART is not recommended for persons with *negligible risk for HIV exposure* (i.e., exposure of vagina, rectum, eye, mouth, or other mucus membrane, intact or non-intact skin, or percutaneous contact with urine, nasal secretions, saliva, sweat, or tears, if not visibly contaminated with blood, regardless of the known or suspected HIV status of the source). There is no evidence indicating any specific antiretroviral medication, or combination of medications is optimal for suppressing local viral replication. There is no evidence to indicate that a 3-drug ART regimen is any more beneficial than a 2-drug regimen. When the source person is available for interview and testing, his or her history of retroviral medication use and most recent/current viral load measurement should be considered when selecting an ART treatment regimen (e.g., to help avoid prescribing an antiretroviral medication to which the source virus is likely to be resistant). Register pregnant patients exposed to antiretroviral agents to the Antiretroviral Pregnancy Registry (APR) at 800-258-4263. The Centers for Disease Control and Prevention recommend that HIV-infected mothers not breastfeed their infants to avoid risking postnatal transmission of HIV infection.

REGIMENS

Nonnucleoside Reverse Transcriptase Inhibitor (NNRTI)-Based Regimen

▷ *efavirenz* <u>plus</u> (*lamivudine* <u>or</u> *emtricitabine*) <u>plus</u> (*zidovudine* <u>or</u> *tenofovir*)

Protease Inhibitor (PI)-Based Regimens

▷ *lopinavir/ritonavir* (co-formulated as **Kaletra**) <u>plus</u> (*lamivudine* <u>or</u> *emtricitabine*) <u>plus</u> *zidovudine*
▷ *darunavir/cobicistat* (co-formulated as **Prezcobix**) <u>plus</u> *other retroviral agents*

ALTERNATIVE REGIMENS

NNRTI-Based Regimen

▷ *efavirenz* <u>plus</u> (*lamivudine* <u>or</u> *emtricitabine*) <u>plus</u> (*abacavir* <u>or</u> *didanosine* <u>or</u> *stavudine*)
Comment: *efavirenz* should be avoided in pregnant women and women of child-bearing potential.

Protease Inhibitor-Based Regimens

Regimen 1

▷ *atazanavir* <u>plus</u> (*lamivudine* <u>or</u> *emtricitabine*) <u>plus</u> (*zidovudine* <u>or</u> *stavudine* <u>or</u> *abacavir* <u>or</u> *didanosine*) <u>or</u> (*tenofovir* <u>plus</u> *ritonavir* (100 mg/day)

Regimen 2

▷ *fosamprenavir* <u>plus</u> (*lamivudine* <u>or</u> *emtricitabine*) <u>plus</u> (*zidovudine* <u>or</u> *stavudine*) <u>or</u> (*abacavir* <u>or</u> *tenofovir* <u>or</u> *didanosine*)

Regimen 3

▷ *fosamprenavir/ritonavir* <u>plus</u> (*lamivudine* <u>or</u> *emtricitabine*) <u>plus</u> (*zidovudine* <u>or</u> *stavudine* <u>or</u> *abacavir* <u>or</u> *tenofovir* <u>or</u> *didanosine*)

Regimen 4

▷ *indinavir/ritonavir* <u>plus</u> (*lamivudine* <u>or</u> *emtricitabine*) <u>plus</u> (*zidovudine* <u>or</u> *stavudine* <u>or</u> *abacavir* <u>or</u> *tenofovir* <u>or</u> *didanosine*)
Comment: Using *ritonavir* with *indinavir* may increase risk for renal adverse events.

Regimen 5

▷ *lopinavir/ritonavir* (co-formulated as **Kaletra**) <u>plus</u> (*lamivudine* <u>or</u> *emtricitabine*) <u>plus</u> (*stavudine* <u>or</u> *abacavir* <u>or</u> *tenofovir* <u>or</u> *didanosine*)

Regimen 6

▷ *nelfinavir* <u>plus</u> (*lamivudine* <u>or</u> *emtricitabine*) <u>plus</u> (*zidovudine* <u>or</u> *stavudine* <u>or</u> *abacavir* <u>or</u> *tenofovir* <u>or</u> *didanosine*)

Regimen 7

▷ *saquinavir/ritonavir* <u>plus</u> (*lamivudine* <u>or</u> *emtricitabine*) <u>plus</u> (*zidovudine* <u>or</u> *stavudine* <u>or</u> *abacavir* <u>or</u> *tenofovir* <u>or</u> *didanosine*)

Triple Nucleoside Reverse Transcriptase Inhibitor (NRTI)-Based Regimen

abacavir plus *lamivudine* plus *zidovudine*
Comment: Triple NRTI therapy should be used only when an NNRTI- or PI-based regimen cannot or should not be used.

BRAND NAMES, DOSING AND DOSE FORMS: SINGLE AGENTS

Integrase Strand Transfer Inhibitor (INSTI)

▷ *dolutegravir* (C) *Treatment naïve or treatment experienced but INSTI naïve:* 50 mg once daily; *Treatment experienced or naïve and co-administered with efavirenz, FPV/r, TPV/r, or rifampin:* 50 mg bid; *INSTI experienced with certain INSTI-associated resistance substitutions:* 50 mg bid
   Pediatric: <12 years, <40 kg: not established; ≥12 years, ≥40 kg: same as adult
      Tivicay *Tab:* 10, 25, 50 mg
▷ *raltegravir (as potassium)* (C) 400 mg (one film-coat tab) bid; take with concomitant *rifampin* 800 mg bid; swallow whole; do not crush or chew
   Pediatric: ≥4 weeks, 3-11 kg [oral suspension] 3-<4 kg: 20 mg bid; 4-<6 kg: 30 mg bid; 6-<8 kg: 40 mg bid; 8-<11 kg: 60 mg bid; ≥11-<25 kg [oral suspension/chewable tab]; 6 mg/kg/dose bid; see mfr pkg insert for dose by weight table; ≥25 kg and unable to swallow tablet use chewable tab; 25-<28 kg: 150 mg bid; 28-<40 kg: 200 mg bid; ≥40 kg: 300 mg bid; 6 years, ≥25 kg, and able to swallow tablets use film-coat tab; 400 mg bid
      Isentress *Tab:* 400 mg film-coat; *Chew tab:* 25, 100*mg (orange banana) (phenylalanine)
      Isentress Oral Suspension *Oral susp:* 100 mg/pkt pwdr for oral susp (banana)
Comment: Oral suspension, chewable tablets and film-coated *raltegravir* tablets are not bioequivalent. Maximum dose for chewable tablets is 300 mg twice daily. Maximum dose for film-coated tabletsis 400 mg twice daily

Nucleoside Reverse Transcriptase Inhibitors (NRTIs)

▷ *abacavir sulfate* (C)(G) 600 mg once daily or 300 mg bid; *Mild hepatic impairment:* use oral solution for titration
   Pediatric: 3 months-16 years: [tablet/oral solution] 16 mg/kg qd or 8 mg/kg bid; max 300 mg bid; >14 kg: see mfr pkg insert for tablet dosing by weight band
      Ziagen (as sulfate) *Tab:* 300*mg
      Ziagen Oral Solution *Oral soln:* 20 mg/ml (240 ml) (strawberry-banana) (parabens, propylene glycol)
▷ *didanosine* (C)
      Videx EC take once daily on an empty stomach; swallow whole; <20 kg: use oral solution; 20-<25 kg: 200 mg; 25-<60 kg: 250 mg; ≥60 kg: 400 mg; *CrCl 30-59 mL/min:* <60 kg: 125 mg; ≥60 kg: 200 mg; *CrCl 10-29 mL/min:* 125 mg; *CrCl<10 mL/min or dialysis:*<60 kg: use oral solution ≥60 kg: 125 mg
         Pediatric: same as adult
            Cap: 125, 200, 250, 400 mg ent-coat del-rel; *Chew tab:* 25, 50, 100, 150, 200 mg (mandarin orange) (buffered with calcium carbonate and magnesium hydroxide, phenylalanine)
      Videx Pediatric Pwdr for Solution <60 kg: 125 mg bid; ≥60 kg: 200 mg bid; *If once daily dosing required:* <60 kg: 250 mg once daily; ≥60 kg: 400 mg once daily; *CrCl 30-59 mL/min:* <60 kg: 150 mg once daily or 75 mg bid; ≥60 kg: 200

mg once daily <u>or</u> 100 mg bid; *CrCl 10-29 mL/min:* <60 kg: 100 mg once daily; ≥60 kg: 150 mg once daily; *CrCl <10 mL/min* <u>or</u> *dialysis:* <60 kg: 75 mg once daily; ≥60 kg: 100 mg once daily; take on an empty stomach

> *Pediatric:* <2 weeks: not recommended; 2 weeks-8 months: 100 mg/m2 bid; >8 months: 120 mg/m2 bid; *Renal impairment:* consider reducing dose <u>or</u> increasing dosing interval; take on an empty stomach

> > *Pwdr for oral soln:* 2, 4 g (120, 240 ml)

Comment: *didanosine* is contraindicated with concomitant ***allopurinal*** <u>or</u> ***ribavirin.***

▷ *emtricitabine* (B) 200 mg once daily; *CrCl 30-49 mL/min:* 200 mg q 48 hours; *CrCl 15-29 mL/min:* 200 mg q 72 hours; *CrCl <15 mL/min* <u>or</u> *dialysis:* 200 mg q 96 hours
Pediatric: <3 months: 3 mg/kg oral soln once daily; 3 months-17 years, 6 mg/kg once daily; ≤33 kg: use oral soln, max 240 mg (24 ml); >33 kg: 200 mg cap once daily; max 240 mg/day; ≥18 years: same as adult

> **Emtriva** *Cap:* 200 mg
> **Emtriva Oral Solution** *Oral soln:* 10 mg/ml (170 ml) (cotton candy)

▷ *lamivudine* (C)(G) *CrCl ≥50 mL/min:* 300 mg qd <u>or</u> 150 mg bid; *CrCl >30-50 mL/min:* 150 mg qd; *CrCl 15-29:* first dose 150 mg, then 100 mg once daily; *CrCl 5-14 mL/min:* first dose 150 mg, then 50 mg qd; *CrCl <5 mL/min:* first dose 50 mg, the 25 mg once daily; max 8mg/kg once daily <u>or</u> 150 mg bid
Pediatric: <3 months: not established; 3 months-16 years: 4 mg/kg oral soln <u>or</u> tab bid; [tab] 14-<20 kg: 150 mg once daily <u>or</u> 75 mg bid; ≥20-<25 kg: 225 mg once daily <u>or</u> 75 mg in the AM and 150 mg in the PM; ≥25 kg: 300 mg once daily <u>or</u> 150 mg bid; max 8 mg/kg once daily <u>or</u> 150 mg bid <u>or</u> 300 mg once daily

> **Epivir** *Tab:* 150*, 300 mg
> **Epivir Oral Solution** *Oral soln:* 10 mg/ml (240 ml) (strawberry-banana) (sucrose 3 g/15 ml)

Comment: With renal impairment reduce ***lamivudine*** dose <u>or</u> extend dosing interval.

▷ *stavudine* (C)(G) ≥60 kg: 40 mg q 12 hours; ≤60 kg: 30 mg q 12 hours; *If peripheral neuropathy develops:* discontinue; *After resolution, ≥60 kg:* may re-start at 20 mg q 12 hours; *After resolution, ≤60 kg:* may restart at 15 mg q 12 hours; *if neuropathy returns:* consider permanent discontinuation; *CrCl 10-50 mL/min, ≥60 kg:* 20 mg q 12 hours; *CrCl 10-50 mL/min, ≥60 kg:* 15 mg q 12 hours; *Hemodialysis, ≥60 kg:* 20 mg q 24 hours; *Hemodialysis, ≤60 kg:* 15 mg q 24 hours; administer at the same time of day; *Hemodialysis:* administer at the end of dialysis
Pediatric: birth-13 days: [tablet/oral solution] 0.5 mg/kg q 12 hours; >14 days, <30 kg: [tablet/oral solution] 1 mg/kg q 12 hours; ≥30-<60 kg: 30 mg q 12 hours; ≥60 kg: 40 mg q 12 hours

> **Zerit** *Cap:* 15, 20, 30, 40 mg
> **Zerit for Oral Solution** *Oral soln:* 1 mg/ml pwdr for reconstitution (fruit) (dye-free)

Comment: Withdraw *stavudine* if peripheral neuropathy occurs. After complete resolution, may restart at half the recommended dose. If peripheral neuropathy recurs consider permanent discontinuation.

▷ *tenofovir disoproxil fumarate* (C) 300 mg once daily; *CrCl 30-49 mL/min:* 300 mg q 48 hours; *CrCl 10-29:* 300 mg q 72-96 hours; *Hemodialysis:* 300 mg once every 7 days <u>or</u> after a total of 12 hours of dialysis; *CrCl <10 mL/min:* not recommended
Pediatric: <2 years: not established; 2-12 years: 8 mg/kg once daily; >12 years, 35 kg: 300 mg once daily; mix oral pwdr with 2-4 oz soft food

> **Viread** *Tab:* 150, 200, 250, 300 mg; *Oral pwdr:* 40 mg/g (60 g w. dosing scoop)

➤ **zidovudine** (C)(G) 600 mg daily divided bid-tid; *ESRD/dialysis:* 100 mg q 6-8 hours;
Vertical transmission, severe anemia, or neutropenia: see mfr pkg insert
Pediatric: Treatment of HIV-1 infection: 4-<9kg: 24 mg/kg/day divided bid or tid;
≥9-<30 kg: 18 mg/kg/day divided bid or tid; ≥30 kg: 600 mg/day divided bid or tid;
Prevention of maternal-fetal neonatal transmission: <12 hours after birth until 6 weeks
of age: [Solution] 2 mg/kg q 6 hours until 6 weeks-of-age; [IV] 1.5 mg/kg infused
over 30 minutes q 6 hours until 6 weeks-of-age; max 200 mg q 8 hours
    Retrovir Tablets *Tab:* 300 mg
    Retrovir Capsules *Cap:* 100 mg
    Retrovir Syrup *Syrup:* 50 mg/5 ml (strawberry)
    Retrovir IV *Vial:* 10 mg/ml after dilution (20 ml) (preservative-free)

Nonnucleoside Reverse Transcriptase Inhibitors (NNRTIs)

➤ **delavirdine mesylate** (C) 400 mg (4 x 100-mg or 2 x 200 mg) tablets tid in combination with other antiretroviral agents
Pediatric: <16 years: not established; ≥16 years: same as adult
    Rescriptor *Tab:* 100, 200 mg
Comment: The 100 mg **Rescriptor** tablets may be dispersed in water prior to
consumption. To prepare a dispersion, add four 100 mg Rescriptor tablets to at least
3 ounces of water, allow to stand for a few minutes, and then stir until a uniform
dispersion occurs. The dispersion should be consumed promptly. The glass should
be rinsed with water and the rinse swallowed to insure the entire dose is consumed.
The 200 mg tablets should be taken as intact tablets, because they are not readily
dispersed in water.
➤ **efavirenz** (D) 600 mg once daily
Pediatric: >3 months, 3.5 kg: [tablet/capsule] 3.5-< 5 kg: 100 mg once daily 5-<7.5
kg: 150 mg once daily; 7.5-<15 kg: 200 mg once daily; 15-<20 kg: 250 mg once daily;
20-<25 kg: 300 mg once daily; 25-<32.5 kg: 350 once daily; 32.5-<40 kg: 400 mg once
daily; >40 kg: 600 mg once daily; max 600 mg once daily
Comment: For children who cannot swallow capsules, the capsule contents can
be administered with a small amount of food or infant formula using the capsule
sprinkle method of administration. See mfr pkg insert for instructions. Tablets
should not be crushed or chewed. Administer at bedtime to limit CNS effects.
    Sustiva *Tab:* 75, 150, 600, 800 mg; *Cap:* 50, 200 mg
➤ **etravirine** (B) 200 mg (1 x 200 mg tablet or 2 x 100 mg tablets) bid following a meal
Pediatric: <3 year: not recommended; ≥**3 years,** >16 kg: 16-< 20 kg: 100 mg bid; **20-**
<25 kg: 125 mg bid; **25-**<30 kg: 150 mg bid; ≥30 kg: 200 mg bid; max 200 mg bid;
take following a mail
    Intelence *Tab:* 25*, 100, 200 mg
➤ **nevirapine** (B)(G) initiatially one 200 mg tablet of immediate-release **Viramune**
once daily for the first 14 days in combination with other antiretroviral agents; then,
one 400 mg tablet of **Viramune XR** once daily
Comment: The 14-day lead-in period has been found to lessen the frequency of
rash.
Pediatric: <6 years: not recommended; 6-<18 years: BSA 0.58-0.83 kg/m2: 200 mg
once daily; BSA 0.84-1.16 kg/m2: 300 mg once daily; BSA ≥1.17 kg/m2: 400 mg;
once daily; max 400 mg once daily
Comment: Children must initiate therapy with immediate-release **Viramune** for the
first 14 days; ≥15 days: [oral suspension/tablet]: 150 mg/m2 once daily for 14 days,
then 150 mg/m2 bid

HIV Exposure, Antiretroviral PEP/nPEP ■ 199

Viramune *Tab:* 200*mg
Viramune Oral Suspension *Oral susp:* 50 mg/5 ml (240 ml)
Viramune XR *Tab:* 100, 400mg ext-rel

▷ *rilpivirine* (D) 25 mg once daily; *If concomitant rifabutin:* 50 mg once daily: *If concomitant rifabutin stopped:* 25 mg once daily
Pediatric: <12 years: not recommended; ≥12 years, >35 kg: same adult
Edurant *Tab:* 25 mg

Nucleoside and Nonnucleoside Reverse Transcriptase Inhibitor (NRTI/NNRTI) Combinations

▷ Atripla (B) *efavirenz/emtricitabine/tenofovir disoproxil fumarate* 1 tab once daily preferably at HS; take on an empty stomach; *Concomitant rifabutin:* >50 kg: take additional *efavirenz* 200 mg/day
Pediatric: <12 years: not recommended; ≥12 years, 40 kg: same as adult
Tab: efa 600 mg/*emtri* 200 mg/*teno dis fum* 300 mg

▷ Complera (B) *emtricitabine/tenofovir disoproxil fumarate/rilpivirine* 1 tab once daily; *CrCl <50 mL/min:* not recommended; *Concomitant rifabutin:* take additional *ribavirin* 25 mg qd
Pediatric: <12 years, <35 kg: not established; ≥12 years, ≥35 kg: same as adult
Tab: emtri 200 mg/*teno dis* 300 mg/*rilpiv 25 mg*

Protease Inhibitors (PIs)

▷ *atazanavir* (B) *Treatment naiive: Recommended regimen:* 300 mg plus *ritonavir* 100 mg once daily; *Unable to tolerate ritonavir:* 400 mg once daily; *Incombination with efavirenz:* 400 mg plus *ritonavir* 100 mg once daily; *Treatment experienced: Recommended regimen:* 300 mg plus *ritonavir* 100 mg once daily; *In combination with both an H2-blocker* or *PPI and tenofovir:* 400 mg plus *ritonavir* 100 mg once daily; take with food
Pediatric: <3 months: not recommended; ≥3 mos, 5 kg: [oral powder] 5-<15 kg: 200 mg (4 packets) plus *ritonavir* 80 mg once daily; 15-<25 kg: 250 mg (5 packets) plus *ritonavir* 80 mg once daily; ≥25 kg, unable to swallow capsules: 300 mg (6 packets) plus *rotinovir* once daily; 6 yrs, <15 kg: [capsule] 15-<20 kg: 150 mg plus *ritonavir* 100 mg once daily; 20-<40 kg: 200 mg plus *ritonavir* 100 mg once daily; ≥40kg: 300 mg plus *ritonavir* 100 mg once daily; [capsule]15-<20 kg: 150 mg plus *ritonavir* 100 mg once daily; 20-<40 kg: 200 mg plus *ritonavir* 100 mg once daily; ≥40kg: 300 mg plus *ritonavir* 100 mg once daily; max dose 400 mg once daily; take with food
Reyataz *Cap:* 100, 150, 200, 300 mg; *Oral pwdr:* 50 mg/pkt (30/carton)
(phenylalanine)
Comment: Administration of *atazanavir* with *rotinavir* is preferred. Dose for treatment-naïve children ≥13 years of age and ≥40 kg unable to tolerate *rotinavir*, administer 400 mg once daily. See mfr pkg insert for special dosing considerations when combining *altazanavir* with other retrovirals.

▷ *darunavir* (C)(G) *Treatment naïve and treatment experienced with no darunavir resistamce associated substitutions:* 800 mg once daily with *ritonavir* 100 mg once daily; *Treatment-experienced with at least one darunavir resistamce associated substitution:* 600 mg bid with ritonavir 100 mg bid; *Severe hepatic impairment:* not recommended

Pediatric: ≥3 yrs, 10 kg [oral solution/tablet/capsule] *Treatment naïve or experienced without darunavir-associated substitutions:* 10-<15 kg: 35 mg/kg once daily plus *ritonavir* 7mg/kg once daily; 15-<30 kg: 600 mg plus *ritonavir* 100 mg once oaily; 30-<40 kg: 675 mg plus *ritonavir* 100 mg once daily; >40 kg: 800 mg plus *ritonavir* 100 mg once daily; *Treatment experienced with ≥1 darunavir-associated substitution(s):* 10-15 kg: 20 mg/kg bid plus *ritonavir* 3 mg/kg bid; 15-<30 kg: 375 mg plus *ritonavir* 48 mg bid; 30-<40 kg: 450 mg plus *ritonavir* 60 mg bid; >40 kg: 600 mg plus *ritonavir* 100 mg bid

> **Prezista** *Tab:* 75, 150, 600, 800 mg film-coat
> **Prezista Oral Suspension** *Susp:* 100 mg/ml (strawberry cream)
> **Comment:** **Prezista** is FDA approved for treatment of HIV-1-infected pregnant women and for the treatment of children >3 years-of-age in combination with *ritonavir* and other antiretrovirals.

▷ *fosamprenavir* **(C)(G)** *Treatment-naïve:* 1,400 mg bid or 1,400 mg once daily plus *ritonavir* 200 mg once daily or 1,400 mg once daily plus *ritonavir* 100 mg once daily or 700 mg bid plus *ritonavir* 100 mg bid; *Protease inhibitor-experienced:* 700 mg bid plus *ritonavir* 100 mg bid

Pediatric: <4 weeks: not recommended; *Protease inhibitor-naïve, ≥4 weeks or protease inhibitor-experienced:* ≥6 Months, <11 kg: 45 mg/kg plus *ritonavir* 7 mg/kg bid; 11-<15 kg: 30 mg/kg plus *ritonavir* 3 mg/kg bid; 15 kg-<20 kg: 23 mg/kg plus *ritonavir* 3 mg/kg bid; ≥20 kg: 18 mg/kg plus *ritonavir* 3 mg/kg bid; *Protease-inhibitor naïve, ≥2 years:* 30 mg/kg bid without *ritonavir*: max dose 700 mg plus *ritonavir* 100 mg bid

> **Lexiva:** *Tab: 700 mg film-coat*
> **Lexiva Oral Suspension** *Oral usp:* 50 mg/ml (225 ml) (grape-bubble gum-peppermint)
> **Comment:** *fosamprenavir* 1 ml is equivalent to approximately 43 mg of *amprenavir* 1 ml.

▷ *indinavir sulfate* **(C)** 800 mg q 8 hours; *Concomitant rifabutin*: 1 g q 8 hours and reduce *rifabutin* dose by half; *Hepatic insufficiency or concomitant ketoconazole, itraconazole, or delavirdine:* 600 mg q 8 hours; take with water on an empty stomach or with a light meal

Pediatric: not established (3-18 years, doses of 500 mg/m2 every 8 hours have been used; see mfr pkg insert)

> **Crixivan** *Cap:* 100, 200, 333, 400 mg

▷ *nelfinavir mesylate* **(B)** 1250 mg (5 x 250 mg tablets or 2 x 625 mg tablets) bid or 750 mg (3 x 250 mg tablets) tid; take with a meal; may dissolve tablets in a small amount of water; max 2500 mg/day

Pediatric: <2 years: not established; 2-13 years: 45-55 mg/kg bid or 25-35 mg/kg tid; take with a meal; max 2500 mg/day; ≥13 years: same as adult

> **Viracept** *Tab:* 250, 625 mg
> **Viracept Oral Powder** *Oral pwdr:* 50 mg/g (144 g) (phenylalanine)
> **Comment:** The 250 mg **Viracept** tabs are interchangeable with oral powder, the 625 mg tabs are not.

▷ *raltegravir (as potassium)* **(B)** 400 mg bid

Pediatric: ≥4 weeks, 3-11 kg: [oral suspension] 3-<4 kg: 20 mg bid; 4-<6 kg: 30 mg bid; 6-<8 kg: 40 mg bid; 8-<11 kg: 60 mg bid; ≥11-<25 kg: [oral suspension/ chewable tablet] 6 mg/kg/dose bid; see mfr pkg insert for dosage by weight; ≥25 kg and unable to swallow tablet: [chewable tablet] 25-<28 kg: 150 mg bid; 28-<40 kg: 200 mg bid; ≥40 kg: 300 mg bid; ≥6 years, ≥25 kg, able to swallow tablets: 400 mg film-coat tablet bid

Comment: Oral suspension, chewable tablets, and film-coated tablets are not bioequivalent. Chewable tablet max dose 300 mg bid. Film-coated tablets max dose 400 mg bid. Oral suspension max dose 100 mg bid

>   Isentress *Tab:* 400 mg film-coat; *Chew tab:* 25, 100*mg (orange-banana) (phenylalanine)

>   **Isentress Oral Suspension** *Oral susp:* 100 mg/pkt pwdr for oral susp (banana)

▷ *ritonavir* (B) initially 300 mg bid; increase at 2-3 day intervals by 100 mg bid; max 600 mg bid

Pediatric: <1 month: not recommended; ≥1 month: 350-400 mg/m2 bid; initiate at 250 mg/m2 bid and titrate upward every 2-3 days by 50 mg/m2 bid; max dose 600 mg bid

Comment: Lower doses of *ritonavir* have been used to boost other protease inhibitors but the *ritonavir* doses used for boosting have not been specifically approved in children.

>   Norvir *Tab:* 100 mg film-coat; *Gel cap:* 100 mg (alcohol)

>   **Norvir Oral Solution** *Oral soln:* 80 mg/ml, 600 mg/7.5 ml (8 oz) (peppermint-caramel) (alcohol)

Comment: **Norvir** tablets should be swallowed whole. Take **Norvir** with meals. Patients may improve the taste of **Norvir Oral Solution** by mixing with chocolate milk, **Ensure,** or **Advera** within one hour of dosing. Dose reduction of **Norvir** is necessary when used with other protease inhibitors (*atazanavir, darunavir, fosamprenavir, saquinavir,* and *tipranavir*). Patients who take the 600 mg gel cap bid may experience more gastrointestinal side effects such as nausea, vomiting, abdominal pain or diarrhea when switching from the gel cap to the tablet because of greater maximum plasma concentration (Cmax) achieved with the tablet. These adverse events (gastrointestinal or paresthesias) may diminish as treatment is continued.

▷ *saquinavir mesylate* (B)

Pediatric: <16 years: not established; >16 years: same as adult

>   **Fortovase** *Tab/Cap:* 200 mg

>   **Invirase** *Tab:* 500 mg; *Cap:* 200 mg

▷ *tipranavir* (C) 500 mg bid plus ritonavir 200 mg bid

Pediatric: <2 years: not recommended; 2-18 yrs: [capsule/oral solution] 14 mg/kg plus *ritonavir* 6 mg/kg bid or 375 mg/m2 plus *ritonavir* 150 mg/m2 bid; max 500 mg plus *ritonavir* 200 mg bid

>   **Aptivus** *Gel cap:* 250 mg (alcohol)

>   **Aptivus Oral Solution** *Oral soln:* 100 mg/ml (buttermint-butter toffee) (Vit E 116 IU/ml)

FUSION INHIBITORS—CCR5 CO-RECEPTOR ANTAGONISTS

▷ *enfuvirtide* (B) 90 mg (1 ml) SC bid; administer in upper arm, abdomen, or anterior thigh; rotate injection sites

Pediatric: <6 years: not established; 6-16 years: administer 2 mg/kg SC bid; max 90 mg SC bid; rotate injection sites

>   **Fuzeon** *Vial:* 90 mg/ml pwdr for SC inj after reconstitution (1 ml, 60 vials/kit) (preservative-free)

▷ *maraviroc* (B) must be administered concomitant with other retrovirals; *Concomitant potent CYP3A inhibitors (with or without a potent CYP3A inducer) including protease inhibitors (except tipranavir/ritonavir), delavirdine, ketoconazole, itraconazole, clarithromycin, other potent CYP3A inhibitors (e.g., nefazodone, telithromycin):*

CrCl ≥30 mL/min: 150 mg bid; *<30 mL/min, dialysis:* not recommended; *Potent CYP3A inducers (without a potent CYP3A inhibitor) including **efavirenz**, **rifampin**, **etravirine**, **carbamazepine**, **phenobarbital**, and **phenytoin**:* 300 mg bid; *CrCl ≥30 mL/min:* 600 mg bid; *<30 mL/min:* not recommended; *Other concomitant agents, including **tipranavir/ritonavir**, **nevirapine**, **raltegravir**, all NRTIs, and **enfuvirtide**:* 300 mg bid
Pediatric: <16 years: not established; ≥16 years: same as adult
> **Selzentry** *Tab:* 150, 300 mg film-coat

BRAND NAMES, DOSING, AND DOSE FORMS: COMBINATION AGENTS

▷ **Atripla (B)** *efavirenz/emtricitabine/tenofovir disoproxil fumarate* 1 tablet once daily on an empty stomach; bedtime dosing may improve the tolerability of nervous system symptoms; *CrCl <50 mL/min:* not recommended
Pediatric: <12 years: not established; ≥12 years, ≥40 kg: same as adult
> *Tab: efa* 600 mg/*emtri* 200 mg/*teno dis fum* 300 mg film-coat

▷ **Combivir (C)(G)** *lamivudine/zidovudine*
Pediatric: <12 years: not recommended; ≥12 years, ≥30 kg: 1 tablet bid with food
> *Tab: lami* 150 mg/*zido* 300 mg

▷ **Complera (B)** *emtricitabine/tenofovir disoproxil fumarate/rilpivirine* 1 tablet once daily; *CrCl <50 mL/min:* not recommended
Pediatric: <12 years, <40 kg: not recommended; ≥12 years, ≥40 kg: same as adult
> *Tab: emtri* 200 mg/*teno dis* 300 mg/*rilpiv 25 mg*

▷ **Descovy (D)** *emtricitabine/tenofovir alafenamide* 1 tablet once daily with or without food; *CrCl <30 mL/min:* not recommended
Pediatric: <12 years, <35 kg: not recommended; ≥12 years, ≥35 kg: same as adult
> *Tab: emtri* 200 mg/*teno ala* 25 mg

Comment: Patients with HIV-1 should be tested for the presence of chronic hepatitis B virus (HBV) before initiating antiretroviral therapy. **Descovy** is not approved for the treatment of chronic HBV infection, and the safety and efficacy of **Descovy** have not been established in patients co-infected with HIV-1 and HBV.

▷ **Epzicom (B)** *abacavir sulfate/lamivudine* 1 tab daily; *Mild hepatic impairment or CrCl<50 mL/min:* not recommended
Pediatric: <25 kg: use individual componbents; ≥25 kg: one tablet once daily; *Mild hepatic impairment or CrCl<50 mL/min:* not recommended
> *Tab: aba* 600 mg/*lami* 300 mg

▷ **Evotaz (B)** *atazanavir/cobicistat* 1 tab once daily
Pediatric: not established
> *Tab: ataz* 600 mg/*cobi* 300 mg

▷ **Genvoya (B)** *elvitegravir/cobicistat/emtricitabine/tenofovir alafenamide* 1 tab once daily; *Severe hepatic impairment or CrCl <30 mL/min:* not recommended; take with food
Pediatric: <12 years: not established; ≥12 years, ≥35 kg: same as adult
> *Tab: elvi* 150 mg/*cobi* 150 mg/*emtri* 200 mg/*teno* 10 mg

▷ **Kaletra, Kaletra Oral Solution (C)** *lopinavir/ritonavir* 800 mg/200 mg (4 tablets or 10 ml) once daily or 400 mg/100 mg (2 tablets or 5 ml) bid; *May administer once daily or bid:* patients with <3 **lopinavir** resistance-associated substitutions; *May dose bid only:* patients with ≥3 resistance-associated substitutions; *Dose must be increased:* when administered in combination with **efavirenz**, **nevirapine**, or **nelfinavir**

(500 mg/125 mg (2 x 200 mg/50 mg tablet <u>plus</u> 1 x 100 mg/25 mg tablet) bid <u>or</u> 520 mg/130 mg (6.5 ml) bid; *Once daily dosing regimen not recommended:* in combination with ≥3 *lopinavir* resistance-associated substitutions <u>or</u> in combination with: *carbamazepine, phenobarbital,* <u>or</u> *phenytoin;* Patients receiving *nevirapine* <u>or</u> *efavirenz* with **Kaletra** should have their **Kaletra** dose increased; swallow whole with <u>or</u> without food

Pediatric: dose calculation is based on the *lopinavir* component; 14 days-6months: 16 mg/kg bid; 6 months-12 years: [tablet/capsule/solution] 7-<15 kg: 12 mg/kg bid (13 mg/kg <u>plus</u> *nevirapine*); 15-40 kg: 10 mg/kg bid (11 mg/kg <u>plus</u> *nevirapine*), >40 kg, >12 years: *lopinavir* 400 mg bid (533 mg <u>plus</u> *nevirapine*); max *lopinavir* 400 mg bid for patients who are not receiving *nevirapine* <u>or</u> *efavirenz;* **Kaletra** should not be used in combination with NNRTIs in children <6 months-of-age; see mfr pkg insert for BSA-based dosing

> *Tab:* **Kaletra 100/25** *lopin* 100 mg/*riton* 25 mg
> **Kaletra 200/50** *lopin* 200 mg/*riton* 50 mg
> *Oral soln:* *lopin* 80 mg/*riton* 20 mg per ml, *lopin* 400 mg/*riton* 500 mg per 5 ml (160 ml) (cotton candy) (alcohol 42.4%)

▷ **Odefsey (D)** *emtricitabine/rilpivirine/tenofovir alafenamide* 1 tab once daily with food; *CrCl <30 mL/min:* not recommended
Pediatric: <12 years, <35 kg: not established; ≥12 years: same as adult
> *Tab:* *emtri* 200 mg/*rilpi* 25 mg/*teno alafen* 25 mg

▷ **Prezcobix (C)** *darunavir/cobicistat* 1 tab once daily; *Treatment naïve and treatment experienced with no darunavir resistance-associated substitution:* 800 mg once daily <u>plus</u> *ritonavir* 100 mg once daily; *Treatment experienced with at least one darunavir resistance associated substitution:* 600 mg bid <u>plus</u> *ritonavir* 100 mg bid; take with food; *CrCl <70 mL/min:* not recommended
Pediatric: not recommended
> *Tab:* *darun* 800 mg/*cobi* 150 mg

▷ **Stribild (B)** *elvitegravir/cobicistat/emtricitabine/tenofovir disoproxil fumarate* 1 tab once daily; *CrCl <70 mL/min:* not recommended; *if CrCl declines to <50 mL/min during treatment:* discontinue; *Severe hepatic impairment:* not recommended
Pediatric: not established
> *Tab:* *elvi* 150 mg/*cobi* 150 mg/*emtri* 200 mg/*teno dis fum* 300 mg

▷ **Triumeq (C)(G)** *abacavir sulfate/dolutegravir/lamivudine* 1 tab once daily
Pediatric: not established
> *Tab:* *aba* 600 mg/*dolu* 50 mg/*lami* 300 mg

▷ **Trizivir (C)(G)** *abacavir sulfate/lamivudine/zidovudine* 1 tab bid
Pediatric: <40 kg: not recommended; ≥40 kg: same as adult
> *Tab:* *aba* 300 mg/*lami* 150 mg/*zido* 300 mg

▷ **Truvada (B)** *emtricitabine/tenofovir disoproxil fumarate*
Pediatric: <17 kg: not established; 17-<22 kg: 100/150 once daily; 22-<28 kg: 133/200 once daily; 28-35 kg: 167/250 once daily; ≥35 kg: 200/300 once daily
> *Tab:* **Truvada 100/150** *emt* 100 mg/*teno* 150 mg
> **Truvada 133/200** *emt* 133 mg/*teno* 200 mg
> **Truvada 167/250** *emt* 167 mg/*teno* 250 mg
> **Truvada 200/300** *emt* 200 mg/*teno* 300 mg

Comment: **Truvada** is indicated for treatment of HIV-1 infection and pre-exposure prophylaxis (PrEP) to reduce the risk of sexually acquired HIV-1 in high risk adults in combination with safe sex practices.

HUMAN PAPILLOMAVIRUS (HPV, VENEREAL WART)

PROPHYLAXIS

Comment: Administer IM in deltoid. Administer a 3-dose series; First dose females (10-25 years of age) and males (9-15 years of age); Second dose: 1-2 months after first dose; Third dose: 6 months after first dose. HPV vaccination is indicated for the prevention of cervical, vulvar, vaginal, and anal cancers. Register pregnant patients exposed to **Gardasil** by calling 800-986-8999.

▶ *bivalent human papillomavirus types 16 and 18 vaccine, aluminum adsorbed* (B)
   Pediatric: <10 years: not recommended
      Cervarix administer in the deltoid; 1st dose 0.5 ml IM on elected date; then, 2nd dose 0.5 ml IM 1 month later; then, 3rd dose 0.5 ml IM 6 months after the first dose
         Vial: susp for IM inj (single-dose; prefilled syringe) (preservative-free)

▶ *quadrivalent human papillomavirus types 6, 11, 16, and 18 vaccine, recombinant, aluminum adsorbed* (B)
   Pediatric: >9 years: not recommended
      Gardasil administer in the deltoid <u>or</u> upper thigh; 1st dose 0.5 ml IM on elected date; then, 2nd dose 0.5 ml IM 2 months later; then, 3rd dose 0.5 ml IM 6 months after the first dose
         Vial: susp for IM inj (single-dose; prefilled syringe w. needles <u>or</u> tip caps) (preservative-free)

▶ *quadrivalent human papillomavirus types 6, 11, 16, 18, 31, 33, 45, 52, and 58 vaccine, recombinant, aluminum adsorbed* (B)
      Gardasil 9 *Adults and Children: 9-26 Years-of-Age:* administer IM in the deltoid or thigh; administer the 1st dose; administer the 2nd dose 2 months after the 1st dose; administer the 3rd dose 6 months after the 1st dose (4 months after the 2nd dose).
         Vial: susp for IM inj (0.5 ml single-dose; prefilled syringe w. needles <u>or</u> tip caps) (preservative-free)

TREATMENT

see **Wart: Venereal** page 460

 HYPERHIDROSIS (PERSPIRATION, EXCESSIVE)

▶ *aluminum chloride* (NE) 20% solution apply q HS; wash treated area the following morning; after 1-2 treatments, may reduce frequency to 1-2 times/week
      Drysol *Soln:* 35, 60 ml (alcohol 93%) cont-rel
Comment: Apply to clean dry skin (e.g., underarms). Do not apply to broken, irritated, <u>or</u> recently shaved skin.

 HYPERHOMOCYSTEINEMIA

Comment: Elevated homocysteine is associated with cognitive impairment, vascular dementia, and dementia of the Alzheimer's type.

HOMOCYSTEINE-LOWERING NUTRITIONAL SUPPLEMENTS

▷ *L-methylfolate calcium (as metafolin)/pyridoxyl 5-phosphate/methyl-cobalamin* (**NE**) take 1 cap daily
Pediatric: not recommended
> **Metanx** *Cap: metafo* 3 mg/*pyrid* 35 mg/*methyl* 2 mg (gluten-free, yeast-free, lactose-free)
> **Comment: Metanx** is indicated as adjunct treatment of endothelial dysfunction and/or hyperhomocysteinemia in patients who have lower extremity ulceration.

▷ *L-methylfolate calcium (as metafolin)/methylcobalamin/N-acetylcysteine* (**NE**) take 1 cap daily
Pediatric: not recommended
> **Cerefolin** *Cap: metafo* 5.6 mg/*methyl* 2 mg/*N-ace* 600 mg (gluten-free, yeast-free, lactose-free)
> **Comment: Cerefolin** is indicated in the dietary management of patients treated for early memory loss, with emphasis on those at risk for neurovascular oxidative stress, hyperhomocysteinemia, mild to moderate cognitive impairment with or without vitamin B-12 deficiency, vascular dementia, or Alzheimer's disease.

◯ HYPERKALEMIA (POTASSIUM EXCESS)

HYPERKALEMIA CATION EXCHANGE RESINS

Comment: Normal serum K^+ range is approximately 3.5-5.5 mEq/L. Hyperkalemia is associated with cardiac dysrhythmias and metabolic acidosis. Risk factors include kidney disease, heart failure, and drugs that inhibit the renin-angiotensin-aldosterone system (RAAS) including ACEIs, ARBs, direct renin inhibitors, and aldosterone antagonists. Cation exchange resins are not for emergency treatment of life-threatening hyperkalemia, severe constipation, bowel obstruction or impaction. May cause GI irritability, ulceration, necrosis, sodium retention, hypocalcemia, hypomagnesemia, fecal impaction, ischemic colitis. Avoid non-absorbable cation-donating antacids and laxatives (e.g., *magnesium hydroxide, aluminum hydroxide*). Concomitant sorbitol should be avoided because it may cause intestinal necrosis.

▷ *patiromer sorbitex calcium* (**B**) initially 8.4 gm once daily; adjust dosage as prescribed based on potassium concentration and target range; may increase dosage at 1-week (or longer) intervals in increments of 8.4 gm; max dose 25.2 gm once daily; prepare immediately prior to administration; do not take in dry form; administer with food; measure 1/3 cup of water and pour half into a glass; then add **Veltassa** and stir; add the remaining water and stir well; the powder will not dissolve and the mixture will look cloudy; add more water as needed for desired consistency; do not heat or mix with heated food or fluids
> **Veltassa** *Pkt:* 8,4, 16.8, 25.2 gm pwdr for oral susp, 30 single-use pkts/carton
> **Comment:** Take **Veltassa** at least 3 hours before or 3 hours after any other medicine taken by mouth. Store packets in the refrigerator. It stored at room temperature, product must be used within 3 months.

▷ *sodium polystyrene sulfonate* (**C**)(**G**)
Pediatrics: Use 1 gm/1 mEq of K^+ as basis of calculation; see mfr literature
> **Kayexalate** *Susp:* 15 gm 1-4 times daily; *Rectal Enema:* 30-50 gm in 100 ml every 6 hours

HYPERPARATHYROIDISM

➤ *calcifediol* **(C)(G)** 1 cap daily
 Pediatric: <18 years: not established
  Rayaldee *Cap:* 30 mcg ext-rel
  Comment: **Rayaldee** is indicated for the prevention and treatment of secondary hyperparathyroidism associated with chronic kidney disease (CKD), stage 3 or 4 and serum total 25-hydroxyvitamin D levels <30 mg/mL.
➤ *paricalcitol* **(C)(G)** administer 0.04-1 mcg/kg (2.8-7 mcg) IV bolus, during dialysis, no more than every other day; may be increased by 2-4 mcg every 2-4 weeks; monitor serum calcium and phosphorus during dose adjustment periods; if Ca x P >75, immediately reduce dose or discontinue until these levels normalize; discard unused portion of single-use vials immediately
 Pediatric: <18 years: not established
  Zemplar *Vial:* 2, 5 mcg/ml soln for inj
  Comment: **Zemplar** is indicated for the prevention and treatment of secondary hyperparathyroidism associated with chronic kidney disease (CKD), stage 5.

 HYPERPHOSPHATEMIA

PHOSPHATE BINDERS

Comment: Monitor for development of hypercalcemia. Normal serum PO_4^- is 2.5-4.5 mg/dL and normal serum calcium is 8.5-10.5 mg/dL.
➤ *calcium acetate* **(C)(G)** initially 2 tabs or caps with each meal; then titrate gradually to keep serum phosphate at <6 mg/dL; usual maintenance is 3-4 tabs or caps with each meal
 Pediatric: not recommended
  PhosLo *Tab:* 667 mg; *Cap:* 667 mg
➤ *lanthanum carbonate* **(C)** initially 750 mg to 1.5 g per day in divided doses; take with meals; titrate at 2-3-week intervals in increments of 750 mg/day based on serum phosphate; usual range 1.5-3 g/day; usual max 3,750 mg/day
 Pediatric: not recommended
  Fosrenol *Chew tab:* 250, 500, 750 mg; 1 g
➤ *sevelamer* **(C)** for patients not taking a phosphate binder, take tid with meals; swallow whole; titrate by 1 tab per meal at 1-week intervals to keep serum phosphorus 3.5-5.5 mg/dL; switching from calcium acetate to *sevelamer,* see mfr pkg insert. *Serum phosphorus >5.5 to >7.5 mg/dL:* 800 mg tid; *Serum phosphorus 7.5-9:* 1.2-1.6 g tid
 Pediatric: not recommended
  Renagel *Tab:* 400, 800 mg
  Renvela *Tab:* 800 mg

 HYPERPIGMENTATION

Comment: Depigmenting agents may be used for hyperpigmented skin conditions including chloasma, melasma, freckles, senile lentigenes. Limit treatments to small areas at one time. Sunscreen ≥30 SPF recommended.

▷ *hydroquinone* (C)(G) apply sparingly to affected area and rub in bid
    Lustra *Crm:* 4% (1, 2 oz) (sulfites)
    Lustra AF *Crm:* 4% (1, 2 oz) (sunscreen, sulfites)
▷ *monobenzone* (C) apply sparingly to affected area and rub in bid-tid; depigmentation
occurs in 1-4 months
    Benoquin *Crm:* 20% (1.25 oz)
▷ *tazarotene* (X)(G) apply daily at HS
  Pediatric: not recommended
    Avage Cream *Crm:* 0.1% (30 g)
    Tazorac Cream *Crm:* 0.05, 0.1% (15, 30, 60 g)
    Tazorac Gel *Gel:* 0.05, 0.1% (30, 100 g)
▷ *tretinoin* (C) apply daily at HS
  Pediatric: <12 years: not recommended; ≥12 years: same as adult
    Avita *Crm/Gel:* 0.025% (20, 45 g)
    Renova *Crm:* 0.02% (40 g); 0.05% (40, 60 g)
    Retin-A Cream *Crm:* 0.025, 0.05, 0.1% (20, 45 g)
    Retin-A Gel *Gel:* 0.01, 0.025% (15, 45 g) (alcohol 90%)
    Retin-A Liquid *Liq:* 0.05% (28 ml) (alcohol 55%)
    Retin-A Micro *Microspheres:* 0.04, 0.1% (20, 45 g)

COMBINATION AGENTS

▷ *hydroquinone/fluocinolone/tretinoin* (C) apply sparingly to affected area and rub in
daily at HS
Pediatric: not recommended
    Tri-Luma *Crm:* hydro 4%/*fluo* 0.01%/*tretin* 0.05% (30 g) (parabens, sulfites)
▷ *hydroquinone/padimate O/oxybenzone/octyl methoxycinnamate* (C) apply sparingly to affected area and rub in bid
Pediatric: <12 years: not recommended; ≥16 years: same as adult
    Glyquin *Crm:* 4% (1 oz jar)
▷ *hydroquinone/ethyl dihydroxypropyl PABA/dioxybenzone/oxybenzone* (C) apply sparingly to affected area and rub in bid; max 2 months
    Pediatric: not recommended
    Solaquin *Crm:* hydro 2%/*PABA* 5%/*dioxy* 3%/*oxy* 2% (1 oz) (sulfites)
▷ *hydroquinone/padimate/dioxybenzone/oxybenzone* (C) apply sparingly to affected
area and rub in bid; max 2 months
Pediatric: not recommended
    Solaquin Forte *Crm:* hydro 4%/*pad* 0.5%/*dioxy* 3%/*oxy* 2% (1oz) (sunscreen, sulfites)
▷ *hydroquinone/padimate/dioxybenzone* (C) apply sparingly to affected area and rub
in bid; max 2 months
Pediatric: not recommended
    Solaquin Forte Gel: hydro 4%/*pad* 0.5%/*dioxy* 3% (1 oz) (alcohol, sulfites)

⊙ HYPERPROLACTINEMIA

DOPAMINE RECEPTOR AGONIST

▷ *dostinex* (B)(G) initial therapy is 0.25 mg twice a week; may increase by 0.25 mg twice
weekly up to 1 mg twice a week according to the patient's serum prolactin level; dose
increases should not occur more than every 4 weeks; after a normal serum prolactin

level has been maintained for 6 months, may be discontinued, with periodic monitoring of serum prolactin level to determine if/when treatment should be reinstituted
Pediatric: not established
> **Cabergoline** *Tab:* 0.5 mg

Comment: **Cabergoline** is indicated to treat hyperprolactinemia disorders due to idiopathic <u>or</u> pituitary adenoma.

 HYPERTENSION: PRIMARY

see JNC-8 Recommendations page 472

BETA-BLOCKERS: CARDIOSELECTIVE

Comment: Cardioselective beta-blockers are less likely to cause bronchospasm, peripheral vasoconstriction, <u>or</u> hypoglycemia than noncardioselective beta-blockers.
➤ *acebutolol* (B)(G) initially 400 mg in 1-2 divided doses; usual range 200-800 mg/day; max 1.2 g/day in 2 divided doses
Pediatric: not recommended
    Sectral *Cap:* 200, 400 mg
➤ *atenolol* (D)(G) initially 50 mg daily; may increase after 1-2 weeks to 100 mg daily; max 100 mg/day
Pediatric: not recommended
    Tenormin *Tab:* 25, 50, 100 mg
➤ *betaxolol* (C) initially 10 mg daily; may increase to 20 mg/day after 7-14 days; usual max 20 mg/day
Pediatric: not recommended
    Kerlone *Tab:* 10*, 20 mg
➤ *bisoprolol* (C) 5 mg daily; max 20 mg daily
Pediatric: not recommended
    Zebeta *Tab:* 5*, 10 mg
➤ *metoprolol succinate* (C)
Pediatric: not recommended
    Toprol-XL initially 25-100 mg in a single dose once daily; increase weekly if needed; max 400 mg/day; as monotherapy or with a diuretic
        Tab: 25*, 50*, 100*, 200*mg ext-rel
➤ *metoprolol tartrate* (C)
Pediatric: not recommended
    Lopressor (G) initially 25-50 mg bid; increase weekly if needed; max 400 mg/day; as monotherapy or with a diuretic
        Tab: 25, 37.5, 50, 75, 100 mg
➤ *nebivolol* (C)(G)
Pediatric: not recommended
    Bystolic initially 5 mg daily; may increase at 2 week intervals; max 40 mg/day
        Tab: 2.5, 5, 10, 20 mg

BETA-BLOCKERS: NONCARDIOSELECTIVE

Comment: Noncardioselective beta-blockers are more likely to cause bronchospasm, peripheral vasoconstriction, <u>and/or</u> hypoglycemia than cardioselective beta-blockers.

▷ *nadolol* (C)(G) initially 40 mg daily; usual maintenance 40-80 mg daily; max 320 mg/day
  Pediatric: not recommended
      Corgard *Tab:* 20*, 40*, 80*, 120*, 160*mg
▷ *penbutolol* (C) 20 mg daily
  Pediatric: not recommended
      Levatol *Tab:* 20*mg
▷ *pindolol* (B)(G) initially 5 mg bid; may increase after 3-4 weeks in 10 mg increments; max 60 mg/day
  Pediatric: not recommended
      Pindolol *Tab:* 5, 10 mg
      Visken *Tab:* 5, 10 mg
▷ *propranolol* (C)(G)
      Inderal initially 40 mg bid; usual maintenance 120-240 mg/day; max 640 mg/day
          Pediatric: initially 1 mg/kg/day; usual range 2-4 mg/kg/day in 2 divided doses; max 16 mg/kg/day
          Tab: 10*, 20*, 40*, 60*, 80*mg
      Inderal LA initially 80 mg daily in a single dose; increase q 3-7 days; usual range 120-160 mg/day; max 320 mg/day in a single dose
          Pediatric: not recommended
          Cap: 60, 80, 120, 160 mg sust-rel
      InnoPran XL initially 80 mg q HS; max 120 mg/day
          Pediatric: not recommended
          Cap: 80, 120 mg ext-rel
▷ *timolol* (C)(G) initially 10 mg bid, increase weekly if needed; usual maintenance 20-40 mg/day; max 60 mg/day in 2 divided doses
  Pediatric: not recommended
      Blocadren *Tab:* 5, 10*, 20*mg

BETA-BLOCKER: (NONCARDIOSELECTIVE)/ALPHA-1 BLOCKER COMBINATIONS

▷ *carvedilol* (C)
  Pediatric: <18 years: not recommended
      Coreg initially 6.25 mg bid; may increase at 1-2-week intervals to 12.5 mg bid; max 25 mg bid
          Tab: 3.125, 6.25, 12.5, 25 mg
      Coreg CR initially 20 mg once daily for 2 weeks; may increase at 1-2-week intervals; max 80 mg once daily
          Tab: 10, 20, 40, 80 mg cont-rel
▷ *carteolol* (C)
  Pediatric: not recommended
      Cartrol initially 2.5 mg daily, gradually increase to 5 or 10 mg daily; usual maintenance 2.5-5 mg daily
          Tab: 2.5, 5 mg
▷ *labetalol* (C)(G) initially 100 mg bid; increase after 2-3 days if needed; usual maintenance 200-400 mg bid; max 2.4 g/day
  Pediatric: not recommended
      Normodyne *Tab:* 100*, 200*, 300 mg
      Trandate *Tab:* 100*, 200*, 300*mg

DIURETICS

Thiazide Diuretics

▷ *chlorthalidone* (B)(G) initially 15 mg daily; may increase to 30 mg once daily based on clinical response; max 45-60 mg/day
  Pediatric: not established
      Chlorthalidone *Tab:* 25, 50 mg
      Thalitone *Tab:* 15 mg
▷ *chlorothiazide* (B)(G) 0.5-1 g/day in a single or divided doses; max 2 g/day
  Pediatric: <6 months: up to 15 mg/lb/day in 2 divided doses; ≥6 months: 10 mg/lb/day in 2 divided doses
      Diuril *Tab:* 250*, 500*mg; *Oral susp:* 250 mg/5 ml (237 ml)
▷ *hydrochlorothiazide* (B)(G)
  Pediatric: not recommended
      Esidrix 25-100 mg once daily
      Tab: 25, 50, 100 mg
      Hydrochlorothiazide *Tab:* 25*, 50*mg
      Microzide 12.5 mg once daily; usual max 50 mg/day
      Cap: 12.5 mg
▷ *methyclothiazide* (B) initially 2.5 mg daily; max 10 mg daily
  Pediatric: not recommended
      Enduronyl *Tab: methy* 5 mg/*deser* 0.25 mg*
      Enduronyl Forte *Tab: methy* 5 mg/*deser* 0.5 mg*
▷ *polythiazide* (C) 2-4 mg once daily
  Pediatric: not recommended
      Renese *Tab:* 1, 2, 4 mg

Potassium-Sparing Diuretics

▷ *amiloride* (B)(C) initially 5 mg; may increase to 10 mg; max 20 mg
  Pediatric: not recommended
      Midamor *Tab:* 5 mg
▷ *spironolactone* (D)(G) initially 50-100 mg in a single or divided doses; titrate at 2-week intervals
  Pediatric: not established
      Aldactone *Tab:* 25, 50*, 100*mg
▷ *triamterene* (B) 100 mg bid; max 300 mg
  Pediatric: not recommended
      Dyrenium
          Cap: 50, 100 mg

Loop Diuretics

▷ *bumetanide* (C)(G) 0.5-2 mg daily; may repeat at 4-5-hour intervals; max 10 mg/day
  Pediatric: <18 years: not recommended
  Tab: 1* mg
  Comment: *bumetanide* is contraindicated with sulfa drug allergy.
▷ *ethacrynic acid* (B)(G) initially 50-200 mg/day
  Pediatric: infant: not recommended; ≥1 month: initially 25 mg/day; then adjust dose in 25-mg increments

Edecrin *Tab:* 25, 50 mg
▷ *ethacrynate sodium* (B)(G) for IV injection
    Sodium Edecrin *Vial:* 50 mg single-dose
    Comment: **Sodium Edecrin** is more potent than more commonly used loop and thiazide diuretics.
▷ *furosemide* (C)(G) initially 40 mg bid
    Pediatric: not recommended
    Lasix *Tab:* 20, 40*, 80 mg; *Oral Soln:* 10 mg/ml (2, 4 oz w. dropper)
    Comment: *furosemide* is contraindicated with sulfa drug allergy.
▷ *torsemide* (B) 5 mg once daily; may increase to 10 mg once daily
    Pediatric: not recommended
    Demadex *Tab:* 5*, 10*, 20*, 100*mg

Other Diuretics

▷ *indapamide* (B) initially 1.25 mg daily; may titrate dosage upward q 4 weeks if needed; max 5 mg/day
    Pediatric: not recommended
    Lozol *Tab:* 1.25, 2.5 mg
    Comment: *indapamide* is contraindicated with sulfa drug allergy.
▷ *metolazone* (B)
    Pediatric: not recommended
    Zaroxolyn 2.5- 5 mg daily
      Tab: 2.5, 5, 10 mg
    Comment: *metolazone* is contraindicated with sulfa drug allergy.

DIURETIC COMBINATIONS

▷ *amiloride/hydrochlorothiazide* (B)(G) initially 1 tab daily; may increase to 2 tabs/day in a single or divided doses
    Pediatric: not recommended
    Moduretic *Tab: amil* 5 mg/*hydro* 50 mg*
▷ *deserpidine/methylchlothiazide* (C) titrate *methylchlothiazide* 2.5-10 mg daily
    Pediatric: not recommended
    Enduronyl
      Tab: Enduronyl **0.25/5** *deser* 0.25 mg/*methylclo* 5 mg*
        Enduronyl **0.5/5** *deser* 0.5 mg/*methylclo* 5 mg*
▷ *spironolactone/hydrochlorothiazide* (D)(G)
    Pediatric: not recommended
    Aldactazide 25 usual maintenance 50-100 mg in a single or divided doses
      Tab: spiro 25 mg/*hctz* 25 mg
    Aldactazide 50 usual maintenance 50-100 mg in a single or divided doses
      Tab: spiro 50 mg/*hydro* 50 mg
▷ *triamterene/hydrochlorothiazide* (C)(G)
    Pediatric: not recommended
    Dyazide 1-2 caps once daily
      Cap: triam 37.5 mg/*hctz* 25 mg
    Maxzide 1 tab once daily
      Tab: triam 75 mg/*hctz* 50 mg*
    Maxzide-25 1-2 tabs once daily
      Tab: triam 37.5 mg/*hctz* 25 mg*

ANGIOTENSIN CONVERTING ENZYME INHIBITORS (ACEIs)

Comment: Black patients receiving ACEI monotherapy have been reported to have a higher incidence of angioedema compared to non-Blacks. Non-Blacks have a greater decrease in BP when ACEIs are used compared to Black patients.

▷ *benazepril* (D)(G) initially 10 mg daily; usual maintenance 20-40 mg/day in 1-2 divided doses; usual max 80 mg/day
  Pediatric: not recommended
  Lotensin *Tab:* 5, 10, 20, 40 mg

▷ *captopril* (D)(G) initially 25 mg bid-tid; after 1-2 weeks increase to 50 mg bid-tid
  Pediatric: not recommended
  Capoten *Tab:* 12.5*, 25*, 50*, 100*mg

▷ *enalapril* (D) initially 5 mg daily; usual dosage range 10-40 mg/day; max 40 mg/day
  Pediatric: not recommended
  Epaned Oral Solution *Oral soln:* 1mg/ml (150 ml) (mixed berry)
  Vasotec (G) *Tab:* 2.5*, 5*, 10, 20 mg

▷ *fosinopril* (D) initially 10 mg daily; usual maintenance 20-40 mg/day in a single <u>or</u> divided doses; max 80 mg/day
  Pediatric: <6 years, <50 kg: not recommended; ≥6-12 years, >50 kg: 5-10 mg once daily
  Monopril *Tab:* 10*, 20, 40 mg

▷ *lisinopril* (D)
  Prinivil initially 10 mg daily; usual range 20-40 mg/day
    Pediatric: not recommended
    Tab: 5*, 10*, 20*, 40 mg
  Qbrelis Oral Solution administer as a single dose once daily
    Pediatric: <6 years, GFR <30 mL/min: not recommended; ≥6 years, GFR >30 mL/min: initially 0.07 mg/kg, max 5 mg; adjust according to BP up to a max 0.61 mg/kg (40 mg) once daily
    Oral soln: 1 mg/ml (150 ml)
  Zestril initially 10 mg daily; usual range 20-40 mg/day
    Pediatric: not recommended
    Tab: 2.5, 5*, 10, 20, 30, 40 mg

▷ *moexipril* (D) initially 7.5 mg daily; usual range 15-30 mg/day in 1-2 divided doses; max 30 mg/day
  Pediatric: not recommended
  Univasc *Tab:* 7.5*, 15*mg

▷ *perindopril* (D) 2-8 mg daily-bid; max 16 mg/day
  Pediatric: not recommended
  Aceon *Tab:* 2*, 4*, 8*mg

▷ *quinapril* (D) initially 10 mg once daily; usual maintenance 20-80 mg daily in 1-2 divided doses
  Pediatric: not recommended
  Accupril *Tab:* 5*, 10, 20, 40 mg

▷ *ramipril* (D)(G) initially 2.5 mg bid; usual maintenance 2.5-20 mg in 1-2 divided doses
  Pediatric: not established
  Altace *Tab/Cap:* 1.25, 2.5, 5, 10 mg

▷ *trandolapril* (C; D in 2nd, 3rd) initially 1-2 mg once daily; adjust at 1-week intervals; usual range 2-4 mg in 1-2 divided doses; max 8 mg/day
  Pediatric: not recommended
  Mavik *Tab:* 1*, 2, 4 mg

ANGIOTENSIN II RECEPTOR BLOCKERS (ARBs)

▷ *azilsartan medoxomil* (D) *Monotherapy, not volume depleted:* 80 mg once daily; *Volume-depleted (concomitant high-dose diuretic):* initially 40 mg once daily
Pediatric: not recommended
    Edarbi *Tab:* 40, 80 mg

▷ *candesartan* (D)(G) initially 16 mg daily; range 8-32 mg in 1-2 divided doses
Pediatric: not recommended
    Atacand *Tab:* 4, 8, 16, 32 mg

▷ *eprosartan* (D)(G) initially 400 mg bid <u>or</u> 600 mg once daily; max 800 mg/day
Pediatric: not established
    Teveten *Tab:* 400, 600 mg

▷ *irbesartan* (D)(G) initially 150 mg daily; titrate up to 300 mg
Pediatric: not recommended
    Avapro *Tab:* 75, 150, 300 mg

▷ *losartan* (D)(G) initially 50 mg daily; max 100 mg/day
Pediatric: not recommended
    Cozaar *Tab:* 25, 50, 100 mg

▷ *olmesartan medoxomil* (D) initially 20 mg once daily; after 2 weeks, may increase to 40 mg daily
Pediatric: <6 years: not recommended; ≥6-16 years: 20-35 kg: initially 10 mg once daily; after 2 weeks, may increase to max 20 mg once daily; ≥6-16 years: >35 kg: initially 20 mg once daily; after 2 weeks, may increase to max 40 mg once daily
    Benicar *Tab:* 5, 20, 40 mg

▷ *telmisartan* (D)(G) initially 40 mg once daily; usual dose 20-80 mg
Pediatric: not recommended
    Micardis *Tab:* 20, 40, 80 mg

▷ *valsartan* (D)(G) initially 80 mg once daily; may increase to 160 <u>or</u> 320 mg once daily after 2-4 weeks; usual range 80-320 mg/day
Pediatric: not recommended
    Diovan *Tab:* 40*, 80, 160, 320 mg

CALCIUM CHANNEL BLOCKERS (CCBs)

Benzothiazepines

▷ *diltiazem* (C)(G)
Pediatric: not established
    Cardizem initially 30 mg qid; may increase gradually every 1-2 days; max 360 mg/day in divided doses
      Tab: 30, 60, 90, 120 mg
    Cardizem CD initially 120-180 mg daily; adjust at 1-2-week intervals; max 480 mg/day
      Cap: 120, 180, 240, 300, 360 mg ext-rel
    Cardizem LA initially 180-240 mg daily; titrate at 2-week intervals; max 540 mg/day
      Tab: 120, 180, 240, 300, 360, 420 mg ext-rel
    Cardizem SR initially 60-120 mg bid; adjust at 2-week intervals; max 360 mg/day
      Cap: 60, 90, 120 mg sust-rel
    Cartia XT initially 180 <u>or</u> 240 mg once daily; max 540 mg once daily
      Cap: 120, 180, 240, 300 mg ext-rel
    Dilacor XR initially 180 <u>or</u> 240 mg in AM; usual range 180-480 mg/day; max 540 mg/day

Cap: 120, 180, 240 mg ext-rel

Tiazac (G) initially 120-240 mg daily; adjust at 2-week intervals; usual max 540 mg/day

Cap: 120, 180, 240, 300, 360, 420 mg ext-rel

▷ *diltiazem maleate* **(C)** initially 120-180 mg daily; adjust at 2-week intervals; usual range 120-480 mg daily

Pediatric: not recommended

Tiamate *Cap:* 120, 180, 240 mg ext-rel

Dihydropyridines

▷ *amlodipine* **(C)** initially 5 mg once daily; max 10 mg/day

Pediatric: not recommended

Norvasc *Tab:* 2.5, 5, 10 mg

▷ *clevidipine butyrate* **(C)** administer by IV infusion; initially 1-2 mg/hour; double dose at 90-second intervals until BP approaches goal; then titrate slower; adjust at 5-10-minute intervals; maintenance 4-6 mg/hour; usual max, 16-32 mg/hour; do not exceed 1,000 ml (21 mg/hour for 24 hours) due to lipid load

Pediatric: <18 years: not recommended

Cleviprex *Vial:* 0.5 mg/ml soln for IV infusion (single use, 50, 100 ml) (lipids)

Comment: Cleviprex is indicated to reduce blood pressure when oral therapy is not feasible or desirable. **Cleviprex** is contraindicated with egg or soy allergy.

▷ *felodipine* **(C)(G)** initially 5 mg daily; usual range 2.5-10 mg daily; adjust at 2-week intervals; max 10 mg/day

Pediatric: not recommended

Plendil *Tab:* 2.5, 5, 10 mg ext-rel

▷ *isradipine* **(C)**

Pediatric: not recommended

DynaCirc initially 2.5 mg bid; adjust in increments of 5 mg/day at 2-4-week intervals; max 20 mg/day

Cap: 2.5, 5 mg

DynaCirc CR initially 5 mg daily; adjust in increments of 5 mg/day at 2-4-week intervals; max 20 mg/day

Tab: 5, 10 mg cont-rel

▷ *nicardipine* **(C)(G)**

Pediatric: <18 years: not recommended

Cardene initially 20 mg tid; adjust at intervals of at least 3 days; max 120 mg/day

Cap: 20, 30 mg

Cardene SR 30-60 mg bid

Cap: 30, 45, 60 mg sust-rel

▷ *nifedipine* **(C)(G)**

Pediatric: not recommended

Adalat initially 10 mg tid; usual range 10-20 mg tid; max 180 mg/day

Cap: 10, 20 mg

Adalat CC initially 10 mg tid; usual range 10-20 mg tid; max 180 mg/day

Cap: 30, 60, 90 mg ext-rel

Afeditab CR initially 30 mg once daily; titrate over 7-14 days; max 90 mg/day

Cap: 30, 60 mg ext-rel

Procardia initially 10 mg tid; titrate over 7-14 days: max 30 mg/dose and 180 mg/day in divided doses

Cap: 10, 20 mg

> **Procardia XL** initially 30-60 mg daily; titrate over 7-14 days; max dose 90 mg/day
>> *Tab:* 30, 60, 90 mg ext-rel

▷ *nisoldipine* (C)
  Pediatric: not recommended
> **Sular** initially 20 mg daily; may increase by 10 mg weekly; usual maintenance 20-40 mg/day; max 60 mg/day
>> *Tab:* 10, 20, 30, 40 mg ext-rel

Diphenylalkylamines

▷ *verapamil* (C)(G)
  Pediatric: not recommended
> **Calan** 80-120 mg tid; may titrate up; usual max 360 mg in divided doses
>> *Tab:* 40, 80*, 120*mg
> **Calan SR** initially 120 mg in the AM; may titrate up; max 480 mg/day in divided doses
>> *Cplt:* 120, 180*, 240*mg sust-rel
> **Covera HS** initially 180 mg q HS; titrate to 240 mg; then to 360 mg; then to 480 mg if needed
>> *Tab:* 180, 240 mg ext-rel
> **Isoptin** initially 80-120 mg tid
>> *Tab:* 40, 80, 120 mg
> **Isoptin SR** initially 120-180 mg in the AM; may increase to 240 mg in the AM; then 180 mg q 12 hours <u>or</u> 240 mg in the AM and 120 mg in the PM; then 240 mg q 12 hours
>> *Tab:* 120, 180*, 240*mg sust-rel
> **Verelan** initially 240 mg once daily; adjust in 120 mg increments; max 480 mg/day
>> *Cap:* 120, 180, 240, 360 mg sust-rel
> **Verelan PM** initially 200 mg q HS; may titrate upward to 300 mg; then 400 mg if needed
>> *Cap:* 100, 200, 300 mg ext-rel

ALPHA-1 ANTAGONISTS

Comment: Educate the patient regarding potential side effects of hypotension when taking an alpha-1 antagonist, especially with first dose ("first dose effect"). Start at lowest dose and titrate upward.

▷ *doxazosin* (C)(G) initially 1 mg once daily at HS; increase dose slowly every 2 weeks if needed; max 16 mg/day
  Pediatric: not recommended
> **Cardura** *Tab:* 1*, 2*, 4*, 8*mg
> **Cardura XL** *Tab:* 4, 8 mg

▷ *prazosin* (C)(G) first dose at HS, 1 mg bid-tid; increase dose slowly; usual range 6-15 mg/day in divided doses; max 20-40 mg/day
  Pediatric: not recommended
> **Minipress** *Cap:* 1, 2, 5 mg

▷ *terazosin* (C) 1 mg q HS, then increase dose slowly; usual range 1-5 mg q HS; max 20 mg/day
  Pediatric: not recommended
> **Hytrin** *Cap:* 1, 2, 5, 10 mg

CENTRAL ALPHA-AGONISTS

▷ *clonidine* (C)
   Pediatric: <12 years: not recommended
     Catapres initially 0.1 mg bid; usual range 0.2-0.6 mg/day in divided doses; max
     2.4 mg/day; *Tab:* 0.1*, 0.2*, 0.3*mg
     Catapres-TTS initially 0.1 mg patch weekly; increase after 1-2 weeks if needed;
     max 0.6 mg/day
       Patch: 0.1, 0.2 mg/day (12/carton); 0.3 mg/day (4/carton)
     Kapvay (G) initially 0.1 mg bid; usual range 0.2-0.6 mg/day in divided doses;
     max 2.4 mg/day; *Tab:* 0.1, 0.2 mg
     Nexiclon XR initially 0.18 mg (2 ml) suspension *or* 0.17 mg tab once daily;
     usual max 0.52 mg (6 ml suspension) once daily
       Tab: 0.17, 0.26 mg ext-rel; *Oral susp:* 0.09 mg/ml ext-rel (4 oz)
▷ *guanabenz* (C)(G) initially 4 mg bid; may increase by 4-8 mg/day every 1-2 weeks;
   max 32 mg/day
   Pediatric: not recommended
     Tab: 4, 8 mg
▷ *guanfacine* (B)(G) initially 1 mg/day q HS; may increase to 2 mg/day q HS; usual
   max 2 mg/day
   Pediatric: not recommended
     Tenex *Tab:* 1, 2 mg
▷ *methyldopa* (B)(G) initially 250 mg bid-tid; titrate at 2-day intervals; usual maintenance 500 mg/day to 2 g/day; max 3 g/day
   Pediatric: initially 10 mg/kg/day in 2-4 divided doses; max 65 mg/kg/day *or* 3 g/day,
   whichever is less
     Aldomet *Tab:* 125, 250, 500 mg; *Oral susp:* 250 mg/5 ml (473 ml)

ALDOSTERONE RECEPTOR BLOCKER

▷ *eplerenone* (B) initially 25-50 mg daily; may increase to 50 mg bid; max 100 mg/day
   Pediatric: not recommended
     Inspra *Tab:* 25, 50 mg
     Comment: Contraindicated with concomitant potent CYP3A4 inhibitors. Risk
     of hyperkalemia with concomitant ACE-I *or* ARB. Monitor serum potassium at
     baseline, 1 week, and 1 month. Caution with serum Cr >2 mg/dL (male) *or* >1.8
     mg/dL (female) *and/or* CrCl <50 mL/min, and DM with proteinuria.

PERIPHERAL ADRENERGIC BLOCKER

▷ *guanethidine* (C) initially 10 mg daily; may adjust dose at 5-7 day intervals; usual
   range 25-50 mg/day
   Pediatric: not recommended
     Ismelin *Tab:* 10, 25 mg

DIRECT RENIN INHIBITOR

▷ *aliskiren* (D) initially 150 mg once daily; max 300 mg/day
   Pediatric: <18 years: not recommended
     Tekturna *Tab:* 150, 300 mg

PERIPHERAL VASODILATORS

▷ *hydralazine* (C)(G) initially 10 mg qid x 2-4 days; then increase to 25 mg qid for
   remainder of 1st week; then increase to 50 mg qid; max 300 mg/day
   Pediatric: initially 0.75 mg/kg/day in 4 divided doses; increase gradually over 3-4
   weeks; max 7.5 mg/kg/day *or* 2,000 mg/day
        Tab: 10, 25, 50, 100 mg
▷ *minoxidil* (C) initially 5 mg daily; may increase at 3-day intervals to 10 mg/day, then
   20 mg/day, then 40 mg/day; usual range 10-40 mg/day; max 100 mg/day
   Pediatric: initially 0.2 mg/kg daily; may increase in 50%-100% increments every 3
   days; usual range 0.25-1 g/kg/day; max 50 mg/day
        Loniten *Tab:* 2.5*, 10*mg

ACEI/DIURETIC COMBINATIONS

▷ *benazepril/hydrochlorothiazide* (D)
        Lotensin HCT 1 tab once daily; titrate individual components
            Pediatric: not recommended
            Tab: **Lotensin HCT 5/6.25** *benaz* 5 mg/*hctz* 6.25 mg*
                Lotensin HCT 10/12.5 *benaz* 10 mg/*hctz* 12.5 mg*
                Lotensin HCT 20/12.5 *benaz* 20 mg/*hctz* 12.5 mg*
                Lotensin HCT 20/25 *benaz* 20 mg/*hctz* 25 mg*
▷ *captopril/hydrochlorothiazide* (D)(G)
   Pediatric: not recommended
        Capozide 1 tab once daily; titrate individual components
            Tab: **Capozide 25/15** *capt* 25 mg/*hctz* 15 mg*
                Capozide 25/25 *capt* 25 mg/*hctz* 25 mg*
                Capozide 50/15 *capt* 50 mg/*hctz* 15 mg*
                Capozide 50/25 *capt* 50 mg/*hctz* 25 mg*
▷ *enalapril/hydrochlorothiazide* (D)
   Pediatric: not recommended
        Vaseretic 1 tab once daily; titrate individual components
            Tab: **Vaseretic 5/12.5** *enal* 5 mg/*hctz* 12.5 mg
                Vaseretic 10/25 *enal* 10 mg/*hctz* 25 mg
▷ *lisinopril/hydrochlorothiazide* (D)
   Pediatric: not recommended
        Prinzide 1 tab once daily; titrate individual components
            Tab: **Prinzide 10/12.5** *lis* 10 mg/*hctz* 12.5 mg
                Prinzide 20/12.5 *lis* 20 mg/*hctz* 12.5 mg
                Prinzide 20/25 *lis* 20 mg/*hctz* 25 mg
        Zestoretic 1 tab once daily; titrate individual components; *CrCl <40 mL/min:*
        not recommended
            Tab: **Zestoretic 10/12.5** *lis* 10 mg/*hctz* 12.5 mg
                Zestoretic 20/12.5 *lis* 20 mg/*hctz* 12.5 mg*
                Zestoretic 20/25 *lis* 20 mg/*hctz* 25 mg
▷ *moexipril/hydrochlorothiazide* (D)
   Pediatric: not recommended
        Uniretic 1 tab once daily; titrate individual components
            Tab: **Uniretic 7.5/12.5** *moex* 7.5 mg/*hctz* 12.5 mg*
                Uniretic 15/12.5 *moex* 15 mg/*hctz* 12.5 mg*
                Uniretic 15/25 *moex* 15 mg/*hctz* 25 mg*

▷ *quinapril/hydrochlorothiazide* (D)
  Pediatric: not recommended
      Accuretic 1 tab once daily; titrate individual components
          Tab: **Accuretic 10/12.5** *quin* 10 mg/*hctz* 12.5 mg*
              Accuretic 20/12.5 *quin* 20 mg/*hctz* 12.5 mg*
              Accuretic 20/25 *quin* 20 mg/*hctz* 25 mg*

ARB/DIURETIC COMBINATIONS

▷ *azilsartan/chlorthalidone* (D)
  Pediatric: <18 years: not recommended
      Edarbyclor 1 tab once daily; titrate individual components
          Tab: **Edarbyclor 40/12.5** *azil* 40 mg/*chlor* 12.5 mg
              Edarbyclor 40/25 *azil* 40 mg/*chlor* 25 mg
▷ *candesartan/hydrochlorothiazide* (D) 1 tab once daily; titrate individual components
  Pediatric: not recommended
      Atacand HCT
          Tab: **Atacand HCT 16/12.5** *cande* 16 mg/*hctz* 12.5 mg
              Atacand HCT 32/12.5 *cande* 32 mg/*hctz* 12.5 mg
▷ *eprosartan/hydrochlorothiazide* (D)
  Pediatric: not recommended
      Teveten HCT 1 tab once daily; titrate individual components
          Tab: **Teveten HCT 600/12.5** *epro* 600 mg/*hctz* 12.5 mg
              Teveten HCT 600/25 *epro* 600 mg/*hctz* 25 mg
▷ *irbesartan/hydrochlorothiazide* (D)
  Pediatric: not recommended
      Avalide 1 tab once daily; titrate individual components
          Tab: **Avalide 150/12.5** *irbes* 150 mg/*hctz* 12.5 mg
              Avalide 300/12.5 *irbes* 300 mg/*hctz* 12.5 mg
▷ *losartan/hydrochlorothiazide* (D)(G)
  Pediatric: not recommended
      Hyzaar 1 tab once daily; titrate individual components
          Tab: **Hyzaar 50/12.5** *losar* 50 mg/*hctz* 12.5 mg
              Hyzaar 100/12.5 *losar* 100 mg/*hctz* 12.5 mg
              Hyzaar 100/25 *losar* 100 mg/*hctz* 25 mg
▷ *olmesartan medoxomil/hydrochlorothiazide* (D)(G)
  Pediatric: not recommended
      Benicar HCT 1 tab once daily; titrate individual components
          Tab: **Benicar HCT 20/12.5** *olmi* 20 mg/*hctz* 12.5 mg
              Benicar HCT 40/12.5 *olmi* 40 mg/*hctz* 12.5 mg
              Benicar HCT 40/25 *olmi* 40 mg/*hctz* 25 mg
▷ *telmisartan/hydrochlorothiazide* (D)(G)
  Pediatric: not recommended
      Micardis HCT 1 tab once daily; titrate individual components
          Tab: **Micardis HCT 40/12.5** *telmi* 40 mg/*hctz* 12.5 mg
              Micardis HCT 80/12.5 *telmi* 80 mg/*hctz* 12.5 mg
              Micardis HCT 80/25 *telmi* 80 mg/*hctz* 25 mg
▷ *valsartan/hydrochlorothiazide* (D)
  Pediatric: not recommended
      Diovan HCT 1 tab once daily; titrate individual components

Tab: **Diovan HCT 80/12.5** *vals* 80 mg/*hctz* 12.5 mg
Diovan HCT 160/12.5 *vals* 160 mg/*hctz* 12.5 mg
Diovan HCT 160/25 *vals* 160 mg/*hctz* 25 mg
Diovan HCT 320/12.5 *vals* 320 mg/*hctz* 12.5 mg
Diovan HCT 320/25 *vals* 320 mg/*hctz* 25 mg

CENTRAL ALPHA-AGONIST/DIURETIC COMBINATIONS

▷ *clonidine/chlorthalidone* (C)
Pediatric: not recommended
Combipres 1 tab daily-bid
Tab: **Combipres 0.1** *clon* 0.1 mg/*chlorthal* 15 mg*
Combipres 0.2 *clon* 0.2 mg/*chlorthal* 15 mg*
Combipres 0.3 *clon* 0.3 mg/*chlorthal* 15 mg*
▷ *methyldopa/hydrochlorothiazide* (C)(G)
Pediatric: not recommended
Aldoril initially **Aldoril 15** bid-tid or **Aldoril 25** bid; titrate individual components
Tab: **Aldoril 15** *meth* 250 mg/*hctz* 15 mg
Aldoril 25 *meth* 250 mg/*hctz* 25 mg
Aldoril D30 *meth* 500 mg/*hctz* 30 mg
Aldoril D50 *meth* 500 mg/*hctz* 50 mg

BETA-BLOCKER (CARDIOSELECTIVE)/DIURETIC COMBINATIONS

▷ *atenolol/chlorthalidone* (D)(G)
Pediatric: not recommended
Tenoretic initially *tenoretic* 50 mg once daily; may increase to *tenoretic* 100 mg once daily
Tab: **Tenoretic 50/25** *aten* 50 mg/*chlor* 25 mg*
Tenoretic 100/25 *aten* 100 mg/*chlor* 25 mg
▷ *bisoprolol/hydrochlorothiazide* (C)
Pediatric: not recommended
Ziac initially one 2.5/6.25 mg tab daily; adjust at 2 week intervals; max two 10/6.25 mg tabs daily
Tab: **Ziac 2.5** *biso* 2.5 mg/*hctz* 6.25 mg
Ziac 5 *biso* 5 mg/*hctz* 6.25 mg
Ziac 10 *biso* 10 mg/*hctz* 6.25 mg
▷ *metoprolol succinate/hydrochlorothiazide* (C)
Pediatric: not recommendxed
Lopressor HCT titrate individual components
Tab: **Lopressor HCT 50/25** *meto succ* 50 mg/*hctz* 25mg*
Lopressor HCT 100/25 *meto succ* 100 mg/*hctz* 25mg*
Lopressor HCT 100/50 *meto succ* 100 mg/*hctz* 50mg*
▷ *metoprolol succinate/ext-rel hydrochlorothiazide* (C)
Pediatric: not established
Dutoprol titrate individual components; may titrate to max 200/25 mg once daily
Tab: **Dutoprol 25/12.5** *meto succ* 25 mg/*ext-rel hctz* 12.5 mg
Dutoprol 50/12.5 *meto succ* 50 mg/*ext-rel hctz* 12.5 mg
Dutoprol 100/12.5 *meto succ* 100 mg/*ext-rel hctz* 12.5 mg

BETA-BLOCKER (NONCARDIOSELECTIVE)/DIURETIC COMBINATIONS

▷ *nadolol/bendroflumethiazide* (C)
  Pediatric: not recommended
     Corzide titrate individual components
        Tab: **Corzide 40/5** *nado* 40 mg/*bend* 5 mg*
              Corzide 80/5 *nado* 80 mg/*bend* 5 mg*
▷ *propranolol/hydrochlorothiazide* (C)(G)
  Pediatric: not recommended
     Inderide titrate individual components
        Tab: **Inderide 40/25** *prop* 40 mg/*hctz* 25 mg*
              Inderide 80/25 prop 80 mg/hctz 25 mg*
              Inderide LA titrate individual components
        Cap: **Inderide LA 80/50** *prop* 80 mg/*hctz* 50 mg sust-rel
              Inderide LA 120/50 *prop* 120 mg/*hctz* 50 mg sust-rel
              Inderide LA 160/50 *prop* 160 mg/*hctz* 50 mg sust-rel
▷ *timolol/hydrochlorothiazide* (C)
  Pediatric: not recommended
     Timolide usual maintenance 2 tabs/day in a single <u>or</u> 2 divided doses
        Tab: *timo* 10 mg/*hctz* 25 mg

BETA-BLOCKER (CARDIOSELECTIVE)/ARB COMBINATION

▷ *nebivolol/valsartan* (X) 1 tab daily; may initiate when inadequately controlled on
  nebivolol 10 mg or *valsartan* 80 mg
  Pediatric: not established
     Byvalson *Tab:* nebi 5 mg/val 80 mg

ALPHA-1 ANTAGONIST/DIURETIC COMBINATIONS

▷ *prazosin/polythiazide* (C)
  Pediatric: not recommended
     Minizide titrate individual components
        Cap: **Minizide 1** *praz* 1 mg/*poly* 0.5 mg
              Minizide 2 *praz* 2 mg/*poly* 0.5 mg
              Minizide 5 *praz* 5 mg/*poly* 0.5 mg

PERIPHERAL ADRENERGIC BLOCKER/HCTZ COMBINATIONS

▷ *guanethidine/hydrochlorothiazide* (C)
  Pediatric: not recommended
     Esmil titrate individual components
        Tab: **Esmil 10/25** *guan* 1 mg/*hctz* 25 mg

ACEI/CCB COMBINATIONS

▷ *amlodipine/benazepril* (D)
  Pediatric: not recommended
     Lotrel titrate individual components
        Cap: **Lotrel 2.5/10** *amlo* 2.5 mg/*benaz* 10 mg
              Lotrel 5/10 *amlo* 5 mg/*benaz* 10 mg
              Lotrel 5/20 *amlo* 5 mg/*benaz* 20 mg

> **Lotrel 10/20** *amlo* 10 mg/*benaz* 20 mg
> **Lotrel 5/40** *amlo* 5 mg/*benaz* 40 mg
> **Lotrel 10/40** *amlo* 10 mg/*benaz* 40 mg

▷ *amlodipine/perindopril* (D)
   Pediatric: not recommended
      Prolastin titrate individual components
         Cap: **Prolastin 2.5/3.5** *amlo* 2.5 mg/*peri* 3.5 mg
            Prolastin 5/7 *amlo* 5 mg/*peri* 7 mg
            Prolastin 5/14 *amlo* 5 mg/*peri* 14 mg

▷ *enalapril/diltiazem* (D)
   Pediatric: not recommended
      Teczem titrate individual components
         Tab: *enal* 5 mg/*dil* 180 mg ext-rel

▷ *enalapril/felodipine* (D)
   Pediatric: <18 years: not recommended
      Lexxel initially 1 tab daily; after 1-2 weeks may increase to 2 tabs/day; titrate
      individual components
         Tab: **Lexxel 5/2.5** *enal* 5 mg/*felo* 2.5 mg ext-rel
            Lexxel 5/5 *enal* 5 mg/*felo* 5 mg ext-rel

▷ *perindopril/amlodipine* (D)
   Pediatric: not established
      Prestalia titrate individual components; max 14/10 once daily
         Tab: **Prestalia 3.5/2.5** *peri* 3.5 mg/*amlo* 2.5 mg
            Prestalia 7/5 *peri* 7 mg/*amlo* 5 mg
            Prestalia 14/10 *peri* 14 mg/*amlo* 10 mg

▷ *trandolapril/verapamil* (D)
   Pediatric: not established
      Tarka titrate individual components
         Tab: **Tarka 1/240** *tran* 1 mg/*ver* 240 mg ext-rel
            Tarka 2/180 *tran* 2 mg/*ver* 180 mg ext-rel
            Tarka 2/240 *tran* 2 mg/*ver* 240 mg ext-rel
            Tarka 4/240 *tran* 4 mg/*ver* 240 mg ext-rel

DRI/HCTZ COMBINATIONS

▷ *aliskiren/hydrochlorothiazide* (D) initially *aliskiren*150 mg once daily; max *aliskiren*
   300 mg/day
   Pediatric: <18 years: not recommended
      Tekturna HCT
         Tab: **Tekturna HCT 150/12.5** *alisk* 150 mg/*hctz* 12.5 mg
            Tekturna HCT 150/25 *alisk* 150 mg/*hctz* 25 mg
            Tekturna HCT 300/12.5 *alisk* 300 mg/*hctz* 12.5 mg
            Tekturna HCT 300/25 *alisk* 300 mg/*hctz* 25 mg

DRI/ARB COMBINATIONS

▷ *aliskiren/valsartan* (D)
   Pediatric: not recommended
      Valturna initially 150/160 once daily; may increase to max 300/320 once daily
         Tab: **Valturna 150/160** *alisk* 150 mg/*vals* 160 mg
            Valturna 300/320 *alisk* 300 mg/*vals* 320 mg

DRI/CCB COMBINATIONS

▷ *aliskiren/amlodipine* (D)
   Pediatric: not recommended
   Tekamlo initially 150/5 once daily; may increase to max 300/10 once daily
   Tab: **Tekamlo 150/5** *alisk* 150 mg/*amlo* 5 mg
   Tekamlo 150/10 *alisk* 150 mg/*amlo* 10 mg
   Tekamlo 300/5 *alisk* 300 mg/*amlo* 5 mg
   Tekamlo 300/10 *alisk* 300 mg/*amlo* 10 mg

DRI/CCB/HCTZ COMBINATIONS

▷ *aliskiren/amlodipine/hydrochlorothiazide* (D)
   Pediatric: not established
   Amturnide initially 150/5/12.5 once daily; may increase to max 300/10/25 once daily
   Tab: **Amturnide 150/5/12.5** *alisk* 150 mg/*amlo* 5 mg/*hctz* 12.5 mg
   Amturnide 300/5/12.5 *alisk* 300 mg/*amlo* 5 mg/*hctz* 12.5 mg
   Amturnide 300/5/25 *alisk* 300 mg/*amlo* 5 mg/*hctz* 25 mg
   Amturnide 300/10/25 *alisk* 300 mg/*amlo* 10 mg/*hctz* 25 mg

◯ HYPERTENSION

ARB/CCB COMBINATIONS

▷ *amlodipine/valsartan medoxomil* (D)(G)
   Pediatric: not recommended
   Exforge 1 tab daily; titrate individual components at 1-week intervals; max 10/320 daily
   Tab: **Exforge 5/160** *amlo* 5 mg/*vals* 160 mg
   Exforge 5/320 *amlo* 5 mg/*vals* 320 mg
   Exforge 10/160 *amlo* 10 mg/*vals* 160 mg
   Exforge 10/320 *amlo* 10 mg/*vals* 320 mg
▷ *amlodipine/olmesartan* (D)
   Pediatric: not established
   Azor titrate individual components
   Tab: **Azor 5/20** *amlo* 5 mg/*olme* 20 mg
   Azor 10/20 *amlo* 10 mg/*olme* 20 mg
   Azor 5/40 *amlo* 5 mg/*olme* 40 mg
   Azor 10/40 *amlo* 10 mg/*olme* 40 mg
▷ *telmisartan/amlodipine* (D)
   Pediatric: not established
   Twynsta initially 40/5 once daily; titrate at 1 week intervals; max 80/10 once daily
   Tab: **Twynsta 40/5** *telmi* 40 mg/*amlo* 5 mg
   Twynsta 40/10 *telmi* 40 mg/*amlo* 10 mg
   Twynsta 80/5 *telmi* 80 mg/*amlo* 5 mg
   Twynsta 80/10 *telmi* 80 mg/*amlo* 10 mg

ARB/CCB/HCTZ COMBINATIONS

▷ *amlodipine/valsartan medoxomil/hydrochlorothiazide* (D)(G)
   Pediatric: not recommended
      Exforge HCT: initially 5/160/12.5 once daily; may titrate at 1-week intervals to
      max 10/320/25 once daily
         Tab: **Exforge HCT 5/160/12.5** *amlo* 5 mg/*vals* 160 mg/*hctz* 12.5 mg
            Exforge HCT 5/160/25 *amlo* 5 mg/*vals* 160 mg/*hctz* 25 mg
            Exforge HCT 10/160/12.5 *amlo* 10 mg/*vals* 160 mg/*hctz* 12.5 mg
            Exforge HCT 10/160/25 *amlo* 10 mg/*vals* 160 mg/*hctz* 25 mg
            Exforge HCT 10/320/25 *amlo* 10 mg/*vals* 320 mg/*hctz* 25 mg
▷ *olmesartan medoxomil/amlodipine/hydrochlorothiazide* (D)
   Pediatric: not recommended
      Tribenzor: initially 40/5/12.5 once daily; may titrate at 1-week intervals to max
      40/10/25 daily
         Tab: **Tribenzor 40/5/12.5** *olme* 40 mg/*amlo* 5 mg/*hctz* 12.5 mg
            Tribenzor 40/5/25 *olme* 40 mg/*amlo* 5 mg/*hctz* 25 mg
            Tribenzor 40/10/12.5 *olme* 40 mg/*amlo* 10 mg/*hctz* 12.5 mg
            Tribenzor 40/10/25 *olme* 40 mg/*amlo* 10 mg/*hctz* 25 mg

OTHER COMBINATION AGENTS

▷ *clonidine/chlorthalidone* (C)
   Pediatric: not recommended
      Clorpres initially 0.1/15 once daily; may titrate to max 0.3/15 bid
         Tab: **Clorpres 0.1/15** *clon* 0.1 mg/*chlor* 15 mg
            Clorpres 0.2/15 *clon* 0.2 mg/*chlor* 15 mg
            Clorpres 0.3/15 *clon* 0.3 mg/*chlor* 15 mg
▷ *reserpine/hydroflumethiazide* (C)
   Pediatric: not recommended
      Salutensin initially 1.25/25 once daily; may titrate to 1.25/25 bid <u>or</u> 1.25/50
      once daily
         Tab: **Salutensin 1.25/25** *enal* 1.25 mg/*hydro* 25 mg
            Salutensin 1.25/50: *enal* 1.25 mg/*hydro* 50 mg

ANTIHYPERTENSION/ANTILIPID COMBINATIONS

CCB/Statin Combinations

▷ *amlodipine/atorvastatin* (X)
   Pediatric: <10 years: not established; ≥10 years (female postmenarche): same as adult
      Caduet select according to blood pressure and lipid values; titrate *amlodipine* over
      7-14 days; titrate **atorvastatin** according to monitored lipid values; max **amlodip-
ine** 10 mg/day and max **atorvastatin** 80 mg/day; refer to contraindications and
      precautions for CCB and statin therapy
         Tab: **Caduet 2.5/10** *amlo* 2.5 mg/*ator* 10 mg
            Caduet 2.5/20 *amlo* 2.5 mg/*ator* 20 mg
            Caduet 5/10 *amlo* 5 mg/*ator* 10 mg
            Caduet 5/20 *amlo* 5 mg/*ator* 20 mg
            Caduet 5/40 *amlo* 5 mg/*ator* 40 mg
            Caduet 5/80 *amlo* 5 mg/*ator* 80 mg
            Caduet 10/10 *amlo* 10 mg/*ator* 10 mg

Caduet 10/20 *amlo* 10 mg/*ator* 20 mg
Caduet 10/40 *amlo* 10 mg/*ator* 40 mg
Caduet 10/80 *amlo* 10 mg/*ator* 80 mg

HYPERTHYROIDISM

▷ *methimazole* **(D)** initially 15-60 mg/day in 3 divided doses; maintenance 5-15 mg/day
Pediatric: initially 0.4 mg/kg/day in 3 divided doses; maintenance 0.2 mg/kg/day <u>or</u> 1/2 initial dose
    Tapazole *Tab:* 5*, 10*mg
Comment: *methimazole* potentiates anticoagulants. Contraindicated in nursing mothers.

▷ *propylthiouracil (ptu)* **(D)(G)**
    Propyl-Thyracil initially 100-900 mg/day in 3 divided doses; maintenance usually 50-600 mg/day in 2 divided doses
        Pediatric: <6 years: not recommended; ≥6-10 years: initially 50-150 mg/day <u>or</u> 5-7 mg/kg/day in 3 divided doses; >10 years: initially 150-300 mg/day <u>or</u> 5-7 mg/kg/day in 3 divided doses; *maintenance:* 0.2 mg/kg/day <u>or</u> 1/2-2/3 of initial dose
        Tab: 50* mg
Comment: Preferred agent in pregnancy. Side effects include dermatitis, nausea, agranulocytosis, and hypothyroidism. Should be taken regularly for 2 years. Do not discontinue abruptly.

BETA-ADRENERGIC BLOCKER

▷ *propranolol* **(C)(G)** 40-240 mg daily
Pediatric: not recommended
    Inderal *Tab:* 10*, 20*, 40*, 60*, 80*mg
    Inderal LA initially 80 mg daily in a single dose; increase q 3-7 days; usual range 120-160 mg/day; max 320 mg/day in a single dose
        Cap: 60, 80, 120, 160 mg sust-rel
    InnoPran XL initially 80 mg q HS; max 120 mg/day
        Cap: 80, 120 mg ext-rel

HYPERTRIGLYCERIDEMIA

OMEGA 3-FATTY ACID ETHYL ESTERS

Comment: *Vascepa*, *Lovaza*, and **Epanova** are indicated for the treatment of TG ≥500 mg/dL.

▷ *icosapent ethyl (omega 3-fatty acid ethyl ester of EPA)* **(C)** 2 caps bid with food; max 4 g/day; swallow whole, do not crush <u>or</u> chew
Pediatric: <18 years: not recommended
    Vascepa sgc: 0.5, 1 g (α-tocopherol 4 mg/cap)

▷ *omega 3-fatty acid ethyl esters* **(C)(G)** 2 g bid <u>or</u> 4 g daily; swallow whole, do not crush <u>or</u> chew

Pediatric: <18 years: not recommended
> **Lovaza** *Gelcap:* 1 g (α-tocopherol 4 mg/cap) *omega 3-carcartonyl acids* (C) take 2-4 gel aps (2-4 g) daily without regard to meals
> **Epanova** *Gelcap:* 1 g

ISOBUTYRIC ACID DERIVATIVE

▷ *gemfibrozil* (C)(G)
Pediatric: not recommended
> **Lopid** 600 mg bid 30 minutes before AM and PM meals
> *Tab:* 600*mg

FIBRATES (FIBRIC ACID DERIVATIVES)

▷ *fenofibrate* (C) take with meals; adjust at 4-8-week intervals; discontinue if inadequate response after 2 months; lowest dose <u>or</u> contraindicated with renal impairment and the elderly
Pediatric: not recommended
> **Antara** 43-130 mg once daily; max 130 mg/day
> *Cap:* 43, 87, 130 mg
> **FibriCor** 30-105 mg once daily; max 105 mg/day
> *Tab:* 30, 105 mg
> **TriCor (G)** 48-145 mg once daily; max 145 mg/day
> *Tab:* 48, 145 mg
> **TriLipix (G)** 45-135 mg once daily; max 135 mg/day
> *Cap:* 45, 135 mg del-rel
> **Lipofen (G)** 50-150 mg once daily; max 150 mg/day
> *Cap:* 50, 150 mg
> **Lofibra** 67-200 mg daily; max 200 mg/day
> *Tab:* 67, 134, 200 mg

NICOTINIC ACID DERIVATIVES

Comment: Contraindicated in liver disease. Decrease total cholesterol, LDL-C, and TG; increase HDL-C. Before initiating and at 4-6 weeks, 3 months, and 6 months of therapy, check fasting lipid profile <u>or</u> as indicated by manufacturer, LFT, glucose, and uric acid. Significant side effect of transient skin flushing. Take with food and take *aspirin* 325 mg 30 minutes before dose to decrease flushing.
▷ *niacin* (C)
> **Niaspan** 375 mg daily for 1st week, then 500 mg daily for 2nd week, then 750 mg daily for 3rd week, then 1 g daily for weeks 4-7; may increase by 500 mg q 4 weeks; usual range 1-3 g/day
> *Tab:* 500, 750, 1,000 mg ext-rel
> **Slo-Niacin** 250 mg <u>or</u> 500 mg <u>or</u> 750 mg q AM <u>or</u> HS
> *Tab:* 250, 500, 750 mg cont-rel

HMG-COA REDUCTASE INHIBITORS

▷ *atorvastatin* (X)(G) initially 10 mg daily; usual range 10-80 mg daily
Pediatric: <10 years: not recommended; ≥10 years (female postmenarche): same as adult
> **Lipitor** *Tab:* 10, 20, 40, 80 mg

▶ *fluvastatin* (X)(G) initially 20-40 mg q HS; usual range 20-80 mg/day
  Pediatric: <18 years: not recommended
      Lescol *Cap:* 20, 40 mg
      Lescol XL *Tab:* 80 mg ext-rel
▶ *lovastatin* (X) initially 20 mg daily at evening meal; may increase at 4 week intervals;
  max 80 mg/day in a single or divided doses; *Concomitant fibrates, niacin,* or *CrCl <40
  mL/min:* usual max 20 mg/day
  Pediatric: <10 years: not recommended; 10-17 years: initially 10-20 mg daily at evening meal; may increase at 4 week intervals; max 40 mg daily; *Concomitant fibrates,
  niacin,* or *CrCl <40 mL/min:* usual max 20 mg/day
      Mevacor *Tab:* 10, 20, 40 mg
▶ *pravastatin* (X)(G) initially 10-20 mg q HS; usual range 10-80 mg/day; may start at
  40 mg/day
  Pediatric: <8 years: not recommended; 8-13 years: 20 mg q HS; 14-17 years: 40 mg q HS
      Pravachol *Tab:* 10, 20, 40, 80 mg
▶ *rosuvastatin* (X) initially 20 mg q HS; usual range 5-40 mg/day; adjust at 4 week intervals
  Pediatric: <10 years: not recommended; 10-17 years: 5-20 mg q HS; max 20 mg q HS
      Crestor *Tab:* 5, 10, 20, 40 mg
▶ *simvastatin* (X)(G) initially 20 mg q HS; usual range 5-80 mg/day; adjust at 4 week intervals
  Pediatric: <10 years: not recommended; 10-17 years: initially 10 mg q HS; may
  increase at 4 week intervals; max 40 mg q HS
      Zocor *Tab:* 5, 10, 20, 40, 80 mg

NICOTINIC ACID DERIVATIVE/HMG-COA REDUCTASE INHIBITOR

▶ *niacin/lovastatin* (X)
      Advicor
      Pediatric: <18 years: not recommended
      Tab: **Advicor 500 mg/20 mg** *niac* 500 mg ext-rel/*lova* 20 mg
            Advicor 750 mg/20 mg *niac* 750 mg ext-rel/*lova* 20 mg
            Advicor 1,000 mg/20 mg *niac* 1,000 mg ext-rel/*lova* 20 mg

⬤ HYPOCALCEMIA

Comment: Hypocalcemia resulting in metabolic bone disease may be secondary
to hyperparathyroidism, pseudoparathyroidism, and chronic renal disease.
Normal serum Ca^{++} range is approximately 8.5-12 mg/dL. Signs and symptoms of
hypocalcemia include confusion, increased neuromuscular excitability, muscle spasms,
paresthesias, hyperphosphatemia, positive Chvostek's sign, and positive Trousseau's
sign. Signs and symptoms of hypercalcemia include fatigue, lethargy, decreased
concentration and attention span, frank psychosis, anorexia, nausea, vomiting,
constipation, bradycardia, heart block, shortened QT interval. Foods high in calcium
include almonds, broccoli, baked beans, salmon, sardines, buttermilk, turnip greens,
collard greens, spinach, pumpkin, rhubarb, and bran. Recommended daily calcium
intake: 1-3 years: 700 mg; 4-8 years: 1,000 mg; 9-18 years: 1,300 mg; 19-50 years:
1,000 mg; 51-70 years (males): 1,000 mg; ≥51 years (females): 1,200 mg; pregnancy or
nursing: 1,000-1,300 mg. Recommended daily vitamin D intake: >1 year: 600 IU; 50+
years: 800-1,000 IU. The American Academy of Rheumatology (AAR) recommends
the following daily doses for anyone on a chronic oral corticosteroid regimen: Calcium
1,200-1,500 mg/day and vitamin D 800-1,000 IU/day.

CALCIUM SUPPLEMENTS

Comment: Take *calcium* supplements after meals to avoid gastric upset. Dosages of *calcium* over 2,000 mg/day have not been shown to have any additional benefit. *Calcium* decreases **tetracycline** absorption. *Calcium* absorption is decreased by corticosteroids.

▷ *calcitonin-salmon* (C)

Miacalcin 200 units (1 spray intranasally) once daily; alternate nostrils each day
Nasal spray: 14 dose (2 ml)
Miacalcin injection 100 units/day SC or IM
Vial: 2 ml

▷ *calcium carbonate* (C)(OTC)(G)

Rolaids chew 2 tabs bid; max 14 tabs/day
Tab: calcium carbonate: 550 mg
Rolaids Extra Strength chew 2 tabs bid; max 8 tabs/day
Tab: 1,000 mg
Tums chew 2 tabs bid; max 16 tabs/day
Tab: 500 mg
Tums Extra Strength chew 2 tabs bid; max 10 tabs/day
Tab: 750 mg
Tums Ultra chew 2 tabs bid; max 8 tabs/day
Tab: 1,000 mg
Os-Cal 500 (OTC) 1-2 tab bid-tid
Tab: elemental calcium carbonate 500 mg

▷ *calcium carbonate/vitamin D* (C)(G)

Os-Cal 250+D (OTC) 1-2 tabs tid
Tab: elemental calcium carbonate 250 mg/*vit d* 125 IU
Os-Cal 500+D (OTC) 1-2 tabs bid-tid
Tab: elemental calcium carbonate 500 mg/*vit d* 125 IU
Viactiv (OTC) 1 tab tid
Chew tab: elemental calcium 500 mg/*vit d and vit a*100 IU/*Vit k* 40 mEq

▷ *calcium citrate*

Citracal (OTC) 1-2 tabs bid
Tab: elemental calcium citrate 200 mg

▷ *calcium citrate/vitamin D* (C)(G)

Citracal+D (OTC) 1-2 cplts bid
Cplt: elemental calcium citrate 315 mg/*vit d* 200 IU
Citracal 250+D (OTC) 1-2 tabs bid
Tab: elemental calcium citrate 250 mg/*vit d* 62.3 IU

VITAMIN D ANALOGS

Comment: Concurrent *vitamin D* supplementation is contraindicated for patients taking *calcitriol* or *doxercalciferol* due to the risk of *vitamin D* toxicity. Symptoms of hypervitaminosis D: hypercalcemia, hypercalciuria, elevated creatinine, erythema multiforme, hyperphosphatemia. Maintain adequate daily calcium and fluid intake. Keep serum calcium times phosphate (Ca x P) product below 70. Monitor serum calcium (esp. during dose titration), phosphorus, other lab values (see literature for frequency).

▷ *calcitriol* (C)(G) *Predialysis:* initially 0.25 mcg daily; may increase to 0.5 mcg daily; *Dialysis:* initially 0.25 mcg daily; may increase by 0.25 mcg/day at 4-8-week intervals; usual maintenance 0.5-1 mcg/day; *Hypoparathyroidism:* initially 0.25 mcg q AM; may increase by 0.25 mcg/day at 4-8 week intervals; usual maintenance 0.5-2 mcg/day

Pediatric: <12 years: *Predialysis:* <3 years: 10-15 ng/kg per day; ≥3 years: initially 0.25 mcg daily; may increase to 0.5mcg daily; *Dialysis:* not recommended; *Hypoparathyroidism:* initially 0.25 mcg daily in the AM; may increase by 0.25 mcg/day at 2-4 week intervals; usual maintenance: (1-5 years): 0.25-0.75 mcg daily; (≥6 years): 0.5-2 mcg daily; *Pseudohypoparathyroidism:* (<6 years): insufficient data, see mfr pkg insert; ≥12 years: *Predialysis:* initially 0.25 mcg daily; may increase to 0.5mcg daily *Dialysis:* initially 0.25 mcg daily; may increase by 0.25 mcg daily at 4-8 week intervals; usual maintenance: 0.5-1 mcg daily.

    Rocaltrol *Cap:* 0.25, 0.5 mcg

    Rocaltrol Solution *Soln:* 1 mcg/ml (15 ml, single-use dispensers)

Comment: *calcitriol* is indicated for the treatment of secondary hyperparathyroidism and resultant metabolic bone disease in predialysis patients (CrCl 15-55 mL/min), hypocalcemia and resultant metabolic bone disease in patients on chronic renal dialysis, hypocalcemia in hypoparathyroidism, and pseudohypoparathyroidism.

▷ *doxecalciferol* (C)(G) *Dialysis:* initially 10mcg 3 x/week at dialysis; adjust to maintain intact parathyroid hormone (iPTH) between 150-300 pg/mL; if iPTH is not lowered by 50% and fails to reach target range, may increase by 2.5 mcg at 8-week intervals; max 20 mcg 3 x/week; if iPTH <100 pg/mL, suspend for 1 week, then resume at a dose that is at least 2.5 mcg lower; *Predialysis:* initially 1mcg once daily; may increase by 0.5 mcg at 2 week intervals to target iPTH levels; max 3.5 mcg/day
Pediatric: <12 years: not established; ≥12 years: same as adult

    Hectorol *Cap:* 0.25, 0.5, 1, 2.5 mcg

    Comment: Oral **Hectorol** is indicated for the treatment of secondary hyperparathyroidism in patients with chronic kidney disease (CKD) on dialysis; Predialysis stage 3 <u>or</u> 4 CKD: use oral form only.

    Hectoral Injection <12 years: not recommended; ≥12 years: 4 mcg 3 x weekly after dialysis; adjust dose to maintain intact parathyroid hormone (iPTH) between 150-300 pg/mL; if iPTH is not lowered by 50% and fails to reach target range, may increase by 1-2 mcg at 8 week intervals; max 18 mcg/week; if iPTH <100 pg/mL, suspend for 1 week, then resume at a dose that is at least 1 mcg lower

      Vial: 2 mcg/ml (1, 2 ml single-dose; 2 ml multi-dose)

    Comment: **Hectorol Injection** is indicated for the treatment of secondary hyperparathyroidism in patients with chronic kidney disease (CKD) on dialysis.

▷ *paricalcitol* (C)(G) administer 0.04-1 mcg/kg (2.8-7 mcg) IV bolus, during dialysis, no more than every other day; may be increased by 2-4 mcg/dose every 2-4 weeks; monitor serum calcium and phosphorus during dose adjustment periods; if Ca x P >75, immediately reduce dose <u>or</u> discontinue until these levels normalize; discard unused portion of single-use vials immediately
Pediatric: <18 years: not established; ≥18 years: same as adult

    Zemplar *Vial:* 2, 5 mcg/ml soln for inj

Comment: *paricalcitol* is indicated for the prevention and treatment of secondary hyperparathyroidism associated with chronic kidney disease (CKD) stage 5.

BIOENGINEERED REPLICA OF HUMAN PARATHYROID HORMONE

▷ *bioengineered replica of human parathyroid hormone* (C) before starting, confirm 25-hydroxyvitamin D stores are sufficient; if insufficient, replace to sufficient levels per standard of care; confirm serum calcium is above 7.5 mg/dL; the goal of treatment is to achieve serum calcium within the lower half of the normal range; administer SC into the thigh once daily; alternate thighs; initially, 50 mcg/day; when initiating, decrease dose of active vitamin D by 50%, if serum calcium is above 7.5 mg/dL; monitor serum calcium levels every 3 to 7 days after starting or adjusting dose and when adjusting either active vitamin D or calcium supplements dose. Abrupt interruption or discontinuation of **Natpara** can result in severe hypocalcemia. Resume treatment with, or increase the dose of, an active form of vitamin D and calcium supplements. Monitor for signs and symptoms of hypocalcemia and monitor serum calcium levels, In the case of a missed dose, the next **Natpara** dose should be administered as soon as reasonably feasible and additional exogenous calcium should be taken in the event of ypocalcemia.

Natpara *Soln for inj:* 25, 50, 75, 100 mcg (2/pkg) multiple dose, dual-chamber glass cartridge containing a sterile powder and diluent

Comment: **Natpara** is indicated as an adjunct to calcium and vitamin D in patients with hypoparathyroidism. Because of a potential risk of osteosarcoma, use **Natpara** only in patients who cannot be well-controlled on calcium and active forms of vitamin D alone and for whom the potential benefits are considered to outweigh the potential risk. Avoid use of **Natpara** in patients who are at increased baseline risk for osteosarcoma, such as patients with Paget's disease of bone or unexplained elevations of alkaline phosphatase, pediatric and young adult patients with open epiphyses, patients with hereditary disorders predisposing to osteosarcoma or patients with a prior history of external beam or implant radiation therapy involving the skeleton. Because of the risk of osteosarcoma, **Natpara** is available only through a restricted program under a Risk Evaluation and Mitigation Strategy (REMS) (www.natparaREMS.com).

◯ HYPOKALEMIA

Comment: Normal serum K^+ range is approximately 3.5-5.5 mEq/L. Signs and symptoms of hypokalemia include neuromuscular weakness, muscle twitching and cramping, hyporeflexia, postural hypotension, anorexia, nausea and vomiting, depressed ST segments, flattened T waves, and cardiac tachyarrhythmias. Signs and symptoms of hyperkalemia include peaked T waves, elevated ST segment, and widened QRS complexes.

PROPHYLAXIS

Comment: Usual dose range is 8-10 mEq/day.

TREATMENT OF HYPOKALEMIA: NONEMERGENCY (K^+ <2.5 mEq/L)

Comment: Usual dose range 40-120 mEq/day in divided doses. Solutions are preferred; potentially serious GI effects may occur with tablet formulations or when taken on an empty stomach.

POTASSIUM SUPPLEMENTS

Comment: Potassium supplements should be taken with food. Solutions are the preferred form. Extended-release and sustained-release forms should be swallowed whole; do not crush or chew. Potassium supplementation is indicated for hypokalemia including that caused by diuretic use, and digitalis intoxication without atrioventricular (AV) block.

▷ *potassium* (C)(G)
  Pediatric: not established
    KCL Solution Oral soln: 10% (30 ml unit dose, 50/case)
    K-Dur (as chloride) *Tab:* 10, 20* mEq sust-rel

K-Lor for Oral Solution (as chloride) *Pkts for reconstitution:* 20 mEq/pkt (fruit)
Klor-Con/25 (as chloride) *Pkts for reconstitution:* 25 mEq/pkt
Klor-Con/EF 25 (as bicarbonate) *Pkts for reconstitution:* 25 mEq/pkt
(effervescent) (fruit)
Klor-Con Extended-Release (as chloride) *Tab:* 8, 10 mEq ext-rel
Klor-Con M (as chloride) *Tab:* 10, 15*, 20* mEq ext-rel
Klor-Con Powder (as chloride) 20, 25 mEq *Pkts for reconstitution:* (30/carton)
(fruit)
Klorvess (as bicarbonate and citrate) *Tab:* 20 mEq effervescent for solution;
Granules: 20 mEq/pkt effervescent for solution; *Oral liq:* 20 mEq/15 ml (16 oz)
Klotrix (as chloride) *Tab:* 10 mEq sust-rel
K-Lyte (as bicarbonate and citrate) *Tab:* 25 mEq effervescent for solution (lime,
orange)
K-Lyte/CL (as chloride) *Tab:* 25 mEq effervescent for solution (citrus, fruit)
K-Lyte/CL 50 (as chloride) *Tab:* 50 mEq effervescent for solution (citrus, fruit)
K-Lyte/DS (as bicarbonate and citrate) *Tab:* 50 mEq effervescent for solution
(lime, orange)
K-Tab (as chloride) *Tab:* 10 mEq sust-rel
Micro-K (as chloride) *Cap:* 8, 10 mEq sust-rel
Potassium Chloride Extended Release Caps *Cap:* 8, 10 mEq ext-rel
Potassium Chloride Sust-Rel Tabs *Tab/Cap:* 10 mEq sust-rel
Potassium Chloride ER *Tab:* 8mEq (600 mg), 10 mEq (750 mg)

 HYPOMAGNESEMIA

Comment: Normal serum Mg^{++} range is approximately 1.2-2.6 mEq/L. Signs and
symptoms of hypomagnesemia include confusion, disorientation, hallucinations,
hyperreflexia, tetany, convulsions, tachyarrhythmia, positive Chvostek's sign,
and positive Trousseau's sign. Signs and symptoms of hypermagnesemia include
drowsiness, lethargy, muscle weakness, hypoactive reflexes, slurred speech,
bradycardia, hypotension, convulsions, and cardiac arrhythmias.

MAGNESIUM SUPPLEMENTS

▷ *magnesium* (B)
    Slow-Mag 2 tabs daily
        Tab: 64 mg (as chloride)/110 mg (as carbonate)
▷ *magnesium oxide* (B)
    Mag-Ox 400 1-2 tabs daily
        Tab: 400 mg

HYPOPARATHYROIDISM

VITAMIN D ANALOGS

Comment: Concurrent vitamin D supplementation is contraindicated for patients
taking *calcitrol* **or** *doxecalciferol* owing to the risk of vitamin D toxicity.
▷ *calcitrol* (C) initially 0.25 mcg q AM; may increase by 0.25 mcg/day at 4-8-week
intervals; usual maintenance 0.5-2 mcg/day

Pediatric: initially 0.25 mcg daily; may increase by 0.25 mcg/day at 2-4-week intervals; usual maintenance (1-5 years) 0.25-0.75 mcg/day, (>6 years) 0.5-2 mcg/day

    Rocaltrol *Cap:* 0.25, 0.5 mcg

    Rocaltrol Solution *Soln:* 1 mcg/ml (15 ml, single-use dispensers)

▶ *doxecalciferol* (C) initially 0.25 mcg q AM; may increase by 0.25 mcg/day at 4-8-week intervals; usual maintenance 0.5-2 mcg/day

Pediatric: initially 0.25 mcg daily; may increase by 0.25 mcg/day at 2-4-week intervals; usual maintenance (1-5 years) 0.25-0.75 mcg/day, (>6 years) 0.5-2 mcg/day

    Hectorol *Cap:* 0.25, 0.5 mcg

HUMAN PARATHYROID HORMONE

▶ *teriparatide* (C) 20 mcg SC daily in the thigh or abdomen; may treat for up to 2 years

Pediatric: not recommended

    Forteo Multidose Pen *Multi-dose pen:* 250 mcg/ml (3 ml)

    Comment: **Forteo** is indicated for the treatment of postmenopausal osteoporosis in women who are at high risk for fracture and to increase bone mass in men with primary or hypogonadal osteoporosis who are at high risk for fracture.

BIOENGINEERED REPLICA OF HUMAN PARATHYROID HORMONE

▶ *bioengineered replica of human parathyroid hormone* (C) initially inject mg IM into the thigh once daily; when initiating, decrease dose of active vitamin D by 50% if serum calcium is above 7.5 mg/dL; monitor serum calcium levels every 3-7 days after starting or adjusting dose and when adjusting either active vitamin D or calcium supplements dose

    Natpara *Soln for inj:* 25, 50, 75, 100 mcg (2/pkg) multiple dose, dual-chamber glass cartridge containing a sterile powder and diluent

    Comment: **Natpara** is indicated as an adjunct to calcium and vitamin D in patients with parathyroidism.

◯ HYPOPHOSPHATASIA (OSTEOMALACIA, RICKETS)

Comment: Hypophosphatasia (HPP) is an inborn error of metabolism marked by abnormally low serum alkaline phosphatase activity and phosphoethanolamine in the urine. It is manifested by osteomalacia in adults and rickets in infants and children. It is most severe in infants under 6 months-of-age. With congenital absence of alkaline phosphatase, an enzyme essential to the calcification of bone tissue, complications include vomiting, growth retardation, and often death in infancy. Surviving children have numerous skeletal abnormalities and dwarfism.

▶ *asfotase alfa* (NE) 6 mg/kg/week SC, administered as 2 mg/kg or 1 mg/kg 6 x/week; max 9 mg/kg/week SC administered as 3 mg/kg 3 x/week

Pediatric: same as adult

    Strensiq *Vial:* 18 mg/0.45 ml, 28 mg/0.7 ml, 40 mg/ml, 80 mg/0.8 ml for SC inj, single-use (1, 12/carton) (preservative-free)

    Comment: **Strensiq** is the first FDA-approved (2015) treatment for perinatal, infantile, and juvenile onset HPP. Prior to the availability of **Strensiq**, there was no effective treatment and patient prognosis was very poor.

HYPOTENSION: NEUROGENIC, ORTHOSTATIC

ALPHA-1 AGONIST

▷ *midodrine* (C)(G) 10 mg tid at 3-4-hour intervals; take while upright; take last dose at least 4 hours before bedtime
Pediatric: not recommended
    ProAmatine *Tab:* 2.5*, 5*, 10*mg

SYNTHETIC AMINO ACID PRECURSOR OF NOREPINEPHRINE

▷ *droxidopa* (C) initially 100 mg, taken 3 times/day (upon arising in the morning, at midday, and in the late afternoon at least 3 hours prior to bedtime (to reduce the potential for supine hypertension during sleep); administer with or without; swallow whole; titrate to symptomatic response, in increments of 100 mg tid every 24-48 hours; max 600 mg tid (max total 1,800 mg/day)
Pediatric: not recommended
    Northera *Cap:* 100, 200, 300 mg
    Comment: **Northera** is indicated for the treatment of orthostatic dizziness, lightheadedness, or feeling about to black out in adult patients with symptomatic neurogenic orthostatic hypotension (NOH) caused by primary autonomic failure [Parkinson's disease (PD), multiple system atrophy (MSA) and pure autonomic failure], dopamine beta-hydroxylase deficiency, and nondiabetic autonomic neuropathy. Effectiveness beyond 2 weeks of treatment has not been established. The continued effectiveness of **Northera** should be assessed. Administering **Northera** in combination with other agents that increase blood pressure (e.g., norepinephrine, ephedrine, midodrine, triptans) would be expected to increase the risk for supine hypertension.

HYPOTHYROIDISM

Comment: Take thyroid replacement hormone in the morning on an empty stomach. For the elderly, start thyroid hormone replacement at 25 mcg/day. Target TSH is 0.4-5.5 mIU/L; target T4 is 4.5-12.5 ng/L. Signs and symptoms of thyroid toxicity include tachycardia, palpitations, nervousness, chest pain, heat intolerance, and weight loss.

ORAL THYROID HORMONE SUPPLEMENTS

T3

▷ *liothyronine* (A) initially 25 mcg daily; may increase by 25 mcg every 1-2 weeks as needed; usual maintenance 25-75 mcg/day
Pediatric: initially 5 mcg/day; may increase by 5 mcg/day every 3-4 days; *Cretinism:* maintenance dose: <1 year: 20 mcg/day; 1-3 years: 50 mcg/day; >3 years: same as adult
    Cytomel *Tab:* 5, 25, 50 mcg

T4

▷ *levothyroxine* (A)(G)
    Levoxyl initially 25-100 mcg/day; increase by 25 mcg/day q 2-3 weeks as needed; maintenance 100-200 mcg/day
        Pediatric: <6 months: 8-10 mcg/kg/day; 6-12 months: 6-8 mcg/kg/day; >1-5 years: 5-6 mcg/kg/day; 6-12 years: 4-5 mcg/kg/day; >12 years: same as adult

Tab: 25*, 50* (dye-free), 75*, 88*, 100*, 112*, 125*, 137*, 150*, 175*, 200*, 300*mcg
Synthroid initially 50 mcg/day; increase by 25 mcg/day q 2-3 weeks as needed; max 300 mcg/day
Pediatric: <6 months: 8-10 mcg/kg/day; 6-12 months: 6-8 mcg/kg/day; >1-5 years: 5-6 mcg/kg/day; 6-12 years: 4-5 mcg/kg/day; >12 years: same as adult
Tab: 25*, 50* (dye-free), 75*, 88*, 100*, 112*, 125*, 137*, 150*, 175*, 200*, 300*mcg
Unithroid initially 50 mcg/day; increase by 25 mcg/day q 2-3 weeks as needed; max 300 mcg/day
Pediatric: 0-3 months: 10-15 mcg/kg/day; 3-6 months: 8-10 mcg/kg/day; 6-12 months: 6-8 mcg/kg/day; 1-5 years: 5-6 mcg/kg/day; 6-12 years: 4-5 mcg/kg/day; >12 years: 2-3 mcg/kg/day; *Growth and puberty complete:* same as adult
Tab: 25*, 50* (dye-free), 75*, 88*, 100*, 112*, 125*, 150*, 175*, 200*, 300*mcg

T3/T4 Combination

▷ *liothyronine/levothyroxine* (A) initially 15-30 mg/day; increase by 15 mg/day q 2-3 weeks to target goal; usual maintenance 60-120 mg/day
Pediatric: <6 months: 4.6-6 mcg/kg/day; 6-12 months: 3.6-4.8 mcg/kg/day; >1-5 years: 3-3.6 mcg/kg/day; 6-12 years: 2.4-3 mcg/kg/day; >12 years: 1.2-1.8 mcg/kg/day; *Growth and puberty complete:* same as adult
Armour Thyroid Tab *Tab:* per grain: T3 9 mcg/T4 38 mcg: 1/4, 1/2, 1, 1, 2, 3*, 4*, 5* gr; 15, 30, 60, 90, 120, 180*, 240*, 300*mg
Thyrolar *Tab:* per grain: T3 12.5 mcg/T4 50 mcg: 1/4, 1/5, 1, 2, 3 gr

PARENTERAL THYROID HORMONE SUPPLEMENT

▷ *levothyroxine sodium* (A)(G) 1/2 oral dose by IV or IM and titrate; *Myxedema Coma:* 200-500 mcg IV x 1 dose; may administer 100-300 mcg (or more) IV on second day if needed; then 50-100 mcg IV daily; switch to oral form as soon as possible
Pediatric: not recommended
T4 *Vial:* 100, 200, 500 mcg (pwdr for IM or IV administration after reconstitution)

◯ IDIOPATHIC PULMONARY FIBROSIS (IPF)

▷ *nintedanib* (D) take with food at the same time each day; take 150 mg bid, 12 hours apart; max 300 mg/day
Pediatric: not established
Ofev *Cap:* 100, 150 mg
Comment: Monitor liver enzymes. If elevated LFTs (3 < AST/ALT <5 XULN) without severe liver damage, interrupt therapy or reduce dose to 100 mg bid. When liver enzymes return to baseline, restart at 100 mg bid and titrate up.
▷ *pirfenidone* (C) take with food at the same time each day; *Days 1-7:* 1 cap tid; *Days 8-14:* 2 caps tid; *Days 15 and ongoing:* 3 caps tid; max 9 caps/day
Pediatric: not established
Esbriet *Gelcap:* 267 mg

◯ IMPETIGO CONTAGIOSA (INDIAN FIRE)

Comment: The most common infectious organisms are *Staphylococcus aureus* and *Streptococcus pyogenes*.

TOPICAL ANTI-INFECTIVES

▷ *mupirocin* (B)(G) apply to lesions bid; apply to walls of nares bid
  Pediatric: same as adult
    Bactroban *Oint:* 2% (22 g); *Crm:* 2% (15, 30 g)
    Centany *Oint:* 2% (15, 30 g)

ORAL ANTI-INFECTIVES

▷ *amoxicillin* (B)(G) 500-875 mg bid <u>or</u> 250-500 mg tid x 10 days
  Pediatric: <40 kg (88 lb): 20-40 mg/kg/day in 3 divided doses x 10 days <u>or</u> 25-45 mg/kg/
  day in 2 divided doses x 10 days; >40 kg: same as adult; *see page 554 for dose by weight*
    Amoxil *Cap:* 250, 500 mg; *Tab:* 875*mg; *Chew tab:* 125, 200, 250, 400 mg (cher-
    ry-banana-peppermint) (phenylalanine); *Oral susp:* 125, 250 mg/5 ml (80, 100,
    150 ml) (strawberry); 200, 400 mg/5 ml (50, 75, 100 ml) (bubble gum); Oral
    drops: 50 mg/ml (30 ml) (bubble gum)
    Moxatag *Tab:* 775 mg ext-rel
    Trimox *Tab:* 125, 250 mg; *Cap:* 250, 500 mg; *Oral susp:* 125, 250 mg/5 ml (80,
    100, 150 ml) (raspberry-strawberry)
▷ *amoxicillin/clavulanate* (B)(G) 500 mg tid <u>or</u> 875 mg bid x 10 days
    Augmentin *Tab:* 250, 500, 875 mg; *Chew tab:* 125, 250 mg (lemon-lime); 200,
    400 mg (cherry-banana) (phenylalanine); *Oral susp:* 125 mg/5 ml (banana), 250
    mg/5 ml (75, 100, 150 ml) (orange); 200, 400 mg/5 ml (50, 75, 100 ml) (orange)
    (phenylalanine)
      Pediatric: 40-45 mg/kg/day divided tid x 10 days <u>or</u> 90 mg/kg/day divided
      bid x 10 days *see page 556 for dose by weight*
    Augmentin ES-600 *Oral susp:* 600 mg/5 ml (50, 75, 100, 125, 150, 200 ml)
    (strawberry cream) (phenylalanine) every 12 hours
      Pediatric: <3 months: not recommended; ≥3 months, <40 kg: 90 mg/kg/day
      in 2 divided doses; ≥40 kg: not recommended
    Augmentin XR 2 tabs q 12 hours x 7-10 days
      Pediatric: <16 years: use other forms; ≥16 years: same as adult
      Tab: 1000*mg ext-rel
▷ *azithromycin* (B) 500 mg <u>x</u> 1 dose on day 1, then 250 mg daily on days 2-5 <u>or</u> 500 mg
  daily <u>x</u> 3 days <u>or</u> 2 g in a single dose
    Zithromax *Tab:* 250, 500, 600 mg; *Oral susp:* 100 mg/5 ml (15 ml); 200 mg/5 ml
    (15, 22.5, 30 ml) (cherry); *Pkt:* 1 g for reconstitution (cherry-banana)
    Zithromax Tri-pak *Tab:* 3 x 500 mg tabs/pck
    Zithromax Z-pak *Tab:* 6 x 250 mg tabs/pck
    Zmax *Oral susp:* 2 g ext-rel for reconstitution (cherry-banana) (148 mg Na$^+$)
▷ *cefaclor* (B)(G) 250-500 mg q 8 hours <u>x</u> 10 days; max 2 g/day
  Pediatric: <1 month: not recommended; 20-40 mg/kg bid <u>or</u> q 12 hours x 10 days;
  max 1 g/day; *see page 560 for dose by weight*
    Tab: 500 mg; *Cap:* 250, 500 mg; *Susp:* 125 mg/5 ml (75, 150 ml) (strawberry); 187
    mg/5 ml (50, 100 ml) (strawberry); 250 mg/5 ml (75, 150 ml) (strawberry); 375
    mg/5 ml (50, 100 ml) (strawberry)
  Pediatric: <16 years: ext-rel not recommended; ≥16 years: same as adult
    Cefaclor Extended Release *Tab:* 375, 500 mg ext-rel
▷ *cefadroxil* (B) 1-2 g in 1-2 divided doses x 10 days
  Pediatric: 30 mg/kg/day in 2 divided doses x 10 days; *see page 561 for dose by
  weight*

Duricef *Cap:* 500 mg; *Tab:* 1 g; *Oral susp:* 250 mg/5 ml (100 ml); 500 mg/5 ml (75, 100 ml) (orange-pineapple)

▷ *cefpodoxime proxetil* (B) 200 mg bid x 10 days
Pediatric: <2 months: not recommended; 2 months-12 years: 10 mg/kg/day (max 400 mg/dose) or 5 mg/kg/day bid (max 200 mg/dose) x 10 days; *see page 564 for dose by weight*
Vantin *Tab:* 100, 200 mg; *Oral susp:* 50, 100 mg/5 ml (50, 75, 100 mg) (lemon creme)

▷ *cefprozil* (B) 500 mg bid x 10 days
Pediatric: ≤6 months: not recommended; 6 months-12 years: *see page 565 for dose by weight*
Cefzil *Tab:* 250, 500 mg; *Oral susp:* 125, 250 mg/5 ml (50, 75, 100 ml) (bubble gum) (phenylalanine)

▷ *ceftaroline fosamil* (B) administer by IV infusion after reconstitution every 12 hours x 5-14 days; *CrCl >50 mL/min:* 600 mg; *CrCl >30-<50 mL/min:* 400 mg; *CrCl >1 5-<30 mL/min:* 300 mg; ESRD: 200 mg
Teflaro *Vial:* 400, 600 mg

▷ *cefuroxime axetil* (B) (G) 250-500 mg bid x 10 days
Pediatric: 15 mg/kg bid x 10 days; *see page 567 for dose by weight*
Ceftin *Tab:* 250, 500 mg; *Oral susp:* 12, 250 mg/5 ml (50, 100 ml) (tutti-frutti)

▷ *cephalexin* (B) (G) 250-500 mg qid or 500 mg bid x 10 days
Pediatric: 25-50 mg/kg/day in 4 divided doses x 10 days; *see page 568 for dose by weight*
Keflex *Cap:* 250, 333, 500, 750 mg; *Oral susp:* 125, 250 mg/5 ml (100, 200 ml) (strawberry)

▷ *clarithromycin* (C)(G) 500 mg or 500 mg ext-rel daily x 7 days
Pediatric: <6 months: not recommended; ≥6 months: 7.5 mg/kg bid x 7 days; *see page 569 for dose by weight*
Biaxin *Tab:* 250, 500 mg
Biaxin Oral Suspension *Oral susp:* 125, 250 mg/5 ml (50, 100 ml) (fruit punch)
Biaxin XL *Tab:* 500 mg ext-rel

▷ *dicloxacillin* (B) (G) 500 mg q 6 hours x 10 days
Pediatric: 12.5-25 mg/kg/day in 4 divided doses x 10 days; *see page 571 for dose by weight*
Dynapen *Cap:* 125, 250, 500 mg; *Oral susp:* 62.5 mg/5 ml (80, 100, 200 ml)

▷ *erythromycin base* (B)(G) 250 mg qid, or 333 mg tid, or 500 mg bid x 7-10 days
Pediatric: ≤45 kg: 30-50 mg in 2-4 divided doses x 7-10 days; ≥45 kg: same as adult
Ery-Tab *Tab:* 250, 333, 500 mg ent-coat
PCE *Tab:* 333, 500 mg
Comment: *erythromycin* may increase INR with concomitant *warfarin*, as well as increase serum level of *digoxin*, benzodiazepines and statins.

▷ *erythromycin ethylsuccinate* (B)(G) 400 mg tid x 7-10 days
Pediatric: 30-50 mg/kg/day in 4 divided doses x 7-10 days; may double dose with severe infection; max 100 mg/kg/day; see page 574 for dose by weight
EryPed *Oral susp:* 200 mg/5 ml (100, 200 ml) (fruit); 400 mg/5 ml (60, 100, 200 ml) (banana); *Oral drops:* 200, 400 mg/5 ml (50 ml) (fruit); *Chew tab:* 200 mg wafer (fruit)
E.E.S. *Oral susp:* 200, 400 mg/5 ml (100 ml) (fruit)
E.E.S. Granules *Oral susp:* 200 mg/5 ml (100, 200 ml) (cherry)
E.E.S. 400 Tablets *Tab:* 400 mg

Comment: *erythromycin* may increase INR with concomitant **warfarin**, as well as increase serum level of **digoxin**, benzodiazepines and statins.

▷ *loracarbef* (B) 200 mg bid x 10 days
  Pediatric: 15 mg/kg/day in 2 divided doses x 10 days; *see page 581 for dose by weight*
  Pediatric: 30 mg/kg/day in 2 divided doses x 7 days
      Lorabid *Pulvule:* 200, 400 mg; *Oral susp:* 100 mg/5 ml (50, 100 ml); 200 mg/5 ml (50, 75, 100 ml) (strawberry bubble gum)

▷ *penicillin G (benzathine)* (B) 1.2 million units IM x 1 dose
  Pediatric: <60 lb: 300,000-600,000 units IM x 1 dose; ≥60 lb: 900,000 units x 1 dose
      Bicillin L-A *Cartridge-needle unit:* 600,000 units (1 ml); 1.2 million units (2 ml)

▷ *penicillin G (benzathine/procaine)* (B) (G) 2.4 million units IM x 1 dose
  Pediatric: <30 lb: 600,000 units IM x 1 dose; 30-60 lb: 900,000-1.2 million units IM x 1 dose
      Bicillin C-R *Cartridge-needle unit:* 600,000 units (1 ml); 1.2 million units (2 ml); 2.4 million units (4 ml)

▷ *penicillin V potassium* (B) 250-500 mg q 6 hours x 10 days
  Pediatric: 50 mg/kg/day in 4 divided doses x 3 days; ≥12 years: same as adult; *see page 583 for dose by weight*
      Pen-Vee K *Tab:* 250, 500 mg; *Oral soln:* 125 mg/5 ml (100, 200 ml); 250 mg/5 ml (100, 150, 200 ml)

◯ INCONTINENCE: FECAL

Comment: Treatment of fecal incontinence in patients who have failed conservative therapy (e.g., diet, fiber therapy, antimotility agents).

▷ *dextranomer microspheres/sodium hyaluronate* (NE)
  Pediatric: ≤18 years: not recommended
      Pretreatment: bowel preparation using enema (required) and prophylactic antibiotics (recommended) prior to injection
      Treatment: inject slowly into the deep submucosal layer in the proximal part of the high pressure zone of the anal canal about 5 mm above the dentate line; four 1-ml injections in the following order: posterior, left lateral, anterior, right lateral; keep needle in place 15-30 seconds to minimize leakage; use a new needle for each syringe and injection site
      Posttreatment: avoid hot baths and physical activity during first 24 hours; avoid antidiarrheal drugs, sexual intercourse, and strenuous activity for 1 week; avoid anal manipulation for 1 month
      Retreatment: may repeat if needed with max 4 ml, no sooner than 4 weeks after the first injection; point of injection should be made in between initial injection sites (i.e., shifted 1/8 of a turn)
      Solesta *dex micro* 50 mg/*sod hyal* 15 mg per ml
          Syringe: 1 ml (4 w. needles)

◯ INCONTINENCE: URINARY (OVERACTIVE BLADDER/ STRESS INCONTINENCE/URGE INCONTINENCE)

See **Enuresis** *page 138*
▷ *estrogen* replacement (X) *see* **Menopause** *page 264*

➤ *pseudoephedrine* (C)(G) 30-60 mg tid
    Sudafed (OTC) *Tab:* 30 mg; *Liq:* 15 mg/5 ml (1, 4 oz)

VASOPRESSIN

➤ *desmopressin acetate (DDAVP)* (B)(G)
    DDAVP usual dosage 0.1-1.2 mg/day in 2-3 divided doses; 0.2 mg q HS prn for nocturnal enuresis
        Pediatric: <6 years: not recommended; ≥6 years: 0.5 mg daily <u>or</u> q HS prn
        Tab: 0.1*, 0.2*mg
    DDAVP Rhinal Tube
        Pediatric: <6 years: not recommended; ≥6 years: 10 mcg <u>or</u> 0.1 ml of soln each nostril (20 mcg total dose) q HS prn; max 40 mcg total dose
        Rhinal tube: 0.1 mg/ml (2.5 ml)

BETA-3 ADRENERGIC AGONIST

➤ *mirabegron* (C) initially 25 mg once daily; max 50 mg once daily; severe renal impairment, 25 mg once daily
    Myrbetriq *Tab:* 25, 50 mg ext-rel

MUSCARINIC RECEPTOR ANTAGONISTS

➤ *fesoterodine* (C)(G) 4 mg daily; max 8 mg/day
    Pediatric: not recommended
        Toviaz *Tab:* 4, 8 mg ext-rel
➤ *tolterodine tartrate* (C)(G)
    Pediatric: not recommended
        Detrol 2 mg bid; may decrease to 1 mg bid
            Tab: 1, 2 mg
        Detrol LA 2-4 mg once daily
            Cap: 2, 4 mg ext-rel

ANTISPASMODIC/ANTICHOLINERGICS

➤ *darifenacin* (C) 7.5-15 mg daily with liquid; max 15 mg/day
    Pediatric: not recommended
        Enablex 7.5-15 mg daily with liquid; max 15 mg/day
            Tab: 7.5, 15 mg ext-rel
➤ *dicyclomine* (B)(G) 10-20 mg qid
    Pediatric: not recommended
        Bentyl *Tab:* 20 mg; *Cap:* 10 mg; *Syr:* 10 mg/5 ml (16 oz)
➤ *flavoxate* (B) 100-200 mg tid-qid
    Pediatric: not recommended
        Urispas *Tab:* 100 mg
➤ *hyoscyamine* (C)(G)
        Anaspaz 1-2 tabs q 4 hours prn; max 12 tabs/day
            Pediatric: <2 years: not recommended; 2-12 years: 0.0625-0.125 mg q 4 hours prn; max 0.75 mg/day
            Tab: 0.125*mg
        Levbid 1-2 tabs q 12 hours prn; max 4 tabs/day
            Pediatric: <12 years: not recommended; ≥12 years: same as adult

Tab: 0.375*mg ext-rel

Levsin 1-2 tabs q 4 hours prn; max 12 tabs/day
> *Pediatric:* <6 years: not recommended; 6-12 years: 1 tab q 4 hours prn
> *Tab:* 0.125*mg

Levsin Drops 1-2 ml q 4 hours prn; max 60 ml/day
> *Pediatric:* 3.4 kg: 4 drops q 4 hours prn; max 24 drops/day; 5 kg: 5 drops q 4 hours prn; max 30 drops/day; 7 kg: 6 drops q 4 hours prn; max 36 drops/day; 10 kg: 8 drops q 4 hours prn; max 40 drops/day
> *Oral drops:* 0.125 mg/ml (15 ml) (orange) (alcohol 5%)

Levsin Elixir 5-10 ml q 4 hours prn
> *Pediatric:* <10 kg: use drops; 10-19 kg: 1.25 ml q 4 hours prn; 20-39 kg: 2.5 ml q 4 hours prn; 40-49 kg: 3.75 ml q 4 hours prn; ≥50 kg: 5 ml q 4 hours prn
> *Elix:* 0.125 mg/5 ml (16 oz) (orange) (alcohol 20%)

Levsinex SL 1-2 tabs q 4 hours SL or PO; max 12 tabs/day
> *Pediatric:* 2-12 years: 1 tab q 4 hours; max 6 tabs/day; >12 years: same as adult
> *Tab:* 0.125 mg sublingual

Levsinex Timecaps 1-2 caps q 12 hours; may adjust to 1 cap q 8 hours
> *Pediatric:* 2-12 years: 1 cap q 12 hours; max 2 caps/day; >12 years: same as adult
> *Cap:* 0.375 mg time-rel

NuLev dissolve 1-2 tabs on tongue, with or without water, q 4 hours prn; max 12 tabs/day
> *Pediatric:* <2 years: not recommended; 2-12 years: dissolve 1 tab on tongue, with or without water, q 4 hours prn; max 6 tabs/day; ≥12 years: same as adult
> *ODT:* 0.125 mg (mint; phenylalanine)

▷ *oxybutynin chloride* (B)

Ditropan 5 mg bid-tid; max 20 mg/day
> *Pediatric:* <5 years: not recommended; 5-12 years: 5 mg bid; max 15 mg/day; ≥16 years: same as adult
> *Tab:* 5*mg; *Syr:* 5 mg/5 ml

Ditropan XL initially 5 mg daily; may increase weekly in 5-mg increments as needed; max 30 mg/day
> *Pediatric:* <6 years: not recommended; ≥6 years: initially 5 mg once daily; may increase weekly in 5-mg increments as needed; max 20 mg/day
> *Tab:* 5, 10, 15 mg ext-rel

GelniQUE 3 mg Pump: apply 3 pumps (84 mg) once daily to clean dry intact skin on the abdomen, upper arm, shoulders, or thighs; rotate sites; wash hands; avoid washing application site for 1 hour after application
> *Pediatric:* not recommended
> *Gel:* 3% (92 g, metered pump dispenser) (alcohol)

GelniQUE 1 g Sachet: apply 1 g gel (1 sachet) once daily to dry intact skin on abdomen, upper arms/shoulders, or thighs; rotate sites; wash hands; avoid washing application site for 1 hour after application
> *Pediatric:* not recommended
> *Gel:* 10%, 1 g/sachet (30/carton) (alcohol)

Oxytrol Transdermal Patch (OTC): apply patch to clean dry area of the abdomen, hip, or buttock; one patch twice weekly; rotate sites
> *Pediatric:* not recommended
> *Transdermal patch:* 3.9 mg/day

▶ *propantheline* (C) 15-30 mg tid
  Pediatric: not recommended
    Pro-Banthine *Tab:* 7.5, 15 mg
▶ *solifenacin* (C)(G) 5-10 mg daily
  Pediatric: not recommended
    VESIcare *Tab:* 5, 10 mg
▶ *trospium chloride* (C)(G)
  Pediatric: not recommended
    Sanctura 20 mg twice daily; ≥75 years: *CrCl ≤30 mL/min:* 20 mg once daily
      Tab: 20 mg
    Sanctura XR 60 mg daily in the morning
      Cap: 60 mg ext-rel
  Comment: Take *trospium chloride* on an empty stomach.

OVERFLOW INCONTINENCE/ATONIC BLADDER

▶ *bethanechol* (C) 10-30 mg tid
    Urecholine *Tab:* 5, 10, 25, 50 mg

OVERFLOW INCONTINENCE/PROSTATIC ENLARGEMENT

Alpha-1 Blockers

Comment: Educate the patient regarding the potential side effect of hypotension when taking an alpha-1 blocker, especially with first dose. Start at lowest dose and titrate upward.
▶ *terazosin* (C) initially 1 mg q HS; titrate to 10 mg q HS; max 20 mg/day
    Hytrin *Cap:* 1, 2, 5, 10 mg
▶ *doxazosin* (C) initially 1 mg q HS; may double dose every 1-2 weeks; max 8 mg/day
    Cardura *Tab:* 1*, 2*, 4*, 8*mg
    Cardura XL *Tab:* 4, 8 mg
▶ *prazosin* (C)(G) 1-15 mg q HS; max 15 mg/day
    Minipress *Tab:* 1, 2, 5 mg
▶ *tamsulosin* (C) initially 0.4 mg daily; may increase to 0.8 mg daily after 2-4 weeks if needed
    Flomax *Cap:* 0.4 mg

5-ALPHA REDUCTASE INHIBITOR

▶ *finasteride* (X)(G) 5 mg daily
    Proscar *Tab:* 5 mg

ALPHA 1A-BLOCKER

▶ *silodosin* (B) take 8 mg with food once daily; *CrCl 30-50 mL/min:* take 4 mg
    Rapaflo *Cap:* 4, 8 mg

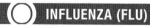 **INFLUENZA (FLU)**

Comment: With the exception of **Flucelvax**, flu vaccine is contraindicated with allergy to egg or chicken proteins, or egg products. All flu vaccines are contraindicated with allergy to latex, active infection, acute respiratory disease, active neurological disorder; history of Guillain-Barre syndrome. Have epinephrine 1:1,000 on hand. Flu vaccine is contraindicated for children under 18 years of age who are taking aspirin and/or an aspirin-containing product due to the risk of developing Reye's syndrome. Under 1 year of age, administer flu vaccine in the vastus lateralis. Over 1 year of age, administer flu vaccine in the deltoid. Flu vaccine formulations change annually. Administer flu vaccine 1 month before flu season. Spray may be administered earlier. The influenza vaccine reduces hospitalization by about 70% and mortality by about 80% in the elderly.

PROPHYLAXIS (NASAL SPRAY)

▷ *trivalent, live attenuated influenza* vaccine, types A and B (C) 1 spray each nostril; ≥50 years not recommended
  Pediatric: ≤5 years: not recommended; ≥5 years: same as adult
    Never vaccinated with **FluMist**: 5-8 years: 2 divided doses 46-74 days apart.
    Previously vaccinated with **FluMist**: 5-8 years: same as adult
    FluMist Nasal Spray 0.5 ml spray annually
      Nasal spray: 0.5 ml (0.25 ml/spray) (10/carton) (preservative-free)

PROPHYLAXIS (INJECTABLE)

▷ *quadrivalent inactivated influenza subvirion vaccine, types A and B* (C)
    Fluad 0.5 ml IM annually
    Comment: **Fluad** is the first seasonal influenza vaccine with adjuvant, indicated for persona ≥65 years-of-age. Adjuvants are incorporated into some vaccine formulations to enhance or direct the immune response.
    Fluarix Quadrivalent 0.5 ml IM annually
      Pediatric: <3 years: not recommended; ≥3 years: same as adult
      Prefilled syringes: 0.5 ml (10/carton; preservative-free, latex-free)
▷ *trivalent inactivated influenza subvirion vaccine, types A and B*
    Fluarix (B) 0.5 ml IM annually
      Pediatric: <3 years: not recommended; 3-9 years (previously unvaccinated or vaccinated for the first time last season with one dose of flu vaccine): 2 doses per season at least 1 month apart; 3-9 years (previously vaccinated with two doses of flu vaccine); and >9 years: 1 dose per season
      Prefilled syringe: 0.5 ml single-dose (5/carton) (may contain trace amounts of hydrocortisone, gentamicin; preservative-free)
    Flublok 0.5 ml IM annually; ≥49 years, not recommended
      Pediatric: <18 years: not recommended
      Vial: 0.5 ml single-dose (10/carton) (preservative-free, egg protein-free, antibiotic-free, latex-free)
    Comment: **Flublok** is a cell culture-derived vaccine and, therefore, is an alternative to the traditional egg-based vaccines. Contains 3 times the amount of active ingredient in traditional flu vaccines **Flucelvax** 0.5 ml IM annually
    Pediatric: <18 years: not recommended
      Prefilled syringes: 0.5 ml (10/carton; preservative-free, latex-free)
    Comment: **Flucelvax** is a cell culture-derived vaccine and, therefore, is an alternative to the traditional egg-based vaccines.
    FluLaval (C) 0.5 ml IM annually
      Pediatric: <6 months: not recommended; ≥6 years: same as adult
      Vial: (5 ml)

FluShield 0.5 ml IM annually
   Pediatric: <6 months: not recommended; *Never vaccinated:* <9 years: 2 doses at least 4 weeks apart; 9-12 years: same as adult; *Previously vaccinated:* 6-35 months: 0.25 ml IM x 1 dose; 3-8 years: same as adult
Fluzone 0.5 ml IM annually
   Vial: 5 ml (thimerosal)
Fluzone Preservative-Free: Adult Dose 0.5 ml IM annually
   Pediatric: <6 months: not recommended; *Not previously vaccinated:* 6 months-8 years: 0.25 ml IM; repeat in 1 month; *Previously vaccinated:* 6-35 months: 0.25 ml IM x 1 dose; >3 years: same as adult
   Prefilled syringe: 0.5 ml (10/carton) (preservative-free, trace thimerosal)
Fluzone Preservative-Free: Pediatric Dose
   Pediatric: <6 months: not recommended; *Not previously vaccinated:* 6 months-8 years: 0.25 ml IM; repeat in 1 month; *Previously vaccinated:* 6-35 months: 0.25 ml IM x 1 dose; ≥3 years: 0.5 ml IM (use **Fluzone for Adult**)
   Prefilled syringe: 0.5 ml (10/carton; preservative-free; trace thimerosal)

PROPHYLAXIS AND TREATMENT

Neuraminidase Inhibitors

Comment: Effective for influenza type A and B. Indicated for treatment of uncomplicated acute illness in patients who have been symptomatic for no more than 2 days; therefore, start within 2 days of symptom onset <u>or</u> exposure. Indicated for influenza prophylaxis in patients ≥3 months of age.

▷ *oseltamivir* phosphate (C)(G)
   Treatment: 75 mg bid x 5 days; initiate treatment only if symptomatic <2 days
     Pediatric: <1 year: not recommended; 1-12 years: <15 kg: 30 mg bid x 5 days; 16-23 kg: 45 mg bid x 5 days; 24-40 kg: 60 mg bid x 5 days; >40 kg: same as adult
   Prophylaxis: 75 mg daily for at least 7 days and up to 6 weeks for community outbreak
     Pediatric: <1 year: not recommended; 1-12 years: <15 kg: 30 mg once daily x 10 days; 16-23 kg: 45 mg once daily x 10 days; 24-40 kg: 60 mg once daily x 10 days; >40 kg: same as adult
   Tamiflu *Cap:* 30, 45, 75 mg; *Oral susp:* 6 mg/ml pwdr for reconstitution (60 ml w. oral dispenser) (tutti-frutti)
   Comment: **Tamiflu** is effective for influenza type A and B.
▷ *zanamivir* (C) 2 inhalations (10 mg) bid x 5 days
  Pediatric: <7 years: not recommended; ≥7 years: same as adult
   Relenza Inhaler *Inhaler:* 5 mg/inh blister; 4 blisters/Rotadisk (5 Rotadisks/carton w. 1 inhaler)
   Comment: **Relenza Inhaler** is effective for influenza type A and B. Use caution with asthma and COPD.
Antipyretics *see **Fever** page* 143

 INSECT BITE/STING

TOPICAL ANESTHETIC

▷ *lidocaine* 3% cream (B) apply bid-tid prn
  Pediatric: reduce dosage commensurate with age, body weight, and physical condition

LidaMantle *Crm:* 3% (1 oz)
Oral Drugs for Allergy, Cough, and Cold *see page* 535
Topical Corticosteroids *see page* 506
Parenteral Corticosteroids *see page* 511
Oral Corticosteroids *see page* 509

OTHER AGENTS

▷ *epinephrine* (C)(G) 1:1,000 0.3-0.5 ml SC
Pediatric: 0.01 ml/kg SC

TETANUS PROPHYLAXIS

▷ *tetanus toxoid* vaccine (C)(G) 0.5 ml IM x 1 dose if previously immunized
Vial: 5 Lf units/0.5 ml (0.5, 5 ml); *Prefilled syringe:* 5 Lf units/0.5 ml (0.5 ml) (For
patients not previously immunized *see* **Tetanus** page 408)

◯ INSOMNIA

MELATONIN RECEPTOR AGONIST

▷ *ramelteon* (C)(IV) 8 mg within 30 minutes of bedtime; delayed effect if taken with
a meal
Pediatric: not recommended
   Rozerem *Tab:* 8 mg

NONBENZODIAZEPINES

▷ *eszopiclone* (C)(IV)(G) (pyrrolopyrazine) 1-3 mg; max 3 mg/day x 1 month; do not
take if unable to sleep for at least 8 hours before required to be active again; delayed
effect if taken with a meal
Pediatric: <18 years: not recommended
   Lunesta *Tab:* 1, 2, 3 mg
▷ *zaleplon* (C)(IV) (imidazopyridine) 5-10 mg at HS or after going to bed if unable to
sleep; do not take if unable to sleep for at least 4 hours before required to be active
again; max 20 mg/day x 1 month; delayed effect if taken with a meal
Pediatric: not recommended
   Sonata *Cap:* 5, 10 mg (tartrazine)
   Comment: Sonata is indicated for the treatment of insomnia when a middle-of-
   the-night awakening is followed by difficulty returning to sleep.
▷ *zolpidem* oral solution spray (C)(IV) (imidazopyridine hypnotic) 2 actuations (10
mg) immediately before bedtime; *Elderly, debilitated*, or *hepatic impairment:* 2 actuations (5 mg); max 2 actuations (10 mg)
Pediatric: not recommended
   ZolpiMist *Oral soln spray:* 5 mg/actuation (60 metered actuations) (cherry)
   Comment: The lowest dose of *zolpidem* in all forms is recommended for women as
   drug elimination is slower than in men.
▷ *zolpidem* tabs (B)(IV)(G) (pyrazolopyrimidine hypnotic) 5-10 mg or 6.25-12.5 ext-
rel q HS prn; max 12.5 mg/day x 1 month; do not take if unable to sleep for at least
8 hours before required to be active again; delayed effect if taken with a meal
Pediatric: ≤18 years: not recommended

Ambien *Tab:* 5, 10 mg
Ambien CR *Tab:* 6.25, 12.5 mg ext-rel
Comment: The lowest dose of *zolpidem* in all forms is recommended for women as drug elimination is slower than in men.

▷ *zolpidem* sublingual tabs **(C)(IV)(G)** (imidazopyridine hypnotic) dissolve 1 tab under the tongue; allow to disintegrate completely before swallowing; take only once per night and only if at least 4 hours of bedtime remain before planned time for awakening
Edluar *SL Tab:* 5, 10 mg
Intermezzo *SL Tab:* 1.75, 3.5 mg
Comment: **Intermezzo** is indicated for the treatment of insomnia when a middle-of-the-night awakening is followed by difficulty returning to sleep. The lowest dose of *zolpidem* in all forms is recommended for women as drug elimination is slower than in men.

OREXIN RECEPTOR ANTAGONIST

▷ *suvorexant* **(C)(IV)** use lowest effective dose; take 30 minutes before bedtime; do not take if unable to sleep for ≥7 hours, max 20 mg
Pediatric: not recommended
Belsomra *Tab:* 5, 10, 15, 20 mg (30/blister pck)

BENZODIAZEPINES

▷ *estazolam* **(X)(IV)(G)** initially 1 mg q HS prn; may increase to 2 mg q HS
Pediatric: ≤18 years: not recommended
ProSom *Tab:* 1*, 2*mg
▷ *flurazepam* **(X)(IV)(G)** 30 mg q HS prn; elderly or debilitated, 15 mg
Pediatric: <15 years: not recommended; ≥15 years: same as adult
Dalmane *Cap:* 15, 30 mg
▷ *temazepam* **(X)(IV)(G)** 7.5-30 mg q HS prn; short term, 7-10 days; max 30 mg; max 1 month
Pediatric: <18 years: not recommended
Restoril *Cap:* 7.5, 15, 22.5, 30 mg
▷ *triazolam* **(X)(IV)** 0.125-0.25 mg q HS prn; short term, 7-10 days; max 0.5 mg; max 1 month
Pediatric: <18 years: not recommended
Halcion *Tab:* 0.125, 0.25*mg
Barbiturates
▷ *pentobarbital* **(D)(II)(G)**
Nembutal 100 mg q HS prn
Cap: 50, 100 mg
Nembutal Suppository 120 or 200 mg suppository rectally q HS prn
Pediatric: 2-12 months (10-20 lb): 30 mg supp; 1-4 years (21-40 lb): 30 or 60 mg supp; 5-12 years (41-80 lb): 60 mg supp; 12-14 years (81-110 lb): 60 or 120 mg sup
Rectal supp: 30, 60, 120, 200 mg

ORAL H₁ RECEPTOR AGONIST (1ST GENERATION ANTIHISTAMINE)

▷ *doxepin* **(C)**
Silenor 3-6 mg q HS prn; *Elderly, hepatic impairment, tendency to urinary retention*: initially 3 mg

Tab: 3, 6 mg
Other Oral 1st Generation Antihistamines *see page* 535

ANALGESIC/1ST GENERATION ANTIHISTAMINE COMBINATIONS

▶ *acetaminophen/diphenhydramine* (B)
> **Excedrin PM** (OTC) 2 tabs q HS prn
>> *Pediatric:* <12 years: not recommended; ≥12 years: same as adult
>> *Tab/Geltab: acet* 500 mg/*diphen* 38 mg
> **Tylenol PM** (OTC) 2 caps q HS prn
>> *Pediatric:* <12 years: not recommended; ≥12 years: same as adult
>> *Tab/Cap/Gel cap: acet* 500 mg/*diphen* 25 mg
> **Tricyclic Antidepressants** *see Depression page* 108

 INTERSTITIAL CYSTITIS

Comment: Avoid peppers and spicy food, citrus, vinegar, caffeine (e.g., coffee, tea, colas), alcohol, carbonated beverages, and other GU tract irritants.

MANAGEMENT OF PAIN AND URINARY URGENCY

Acetaminophen for IV Infusion *see Pain page* 306
Oral Prescription NSAIDs *see page* 501
▶ *phenazopyridine* (B)(G) 95-200 mg q 6 hours prn; max 2 days
> *Pediatric:* not recommended
>> **AZO Standard, Prodium, Uristat** (OTC) *Tab:* 95 mg
>> **AZO Standard Maximum Strength** (OTC) *Tab:* 97.5 mg
>> **Pyridium, Urogesic** *Tab:* 100, 200 mg *phenazopyridine* (B)(G) 190-200 mg tid; max 2 days
> *Pediatric:* not recommended
>> **Azo Standard** (OTC) *Tab:* 95 mg
>> **Azo Standard Maximum Strength** (OTC) *Tab:* 97.5 mg
>> **Pyridium** *Tab:* 100, 200 mg ent-coat
>> **Uristat** (OTC) *Tab:* 95 mg
>> **Urogesic** *Tab:* 100, 200 mg
▶ *hyoscyamine* (C)(G)
> **Anaspaz** 1-2 tabs q 4 hours prn; max 12 tabs/day
>> *Pediatric:* <2 years: not recommended; 2-12 years: 0.0625-0.125 mg q 4 hours prn; max 0.75 mg/day; ≥12 years: same as adult
>> *Tab:* 0.125*mg
> **Levbid** 1-2 tabs q 12 hours prn; max 4 tabs/day
>> *Pediatric:* <12 years: not recommended; ≥12 years: same as adult
>> *Tab:* 0.375*mg ext-rel
> **Levsin** 1-2 tabs q 4 hours prn; max 12 tabs/day
>> *Pediatric:* <6 years: not recommended; 6-12 years: 1 tab q 4 hours prn; ≥12 years: same as adult
>> *Tab:* 0.125*mg
> **Levsin Drops** 1-2 ml q 4 hours prn; max 60 ml/day
>> *Pediatric:* 3.4 kg: 4 drops q 4 hours prn; max 24 drops/day; 5 kg: 5 drops q 4 hours prn; max 30 drops/day; 7 kg: 6 drops q 4 hours prn; max 36 drops/day; 10 kg: 8 drops q 4 hours prn; max 40 drops/day

Oral drops: 0.125 mg/ml (15 ml) (orange) (alcohol 5%)

Levsin Elixir 5-10 ml q 4 hours prn
> *Pediatric:* <10 kg: use drops; 10-19 kg: 1.25 ml q 4 hours prn; 20-39 kg: 2.5 ml
> q 4 hours prn; 40-49 kg: 3.75 ml q 4 hours prn; ≥50 kg: 5 ml q 4 hours prn; *Elix:*
> 0.125 mg/5 ml (16 oz) (orange) (alcohol 20%)

Levsinex SL 1-2 tabs q 4 hours SL or PO; max 12 tabs/day
> *Pediatric:* <2 years: not recommended; 2-12 years: 1 tab q 4 hours; max 6 tabs/
> day; ≥12 years: same as adult
> *SL tab:* 0.125 mg

Levsinex Timecaps 1-2 caps q 12 hours; may adjust to 1 cap q 8 hours
> *Pediatric:* <2 years: not recommended; 2-12 years: 1 cap q 12 hours; max 2
> caps/day; ≥12 years: same as adult
> *Cap:* 0.375 mg time-rel

NuLev dissolve 1-2 tabs on tongue, with or without water, q 4 hours prn; max
12 tabs/day
> *Pediatric:* <2 years: not recommended; 2-12 years: dissolve 1 tab on tongue,
> with or without water, q 4 hours prn; max 6 tabs/day; ≥12 years: same as
> adult
> *ODT:* 0.125 mg (mint; phenylalanine)

▷ *methenamine/na phosphate monobasic/phenyl salicylate/methylene blue/hyoscyam-*
ine sulfate (C) 1 cap qid
Pediatric: <6 years: not recommended; ≥6 years: individualize dose
> **Uribel** *Cap: meth* 118 mg/*na phos* 40.8 mg/*phenyl sal* 36 mg/*meth blue* 10 mg/
> *hyoscy* 0.12 mg

▷ *methenamine/phenyl salicylate/methylene blue/benzoic acid/atropine sulfate/hyos-*
cyamine sulfate (C)(G) 2 tabs qid
Pediatric: <6 years: not recommended; ≥6 years: same as adult
> **Urised** *Tab: meth* 40.8 mg/*phenyl sal* 18.1 mg/*meth blue* 5.4 mg/*benz acid* 4.5
> mg/*atro sul* 0.03 mg/*hyoscy* 0.03 mg
>
> **Comment:** **Urised** imparts a blue-green color to urine which may stain fabrics.

▷ *oxybutynin chloride* (B)
> **Ditropan** 5 mg bid-tid; max 20 mg/day
> > *Pediatric:* <5 years: not recommended; 5-12 years: 5 mg bid; max 15 mg/day;
> > ≥12 years: same as adult
> > *Tab:* 5*mg; *Syr:* 5 mg/5 ml
>
> **Ditropan XL** initially 5 mg daily; may increase weekly in 5-mg increments as
> needed; max 30 mg/day
> > *Tab:* 5, 10, 15 mg ext-rel

▷ *pentosan* (B) 100 mg tid; reevaluate at 3 and 6 months
Pediatric: <16 years: not recommended; ≥16 years: same as adult
> **Elmiron** *Cap:* 100 mg

URINARY TRACT ANALGESIA

▷ *phenazopyridine* (B)(G) 95-200 mg q 6 hours prn; max 2 days
Pediatric: not recommended
> **AZO Standard, Prodium, Uristat** (OTC) *Tab:* 95 mg
> **AZO Standard Maximum Strength** (OTC) *Tab:* 97.5 mg
> **Pyridium, Urogesic** *Tab:* 100, 200 mg
> > *Pediatric:* not recommended

Azo Standard (OTC) *Tab:* 95 mg
Azo Standard Maximum Strength (OTC) *Tab:* 97.5 mg
Pyridium *Tab:* 100, 200 mg ent-coat
Uristat (OTC) *Tab:* 95 mg
Urogesic *Tab:* 100, 200 mg

Comment: *Phenazopyridine* imparts an orange-red color to urine which may stain fabrics.

▷ *propantheline* (C) 15-30 mg tid
 Pro-Banthine *Tab:* 7.5, 15 mg
▷ *tolterodine tartrate* (C)(G) 2 mg bid; may decrease to 1 mg bid
 Detrol 2 mg bid; may decrease to 1 mg bid
  Tab: 1, 2 mg
 Detrol XL 2-4 mg daily
  Cap: 2, 4 mg ext-rel

ANTICHOLINERGIC/SEDATIVE COMBINATION

▷ *chlordiazepoxide/clidinium* (D)(IV) 1-2 caps ac and HS; max 8 caps/day
 Pediatric: not recommended
  Librax *Cap: chlor* 5 mg/*clid* 2.5 mg

TRICYCLIC ANTIDEPRESSANTS (TCAS)

▷ *amitriptyline* (C)(G) 25-50 mg q HS
 Pediatric: not recommended
  Tab: 10, 25, 50, 75, 100, 150 mg
▷ *imipramine* (C)(G)
 Pediatric: not recommended
  Tofranil initially 75 mg daily (max 200 mg); adolescents initially 30-40 mg daily (max 100 mg/day); if maintenance dose exceeds 75 mg daily, may switch to **Tofranil PM** for divided <u>or</u> bedtime dose
   Tab: 10, 25, 50 mg
  Tofranil PM initially 75 mg daily 1 hour before HS; max 200 mg
   Cap: 75, 100, 125, 150

◯ INTERTRIGO

Comment: Intertrigo is an irritation and rash secondary to adjacent skin surfaces rubbing together. Treatment is dependent on symptoms and presence of infection.
Topical Corticosteroids *see page* 506
Topical Antifungals *see Tinea Corporis page* 410
Topical Anti-infectives *see Skin Infection: Bacterial page* 396

◯ IRITIS: ACUTE

▷ *loteprednol etabonate* (C) 1-2 drops qid; may increase to 1 drop hourly as needed
 Pediatric: not recommended
  Lotemax Ophthalmic Solution *Ophth soln:* 0.3% (2.5, 5, 10, 15 ml)

▷ *prednisone acetate* (C) 1 drop q 1 hour x 24-48 hours, then 1 drop q 2 hours while awake x 24-48 hours, then 1 drop bid-qid until resolved
Pediatric: not recommended
   Pred Forte *Ophth soln:* 1% (1, 5, 10, 15 ml)

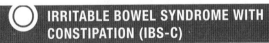

IRON OVERLOAD

IRON CHELATING AGENTS

▷ *deferasirox* (***tridentate ligand***) (C)(G) initially 20 mg/kg/day; titrate; may increase 5-10 mg/kg q 3-6 months based on serum ferritin trends; max 30 mg/kg/day
Pediatric: <2 years: not recommended; ≥2 years: same as adult
   Exjade *Tab for oral soln:* 125, 250, 500 mg
   Jadenu *Tab:* 90, 180, 360 mg film-coat
Comment: *deferasirox* is an orally active chelator selective for iron. It is indicated for the treatment of chronic iron overload due to blood transfusions (transfusional hemosiderosis). Monitor serum ferritin monthly. Consider interrupting therapy if serum ferritin falls below 500 mcg/L. Take *deferasirox* (**Jadenu, Exjade**) on an empty stomach. Completely disperse tablet(s) for oral solution in 3.5 oz liquid if dose is ≤1 g or 7 oz liquid if dose is ≥1 g.

▷ *Succimer* (C) initially 10 mg/kg q 8 hours x 5 days; then, reduce frequency to every 12 hours x 14 more days; allow at least 14 days between courses unless blood lead levels indicate need for prompt treatment
Pediatric: <12 months: not recommended; ≥12 monhs: same as adult
   Chemet *Cap:* 100 mg
Comment: *Chemet is* indicated for the treatment of lead poisoning when blood lead level 45 mcg/dL. Treatment for more than 3 consecutive weeks is not recommended. Monitor hydration, renal, and hepatic function.

IRRITABLE BOWEL SYNDROME WITH CONSTIPATION (IBS-C)

Bulk-Producing Agents, Laxatives, Stool Softeners *see **Constipation** page* 95

GUANYLATE CYCLASE-C AGONIST

▷ *linaclotide* (C) 290 mcg once daily; take on an empty stomach at least 30 minutes before the first meal of the day; swallow whole
Pediatric: <6 years: not recommended; 6-17 years: avoid
   Linzess *Cap:* 145, 290 mcg
   Comment: May open **Linzess** cap and sprinkle on applesauce or in water for administration

▷ *lubiprostone* (C) 8 mcg bid; take with food and water; *Severe hepatic impairment (Child-Pugh Class C):* 8 mcg once daily
Pediatric: <18 years: not recommended
   Amitiza *Cap:* 8, 24 mcg

IRRITABLE BOWEL SYNDROME WITH DIARRHEA (IBS-D)

Bulk-Producing Agents *see Constipation page* 95

CONSTIPATING AGENTS

➤ *difenoxin/atropine* (C) 2 tabs, then 1 tab after each loose stool <u>or</u> 1 tab q 3-4 hours as needed; max 8 tab/day x 2 days
Pediatric: <12 years: not recommended; ≥12 years: same as adult
 Motofen *Tab: difen* 1 mg/*atro* 0.025 mg

➤ *diphenoxylate/atropine* (C)(G) 2 tabs <u>or</u> 10 ml qid
Pediatric: <2 years: not recommended; 2-12 years: initially 0.3-0.4 mg/kg/day in 4 divided doses; ≥12 years: same as adult
 Lomotil *Tab: difen* 2.5 mg/*atro* 0.025 mg; *Liq: difen* 2.5 mg/*atro* 0.025 mg per 5 ml (2 oz)

➤ *eluxadoline* (NA)(IV) 100 mg bid; 75 mg bid if unable to tolerate 100 mg, <u>or</u> without a gall bladder, <u>or</u> mild-to-moderate hepatic impairment, <u>or</u> receiving concomitant OATP1B1 inhibitors
Pediatric: not established
 Viberzi 4 mg initially, then 2 mg after each loose stool; max 16 mg/day
  Tab: 75, 100 mg film-coat
Comment: *Eluxadoline* is a mu-opioid receptor agonist. It is contraindicated with biliary obstruction, Sphincter of Oddi disease <u>or</u> dysfunction, alcohol abuse <u>or</u> addiction, pancreatitis, pancreatic duct obstruction, severe hepatic impairment, and mechanical GI obstruction.

➤ *loperamide* (B)(G)
 Imodium (OTC) 4 mg initially, then 2 mg after each loose stool; max 16 mg/day
  Pediatric: <5 years: not recommended; ≥5 years: same as adult
  Cap: 2 mg
 Imodium A-D (OTC) 4 mg initially, then 2 mg after each loose stool; usual max 8 mg/day x 2 days
  Pediatric: <2 years: not recommended; 2-5 years (24-47 lb): 1 mg up to tid x 2 days; 6-8 years (48-59 lb): 2 mg initially, then 1 mg after each loose stool; max 4 mg/day x 2 days; 9-11 years (60-95 lb): 2 mg initially, then 1 mg after each loose stool; max 6 mg/day x 2 days; ≥12 years: same as adult
  Cplt: 2 mg; *Liq:* 1 mg/5 ml (2, 4 oz)

➤ *loperamide/simethicone* (B)(G)
 Imodium Advanced (OTC) 2 tabs chewed after loose stool, then 1 after the next loose stool; max 4 tabs/day
  Pediatric: <6 years: not recommended; 6-8 years: 1 tab chewed after loose stool, then 1/2 after next loose stool; max 2 tabs/day; 9-11 years: 1 tab chewed after loose stool, then 1/2 after next loose stool; max 3 tabs/day; ≥12 years: same as adult
  Chew tab: lop 2 mg/*sim* 125 mg

5-HT3 RECEPTOR ANTAGONIST

➤ *alosetron* (B)(G) initially 0.5 mg bid; may increase to 1 mg bid after 4 weeks if starting dose is tolerated but inadequate
Pediatric: not recommended
 Lotronex *Tab:* 0.5, 1 mg

ANTISPASMODIC/ANTICHOLINERGIC COMBINATIONS

▷ *dicyclomine* (B)(G) initially 20 mg bid-qid; may increase to 40 mg qid PO; usual IM dose 80 mg/day divided qid; do not use IM route for more than 1-2 days
  Pediatric: not recommended
  Bentyl *Tab:* 20 mg; *Cap:* 10 mg; *Syr:* 10 mg/5 ml (16 oz); *Vial:* 10 mg/ml (10 ml); *Amp:* 10 mg/ml (2 ml)

▷ *methscop olamine bromide* (B) 1 tab q 6 hours prn
  Pediatric: not recommended
  Pamine *Tab:* 2.5 mg
  Pamine Forte *Tab:* 5 mg

ANTICHOLINERGICS

▷ *hyoscyamine* (C)(G)
  Anaspaz 1-2 tabs q 4 hours prn; max 12 tabs/day
    Pediatric: <2 years: not recommended; 2-12 years: 0.0625-0.125 mg q 4 hours prn; max 0.75 mg/day; ≥12 years: same as adult
    Tab: 0.125*mg
  Levbid 1-2 tabs q 12 hours prn; max 4 tabs/day
    Pediatric: <12 years: not recommended; ≥12 years: same as adult
    Tab: 0.375*mg ext-rel
  Levsin 1-2 tabs q 4 hours prn; max 12 tabs/day
    Pediatric: <6 years: not recommended; 6-12 years: 1 tab q 4 hours prn; >12 years: same as adult
    Tab: 0.125*mg
  Levsinex SL 1-2 tabs q 4 hours SL o̱r PO; max 12 tabs/day
    Pediatric: <2 years: not recommended; 2-12 years: 1 tab q 4 hours; max 6 tabs/day; >12 years: same as adult
    Tab: 0.125 mg sublingual
  Levsinex Timecaps 1-2 caps q 12 hours; may adjust to 1 cap q 8 hours
    Pediatric: <2 years: not recommended; 2-12 years: 1 cap q 12 hours; max 2 caps/day; >12 years: same as adult
    Cap: 0.375 mg time-rel
  NuLev dissolve 1-2 tabs on tongue, with o̱r without water, q 4 hours prn; max 12 tabs/day
    Pediatric: <2 years: not recommended; 2-12 years: dissolve 1 tab on tongue, with o̱r without water, q 4 hours prn; max 6 tabs/day; >12 years: same as adult
    ODT: 0.125 mg (mint; phenylalanine)

▷ *simethicone* (C)(G) 0.3 ml qid pc and HS
  Mylicon Drops (OTC) *Oral drops:* 40 mg/0.6 ml (30 ml)

▷ *phenobarbital/hyoscyamine/atropine/scopolamine* (C)(IV)(G)
  Donnatal 1-2 tabs ac and HS
    Pediatric: not recommended
    Tab: pheno 16.2 mg/*hyo* 0.1037 mg/*atro* 0.0194 mg/*scop* 0.0065 mg
  Donnatal Elixir 1-2 tsp ac and HS
    Pediatric: 20 lb: 1 ml q 4 hours o̱r 1.5 ml q 6 hours; 30 lb: 1.5 ml q 4 hours o̱r 2 ml q 6 hours; 50 lb: 1/2 tsp q 4 hours o̱r 3/4 tsp q 6 hours; 75 lb: 3/4 tsp q 4 hours o̱r 1 tsp q 6 hours; 100 lb: 1 tsp q 4 hours o̱r 1 tsp q 6 hours
    Elix: pheno 16.2 mg/*hyo* 0.1037 mg/*atro* 0.0194 mg/*scop* 0.0065 mg per 5 ml (4, 16 oz)

Donnatal Extentabs 1 tab q 12 hours
Pediatric: not recommended
Tab: pheno 48.6 mg/*hyo* 0.3111 mg/*atro* 0.0582 mg/*scop* 0.0195 mg ext-rel

ANTICHOLINERGIC/SEDATIVE COMBINATION

▷ *chlordiazepoxide/clidinium* (D)(IV) 1-2 caps ac and HS: max 8 caps/day
Pediatric: not recommended
Librax *Cap: chlor* 5 mg/*clid* 2.5 mg

TRICYCLIC ANTIDEPRESSANTS (TCAs)

▷ *amitriptyline* (C)(G) 25-50 mg q HS
Pediatric: not recommended
Tab: 10, 25, 50, 75, 100, 150 mg
▷ *imipramine* (C)(G) 25-50 mg tid
Pediatric: not recommended
Tofranil initially 75 mg daily (max 200 mg); adolescents initially 30-40 mg daily
(max 100 mg/day); if maintenance dose exceeds 75 mg daily, may switch to
Tofranil PM for divided <u>or</u> bedtime dose
Tab: 10, 25, 50 mg
Tofranil PM initially 75 mg daily 1 hour before HS; max 200 mg
Cap: 75, 100, 125, 150
Tofranil Injection 50 mg IM; lower dose for adolescents; switch to oral form as
soon as possible
Amp: 25 mg/2 ml (2 ml)

◯ JUVENILE RHEUMATOID ARTHRITIS (JRA)

Acetaminophen for IV Infusion *see Pain page* 306
Oral Prescription NSAIDs *see page* 501
Other Oral Analgesics *see Pain page* 308
Topical/Transdermal NSAIDs *see Pain page* 307
Parenteral Corticosteroids *see page* 511
Oral Corticosteroids *see page* 509
Topical Analgesic and Anesthetic Agents *see page* 499

TOPICAL ANALGESICS

▷ *capsaicin* (B)(G) apply tid-qid prn to intact skin
Pediatric: <2 years: not recommended; ≥2 years: same as adult
Axsain *Crm:* 0.075% (1, 2 oz)
Capsin *Lotn:* 0.025, 0.075% (59 ml)
Capzasin-P (OTC) *Crm:* 0.025% (1.5 oz); *Lotn:* 0.025% (2 oz)
Dolorac *Crm:* 0.025% (28 g)
Double Cap (OTC) *Crm:* 0.05% (2 oz)
R-Gel *Gel:* 0.025% (15, 30 g)
Zostrix (OTC) *Crm:* 0.025% (0.7, 1.5, 3 oz)
Zostrix HP (OTC) *Emol crm:* 0.075% (1, 2 oz)
Comment: Provides some relief by 1-2 weeks; optimal benefit may take 4-6 weeks.

ORAL SALICYLATE

▷ *indomethacin* (C) initially 25 mg bid-tid, increase as needed at weekly intervals by 25-50 mg/day; max 200 mg/day
Pediatric: <14 years: usually not recommended; ≥2 years, if risk warranted: 1-2 mg/kg/day in divided doses; max 3-4 mg/kg/day (or total 150-200 mg/day, whichever is less); ≤14 years, ER cap not recommended
Cap: 25, 50 mg; Susp: 25 mg/5 ml (pineapple-coconut, mint; alcohol 1%); Supp: 50 mg; ER Cap: 75 mg ext-rel
Comment: *Indomethacin* is indicated only for acute painful flares. Administer with food and/or antacids. Use lowest effective dose for shortest duration.

▷ *methotrexate* (X) 7.5 mg x 1 dose per week or 2.5 mg x 3 at 12-hour intervals once a week; max 20 mg/week; therapeutic response begins in 3-6 weeks; administer methotrexate injection SC only into the abdomen or thigh
Pediatric: <2 years: not recommended; ≥2 years: 10 mg/m² once weekly; max 20 mg/m²
  Rasuvo *Autoinjector:* 7.5 mg/0.15 ml, 10 mg/0.20 ml, 12.5 mg/0.25 ml, 15 mg/0.30 ml, 17.5 mg/0.35 ml, 20 mg/0.40 ml, 22.5 mg/0.45 ml, 25 mg/0.50 ml, 27.5 mg/0.55 ml, 30 mg/0.60 ml (solution concentration for SC injection is 50 mg/ml)
  Rheumatrex *Tab:* 2.5*mg (5, 7.5, 10, 12.5, 15 mg/week, 4/card unit-of-use dose pack)
  Trexall *Tab:* 5*, 7.5*, 10*, 15*mg (5, 7.5, 10, 12.5, 15 mg/week, 4/card unit-of-use dose pack)
Comment: *methotrexate* (MTX) is contraindicated with immunodeficiency, blood dyscrasias, alcoholism, and chronic liver disease.

 ## KERATITIS/KERATOCONJUNCTIVITIS: HERPES SIMPLEX

▷ *ganciclovir* (C) instill 1 drop 5 times per day (every 3 hours) while awake until corneal ulcer heals; then 1 drop tid x 7 days
Pediatric: <2 years: not recommended; ≥2 years: same as adult
  Zirgan *Ophth gel:* 0.15% (5 gm)(benzalkonium chloride)

▷ *idoxuridine* (C) instill 1 drop q 1 hour during day and every other hour at night or 1 drop every minute for 5 minutes and repeat q 4 hours during day and night
  Herplex *Ophth soln:* 0.1% (15 ml)

▷ *trifluridine* (C) instill 1 drop q 2 hours while awake (max 9 drops/day until reepithelialization; then 1 drop q 4 hours x 7 more days (at least 5 drops/day); max 21 days
Pediatric: <6 years: not recommended; ≥6 years: same as adult
  Viroptic *Ophth soln:* 1% (7.5 ml) (thimerosal)

▷ *vidarabine* (C) apply 1/2 inch in lower conjunctival sac 5 times/day q 3 hours until reepithelialization occurs, then bid x 7 more days
Pediatric: <2 years: not recommended; ≥2 years: same as adult
  Vira-A *Ophth oint:* 3% (3.5 g)

KERATITIS/KERATOCONJUNCTIVITIS: VERNAL

OPHTHALMIC MAST CELL STABILIZERS

Comment: Contact lens wear is contraindicated

▷ *cromolyn sodium* (B) 1-2 drops 4-6 times/day
   Pediatric: <4 years: not recommended; ≥4 years: same as adult
      Crolom, Opticrom *Ophth soln:* 4% (10 ml) (benzalkonium chloride)
▷ *lodoxamide tromethamine* (B) 1-2 drops qid; max 3 months
   Pediatric: <2 years: not recommended; ≥2 years: same as adult
      Alomide *Ophth susp:* 0.1% (10 ml)

◯ LABYRINTHITIS

▷ *meclizine* (B) 25 mg tid
   Pediatric: not recommended
      Antivert *Tab:* 12.5, 25, 50*mg
      Bonine (OTC) *Cap:* 15, 25, 30 mg; *Tab:* 12.5, 25, 50 mg; *Chew tab/Film-coated tab:* 25 mg
      Dramamine II (OTC) *Tab:* 25*mg
      Zentrip *Strip:* 25 mg orally disintegrating
▷ *promethazine* (C)(G) 25 mg tid
   Pediatric: <2 years: not recommended; ≥2 years: 0.5 mg/lb or 6.25-25 mg tid
      Phenergan *Tab:* 12.5*, 25*, 50 mg; *Plain syr:* 6.25 mg/5 ml; *Fortis syr:* 25 mg/5 ml; *Rectal supp:* 12.5, 25, 50 mg
▷ *scopolamine* (C)
      Transderm Scop 1 patch behind ear at least 4 hours before travel; each patch is effective for 3 days
         Transdermal patch: 1.5 mg (4/carton)

◯ LACTOSE INTOLERANCE

▷ *lactase* enzyme (NE) 9,000 FCC units taken with dairy food; adjust based on abatement of symptoms; usual max 18,000 units/dose
   Pediatric: same as adult
      Lactaid Drops (OTC) 5-7 drops to each quart of milk and shake gently; may increase to 10-15 drops if needed; hydrolyzes 70%-99% of lactose at refrigerator temperature in 24 hours
         Oral drops: 1,250 units/5 gtts (7 ml w. dropper)
      Lactaid Extra (OTC) *Cplt:* 4,500 FCC units
      Lactaid Fast ACT (OTC) *Cplt:* 9,000 FCC units; *Chew tab:* 9,000 FCC units (vanilla twist)
      Lactaid Original (OTC) *Cplt:* 3,000 FCC units
      Lactaid Ultra (OTC) *Cplt:* 9,000 FCC units; *Chew tab:* 9,000 FCC units (vanilla twist)

◯ LARVA MIGRANS: CUTANEOUS/VISCERAL

▷ *thiabendazole* (C) Adult and pediatric dosing schedules are the same; dosing is bid, is based on weight in pounds, and must be taken with meals.
      Cutaneous Larva Migrans: treat bid x 2 days
      Visceral Larva Migrans: treat bid x 7 days
         <30 lbs: consult mfr pkg insert; 30 lbs: 250 mg bid; 50 lbs: 500 mg bid; 75 lbs: 750 mg bid; 100 lbs: 1000 mg bid; 125 lbs: 1250 mg bid; ≥150 lbs: 1500 mg bid; max 3000 mg/day.

Mintezol *Chew tab:* 500*mg (orange); *Oral susp:* 500 mg/5 ml (120 ml) (orange)
Comment: *thiabendazole* is not for prophylaxis. May impair mental alertness.

LEAD POISONING

Comment: Chelation therapy for lead poisoning requires maintenance of adequate hydration, close monitoring of renal and hepatic function, and monitoring for neutropenia; discontinue therapy at first sign of toxicity. Contraindicated with severe renal disease or anuria.

CHELATING AGENTS

▷ *deferoxamine mesylate* (C) initially 1 g IM, followed by 500 mg IM every 4 hours x 2 doses; then repeat every 4-12 hours if needed; max 6 g/day
Pediatric: <3 months: not recommended; ≥3 months: same as adult
   Desferal *Vial:* 250 mg/ml after reconstitution (500 mg)
▷ *edetate calcium disodium (EDTA)* (B) administer IM or IV; use IM route of administration for children and overt lead encephalopathy
Pediatric: same as adult; *Serum lead level:* 20-70 mcg/dL: 1 g/m^2 per day; *IV:* infuse over 8-12 hours; *IM:* divided doses q 8-12 hours; Treat for 5 days; then stop for 2-4 days; may repeat if serum lead level is >70 mcg/dL
   Calcium Disodium Versenate *Amp:* 200 mg/ml (5 ml)
▷ *succimer* (C) may swallow caps whole or put contents onto a small amount of soft food or a spoon and swallow, followed by a fruit drink
Pediatric: <12 months: not recommended; ≥12 months: same as adult; *Serum lead level:* >45 *mcg/dL:* initially 10 mg/kg (or 350 mg/m^2) every 8 hours for 5 days; then reduce frequency to every 12 hours for 14 more days; allow at least 14 days between courses unless serum lead levels indicate a need for more prompt treatment; for more than 3 consecutive weeks not recommended
   Chemet *Cap:* 100 mg

LEG CRAMPS: NOCTURNAL, RECUMBENCY

▷ *quinine sulfate* (C)(G) 1 tab or cap q HS
Pediatric: <16 years: not recommended; ≥16 years: same as adult
   Qualaquin *Tab:* 260 mg; *Cap:* 260, 300, 325 mg
Comment: If hypokalemia is the cause of leg cramps, treat with potassium supplementation (*see page 229*).

LEISHMANIASIS: CUTANEOUS, MUCOSAL, VISCERAL

Comment: The leishmanial parasite species addressed in this section are: **cutaneous leishmaniasis** (due to *Leishmania braziliensis, Leishmania guyanensis, Leishmania panamensis*), **mucosal leishmaniasis** (due to *Leishmania braziliensis*), and **visceral leishmaniasis** (due to *Leishmania donovani*). The weight-based treatment for adults and adolescents is the same for each of the species, the anti-leishmanial drug *miltefosone* (**Impavido**). Contraindications to this drug include pregnancy, lactation, and Sjogren-Larsson-Syndrome. The contraindication in pregnancy is due to embryo-fetal toxicity, teratogenicity, and fetal death. Obtain a serum or urine pregnancy test for females of reproductive potential and advise females to use effective contraception during therapy and for 5 months following treatment. Breastfeeding is contraindicated while taking this drug and for 5 months following termination of breastfeeding. Potential ASEs include loss of appetite, abdominal pain, nausea, vomiting, diarrhea, headache, dizziness, pruritis, somnolence, elevated liver transaminases, bilirubin, and serum creatinine and thrombocytopenia. Miltefosine is associated with impaired fertility in females and males in animal studies. To report a suspected adverse reaction to this drug, call 888-550-6060 or the FDA at 800-FDA-1088 or visit www.fda.gov/medwatch

▷ *miltefosine* (D)(G) 30-44 kg: one cap bid x 28 consecutive days; ≥45 kg: one cap tid x 28 consecutive days; take with a full meal
   Pediatric: <12 years, <30 kg (60 lbs): not established
      Impavido *Cap:* 50 mg

⬤ LENTIGINES: BENIGN, SENILE

Comment: Wash affected area with a soap-free cleanser; pat dry and wait 20-30 minutes; then apply agent sparingly to affected area; use only once daily in PM. Avoid eyes, ears, nostrils, mouth, and healthy skin. Avoid sun exposure. Cautious use of concomitant astringents, alcohol-based products, sulfur-containing products, salicylic acid-containing products, soap, and other topical agents.

TOPICAL RETINOIDS

▷ *tazarotene* (X) apply daily at HS
   Pediatric: not recommended
      Avage Cream *Crm:* 0.1% (30 g)
      Tazorac Cream *Crm:* 0.05, 0.1% (15, 30, 60 g)
      Tazorac Gel *Gel:* 0.05, 0.1% (30, 100 g)
▷ *tretinoin* (C)(G) apply daily at HS
   Pediatric: <12 years: not recommended; ≥12 years: same as adult
      Avita *Crm:* 0.025% (20, 45 g); *Gel:* 0.025% (20, 45 g)
      Renova *Crm:* 0.02% (40 g); 0.05% (40, 60 g)
      Retin-A Cream *Crm:* 0.025, 0.05, 0.1% (20, 45 g)
      Retin-A Gel *Gel:* 0.01, 0.025% (15, 45 g) (alcohol 90%)
      Retin-A Liquid *Liq:* 0.05% (28 ml; alcohol 55%)
      Retin-A Micro *Microspheres:* 0.04, 0.1% (20, 45 g)
      Retin-A Micro Gel *Gel:* 0.04, 0.1% (20, 45 g)

⬤ LISTERIOSIS

▷ *erythromycin base* (B)(G) 500 mg qid x 10 days
   Pediatric: <45 kg: 30-40 mg/kg/day in 4 divided doses x 10 days; ≥45 kg: same as adult
      Ery-Tab *Tab:* 250, 333, 500 mg ent-coat
      PCE *Tab:* 333, 500 mg
   Comment: *erythromycin* may increase INR with concomitant *warfarin*, as well as increase serum level of *digoxin*, benzodiazepines and statins.

▶ *erythromycin ethylsuccinate* (B)(G) 400 mg PO qid x 10 days
Pediatric: 30-50 mg/kg/day in 4 divided doses x 10 days; may double dose with severe infection; max 100 mg/kg/day; *see page 574 for dose by weight*
   EryPed *Oral susp:* 200 mg/5 ml (100, 200 ml) (fruit); 400 mg/5 ml (60, 100, 200 ml; banana); *Oral drops:* 200, 400 mg/5 ml (50 ml) (fruit); *Chew tab:* 200 mg wafer (fruit)
   E.E.S. *Oral susp:* 200, 400 mg/5 ml (100 ml) (fruit)
   E.E.S. Granules *Oral susp:* 200 mg/5 ml (7.5 ml) (thimerosal)
   E.E.S. 400 Tablets *Tab:* 400 mg
   Comment: *erythromycin* may increase INR with concomitant *warfarin*, as well as increase serum level of *digoxin*, benzodiazepines and statins.

LOW BACK STRAIN

Acetaminophen for IV Infusion *see Pain page 306*
Oral Prescription NSAIDs *see page 501*
Other Oral Analgesics *see Pain page 308*
Topical/Transdermal NSAIDs *see Pain page 307*
Parenteral Corticosteroids *see page 511*
Oral Corticosteroids *see page 509*
Topical Analgesic and Anesthetic Agents *see page 499*

LOW LIBIDO, HYPOACTIVE SEXUAL DESIRE DISORDER (HSDD)

5-HT1A AGONIST/5-HT2A

▶ *flibanserin* (NE) 1 tab once daily at bedtime; discontinue if no improvement in 8 weeks
Pediatric: <18 years: not recommended
   Tab: 100 mg
   Comment: **Addyi** is for use in premenopausal women. **Addyi** is not for use in men, postmenopausal women, and is not recommended in pregnancy, or lactation. Potential ASEs include dry mouth, nausea, hypotension, dizziness, syncope, fatigue, somnolence, and insomnia.

LYME DISEASE (ERYTHEMA CHRONICUM MIGRANS)

Comment: The bite of the deer tick (*Ioxodes scapularis*) carries the *Borrelia burgdorferi* organism causing Lyme disease. Proper removal of the tick, and early diagnosis and treatment are essential to effective management of this disease.

STAGE 1

▶ *amoxicillin* (B)(G) 500-875 mg bid or 250-500 mg tid x 10 days
Pediatric: <40 kg (88 lb): 20-40 mg/kg/day in 3 divided doses x 10 days or 25-45 mg/kg/day in 2 divided doses x 10 days; ≥40 kg: same as adult; *see page 554 for dose by weight*

Amoxil *Cap:* 250, 500 mg; *Tab:* 875*mg; *Chew tab:* 125, 200, 250, 400 mg (cherry-banana-peppermint) (phenylalanine); *Oral susp:* 125, 250 mg/5 ml (80, 100, 150 ml) (strawberry); 200, 400 mg/5 ml (50, 75, 100 ml) (bubble gum); *Oral drops:* 50 mg/ml (30 ml) (bubble gum)

Moxatag *Tab:* 775 mg ext-rel

Trimox *Tab:* 125, 250 mg; *Cap:* 250, 500 mg; *Oral susp:* 125, 250 mg/5 ml (80, 100, 150 ml) (raspberry-strawberry)

▷ *cefuroxime axetil* (B)(G) 500 mg bid x 20 days
Pediatric: <3 months: not recommended; ≥3 months: 15 mg/kg bid x 20 days

Ceftin *Tab:* 250, 500 mg; *Oral susp:* 125, 250 mg/5 ml (50, 100 ml) (tutti-frutti)

▷ *clarithromycin* (C)(G) 500 mg bid or 500 mg ext-rel daily x 14-21 days
Pediatric: <6 months: not recommended; ≥6 months: 7.5 mg/kg bid x 7 days; *see page 569 for dose by weight*

Biaxin *Tab:* 250, 500 mg

Biaxin Oral Suspension *Oral susp:* 125, 250 mg/5 ml (50, 100 ml)

Biaxin XL *Tab:* 500 mg ext-rel

▷ *doxycycline* (D)(G) 100 mg bid x 14-21 days
Pediatric: <8 years: not recommended; ≥8 years, ≤100 lb: 2 mg/lb on first day in 2 divided doses, followed by 1 mg/lb/day in 1-2 divided doses; ≥8 years, >100 lb: same as adult; *see page 572 for dose by weight*

Actilate *Tab:* 75, 150** mg

Adoxa *Tab:* 50, 75, 100, 150 mg ent-coat

Doryx *Tab:* 50, 75, 100, 150, 200 mg del-rel

Monodox *Cap:* 50, 75, 100 mg

Oracea *Cap:* 40 mg del-rel

Vibramycin *Tab:* 100 mg; *Cap:* 50, 100 mg; *Syr:* 50 mg/5 ml (raspberry-apple) (sulfites); *Oral susp:* 25 mg/5 ml (raspberry)

Vibra-Tab *Tab:* 100 mg film-coat

Comment: *doxycycline* is contraindicated <8-years-of-age, in pregnancy, and lactation (discolors developing tooth enamel). A side effect may be photosensitivity (photophobia). Do not give with antacids, calcium supplements, milk or other dairy, or within two hours of taking another drug.

▷ *minocycline* (D)(G) 200 mg on first day; then 100 mg q 12 hours x 9 more days
Pediatric: ≤8 years: not recommended; ≥8 years, <100 lb: 2 mg/lb on first day in 2 divided doses, followed by 1 mg/lb q 12 hours x 9 more days; ≥8 years, >100 lb: same as adult

Dynacin *Cap:* 50, 100 mg

Minocin *Cap:* 50, 75, 100 mg; *Oral susp:* 50 mg/5 ml (60 ml) (custard) (sulfites, alcohol 5%)

Comment: *minocycline* is contraindicated <8-years-of-age, in pregnancy, and lactation (discolors developing tooth enamel). A side effect may be photosensitivity (photophobia). Do not give with antacids, calcium supplements, milk or other dairy, or within two hours of taking another drug.

▷ *tetracycline* (D)(G) 250-500 mg qid ac x 21 days
Pediatric: <8 years: not recommended; ≥8 years, ≤100 lb: 25-50 mg/kg/day in 2-4 divided doses x 7 days; ≥8 years, >100 lb: same as adult; *see page 585 for dose by weight*

Achromycin V *Cap:* 250, 500 mg

Sumycin *Tab:* 250, 500 mg; *Cap:* 250, 500 mg; *Oral susp:* 125 mg/5 ml (100, 200 ml) (fruit) (sulfites)

Comment: *tetracycline* is contraindicated <8 years-of-age, in pregnancy, and lactation (discolors developing tooth enamel). A side effect may be photo-sensitivity (photophobia). Do not give with antacids, calcium supplements, milk or other dairy, or within two hours of taking another drug.

◯ LYMPHADENITIS

Comment: Therapy should continue for no less than 5 days after resolution of symptoms.
➤ *amoxicillin/clavulanate* (B)(G) 500 mg tid or 875 mg bid x 10 days
    Augmentin *Tab:* 250, 500, 875 mg; *Chew tab:* 125, 250 mg (lemon-lime); 200, 400 mg (cherry-banana) (phenylalanine); *Oral susp:* 125 mg/5 ml (banana), 250 mg/5 ml (75, 100, 150 ml) (orange); 200, 400 mg/5 ml (50, 75, 100 ml) (orange) (phenylalanine)
      Pediatric: 40-45 mg/kg/day divided tid x 10 days or 90 mg/kg/day divided bid x 10 days *see pages 556-557 for dose by weight*
    Augmentin ES-600 *Oral susp:* 600 mg/5 ml (50, 75, 100, 125, 150, 200 ml) (strawberry cream) (phenylalanine) every 12 hours
      Pediatric: <3 months: not recommended; ≥3 months, <40 kg: 90 mg/kg/day in 2 divided doses; ≥40 kg: not recommended
    Augmentin XR 2 tabs q 12 hours x 7-10 days
      Pediatric: <16 years: use other forms; ≥16 years: same as adult
      Tab: 1000*mg ext-rel
➤ *cephalexin* (B)(G) 500 mg bid x 10 days
  Pediatric: 25-50 mg/kg/day in 4 divided doses x 10 days; *see page 568 for dose by weight*
    Keflex *Cap:* 250, 333, 500, 750 mg; *Oral susp:* 125, 250 mg/5 ml (100, 200 ml) (strawberry)
➤ *dicloxacillin* (B) 500 mg qid x 10 days
  Pediatric: 12.5-25 mg/kg/day in 4 divided doses x 10 days; *see page 571 for dose by weight*
    Dynapen *Cap:* 125, 250, 500 mg; *Oral susp:* 62.5 mg/5 ml (80, 100, 200 ml)

◯ LYMPHOGRANULOMA VENEREUM

Comment: The following treatment regimens are published in the **2015 CDC Sexually Transmitted Diseases Treatment Guidelines**. This section contains treatment regimens for adults only; consult a specialist for treatment of patients less than 18 years of age. Treatment regimens are presented in alphabetical order by generic drug name, followed by brands and dose forms. Treat all sexual contacts. Persons with both LGV and HIV infection should receive the same treatment regimens as those who are HIV-negative; however, prolonged treatment may be required and delay in resolution of symptoms may occur.

RECOMMENDED REGIMEN

Regimen 1

➤ *doxycycline* 100 mg bid x 21 days

ALTERNATIVE REGIMEN

Regimen 1

▷ *erythromycin base* 500 mg qid x 21 days or *erythromycin ethylsuccinate* 400 mg qid x 21 days

RECOMMENDED REGIMENS FOR THE MANAGEMENT OF SEXUAL CONTACTS

Comment: LGV is caused by *C. trachomatis* serovars L1, L2, or L3. Persons who have had sexual contact with a patient who has LGV within 60 days before onset of the patient's symptoms should be examined, tested for urethral or cervical chlamydial infection, and treated with a chlamydia regimen.

Regimen 1

▷ *azithromycin* 1 g in a single dose

Regimen 2

▷ *doxycycline* 100 mg bid x 7 days

DRUG BRANDS AND DOSE FORMS

▷ *azithromycin* (B)
   Zithromax *Tab:* 250, 500, 600 mg; *Oral susp:* 100 mg/5 ml (15 ml);
   200 mg/5 ml (15, 22.5, 30 ml) (cherry); *Pkt:* 1 g for reconstitution (cherry-banana)
   Zithromax Tri-pak *Tab:* 3 x 500 mg tabs/pck
   Zithromax Z-pak *Tab:* 6 x 250 mg tabs/pck
   Zmax *Oral susp:* 2 g ext-rel for reconstitution (cherry-banana) (148 mg Na⁺)

▷ *doxycycline* (D)(G)
   Actilate *Tab:* 75, 150** mg
   Adoxa *Tab:* 50, 75, 100, 150 mg ent-coat
   Doryx *Tab:* 50, 75, 100, 150, 200 mg del-rel
   Monodox *Cap:* 50, 75, 100 mg
   Vibramycin *Tab:* 100 mg; *Cap:* 50, 100 mg; *Syr:* 50 mg/5 ml (raspberry-apple)
   (sulfites); *Oral susp:* 25 mg/5 ml (raspberry)
   Vibra-Tab *Tab:* 100 mg film-coat

   Comment: *doxycycline* is contraindicated <8 years-of-age, in pregnancy, and lactation (discolors developing tooth enamel). A side effect may be photosensitivity (photophobia). Do not give with antacids, calcium supplements, milk or other dairy, or within two hours of taking another drug.

▷ *erythromycin base* (B)(G)
   Ery-Tab *Tab:* 250, 333, 500 mg ent-coat
   PCE *Tab:* 333, 500 mg

   Comment: *erythromycin* may increase INR with concomitant *warfarin*, as well as increase serum level of *digoxin*, benzodiazepines and statins.

▷ *erythromycin ethylsuccinate* (B)(G)
   EryPed *Oral susp:* 200 mg/5 ml (100, 200 ml) (fruit); 400 mg/5 ml (60, 100, 200 ml) (banana); *Oral drops:* 200, 400 mg/5 ml (50 ml) (fruit); *Chew tab:* 200 mg wafer (fruit)
   E.E.S. *Oral susp:* 200, 400 mg/5 ml (100 ml) (fruit)
   E.E.S. Granules *Oral susp:* 200 mg/5 ml (100, 200 ml) (cherry)

E.E.S. 400 Tablets *Tab:* 400 mg

Comment: *erythromycin* may increase INR with concomitant *warfarin*, as well as increase serum level of *digoxin*, benzodiazepines and statins.

◯ MALARIA (*PLASMODIUM FALCIPARUM, PLASMODIUM VIVAX*)

➤ *doxycycline* (D)(G) 100 mg daily; initiate 1-2 days prior to travel; take during travel; continue for 4 weeks after leaving the endemic area
Pediatric: ≤8 years: not recommended; ≥8 years, ≤100 lb: 1 mg/lb/day prior to travel; take during travel; continue for 4 weeks after leaving the endemic area; ≥8 years, ≥100 lb: same as adult; *see page 572 for dose by weight*

Actilate *Tab:* 75, 150** mg
Adoxa *Tab:* 50, 75, 100, 150 mg ent-coat
Doryx *Tab:* 50, 75, 100, 150, 200 mg del-rel
Monodox *Cap:* 50, 75, 100 mg
Vibramycin *Tab:* 100 mg; *Cap:* 50, 100 mg; *Syr:* 50 mg/5 ml (raspberry-apple) (sulfites); *Oral susp:* 25 mg/5 ml (raspberry)
Vibra-Tab *Tab:* 100 mg film-coat

Comment: *doxycycline* is contraindicated <8 years-of-age, in pregnancy, and lactation (discolors developing tooth enamel). A side effect may be photosensitivity (photophobia). Do not give with antacids, calcium supplements, milk or other dairy, or within two hours of taking another drug.

➤ *minocycline* (D)(G) 100 mg daily; initiate 1-2 days prior to travel; take during travel; continue for 4 weeks after leaving the endemic area
Pediatric: <8 years: not recommended; ≥8 years, ≤100 lb: 2 mg/lb on first day in 2 divided doses, followed by 1 mg/lb q 12 hours x 9 more days; ≥8 years, >100 lb: same as adult

Dynacin *Cap:* 50, 100 mg
Minocin *Cap:* 50, 75, 100 mg; *Oral susp:* 50 mg/5 ml (60 ml) (custard) (sulfites, alcohol 5%)

Comment: *minocycline* is contraindicated <8 years-of-age, in pregnancy, and lactation (discolors developing tooth enamel). A side effect may be photosensitivity (photophobia). Do not give with antacids, calcium supplements, milk or other dairy, or within 2 hours of taking another drug.

➤ *tetracycline* (D) 250 mg daily; initiate 1-2 days prior to travel; take during travel; continue for 4 weeks after leaving the endemic area
Pediatric: <8 years: not recommended; ≥8 years, ≤100 lb: 25-50 mg/kg/day in 4 divided doses x 10 days; ≥8 years, >100 lb: same as adult; *see page 585 for dose by weight*

Achromycin V *Cap:* 250, 500 mg
Sumycin *Tab:* 250, 500 mg; *Cap:* 250, 500 mg; *Oral susp:* 125 mg/5 ml (100, 200 ml) (fruit) (sulfites)

Comment: *tetracycline* is contraindicated <8 years-of-age, in pregnancy, and lactation (discolors developing tooth enamel). A side effect may be photosensitivity (photophobia). Do not give with antacids, calcium supplements, milk or other dairy, or within 2 hours of taking another drug.

ANTIMALARIALS

➤ *quinine sulfate* (C)(G) 1 tab <u>or</u> cap every 8 hours x 7 days
Pediatric: <16 years: not recommended; ≥16 years: same as adult

Tab: 260 mg; *Cap:* 260, 300, 325 mg

Qualaquin *Cap:* 324 mg

Comment: *Qualaquin* is indicated in the treatment of uncomplicated *P. falciparum* malaria (including chloroquine-resistant strains).

▷ *atovaquone* (C)(G) take as a single dose with food <u>or</u> a milky drink at the same time each day; repeat dose if vomited within 1 hour; *Prophylaxis:* 1,500 mg once daily; *Treatment:* 750 mg bid x 21 days

Mepron *Susp:* 750 mg/5 ml

▷ *atovaquone/proguanil* (C)(G) take as a single dose with food <u>or</u> a milky drink at the same time each day; repeat dose if vomited within 1 hour; *Prophylaxis:* 1 tab daily starting 1-2 days before entering endemic area, during stay, and for 7 days after return; *Treatment (acute, uncomplicated):* 4 tabs daily x 3 days

Pediatric: <5 kg: not recommended; 5-40 kg

Prophylaxis: daily dose starting 1-2 days before entering endemic area, during stay, and for 7 days after return; 5-20 kg: 1 ped tab; 21-30 kg: 2 ped tabs; 31-40 kg: 3 ped tabs; ≥40 kg: same as adult; *Treatment (acute, uncomplicated):* daily dose x 3 days; 5-8 kg: 2 ped tabs; 9-10 kg: 3 ped tabs; 11-20 kg: 1 adult tab; 21-30 kg: 2 adult tabs; 31-40 kg: 3 adult tabs; >40 kg: same as adult

Malarone *Tab: atov* 250 mg/*prog* 100 mg

Malarone Pediatric *Tab: atov* 62.5 mg/*prog* 25 mg

Comment: *atovaquone* is antagonized by *tetracycline* and *metoclopramide*. Concomitant *rifampin* is not recommended (may elevate LFTs).

▷ *chloroquine* (C)(G) *Prophylaxis:* 500 mg once weekly (on the same day of each week); start 2 weeks prior to exposure, continue while in the endemic area, and continue 4 weeks after departure; *Treatment:* initially 1 g; then 500 mg 6 hours, 24 hours, and 48 hours after initial dose <u>or</u> initially 200-250 mg IM; may repeat in 6 hours; max 1 g in first 24 hours; continue to 1.875 g in 3 days

Pediatric: Suppression: 8.35 mg/kg (max 500 mg) weekly (on the same day of each week); *Treatment:* initially 16.7 mg/kg (max 1 g); then 8.35 mg/kg (max 500 mg) 6 hours, 24 hours, and 48 hours after initial dose, <u>or</u> initially 6.25 mg/kg IM; may repeat in 6 hours; max 12.5 mg/kg/day

Aralen *Tab:* 500 mg; *Amp:* 50 mg/ml (5 ml)

▷ *hydroxychloroquine* (C)(G) *Prophylaxis:* 400 mg once weekly (on the same day of each week); start 2 weeks prior to exposure, continue while in the endemic area, and continue 8 weeks after departure; *Treatment:* initially 800 mg; then 400 mg 6 hours, 24 hours, and 48 hours after initial dose

Pediatric: Suppression: 6.45 mg/kg (max 400 mg) weekly (on the same day of each week) beginning 2 weeks prior to arrival, continuing while in endemic area, and continuing 4 weeks after departure; *Treatment:* initially 12.9 mg/kg (max 800 mg); then 6.45 mg/kg (max 400 mg) 6 hours, 24 hours, and 48 hours after initial dose hours after initial dose

Plaquenil *Tab:* 200 mg

▷ *mefloquine* (C) *Prophylaxis:* 250 mg once weekly (on the same day of each week); start 1 week prior to exposure, continue while in the endemic area, and continue for 4 weeks after departure; *Treatment:* 1,250 mg as a single dose

Pediatric: <6 months: not recommended; *Prophylaxis:* ≥6 months: 3-5 mg/kg (max 250 mg) weekly (on the same day of each week); start 1 week prior to exposure, continue while in the endemic area, and continue for 4 weeks after departure; *Treatment:* ≥6 months: 25-50 mg/kg as a single dose; max 250 mg

Lariam *Tab:* 250*mg

Comment: *mefloquine* is contraindicated with active or recent history of depression, generalized anxiety disorder, psychosis, schizophrenia or any other psychiatric disorder or history of convulsions.

◯ MASTITIS (BREAST ABSCESS)

ANTI-INFECTIVES

▷ *amoxicillin/clavulanate* (B)(G) 500 mg tid or 875 mg bid x 10 days
  Augmentin *Tab:* 250, 500, 875 mg; *Chew tab:* 125, 250 mg (lemon-lime); 200, 400 mg (cherry-banana) (phenylalanine); *Oral susp:* 125 mg/5 ml (banana), 250 mg/5 ml (75, 100, 150 ml) (orange); 200, 400 mg/5 ml (50, 75, 100 ml) (orange) (phenylalanine)
    Pediatric: 40-45 mg/kg/day divided tid x 10 days or 90 mg/kg/day divided bid x 10 days *see pages 556-557 for dose by weight*
  Augmentin ES-600 *Oral susp:* 600 mg/5 ml (50, 75, 100, 125, 150, 200 ml) (strawberry cream) (phenylalanine) every 12 hours
    Pediatric: <3 months: not recommended; ≥3 months, <40 kg: 90 mg/kg/day in 2 divided doses; ≥40 kg: not recommended
  Augmentin XR 2 tabs q 12 hours x 7-10 days
    Pediatric: <16 years: use other forms; ≥16 years: same as adult
    Tab: 1000*mg ext-rel
▷ *cefaclor* (B)(G) 250-500 mg q 8 hours x 10 days; max 2 g/day
  Pediatric: <1 month: not recommended; 20-40 mg/kg bid or q 12 hours x 10 days; max 1 g/day; *see page 560 for dose by weight*
  Tab: 500 mg; *Cap:* 250, 500 mg; *Susp:* 125 mg/5 ml (75, 150 ml) (strawberry); 187 mg/5 ml (50, 100 ml) (strawberry); 250 mg/5 ml (75, 150 ml) (strawberry); 375 mg/5 ml (50, 100 ml) (strawberry)
  Pediatric: <16 years: ext-rel not recommended; ≥12 years: same as adult
    Cefaclor Extended Release *Tab:* 375, 500 mg ext-rel
▷ *ceftriaxone* (B)(G) 1-2 grams IM daily continued 2 days after signs of infection have disappeared; max 4 g/day
  Pediatric: 50 mg/kg IM daily continued 2 days after signs of infection have disappeared
    Rocephin *Vial:* 250, 500 mg; 1, 2 g
▷ *cephalexin* (B)(G) 500 mg bid x 10 days
  Pediatric: 25-50 mg/kg/day in 4 divided doses x 10 days; *see page 568 for dose by weight*
    Keflex *Cap:* 250, 333, 500, 750 mg; *Oral susp:* 125, 250 mg/5 ml (100, 200 ml) (strawberry)
▷ *clindamycin* (B)(G) 300 mg tid x 10 days
  Pediatric: not recommended
    Cleocin *Cap:* 75 (tartrazine), 150 (tartrazine), 300 mg
    Cleocin Pediatric Granules *Oral susp:* 75 mg/5 ml (100 ml) (cherry)
▷ *erythromycin base* (B)(G) 250-500 mg qid x 10 days
  Pediatric: <45 kg: 30-40 mg/kg/day in 4 divided doses x 10 days; ≥45 kg: same as adult
    Ery-Tab *Tab:* 250, 333, 500 mg ent-coat
    PCE *Tab:* 333, 500 mg
Comment: *erythromycin* may increase INR with concomitant *warfarin*, as well as increase serum level of *digoxin*, benzodiazepines and statins.

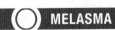

MELASMA

SKIN DEPIGMENTING AGENTS

▷ *hydroquinone* (C) apply a thin film to clean dry affected areas bid; discontinue if lightening does not occur after 2 months
Pediatric: not recommended

    Lustra *Crm:* hydro 4% (1, 2 oz) (sulfites)

    Lustra AF *Crm:* hydro 4% (1, 2 oz) (sunscreens, sulfites)

▷ *hydroquinone/fluocinolone acetonide/tretinoin* (C) apply a thin film to clean dry affected areas once daily at least 30 minutes before bedtime
Pediatric: not recommended

    Tri-Luma *Crm:* hydro 4%/fluo acet 0.01%/tret 0.05% (30 g) (sulfites, parabens)

MENIERE'S DISEASE

▷ *diazepam* (D)(IV)(G) initially 1-2.5 mg tid-qid; may increase gradually
Pediatric: <6 months: not recommended; ≥6 months: same as adult

    Diastat *Rectal gel delivery system:* 2.5 mg

    Diastat AcuDial *Rectal gel delivery system:* 10, 20 mg

    Valium *Tab:* 2*, 5*, 10*mg

    Valium Intensol Oral Solution *Conc oral soln:* 5 mg/ml (30 ml w. dropper) (alcohol 19%)

    Valium Oral Solution *Oral soln:* 5 mg/5 ml (500 ml) (wintergreen-spice)

▷ *dimenhydrinate* (B) 50 mg q 4-6 hours
Pediatric: <2 years: not recommended; 2-6 years: 12.5-25 mg q 6-8 hours; max 75 mg/day; >6-11 years: 25-50 mg q 6-8 hours; max 150 mg/day; >11 years: same as adult

    Dramamine (OTC) *Tab:* 50*mg; *Chew tab:* 50 mg (phenylalanine, tartrazine); *Liq:* 12.5 mg/5 ml (4 oz)

▷ *diphenhydramine* (B)(OTC)(G) 25-50 mg q 6-8 hours; max 100 mg/day
Pediatric: <2 years: not recommended; 2-6 years: 6.25 mg q 4-6 hours; max 37.5 mg/day; >6-12 years: 12.5-25 mg q 4-6 hours; max 150 mg/day; >12 years: same as adult

    Benadryl (OTC) *Chew tab:* 12.5 mg (grape; phenylalanine); *Liq:* 12.5 mg/5 ml (4, 8 oz); *Cap:* 25 mg; *Tab:* 25 mg; *dye-free softgel:* 25 mg; Dye-free liq: 12.5 mg/5 ml (4, 8 oz)

▷ *meclizine* (B)(G) 25-100/day in divided doses
Pediatric: not recommended

    Antivert *Tab:* 12.5, 25, 50*mg; *Amp:* 50 mg/ml (1 ml); *Vial:* 50 mg/ml (1 ml single-use); 50 mg/ml (10 ml multi-dose)

    Bonine (OTC) *Cap:* 15, 25, 30 mg; *Tab:* 12.5, 25, 50 mg; *Chew tab/Film-coat tab:* 25 mg

    Dramamine II 25 mg bid; max 50 mg/day

        Tab: 25*mg

    Zentrip *Strip:* 25 mg orally disintegrating

▷ *promethazine* (C) 12.5-25 q 4-6 hours PO or rectally
Pediatric: <2 years: not recommended; ≥2 years: 0.5 mg/lb or 6.25-25 mg q 4-6 hours PO or rectally

Phenergan *Tab:* 12.5*, 25*, 50 mg; *Plain syr:* 6.25 mg/5 ml; *Fortis syr:* 25 mg/5 ml; *Rectal supp:* 12.5, 25, 50 mg

▷ *scopolamine* transdermal patch **(C)** 1 patch behind ear; each patch is effective for 3 days; change patch every 4th day; alternate sites
Pediatric: not recommended
Transderm Scop *Patch:* 1.5 mg (4/carton)

MENINGITIS (*NEISSERIA MENINGITIDIS*)

PROPHYLAXIS

Comment: Meningitis vaccine is a 3-dose series (0, 2, 6 month schedule) indicated for persons age ≥10-25 years. Have epinephrine 1:1,000 readily available and monitor for 15 minutes post-dose of meningitis vaccine.

▷ *Meningococcal group b vaccine [recombinant, absorbed]* administer first dose IM in the deltoid; administer second dose 2 months later; administer the third dose 6 months from the first dose;
Pediatric: <10 years: not established; ≥10 years: same as adult
Bexsero *Susp for IM inj:* 0.5 ml single-dose prefilled syringes (1, 10/carton)
Trumenba *Susp for IM inj:* 0.5 ml single-dose prefilled syringes (5, 10/carton)

▷ *Neisseria meningitides oligosaccharide conjugate* quadrivalent meningonococcal vaccine **(B)** contains *Corynebacterium diphtheria* CRM197 protein; 10 mcg of Group A + 5 mcg each of Group C, Y, and W-135 + 32.7-64.1 mcg of diphtheria CRM 197 protein per 0.5 m.
Pediatric: <11 years: not recommended; ≥11-55 years: 0.5 ml IM x 1 dose in the deltoid
Menveo *Vial multi-dose:* 5 doses/vial (MenA conjugate component pwdr for reconstitution + 1 vial liquid MenCWY conjugate component for reconstitution) (preservative-free)

▷ *Neisseria meningitidis polysaccharides* vaccine **(C)** 0.5 ml SC x 1 dose; if at high risk, may revaccinate after 3-5 years; age ≥55 years contact mfr
Menactra (A/C/Y/W-135)
Pediatric: <2 years: see mfr pkg insert; ≥2 years: same as adult; if at high risk, may revaccinate children first vaccinated ≤4 years-of-age after 2-3 years
Vial (single-dose): 4 mcg each of group A, C, Y, and W-135 per 0.5 ml (pwdr for SC inj after reconstitution) (preservative-free diluent); *Vial (multi-dose):* 4 mcg each of group A, C, Y, and W-130 per 0.5 ml [pwdr for SC inj after reconstitution (5 doses/vial) (preservative-free)]
Comment: Latex allergy is a contraindication to **Menactra**.
Menomune-A/C/Y/W-135
Pediatric: <2 years: not recommended (except ≥3 months of age as short-term protection against group A); ≥2 years: same as adult; if at high risk, may revaccinate children first vaccinated ≤4 years of age after 2-3 years (older children after 3-5 years)
Vial (single-dose): 50 mcg each of group A, C, Y, and W-135 per 0.5 ml (pwdr for SC inj after reconstitution; preservative-free diluent); *Vial (multi-dose):* 50 mcg each of group A, C, Y, and W-130 per 0.5 ml [pwdr for SC inj after reconstitution (10 doses/vial) (thimerosal-preserved diluent)]
Comment: Use precaution with latex allergy.

◯ MENOPAUSE

Comment: *Estrogen* replacement lowers LDL and raises HDL. *Estrogen* replacement is indicated for osteoporosis prevention. Exogenous *estrogen* administration increases risk for endometrial cancer, MI, stroke, invasive breast cancer, pulmonary embolism, and DVT. *Estrogen* replacement is contraindicated in known or suspected pregnancy, known or suspected cancer of the breast, known or suspected *estrogen*-dependent neoplasia, undiagnosed genital bleeding, and active thrombo-phlebitis or thromboembolic disorders. Use HRT with caution in patients with cardiovascular or peripheral vascular disease.

VAGINAL RINGS

▷ *estradiol, acetate* (X)
   Femring Vaginal Ring insert high into vagina; replace every 90 days
▷ *estradiol, micronized* (X)
   Estring Vaginal Ring insert high into vagina; replace every 90 days
      Vag ring: 7.5 mcg/24 hours (1/pck)

REGIMENS FOR PATIENTS WITH INTACT UTERUS

Vaginal Preparations (With Uterus)

Comment: Vaginal preparations provide relief from vaginal and urinary symptoms only (i.e., atrophic vaginitis, dyspareunia, dysuria, and urinary frequency).
▷ *estradiol* (X)(G)
   Vagifem Tabs insert one 10 mcg or 25 mcg vaginal tablet once daily x 2 weeks; then twice weekly for 2 weeks (e.g., tues/fri); consider the addition of a progestin
      Vag tab: 10, 25 mcg (8, 18/blister pck with applicator)
   Yuvafem Vaginal Tablet 1 tab intravaginally daily x 2 weeks; then 1 tab intra-vaginally twice weekly
      Vag tab: 10 mcg (15 tabs w. applicators)
▷ *estradiol, micronized* (X) **Estrace Vaginal Cream** 2-4 g daily x 1-2 weeks, then grad-ually reduced to 1/2 initial dose x 1-2 weeks, then maintenance dose of 1 g 1-3 times/week
      Vag crm: 0.01% (12, 42.5 g w. calib applicator)
▷ *estrogen, conjugated equine* (X)
   Premarin Vaginal Cream 0.5-2 g/day intravaginally; cyclically (3 weeks on, 1 week off)
      Vag crm: 1.5 oz w. applicator marked in 1/2 g increments to max of 2 g

Transdermal Systems (With Uterus)

Comment: Alternate sites. Do not apply patches on or near breasts.
▷ *estradiol* (X)
   Climara initially 0.025 mg/day patch once/week to trunk (3 weeks on and 1 week off)
      Transdermal patch: 0.025, 0.0375, 0.05, 0.075, 0.1 mg/day (4/pck)
   Esclim apply twice weekly x 3 weeks, then 1 week off; use with an oral progestin to prevent endometrial hyperplasia
      Transdermal patch: 0.025, 0.0375, 0.05, 0.075, 0.1 mg/day (8, 48/pck)

Vivelle initially one 0.0375 mg/day patch twice weekly to trunk area; use with an oral progestin to prevent endometrial hyperplasia
Transdermal patch: 0.025, 0.0375, 0.05, 0.075, 0.1 mg/day (8, 48/pck)

Vivelle-Dot initially one 0.05 mg/day patch twice weekly to lower abdomen, below the waist; use with an oral progestin to prevent endometrial hyperplasia
Transdermal patch: 0.025, 0.0375, 0.05, 0.075, 0.1 mg/day (8, 24/pck)

▷ *estradiol/levonorgestrel* (X) apply 1 patch weekly to lower abdomen; avoid waistline; alternate sites
Climara Pro *Transdermal patch: estra* 0.045 mg/*levo* 0.015 mg per day (4/pck)

▷ *estradiol/norethindrone* (X)
CombiPatch apply twice weekly <u>or</u> q 3-4 days
Transdermal patch: 9 cm^2: *estra* 0.05 mg/*noreth* 0.14 mg; 16 cm^2: *estra* 0.05 mg/*noreth* 0.25 mg

Comment: May cause irregular bleeding in first 6 months of therapy, but usually decreases over time (often to amenorrhea).

ORAL AGENTS (WITH UTERUS)

▷ *estradiol* (X)(G)
Estrace 1-2 mg daily cyclically (3 weeks on and 1 week off)
Tab: 0.5, 1, 2*mg (tartrazine)

▷ *estradiol/drospirenone* (X)
Angeliq 1 tab daily
Tab: **Angeliq 0.5/0.25:** *estra* 0.5 mg/*dros* 0.25 mg
Angeliq 1/0.5: *estra* 1 mg/*dros* 0.5 mg

▷ *estradiol/norethindrone* (X) 1 tab daily
Activella (G) *Tab: estra* 1 mg/*noreth* 0.5 mg
FemHRT (G) **1/5** *Tab: estra* 5 mcg/*noreth* 1 mg
Fyavolv (G) *Tab: estra* 0.25 mg/*noreth* 1 mg; *Tab: estra* 0.5 mg/*noreth* 1 mg
Mimvey LO *Tab: estra* 0.5 mg/*noreth* 0.1 mg

▷ *estradiol/norgestimate* (X) 1 x *estradiol* 1 mg tab once daily x 3 days, then 1 x *estradiol* 1 mg/*norgestimate* 0.09 mg tab daily x 3 days; repeat this pattern continuously
Ortho-Prefest *Tab: estra* 1 mg/*norgest* 0.09 mg (30/blister pck)

▷ *estrogen, conjugated/medroxyprogesterone* (X)
Prempro 1 tab daily
Tab: **Prempro 0.3/1.5:** *conj estra* 0.3 mg/*medroxy* 1.5 mg
Prempro 0.45/1.5: *conj estra* 0.45 mg/*medroxy* 1.5 mg
Prempro 0.625/2.5: *conj estra* 0.625 mg/*medroxy* 2.5 mg
Prempro 0.625/5: *conj estra* 0.625 mg/*medroxy* 5 mg
Premphase 0.625 *estrogen* on days 1-14, then 0.625 mg *estrogen*/5 mg *medroxyprogesterone* on days 15-28
Tab (in dial dispenser): conj estra 0.625 mg (14 maroon tabs) + *medroxy* 5 mg (14 blue tabs)

▷ *estrogen, esterified (plant derived)* (X)
Menest 0.3-2.5 mg daily cyclically, 3 weeks on and 1 week off (with progestins in the latter part of the cycle to prevent endometrial hyperplasia)
Tab: 0.3, 0.625, 1.25, 2.5 mg

▷ *estrogen, esterified/methyltestosterone* (X)
Estratest 1 tab daily cyclically, 3 weeks on and 1 week off
Tab: ester estra 1.25 mg/*meth* 2.5 mg

Estratest HS 1-2 tabs daily cyclically, 3 weeks on and 1 week off
Tab: ester estra 0.625 mg/*meth* 1.25 mg
▷ *ethinyl estradiol* (X) 0.02-0.05 mg q 1-2 days cyclically, 3 weeks on and 1 week off
(with progestins in the latter part of the cycle to prevent endometrial hyperplasia)
Estinyl *Tab:* 0.02 (tartrazine), 0.05 mg
▷ *estropipate, piperazine estrone sulfate* (X)(G)
Ogen 0.625-1.25 mg daily cyclically (3 weeks on and 1 week off)
Tab: 0.625, 1.25, 2.5 mg
Ortho-Est 0.75-6 mg daily cyclically (3 weeks on and 1 week off)
Tab: 0.625, 1.25 mg
▷ *medroxyprogesterone* (X) 5-10 mg daily for 12 sequential days of each 28-day cycle
to prevent endometrial hyperplasia in the postmenopausal women with an intact
uterus receiving conjugated estrogens
Provera *Tab:* 2.5, 5, 10 mg
▷ *norethindrone acetate* (X) 2.5-10 mg daily x 5-10 days during second half of menstrual cycle
Aygestin *Tab:* 5*mg
▷ *progesterone, micronized* (X)(G)
Prometrium 200 mg daily in the PM for 12 sequential days of each 28-day cycle
to prevent endometrial hyperplasia in the postmenopausal woman with an
intact uterus receiving conjugated estrogens
Cap: 100, 200 mg (peanut oil)

ESTROGENS, CONJUGATED/ESTROGEN AGONIST-ANTAGONIST

▷ *estrogen, conjugated/bazedoxifene* (X)
Duavee 1 tab daily
Tab: conj estra 0.45 mg/*baze* 20 mg

REGIMENS FOR PATIENTS WITHOUT UTERUS

Oral Agents (Without Uterus)

▷ *estradiol* (X)(G)
Estrace 1-2 mg daily
Tab: 0.5*, 1*, 2*mg (tartrazine)
▷ *estrogen, conjugated (equine)* (X)
Premarin 1 tab daily
Tab: 0.3, 0.45, 0.625, 0.9, 1.25, 2.5 mg
▷ *estrogen, conjugated (synthetic)* (X) 1 tab daily; may titrate up to max 1.25 mg/day
Cenestin *Tab:* 0.3, 0.625, 0.9, 1.25 mg
Enjuvia *Tab:* 0.3, 0.45, 0.625 mg
▷ *estrogen, esterified (plant derived)* (X) 1 tab daily
Estratab *Tab:* 0.3, 0.625, 2.5 mg
Menest *Tab:* 0.3, 0.625, 1.25, 2.5 mg
▷ *ethinyl estradiol* (X) 0.02-0.05 mg q 1-2 days
Estinyl *Tab:* 0.02 (tartrazine), 0.05 mg

Vaginal Preparations (Without Uterus)

Comment: Vaginal preparations provide relief from vaginal and urinary symptoms
only (i.e., atrophic vaginitis, dyspareunia, dysuria, and urinary frequency).

▷ *estradiol* (X)(G)

Vagifem Tabs insert one 10 mcg or 25 mcg vaginal tablet once daily x 2 weeks; then twice weekly for 2 weeks (e.g., tues/fri); consider the addition of a progestin

Vag tab: 10, 25 mcg (8, 18/blister pck with applicator)

Yuvafem Vaginal Tablet 1 tab intravaginally daily x 2 weeks; then 1 tab intravaginally twice weekly

Vag tab: 10 mcg (15 tabs w. applicators)

Topical Agents (Without Uterus)

▷ *estradiol* (X)

Estrasorb apply 3.48 g (2 pouches) every morning; apply one pouch to each leg from the upper thigh to the calf; rub in for 3 minutes; rub excess on hands onto buttocks

Emul: 0.025 mg/day/pouch (2.5 mg/g; 1.74 g/pouch)

EstroGel apply 1.25 g (one compression) to one arm from wrist to shoulder once daily at the same time each day

Gel: 0.06% per compression (93 g)

Transdermal Systems (Without Uterus)

Comment: Do not apply patches on or near breasts. Alternate sites.

▷ *estradiol* (X)

Alora initially 0.05 mg/day apply patch twice weekly to lower abdomen, upper quadrant of buttocks or outer aspect of hip

Transdermal patch: 0.025, 0.05, 0.075, 0.1 mg/day (8, 24/pck)

Climara initially 0.025 mg/day patch once/week to trunk

Transdermal patch: 0.025, 0.0375, 0.05, 0.075, 0.1 mg/day (4, 8, 24/pck)

Esclim initially 0.025 mg/day apply patch twice weekly to buttocks, femoral triangle, or upper arm

Transdermal patch: 0.025, 0.0375, 0.05, 0.075, 0.1 mg/day (8/pck)

Estraderm initially apply one 0.05 mg/day patch twice weekly to trunk

Transdermal patch: 0.05, 0.1 mg/day (8, 24/pck)

Menostar apply one patch weekly to lower abdomen, below the waist; avoid the breasts; alternate sites

Transdermal patch: 14 mcg/day (4/pck)

Minivelle initially one 0.0375 mg/day patch twice weekly to trunk area; adjust after one month of therapy

Transdermal patch: 0.025, 0.0375, 0.05, 0.075, 0.1 mg/day (8/pck)

Vivelle initially one 0.0375 mg/day patch twice weekly to trunk area; adjust after one month of therapy

Transdermal patch: 0.025, 0.0375, 0.05, 0.075, 0.1 mg/day (8, 48/pck)

Vivelle-Dot initially apply one 0.05 mg/day patch twice weekly to lower abdomen, below the waist; adjust after one month of therapy

Transdermal patch: 0.025, 0.0375, 0.05, 0.075, 0.1 mg/day (8, 24/pck)

Comment: The *estrogens* in **Alora**, **Climara**, **Estraderm**, and **Vivelle-Dot** are plant derived.

MENOMETORRHAGIA: IRREGULAR HEAVY MENSTRUAL BLEEDING/MENORRHAGIA: HEAVY CYCLICAL MENSTRUAL BLEEDING

ANTIFIBROLYTIC AGENT

▷ *tranexamic acid* (B)(G) 1,300 mg tid; treat for up to 5 days during menses; *Normal renal function (SCr ≤1.4 mg/dL):* 1,300 mg tid; *SCr ≥1.4-2.8 mg/dL:* 1,300 mg bid; *SCr ≥2.8-5.7 mg/dL:* 1,300 mg once daily; *SCr ≥5.7 mg/dL:* 650 mg once daily
Pediatric: <18 years: not recommended
   Lysteda *Tab:* 650 mg

Injectible Progesterone Only Contraceptives

▷ *medroxyprogesterone* (X)(G)
   Depo-Provera 150 mg deep IM q 3 months
   Vial: 150 mg/ml (1 ml)
      Prefilled syringe: 150 mg/ml
   Depo-SubQ 104 mg SC q 3 months
      Prefilled syringe: 104 mg/ml (0.65 ml; parabens)
Comment: Administer first dose within 5 days of onset of normal menses, within 5 days postpartum if not breastfeeding, or at 6 weeks postpartum if breastfeeding exclusively. Do not use for >2 years unless other methods are inadequate.
Combined Oral Contraceptives *see page* 585
Intrauterine Devices *see page* 497

 MITRAL VALVE PROLAPSE (MVP)

▷ *propranolol* (C)(G)
   Inderal 10-30 mg tid-qid
   Tab: 10*, 20*, 40*, 60*, 80*mg
   Inderal LA initially 80 mg daily in a single dose; increase q 3-7 days; usual range 120-160 mg/day; max 320 mg/day in a single dose
   Cap: 60, 80, 120, 160 mg sust-rel
   InnoPran XL initially 80 mg q HS; max 120 mg/day
   Cap: 80, 120 mg ext-rel

MONONUCLEOSIS (MONO)

ANALGESICS

▷ *acetaminophen* (B) *see Fever page* 143
   Acetaminophen for IV Infusion *see page* 501
   Other Oral Analgesics *see Pain page* 308
   Parenteral Corticosteroids *see page* 511
   Oral Corticosteroids *see page* 509
▷ *prednisone* (C) initially 40-80 mg/day, then taper off over 5-7 days
Comment: Corticosteroids recommended in patients with significant pharyngeal edema.

MOTION SICKNESS

▶ *dimenhydrinate* (B)(OTC) 50-100 mg q 4-6 hours; start 1 hour before travel; max 400 mg/day
Pediatric: <2 years: not recommended; 2-6 years: 12.5-25 mg; max 75 mg/day; start 1 hour before travel; may repeat q 6-8 hours; 6-11 years: 25-50 mg; max 150 mg/day; start 1 hour before travel; may repeat q 6-8 hours; ≥12 years: same as adult
    Dramamine
    Tab: 50*mg; *Chew tab:* 50 mg (phenylalanine, tartrazine); *Liq:* 12.5 mg/5 ml (4 oz)

▶ *meclizine* (B)(G) 25-50 mg 1 hour before travel; may repeat q 24 hours as needed; max 50 mg/day
Pediatric: not recommended
    Antivert *Tab:* 12.5, 25, 50*mg
    Bonine (OTC) *Cap:* 15, 25, 50 mg; *Tab:* 12.5, 25, 50 mg;
    Chew tab/Film-coat tab: 25 mg
    Dramamine II (OTC) *Tab:* 25 mg
    Zentrip *Strip:* 25 mg orally-disint

▶ *prochlorperazine* (C)(G)
    Compazine 5-10 mg q 4 hours as needed
        Pediatric: not recommended
        Tab: 5 mg; *Syr:* 5 mg/5 ml (4 oz; fruit); *Rectal supp:* 2.5, 5, 25 mg
    Compazine Spansule 15 mg q AM or 10 mg q 12 hours
        Spansules: 10, 15 mg sust-rel

▶ *promethazine* (C)(G) 25 mg 30-60 minutes before travel; may repeat in 8-12 hours
Pediatric: <2 years: not recommended; ≥2 years: 12.5-25 mg 30-60 minutes before travel; may repeat in 8-12 hours
    Phenergan *Tab:* 12.5*, 25*, 50 mg; *Plain syr:* 6.25 mg/5 ml; *Fortis syr:* 25 mg/5 ml; *Rectal supp:* 12.5, 25, 50 mg

▶ *scopolamine* (C)
    Scopace 0.4-0.8 mg 1 hour before travel; may repeat in 8 hours
        Pediatric: not recommended
        Tab: 0.4 mg
    Transderm Scop 1 patch behind ear at least 4 hours before travel; each patch is effective for 3 days
        Pediatric: not recommended
        Transdermal patch: 1.5 mg (4/carton)

MULTIPLE SCLEROSIS (MS)

NICOTINIC ACID RECEPTOR AGONIST

▶ *dimethyl fumarate* (C) initially 120 mg bid x 7 days; then maintenance 240 mg bid
Pediatric: <18 years: not recommended
    Tecfidera *Cap:* 120, 240 mg del-rel; *Starter Pack:* 14 x 120 mg, 46 x 240 mg
Comment: The mechanism by which *dimethyl fumarate* (DMF) exerts its therapeutic effect in multiple sclerosis is unknown. DMF and the metabolite, *mono-methyl fumarate* (MMF), have been shown to activate the nuclear factor (erythroid-derived 2)-like 2 (Nrf2) pathway in vitro and in vivo in animals and humans. The Nrf2 pathway is involved in the cellular response to oxidative stress. MMF has been identified as a nicotinic acid receptor agonist in vitro.

POTASSIUM CHANNEL BLOCKER

▷ *dalfampridine* (C) 10 mg q 12 hours
  Pediatric: <18 years: not recommended
      Ampyra *Tab:* 10 mg ext-rel
  Comment: *dalfampridine* is indicated to improve walking speed.

PYRIMIDINE SYNTHESIS INHIBITOR (DMARD)

▷ *teriflunomide* (X) 7 mg or 14 mg once daily
  Pediatric: not recommended
      Aubagio *Tab:* 7, 14 mg
  Comment: Contraindicated with severe hepatic impairment and women
  of childbearing potential not using reliable contraception. Co-administer
  teriflunomide with the DMARD *leflunomide* (**Arava**).

IMMUNOMODULATORS

Comment: The role of immunomodulators in the treatment of MS is to slow the
progression of physical disability and to decrease frequency of clinical exacerbations.

▷ *alemtuzumab* (C) administer two treatment courses:
  First treatment course: 12 mg/day x 5 days (total 60 mg); *Second treatment course:* 12
  months later, administer 12 mg/day x 3 days (total 36 mg); complete all immunizations 6 weeks prior to the first treatment; premedicate with 1000 mg methylprednisolone or equivalent immediately prior to the first 3 treatment days in each
  treatment course
  Pediatric: <18 years: not recommended
      Lemtrada *Vial:* 12 mg/1.2 ml soln for IV infusion, single-use vial
      Comment: **Lemtrada** is indicated for the treatment of patients with relapsing
      forms of MS. Because of its safety profile, the use of **Lemtrada** should generally
      be reserved for patients who have had an inadequate response to two or more
      drugs indicated for the treatment of MS. **Lemtrada REMS** is a restricted
      distribution program, which allows early detection and management of some of
      the serious risks associated with its use.
▷ *fingolimod* (C) 0.5 mg once daily
  Pediatric: <18 years: not recommended
      Gilenya *Cap:* 0.5 mg
  Comment: First-dose monitoring for bradycardia. In the first 2 weeks, first-dose
  monitoring is recommended after an interruption of 1 day or more. During weeks
  3 and 4, first-dose monitoring is recommended after an interruption of more than
  7 days.
▷ *glatiramer acetate* (B)(G) 20-40 mg SC daily
  Pediatric: <18 years: not recommended
      Copaxone *Prefilled syringe:* 20, 40 mg/ml (mannitol, preservative-free)
▷ *interferon beta-1a* (C)
  Pediatric: <18 years: not recommended
      Avonex 30 mcg IM weekly; rotate sites; may titrate to reduce flu-like symp-
      toms; may use concurrent analgesics/antipyretics on treatment days; *Titration
      Schedule:* 7.5 mcg week 1; 15 mcg week 2; 22.5 mcg week 3; 30 mcg week 4 and
      ongoing

Vial: 30 mcg/vial pwdr for reconstitution (single-dose w. diluent, 4 vials/kit) (albumin [human], preservative-free); *Prefilled syringe:* 30 mcg single-dose (0.5 ml) (4/dose pck)

Rebif, administer SC 3x/week (at least 48 hours apart and preferably in the late afternoon <u>or</u> evening); increase over 4 weeks to usual dose 22-44 mcg 3x/week; *Titration Schedule (22 mcg prescribed dose):* 4.4 mcg week 1 & 2; 11 mcg week 3 & 4; 22 mcg week 5 and ongoing; *Titration Schedule (44 mcg prescribed dose):* 8.8 mcg week 1 & 2; 22 mcg week 3 & 4; 44 mcg week 5 and ongoing

Prefilled syringe: 22, 44 mcg/0.5 ml w. needle (12/carton) (albumin [human], preservative-free); (titration pack, 6 doses of 8.8 mcg [0.2 ml] w. needle per carton) (albumin [human], preservative-free)

Comment: Only prefilled syringes (**Rebif**) can be used to titrate to the 22 mcg prescribed dose. Prefilled syringes <u>or</u> autoinjectors (**Rebif Rebidose**) can be used to titrate to the 44 mcg prescribed dose.

Rebif Rebidose administer SC 3x/week (at least 48 hours apart and preferably in the late afternoon <u>or</u> evening) after titration to 22 mcg <u>or</u> 44 mcg

Titration Schedule: *see* **Rebif.**

Prefilled autoinjector: 22, 44 mcg/0.5 ml (0.5ml, 12/carton) (titration pack, 6 doses of 8.8 mcg [0.2 ml] per carton (albumin [human], preservative-free)

Comment: Only prefilled syringes (**Rebif**) can be used to titrate to the 22 mcg prescribed dose. Prefilled syringes <u>or</u> autoinjectors (**Rebif Rebidose**) can be used to titrate to the 44 mcg prescribed dose.

▷ *interferon beta-1b* (C)

Pediatric: <18 years: not recommended

Actimmune *BSA ≤0.5m²:* 1.5 mgc/kg SC in a single dose 3 times weekly; *BSA ≥0.5/m²:* 50 mgc/m² SC in a single dose 3 times weekly *Vial:* 100 mcg/0.5 ml single-dose for SC injection

Betaseron, Extavia 0.0625 mg (0.25 ml) SC every other day; increase over 6 weeks to 0.25 mg (1 ml) SC every other day

Vial: 0.3 mg/vial pwdr for reconstitution (single-dose w. prefilled diluents syringes) (albumin [human], mannitol, preservative-free)

▷ *natalizumab* (C) administer 300 mg by IV infusion over 1 hour every 4 weeks; monitor during infusion and for 1 hour postinfusion

Pediatric: <18 years: not recommended

Tysabri *Vial:* 300 mg/15 ml (15 ml)

⭕ MUMPS (INFECTIOUS PAROTITIS)

PROPHYLAXIS

▷ *measles, mumps, rubella, live, attenuated, neomycin vaccine* (C)

MMR II 25 mcg SC (preservative-free)

Comment: Contraindications: hypersensitivity to *neomycin* <u>or</u> eggs, primary <u>or</u> acquired immune deficiency, immunosuppressant therapy, bone marrow <u>or</u> lymphatic malignancy, and pregnancy (within 3 months after vaccination).

see **Childhood Immunizations** *page* 574

Parenteral Corticosteroids *see page* 511

Oral Corticosteroids *see page* 509

Antipyretics *see* **Fever** *page* 143

MUSCLE STRAIN

Comment: Usual length of treatment for acute injury is approximately 5 days.
Acetaminophen for IV Infusion *see Pain page* 306
Narcotic Analgesics *see Pain page* 308
Parenteral Corticosteroids *see page* 511
Oral Corticosteroids *see page* 509

SKELETAL MUSCLE RELAXANTS

▷ *baclofen* (C)(G) 5 mg tid; titrate up by 5 mg every 3 days to 20 mg tid; max 80 mg/day
   Pediatric: not recommended
       Lioresal *Tab:* 10*, 20*mg
   Comment: *baclofen* is indicated for muscle spasm pain and chronic spasticity associated with multiple sclerosis and spinal cord injury or disease. Potential for seizures or hallucinations on abrupt withdrawal.
▷ *carisoprodol* (C)(G) 1 tab tid or qid
   Pediatric: not recommended
       Soma *Tab:* 350 mg
▷ *chlorzoxazone* (NE)(G) 1 caplet qid; max 750 mg qid
   Pediatric: not recommended
       Parafon Forte DSC *Cplt:* 500*mg
▷ *cyclobenzaprine* (B)(G) 10 mg tid; usual range 20-40 mg/day in divided doses; max 60 mg/day x 2-3 weeks or 15 mg ext-rel once daily; max 30 mg ext-rel/day x 2-3 weeks
   Pediatric: <15 years: not recommended
       Amrix *Cap:* 15, 30 mg ext-rel
       Fexmid *Tab:* 7.5 mg
       Flexeril *Tab:* 5, 10 mg
▷ *dantrolene* (C) 25md daily x 7 days; then 25 mg tid x 7 days; then 50 mg tid x 7 days; max 100 mg qid
   Pediatric: 0.5 mg/kg daily x 7 days; then 0.5 mg/kg tid x 7 days; then 1 mg/kg tid x 7 days; then 2 mg/kg tid; max 100 mg qid
       Dantrium *Tab:* 25, 50, 100 mg
   Comment: *dantrolene* is indicated for chronic spasticity associated with multiple sclerosis and spinal cord injury or disease.
▷ *diazepam* (C)(IV) 2-10 mg bid-qid; may increase gradually
   Pediatric: <6 months: not recommended; >6 months: initially 1-2.5 mg bid-qid; may increase gradually
       Diastat *Rectal gel delivery system:* 2.5 mg
       Diastat AcuDial *Rectal gel delivery system:* 10, 20 mg
       Valium *Tab:* 2, 5, 10 mg
       Valium Intensol Oral Solution *Conc oral soln:* 5 mg/ml (30 ml w. dropper) (alcohol 19%)
       Valium Oral Solution *Oral soln:* 5 mg/5 ml (500 ml) (wintergreen spice)
▷ *metaxalone* (B) 1 tab tid-qid
   Pediatric: not recommended
       Skelaxin *Tab:* 800*mg

➤ *methocarbamol* (C)(G) initially 1.5 g qid x 2-3 days; maintenance, 750 mg every 4 hours <u>or</u> 1.5 g 3 times daily; max 8 g/day
  Pediatric: <16 years: not recommended
      Robaxin *Tab:* 500 mg
      Robaxin 750 *Tab:* 750 mg
      Robaxin Injection 10 ml IM <u>or</u> IV; max 30 ml/day; max 3 days; max 5 ml/ gluteal injection q 8 hours; max IV rate 3 ml/min
        Vial: 100 mg/ml (10 ml)
➤ *nabumetone* (C)
  Pediatric: not recommended
      Relafen *Tab:* 500, 750 mg
      Relafen 500 *Tab:* 500 mg
➤ *orphenadrine citrate* (C)(G) 1 tab bid
  Pediatric: not recommended
      Norflex *Tab:* 100 mg sust-rel
➤ *tizanidine* (C) 1-4 mg q 6-8 hours; max 36 mg/day
  Pediatric: not recommended
      Zanaflex *Tab:* 2*, 4**mg; *Cap:* 2, 4, 6 mg

SKELETAL MUSCLE RELAXANT/NSAID COMBINATIONS

Comment: *aspirin*-containing medications are contraindicated with history of allergic-type reaction to *aspirin*, children and adolescents with *Varicella* <u>or</u> other viral illness, and 3rd trimester pregnancy.
➤ *carisoprodol/aspirin* (C)(III)(G) 1-2 tabs qid
  Pediatric: not recommended
      Soma Compound *Tab: caris* 200 mg/*asa* 325 mg (sulfites)
➤ *meprobamate/aspirin* (D)(IV) 1-2 tabs tid <u>or</u> qid
  Pediatric: not recommended
      Equagesic *Tab: mepro* 200 mg/*asa* 325*mg

SKELETAL MUSCLE RELAXANT/NSAID/CAFFEINE COMBINATIONS

➤ *orphenadrine/aspirin/caffeine* (D)(G)
  Pediatric: not recommended
      Norgesic 1-2 tabs tid-qid
        Tab: orphen 25 mg/*asa* 385 mg/*caf* 30 mg
      Norgesic Forte 1 tab tid <u>or</u> qid; max 4 tabs/day
        Tab: orphen 50 mg/*asa* 770 mg/*caf* 60*mg

SKELETAL MUSCLE RELAXANT/NSAID/CODEINE COMBINATIONS

➤ *carisoprodol/aspirin/codeine* (D)(III)(G)
  Pediatric: not recommended
      Soma Compound w. Codeine 1-2 tabs qid
        Tab: caris 200 mg/*asa* 325 mg/*cod* 16 mg (sulfites)

TOPICAL/TRANSDERMAL NSAIDs

➤ *capsaicin* (B)(G) apply tid-qid prn to intact skin
  Pediatric: <2 years: not recommended; ≥2 years: apply sparingly tid-qid prn
      Axsain *Crm:* 0.075% (1, 2 oz)
      Capsin *Lotn:* 0.025, 0.075% (59 ml)

Capzasin-P (OTC) *Crm:* 0.025% (1.5 oz); *Lotn:* 0.025% (2 oz)
Dolorac *Crm:* 0.025% (28 g)
Double Cap (OTC) *Crm:* 0.05% (2 oz)
R-Gel *Gel:* 0.025% (15, 30 g)
Zostrix (OTC) *Crm:* 0.025% (0.7, 1.5, 3 oz)
Zostrix HP (OTC) *Emol crm:* 0.075% (1, 2 oz)

▷ *capsaicin* 8% patch **(B)** apply up to 4 patches for one 60-minute application to clean dry skin; may prep area with topical anesthetic; wear nonlatex gloves; patches may be cut to size/shape; treatment may be repeated every 3 months; remove with cleansing gel after treatment
Pediatric: <18 years: not recommended
    Qutenza *Patch:* 8% 1640 mcg/cm (179 mg; 1 or 2 patches, each w. 1-50 g tube cleansing gel/carton)

▷ *diclofenac epolamine transdermal patch* **(C; D ≥30 wks)** apply one patch to affected area bid; remove during bathing; avoid non-intact skin
Pediatric: not recommended
    Flector Patch *Patch:* 180 mg/patch (30/carton)

ORAL NSAIDs

▷ *diclofenac* **(C)**
Pediatric: <18 years: not recommended
    Zorvolex take on empty stomach; 35 mg tid; *Hepatic impairment:* use lowest dose
        Gelcap: 18, 35 mg

▷ *diclofenac sodium* **(C)**
Pediatric: <18 years: not recommended
    Voltaren 50 mg bid-qid or 75 mg bid or 25 mg qid with an additional 25 mg at HS if necessary
        Tab: 25, 50, 75 mg ent-coat
    Voltaren XR 100 mg once daily; rarely, 100 mg bid may be used
        Tab: 100 mg ext-rel

For an expanded list of Oral Prescription NSAIDs *see page* 501

ORAL NSAIDS/PPI COMBINATIONS

▷ *esomeprazole/naproxen* **(C)(G)** 1 tab bid; use lowest effective dose for the shortest duration swallow whole; take at least 30 minutes before a meal
Pediatric: <18 years: not recommended
    Vimovo *Tab: nap* 375 mg/*eso* 20 mg ext-rel; *nap* 500 mg/*eso* 20 mg ext-rel
    Comment: Vimovo is indicated to improve signs/symptoms, and risk of gastric ulcer in patients at risk of developing NSAID-associated gastric ulcer.

COX-2 INHIBITORS

Comment: Cox-2 inhibitors are contraindicated with history of asthma, urticaria, and allergic-type reactions to *aspirin*, other NSAIDs, and sulfonamides, 3rd trimester of pregnancy, and coronary artery bypass graft (CABG) surgery.

▷ *celecoxib* **(C)(G)** 100-400 mg daily bid; max 800 mg/day
Pediatric: <18 years: not recommended
    Celebrex *Cap:* 50, 100, 200, 400 mg

▷ *meloxicam* **(C)(G)** initially 7.5 mg once daily; max 15 mg once daily
Pediatric: <2 years: not recommended; ≥2 years: 0.125 mg/kg; max 7.5 mg once daily

Mobic *Tab:* 7.5, 15 mg; *Oral susp:* 7.5 mg/5 ml (100 ml) (raspberry)
Vivlodex *Cap:* 5, 10 mg

TOPICAL/TRANSDERMAL NSAIDs

▷ *capsaicin* (B)(G) apply tid-qid prn to intact skin
   Pediatric: <2 years: not recommended; ≥2 years: apply sparingly tid-qid prn
      Axsain *Crm:* 0.075% (1, 2 oz)
      Capsin *Lotn:* 0.025, 0.075% (59 ml)
      Capzasin-P (OTC) *Crm:* 0.025% (1.5 oz); *Lotn:* 0.025% (2 oz)
      Dolorac *Crm:* 0.025% (28 g)
      Double Cap (OTC) *Crm:* 0.05% (2 oz)
      R-Gel *Gel:* 0.025% (15, 30 g)
      Zostrix (OTC) *Crm:* 0.025% (0.7, 1.5, 3 oz)
      Zostrix HP (OTC) *Emol crm:* 0.075% (1, 2 oz)
▷ *capsaicin* 8% patch (B) apply up to 4 patches for one 60-minute application to clean
   dry skin; may prep area with topical anesthetic; wear nonlatex gloves; patches may be
   cut to size/shape; treatment may be repeated every 3 months; remove with cleansing
   gel after treatment
   Pediatric: <18 years: not recommended
      Qutenza *Patch:* 8% 1640 mcg/cm (179 mg; 1 or 2 patches, each w. 1-50 g tube
      cleansing gel/carton)
▷ *diclofenac epolamine transdermal patch* (C; D ≥30 wks) apply one patch to affected
   area bid; remove during bathing; avoid nonintact skin
   Pediatric: not recommended
      Flector Patch *Patch:* 180 mg/patch (30/carton)
▷ *diclofenac sodium* (C; D ≥30 wks)(G) apply gel qid prn; avoid non-intact skin
   Pediatric: not recommended
      Voltaren Gel *Gel:* 1% (100 g)

TOPICAL/TRANSDERMAL LIDOCAINE

▷ *lidocaine* transdermal patch (C)(G) apply one patch to affected area for 12 hours
   (then off for 12 hours); remove during bathing; avoid non-intact skin
   Pediatric: not recommended
      Lidoderm *Patch:* 5% (10 cm x14 cm; 30/carton)

 NARCOLEPSY

STIMULANTS

▷ *amphetamine sulfate* (C)(II) administer first dose on awakening, and additional doses at 4- to 6-hour intervals; usual range 5-60 mg/day
   Pediatric: <6 years: not recommended; 6-12 years: 5 mg daily in the AM; may increase by 5 mg/day at weekly intervals; >12-18 years: initially 10 mg in the AM; may
   increase by 10 mg daily at weekly intervals
      Evekeo initially 10 mg once or twice daily at the same time(s) each day; may
      increase by 10 mg/day at weekly intervals; max 40 mg/day
      Pediatric: <6 years: not recommended; 6-12 years: initially 5 mg once or
      twice daily at the same time(s) each day; may increase by 5 mg/day at weekly
      intervals; max 40 mg/day; >12 years: same as adult
      Tab: 5, 10 mg

▷ *armodafinil* (C)(IV)(G) *OSAHS:* 50-250 mg once daily in the AM; *SWSD:* 150 mg 1 hour before starting shift; reduce dose with severe hepatic impairment
Pediatric: <17 years: not recommended
    Nuvigil *Tab:* 50, 150, 200, 250 mg
▷ *modafinil* (C)(IV)(G) 100-200 mg q AM; max 400 mg/day
Pediatric: <17 years: not recommended
    Provigil *Tab:* 100, 200*mg
    Comment: **Provigil** also promotes wakefulness in patients with shift work sleep disorder and excessive sleepiness due to obstructive sleep apnea/hypopnea syndrome.
▷ *sodium oxybate* (B) take dose at bedtime while in bed and repeat 2.5-4 hours later; titrate to effect; initially 4.5 grams/night in 2 divided doses; may increase by 1.5 g/night in 2 divided doses; max 9 g/night
Pediatric: <16 years: not recommended; ≥16 years: same as adult
    Xyrem *Oral soln:* 100, 200*mg
    Comment: **Xyrem** is used to reduce the number of cataplexy attacks (sudden loss of muscle strength) and reduce daytime sleepiness in patients with narcolepsy. Contraindicated with *alcohol* or CNS depressant (may impair consciousness; may lead to respiratory depression, coma, or death). Prepare both doses prior to bedtime and do not attempt to get out of bed after taking the first dose. Place both doses within reach at the bedside. Set the bedside clock to awaken for the second dose. Dilute each dose in 60 ml (1/4 cup, 4 tblsp) water in child resistant dosing containers. Food significantly reduces the bioavailability of *sodium oxybate*; take at least 2 hours after ingesting food.

STIMULANTS

▷ *dextroamphetamine sulfate* (C)(II)(G) initially start with 10 mg daily; increase by 10 mg at weekly intervals if needed; may switch to daily dose with sust-rel spansules when titrated
Pediatric: <3 years: not recommended; 3-5 years: 2.5 mg daily; may increase by 2.5 mg daily at weekly intervals if needed; 6-12 years: initially 5 mg daily-bid; may increase by 5 mg/day at weekly intervals; usual max 40 mg/day; >12 years: initially 10 mg daily; may increase by mg/day at weekly intervals; max 40 mg/day 10
    Dexedrine *Tab:* 5*mg (tartrazine)
    Dexedrine Spansule *Cap:* 5, 10, 15 mg sust-rel
    Dextrostat *Tab:* 5, 10 mg (tartrazine)
▷ *dextroamphetamine saccharate/dextroamphetamine sulfate/amphetamine aspartate/amphetamine sulfate* (C)(II)(G)
    Adderall initially 10 mg daily; may increase weekly by 10 mg/day; usual max 60 mg/day in 2-3 divided doses; first dose on awakening and then q 4-6 hours prn
        Pediatric: <6 years: not indicated; 6-12 years: initially 5 mg daily; may increase weekly by 5 mg/day; usual max 40 mg/day in 2-3 divided doses; >12 years: same as adult
        Tab: 5**, 7.5**, 10**, 12.5**, 15**, 20**, 30**mg
    Adderall XR
        Pediatric: <6 years: not recommended; 6-12 years: initially 10 mg daily in the AM; may increase by 10 mg weekly; max 30 mg/day; 13-17 years: initially 10 mg daily; may increase to 20 mg/day after 1 week; max 30 mg/day; Do not chew; may sprinkle on apple sauce

Cap: 5, 10, 15, 20, 25, 30 mg ext-rel

Comment: **Adderall** is also indicated to improve wakefulness in patients with shift-work sleep disorder and excessive sleepiness due to obstructive sleep apnea/hypopnea syndrome.

▷ *dexmethylphenidate* (C)(II)(G) take once daily in the AM

Pediatric: <6 years: not recommended; ≥6 years: same as adult

Focalin initially 2.5 mg bid; allow at least 4 hours between doses; may increase at 1 week intervals; max 40 mg/day

Tab: 2.5, 5, 10*mg (dye-free)

Focalin XR 20-40 mg q AM; max 40 mg/day

Tab: 5, 10, 15, 20, 30, 40 mg ext-rel (dye-free)

▷ *methamphetamine* (C)(II)(G)

Desoxyn Granumets

Pediatric: <6 years: not recommended; ≥6 years: initially 5 mg daily bid; may increase by 5 mg/day at weekly intervals; usual effective dose; 20-25 mg/day

Tab: 5, 10, 15 mg sust-rel

▷ *methylphenidate (regular-acting)* (C)(II)(G)

Methylin, Methylin Chewable, Methylin Oral Solution usual dose 20-30 mg/day in 2-3 divided doses 30-45 minutes before a meal; may increase to 60 mg/day

Pediatric: <6 years: not recommended; ≥6 years: initially 5 mg twice daily before breakfast and lunch; may increase 5-10 mg/week; max 60 mg/day

Tab: 5, 10*, 20*mg; *Chew tab:* 2.5, 5, 10 mg (grape) (phenylalanine); *Oral soln:* 5, 10 mg/5 ml) (grape)

Ritalin 10-60 mg/day in 2-3 divided doses 30-45 minutes ac; max 60 mg/day

Pediatric: <6 years: not recommended; ≥6 years: initially 5 mg bid ac (before breakfast and lunch); may gradually increase by 5-10 mg at weekly intervals as needed; max 60 mg/day

Tab: 5, 10*, 20*mg

▷ *methylphenidate (long-acting)* (C)(II)

Concerta initially 18 mg q AM; may increase in 18 mg increments as needed; max 54 mg/day; do not crush or chew

Tab: 18, 27, 36, 54 mg sust-rel

Metadate CD (G) 1 cap daily in the AM; may sprinkle on food; do not crush or chew

Pediatric: <6 years: not recommended; ≥6 years: initially 20 mg daily; may gradually increase by 20 mg/day at weekly intervals as needed; max 60 mg/day

Cap: 10, 20, 30, 40, 50, 60 mg immed- and ext-rel beads

Metadate ER 1 tab daily in the AM; do not crush or chew

Pediatric: <6 years: not recommended; ≥6 years: use in place of regular-acting *methylphenidate* when the 8-hour dose of **Metadate-ER** corresponds to the titrated 8-hour dose of regular-acting *methylphenidate*

Tab: 10, 20 mg ext-rel (dye-free)

Ritalin LA 1 cap daily in the AM

Pediatric: <6 years: not recommended; ≥6 years: use in place of regular-acting *methylphenidate* when the 8-hour dose of **Ritalin LA** corresponds to the titrated 8-hour dose of regular-acting *methylphenidate*; max 60 mg/day

Cap: 10, 20, 30, 40 mg ext-rel (immed- and ext-rel beads)

Ritalin SR 1 cap daily in the AM
> *Pediatric:* <6 years: not recommended; ≥6 years: use in place of regular-acting ***methylphenidate*** when the 8-hour dose of **Ritalin SR** corresponds to the titrated 8-hour dose of regular-acting ***methylphenidate***; max 60 mg/day
> *Tab:* 20 mg sust-rel (dye-free)

▷ ***methylphenidate (transdermal patch)*** (C)(II)(G) 1 patch daily in the AM
Pediatric: <6 years: not recommended; ≥6 years: initially 10 mg patch daily in the AM; may increase by 5-10 mg/week; max 60 mg/day
Transdermal patch: 10, 15, 20, 30 mg

▷ ***pemoline*** (B)(IV) 18.75-112.5 mg/day; usually start with 37.5 mg in AM; increase weekly by 18.75 mg/day if needed; max 112.5 g/day
Pediatric: <6 years: not recommended; ≥6 years: same as adult
> **Cylert** *Tab:* 18.75*, 37.5*, 75*mg
> **Cylert Chewable** *Chew tab:* 37.5*mg

Comment: Monitor baseline serum ALT and repeat every 2 weeks thereafter.

◯ NAUSEA/VOMITING

PROPHYLAXIS (FOR PREVENTION OF MOTION SICKNESS AND POST-OP NAUSEA AND VOMITING)

Anticholinergic Agents

▷ ***scopolamine*** (C)
> **Scopace** 0.4-0.8 mg 1 hour before travel; may repeat in 8 hours
> *Pediatric:* not recommended
> *Tab:* 0.4 mg
> **Transderm Scop** 1 patch behind ear at least 4 hours before travel; each patch is effective for 3 days
> *Pediatric:* not recommended
> *Transdermal patch:* 1.5 mg (4/carton)

MILD NAUSEA

▷ ***phosphorylated carbohydrate*** solution (C)(G) 1-2 tblsp q 15 minutes until nausea subsides; max 5 doses/day
Pediatric: 1-2 tsp q 15 minutes until nausea subsides; max 5 doses/day
> **Emetrol (OTC)** *Soln:* dextrose 1.87 g/fructose 1.87 g/phosphoric acid 21.5 mg per 5 ml (4, 8, 16 oz)

Cannabinoid

▷ ***dronabinol*** (C)(III) initially 5 mg/m² 1-3 hours before chemotherapy; then q 2-4 hours prn; max 4-6 doses/day, 15 mg/m²
> **Marinol** *Cap:* 2.5, 5, 10 mg (sesame seed oil)

▷ ***nabilone*** (C)(II) 1-2 mg bid; max 6 mg/day in 3 divided doses; initially 1-3 hours before chemotherapy; may give 1-2 mg the night before chemo; may continue 48 hours after each chemo cycle
> **Cesamet** *Cap:* 1 mg (sesame seed oil)

Antihistamines

▷ *diphenhydramine* (C)(G) 10-50 mg IV or deep IM q 6-8 hours prn; max 400 mg/day
  Pediatric: 5 mg/kg/day in 4 divided doses; max 300 mg/day
    Benadryl *Vial:* 50 mg/ml (1 ml single-use); 50 mg/ml (10 ml multi-dose); *Amp:*
    50 mg/ml (1 ml); *Prefilled syringe:* 50 mg/ml (1 ml)
▷ *meclizine* (C)(G) *Travel:* 25-50 mg 1 hour prior to travel; repeat every 24 hours;
  Vertigo of vestibular origin: 25-100 mg/day in divided doses
  Pediatric: 5 mg/kg/day in 4 divided doses; max 300 mg/day
    Antivert *Tab:* 12.5, 25, 50*mg; *Amp:* 50 mg/ml (1 ml)
      Vial: 50 mg/ml (1 ml single-use); 50 mg/ml (10 ml multi-dose)
    Bonine (OTC) *Cap:* 15, 25, 50 mg; *Tab:* 12.5, 25, 50 mg;
      Chew tab/Film-coat tab: 25 mg
    Dramamine II (OTC) *Tab:* 25 mg
    Zentrip *Strip:* 25 mg orally-disint

MODERATE TO SEVERE NAUSEA

Phenothiazines

▷ *chlorpromazine* (C)(G) 10-25 mg PO q 4 hours prn or 50-100 mg rectally q 6-8 hours
  prn
  Pediatric: <6 months: not recommended; ≥6 months: 0.25 mg/lb orally q 4-6 hours
  prn or 0.5 mg/lb rectally q 6-8 hours prn
    Thorazine *Tab:* 10, 25, 50, 100, 200 mg; *Spansule:* 30, 75, 150 mg sust-rel; *Syr:*
    10 mg/5 ml (4 oz; orange custard); *Conc:* 30 mg/ml (4 oz); 100 mg/ml (2, 8 oz);
    Supp: 25, 100 mg
▷ *perphenazine* (C) 5 mg IM (may repeat in 6 hours) or 8-16 mg/day PO in divided
  doses; max 15 mg/day IM; max 24 mg/day PO
  Pediatric: not recommended
    Trilafon *Tab:* 2, 4, 8, 16 mg; *Oral conc:* 16 mg/5 ml (118 ml); *Amp:* 5 mg/ml (1 ml)
▷ *prochlorperazine* (C)(G) 5-10 mg tid-qid prn; usual max 40 mg/day
    Compazine
      Pediatric: <2 years or <20 lb: not recommended; 20-29 lb: 2.5 mg daily bid prn;
      max 7.5 mg/day; 30-39 lb: 2.5 mg bid-tid prn; max 10 mg/day; 40-85 lb: 2.5
      mg tid or 5 mg bid prn; max 15 mg/day
      Tab: 5, 10 mg; *Syr:* 5 mg/5 ml (4 oz) (fruit)
    Compazine Suppository 25 mg rectally bid prn; usual max 50 mg/day
      Pediatric: <2 years or <20 lb: not recommended; 20-29 lb: 2.5 mg daily-bid
      prn; max 7.5; mg/day; 30-39 lb: 2.5 mg bid-tid prn; max 10 mg/day; 40-85 lb:
      2.5 mg tid or 5 mg bid prn; max 15 mg/day
      Rectal supp: 2.5, 5, 25 mg
    Compazine Injectable 5-10 mg tid or qid prn
      Pediatric: <2 years or <20 lb: not recommended; ≥2 years or ≥20 lb: 0.06 mg/
      kg x 1 dose
      Vial: 5 mg/ml (2, 10 ml)
    Compazine Spansule 15 mg q AM prn or 10 mg q 12 hours prn usual max 40
    mg/day
      Pediatric: not recommended
      Spansule: 10, 15 mg sust-rel

▷ *promethazine* (C)(G) 25 mg PO or rectally q 4-6 hours prn
  Pediatric: <2 years: not recommended; ≥2 years: 0.5 mg/lb or 6.25-25 mg q 4-6
  hours prn
    Phenergan *Tab:* 12.5*, 25*, 50 mg; *Plain syr:* 6.25 mg/5 ml; *Fortis syr:* 25 mg/5
    ml; *Rectal supp:* 12.5, 25, 50 mg

Substance P/Neurokinin 1 Receptor Antagonist

▷ *aprepitant* (B)(G) administer with corticosteroid and 5-HT-3 receptor antagonist;
  Day 1 of chemotherapy cycle: 125 mg 1 hour prior to chemotherapy *Day 2 & 3:* 80
  mg in the morning
  Pediatric: <6 months: years: not recommended; ≥6 months: use oral suspension (see
  mfr pkg insert for dose by weight
    Emend *Cap:* 40, 80, 125 mg (2 x 80 mg bifold pck; 1 x 25 mg/2 x 80 mg tri-
    fold pck); *Oral susp:* 125 mg pwdr for oral suspension, single dose pouch w
    dispenser; *Vial:* 150 mg pwdr for reconstitution and IV infusion

5-HT-3 Receptor Antagonists

Comment: The selective 5-HT-3 receptor antagonists indicated for prevention of
nausea and vomiting associated with moderately to highly emetogenic chemotherapy.
▷ *dolasetron* (B) administer 100 mg IV over 30 seconds, 30 min prior to administration of chemotherapy or 2 hours before surgery; max 100 mg/dose
  Pediatric: <2 years: not recommended; 2-16 years: 1.8 mg/kg; >16 years: same as
  adult
    Anzemet *Tab:* 50, 100 mg; *Amp:* 12.5 mg/0.625 ml; *Prefilled carpuject syringe:*
    12.5 mg (0.625 ml); *Vial:* 100 mg/5 ml (single- use); *Vial:* 500 mg/25 ml (multi-
    dose)
▷ *granisetron*
    Kytril (B) administer IV over 30 seconds, 30 min prior to administration of
    chemotherapy; max 1 dose/week
      Pediatric: <2 years: not recommended; ≥2 years: 10 mcg/kg
      Tab: 1 mg; *Oral soln:* 2 mg/10 ml (30 ml; orange); *Vial:* 1 mg/ml (1 ml single-
      dose; preservative-free); 1 mg/ml (4 ml multi-dose) (benzyl alcohol)
    Sancuso (B) apply 1 patch 24-48 hours before chemo; remove 24 hours (mini-
    mum) to 7 days (maximum) after completion of treatment
      Transdermal patch: 3.1 mg/day
▷ **Sustol** (NE) administer SC over 20-30 seconds (due to drug viscosity) on Day 1 of
  chemotherapy and not more frequently than once every 7 days; *CrCl 30-59 mL/min:*
  repeat dose no more than every 14th day; *CrCl <30 mL/min:* not recommended; for
  patients receiving MEC, the recommended *dexamethasone* dosage is 8 mg IV on Day
  1; for patients receiving AC combination chemotherapy regimens, the recommended
  dexamethasone dosage is 20 mg IV on Day 1, followed by 8 mg PO bid on Days 2, 3
  and 4; if **Sustol** is administered with an NK_1 receptor antagonist, see that drug's mfr
  pkg insert for the recommended *dexamethasone* dosing
  Pediatric: <18 years: not established
    Syringe: 10 mg/0.4 ml ext-rel; prefilled single-dose/kit
  Comment: At least 60 minutes prior to administration, remove the **Sustol** kit from
  refrigeration; activate a warming pouch and wrap the syringe in the warming pouch
  for 5-6 minutes to warm it to room temperature.

▷ *ondansetron* (C)(G)
   Oral Forms: *Highly emetogenic chemotherapy:* 24 mg x 1 dose 30 min prior to start of single-day chemotherapy; *Moderately emetogenic chemotherapy:* 8 mg q 8 hours x 2 doses beginning 30 minutes prior to start of chemotherapy; then 8 mg q 12 hours x 1-2 days following
   Pediatric: <4 years: not recommended; 4-11 years, moderately emetogenic chemotherapy: 4 mg q 4 hours x 3 doses beginning 30 min prior to start; then 4 mg q 8 hours x 1-2 days following
   Zofran *Tab:* 4, 8, 24 mg
   Zofran ODT *ODT:* 4, 8 mg (strawberry) (phenylalanine)
   Zofran Oral Solution *Oral soln:* 4 mg/5 ml (50 ml) (strawberry) (phenylalanine); *Parenteral form:* see mfr pkg insert
   Zofran Injection *Vial:* 2 mg/ml (2 ml single-dose); 2 mg/ml (20 ml multidose); 32 mg/50 ml (50 ml multi-dose); *Prefilled syringe:* 4 mg/2 ml, single-use (24/carton)
   Zuplenz Oral Soluble Film: 4, 8 mg oral-dis (10/carton) (peppermint)
▷ *palonosetron* (B)(G) *Chemotherapy:* administer 0.25 mg IV over 30 seconds, 30 min prior to administration of chemo; max 1 dose/week or 1 cap 1 hour before chemo; *Postop:* administer 0.075 mg IV over 10 seconds immediately before induction of anesthesia
   Pediatric: <1 month: not recommended; 1 month to 17 years: 20 mcg/kg; max 1.5 mg single-dose; infuse over 15 minutes beginning 30 minutes prior to administration of chemo
   Aloxi *Vial (single-use):* 0.075 mg/1.5 ml; 0.25 mg/5 ml (mannitol)

ANTI-DOPAMINERGIC (PROMOTILITY) AGENTS

▷ *metoclopramide* (B)(G) 10 mg 30 minutes before each meal and at HS for 2-8 weeks
   Metozolv ODT *ODT:* 5, 10 mg (mint)
   Reglan *Tab:* 5, 10*mg
   Comment: *metoclopramide* is contraindicated when stimulation of GI motility may be dang6erous. Observe for tardive dyskinesia and Parkinsonism.
   Avoid concomitant drugs which may cause an extrapyramidal reaction (e.g., phenothiazines, *haloperidol*).
   Substance P/Neurokinin-1 (NK-1) Receptor Antagonist
▷ *rolapitant* (NE) take 180 mg in a single dose 1-2 hours before chemotherapy treatment; administer in combination with dexamethasone and 5-HT3 receptor antagonist
   Pediatric: not established
   Varubi *Tab:* 90 mg film-coat
   Comment: **Varubi is** indicated in combination with other antiemetic agents in adults for the prevention of delayed nausea and vomiting associated with emetogenic cancer chemotherapy.

SUBSTANCE P/NEUROKININ-1 (NK-1) RECEPTOR ANTAGONIST/5-HT-3 RECEPTOR ANTAGONIST COMBINATION

▷ *netupitant/palonosetron* (C) take one cap approximately 1 hour prior to chemotherapy; administer in combination with dexamethasone
   Pediatric: not established
   Akynzeo *Gelcap: netu* 300 mg/*palo* 0.5 mg

Comment: **Akynzeo is** indicated in combination with other antiemetic agents in adults for the prevention of delayed nausea and vomiting associated with emetogenic cancer chemotherapy.

 NERVE AGENT POISONING

▷ *atropine sulfate* **(NE)(G)** 2 mg IM
Pediatric: <15 lb: not recommended; ≥15-40 lb: 0.5 mg IM; ≥40-90 lb: 1 mg IM; >90 lb: same as adult
   AtroPen *Pen (single-use):* 0.5, 1, 2 mg (0.5 ml)

 NON-24 SLEEP-WAKE DISORDER

Comment: For other drug options (stimulants, sedative hypnotics), *see* **Insomnia** *page* 242, **Sleepiness: Excessive, Shift Work Sleep Disorder** *page* 400

MELATONIN RECEPTOR AGONIST

▷ *tasimelteon* **(C)** take 1 gelcap before bedtime at the same time every night; do not take with food
Pediatric: not established
   Hetlioz *Gel cap:* 20 mg

OREXIN RECEPTOR ANTAGONIST

▷ *suvorexant* **(C)(IV)** use lowest effective dose; take 30 minutes before bedtime; do not take if unable to sleep for ≥7 hours; max 20 mg
Pediatric: not recommended
   Belsomra *Tab:* 5, 10, 15, 20 mg (30/blister pck)

 OBESITY

Comment: Target BMI is 25-30 (≤27 preferred).

STIMULANTS

▷ *amphetamine sulfate* **(C)(II)**
   Evekeo initially 5 mg 30-60 minutes before meals; usually up to 30 mg/day
Pediatric: <12 years: not recommended; ≥12 years: same as adult
Tab: 5, 10 mg

LIPASE INHIBITOR

▷ *orlistat* **(X)(G)** 1 cap tid 1 hour before <u>or</u> during each main meal containing fat
Pediatric: <12 years: not recommended; ≥12 years: same as adult
   Alli (OTC) *Cap:* 60 mg
   Xenical *Cap:* 120 mg
Comment: For use when BMI >30 kg/m² <u>or</u> BMI >27 kg/m² in the presence of other risk factors (i.e., HTN, DM, dyslipidemia).

ANOREXIGENICS

Sympathomimetics

Comment: Side effects include hypertension, tachycardia, restlessness, insomnia, and dry mouth.

▷ *benzphetamine* (X)(III) initially 25-50 mg daily in the mid-morning or mid-afternoon; may increase to bid-tid as needed
Pediatric: not recommended
  Didrex *Tab:* 50*mg

▷ *naltrexone/bupropion* (X) swallow whole; avoid high-fat meals; initially 10 mg bid; evaluate weight loss after 12 weeks; discontinue if less than 5% weight loss
Pediatric: <18 years: not recommended
    Contrave *Tab:* nal 8 mg/*bup* 900 mg ext-rel

▷ *methamphetamine* (C)(II) 10-15 mg q AM
Pediatric: <12 years: not recommended; ≥12 years: same as adult
    Desoxyn *Tab:* 5, 10, 15 mg sust-rel

▷ *phendimetrazine* (C)(III)
Pediatric: <12 years: not recommended; ≥12 years: same as adult
    Bontril PDM 35 mg bid-tid 1 hour ac; may reduce to 17.5 mg (1/2 tab)/dose; max 210 mg/day in 3 divided doses
      Tab: 35*mg
    Bontril Slow-Release 105 mg in the AM 30-60 minutes before breakfast
      Cap: 105 mg slow-rel

▷ *phentermine* (C)(IV)
Pediatric: <16 years: not recommended; ≥16 years: same as adult
    Adipex-P (G) 1 cap or tab before breakfast or 1/2 tab bid ac
      Cap: 37.5 mg; *Tab:* 37.5*mg
    Fastin (G) 1 cap before breakfast
      Cap: 30 mg
    Ionamin (G) 1 cap before breakfast or 10-14 hours prior to HS
      Cap: 15, 30 mg
    Suprenza ODT (X)(IV) dissolve 1 tab on top of tongue once daily in the morning, with or without food; use lowest effective dose
      Tab: 15, 30, 37.5 mg orally-disint

Comment: Contraindicated with history of cardiovascular disease (e.g., coronary artery disease, stroke, arrhythmias, congestive heart failure, uncontrolled hypertension, during or within 14 days following the administration of an MAOI, hyperthyroidism, glaucoma, agitated states, history of drug abuse, pregnancy, nursing).

Sympathomimetic/Antiepileptic Combination

▷ *phentermine/topiramate ext-rel* (X)(IV)(G) initially 3.75 mg/23 mg daily in the AM x 14 days; then increase to 7.5 mg/46 mg and evaluate weight loss on this dose after 12 weeks; if ≤3% weight loss from baseline, discontinue or increase dose to 11.25 mg/69 mg x 14 days; then increase to 15 mg/92 mg and evaluate weight loss on this dose after 12 weeks; if ≤5% weight loss from baseline, discontinue by taking a dose every other day for at least one week prior to stopping; max 7.5 mg/46 mg for moderate to severe renal impairment or moderate hepatic impairment.
Pediatric: <16 years: not established; ≥16 years: same as adult

Qsymia
    Cap: **Qsymia 3.75/23**: *phen* 3.75 mg/*topir* 23 mg ext-rel
          Qsymia 7.5/46: *phen* 7.5 mg/*topir* 46 mg ext-rel
          Qsymia 11.25/69: *phen* 11.25 mg/*topir* 69 mg ext-rel
          Qsymia 15/92: *phen* 15 mg/*topir* 92 mg ext-rel
Comment: Side effects include hypertension, tachycardia, restlessness, insomnia, and dry mouth. Contraindicated with glaucoma, hyperthyroidism, and within 14 days of taking an MAOI. **Qsymia 3.75/23** and **Qsymia 11.25/69** are for titration purposes only.

Serotonin 2C Receptor Agonist

▷ *lorcaserin* (X)(G) 10 mg bid; discontinue if 5% weight loss is not achieved by week 12
    Pediatric: <18 years: not recommended
    Belviq *Tab:* 10 mg film-coat
    Comment: **Belviq** is indicated as an adjunct to a reduced-calorie diet and increased physical activity for chronic weight management in adults with an initial body mass index (BMI) of 30 kg/m² <u>or</u> greater (obese) <u>or</u> 27 kg/m² <u>or</u> greater (overweight) in the presence of at least one weight-related comorbid condition (e.g., hypertension, dyslipidemia, type 2 diabetes). Serotonin 2C receptor agonists interact with serotonergic drugs (selective serotonin reuptake inhibitors (SSRIs), serotonin-norepinephrine reuptake inhibitors (SNRIs), monoamine oxidase inhibitors (MAOIs), triptans, *bupropion, dextromethorphan, St. John's wort*); therefore, use with extreme caution due to the risk of serotonin syndrome.

GLUCAGON-LIKE PEPTIDE-1 (GLP-1) RECEPTOR AGONIST

▷ *liraglutide* (C) administer SC in the upper arm, abdomen, <u>or</u> thigh once daily; escalate dose gradually over 5 weeks to 3 mg SC daily; *Week 1:* 0.6 mg SC daily; *Week 2:* 1.2 mg SC daily; *Week 3:* 1.8 mg SC daily; *Week 4:* 2.4 mg SC daily; *Week 5:* 3 mg SC daily; *Pediatric:* <18 years: not recommended
    Saxenda Soln for SC inj: 6 mg/ml multi-dose prefilled pen (3 ml; 3, 5 pens/carton)
    Comment: **Saxenda** is indicated as an adjunct to a reduced-calorie diet and increased physical activity for chronic weight management in adults with an initial body mass index (BMI) of 30 kg/m² <u>or</u> greater (obese) <u>or</u> 27 kg/m² <u>or</u> greater overweight) in the presence of at least one weight-related comorbid condition (e.g., hypertension, dyslipidemia, type 2 diabetes). Not indicated for treatment of T2DM. Do not use with **Victoza**, other GLP-1 receptor agonists, <u>or</u> insulin. Contraindicated with personal <u>or</u> family history of medullary thyroid carcinoma (MTC) and multiple endocrine neoplasia syndrome (MENS) type 2. Monitor for signs/symptoms pancreatitis. Discontinue if gastroparesis, renal, <u>or</u> hepatic impairment.

 OBSESSIVE-COMPULSIVE DISORDER (OCD)

SELECTIVE SEROTONIN REUPTAKE INHIBITORS (SSRIs)

Comment: Co-administration of SSRIs with TCAs requires extreme caution. Concomitant use of MAOIs and SSRIs is absolutely contraindicated. Avoid other serotonergic drugs. A potentially fatal adverse event is *Serotonin Syndrome*, caused by serotonin excess. Milder symptoms require HCP intervention to avert severe symptoms which can be rapidly fatal without urgent/emergent medical care. Symptoms include restlessness, agitation, confusion, hallucinations, tachycardia, hypertension, dilated pupils, muscle twitching, muscle rigidity, loss of muscle coordination, diaphoresis, diarrhea, headache, shivering, piloerection, hyperpyrexia, cardiac arrhythmias, seizures, loss of consciousness, coma, death. Abrupt withdrawal or interruption of treatment with an antidepressant medication is sometimes associated with an *Antidepressant Discontinuation Syndrome* which may be mediated by gradually tapering the drug over a period of two weeks or longer, depending on the dose strength and length of treatment. Common symptoms of the *Serotonin Discontinuation Syndrome* include flu-like symptoms (nausea, vomiting, diarrhea, headaches, sweating), sleep disturbances (insomnia, nightmares, constant sleepiness), mood disturbances (dysphoria, anxiety, agitation), cognitive disturbances (mental confusion, hyperarousal), sensory and movement disturbances (imbalance, tremors, vertigo, dizziness, electric-shock-like sensations in the brain, often described by sufferers as "brain zaps."

▷ *fluoxetine* (C)(G)

Prozac initially 20 mg daily; may increase after 1 week; doses >20 mg/day may be divided into AM and noon doses; max 80 mg/day

Pediatric: <7 years: not recommended; 7-17 years: initially 10 mg/day; may increase after 2 weeks to 20 mg/day; range 20-60 mg/day; range for lower weight children 20-30 mg/day

Cap: 10, 20, 40 mg; *Tab:* 30*, 60*mg; *Oral soln:* 20 mg/5 ml (4 oz) (mint)

Prozac Weekly following daily *fluoxetine* therapy at 20 mg/day for 13 weeks, may initiate **Prozac Weekly** 7 days after the last 20 mg *fluoxetine* dose

Pediatric: not recommended

Cap: 90 mg ent-coat del-rel pellets

▷ *fluvoxamine* (C)(G)

Luvox initially 50 mg q HS; adjust in 50 mg increments at 4-7 day intervals; range 100-300 mg/day; over 100 mg/day, divide into 2 doses giving the larger dose at HS

Pediatric: <8 years: not recommended; 8-17 years: initially 25 mg q HS; adjust in 25 mg increments q 4-7 days; usual range 50-200 mg/day; over 50 mg/day, divide into 2 doses giving the larger dose at HS

Tab: 25, 50*, 100*mg

Luvox CR initially 100 mg once daily at HS; may increase by 50 mg increments at 1 week intervals; max 300 mg/day; swallow whole

Pediatric: <18 years: not recommended

Cap: 100, 150 mg ext-rel

▷ *paroxetine maleate* (D)(G)

Pediatric: not recommended

Paxil initially 20 mg daily in AM; may increase by 10 mg/day at weekly intervals as needed; max 60 mg/day

Tab: 10*, 20*, 30, 40 mg

Paxil CR initially 25 mg daily in AM; may increase by 12.5 mg at weekly intervals as needed; max 62.5 mg/day

Tab: 12.5, 25, 37.5 mg cont-rel ent-coat

Paxil Suspension initially 20 mg daily in AM; may increase by 10 mg/day at weekly intervals as needed; max 60 mg/day

Oral susp: 10 mg/5 ml (250 ml) (orange)

▷ *sertraline* (C) initially 50 mg daily; increase at 1 week intervals if needed; max 200 mg daily
Pediatric: <6 years: not recommended; 6-12 years: initially 25 mg daily; max 200 mg/day; 13-17 years: initially 50 mg daily; max 200 mg/day
   Zoloft *Tab:* 15*, 50*, 100*mg; *Oral conc:* 20 mg per ml (60 ml [dilute just before administering in 4 oz water, ginger ale, lemon-lime soda, lemonade, <u>or</u> orange juice]) (alcohol 12%)

TRICYCLIC ANTIDEPRESSANT (TCA) COMBINATIONS

▷ *clomipramine* (C)(G) initially 25 mg daily in divided doses; gradually increase to 100 mg during first 2 weeks; max 250 mg/day; total maintenance dose may be given at HS
Pediatric: <10 years: not recommended; ≥10 years: initially 25 mg daily in divided doses; gradually increase; max 3 mg/kg <u>or</u> 100 mg, whichever is smaller
   Anafranil *Cap:* 25, 50, 75 mg
▷ *imipramine* (C)(G)
   Tofranil initially 75 mg/day; max 200 mg/day
      Pediatric: adolescents initially 30-40 mg/day; max 100 mg/day
      Tab: 10, 25, 50 mg
   Tofranil PM initially 75 mg/day; max 200 mg/day
      Pediatric: not recommended
      Cap: 75, 100, 125, 150 mg

◯ ONYCHOMYCOSIS (FUNGAL NAIL)

ORAL AGENTS

▷ *griseofulvin, microsize* (C)(G) 1 g daily for at least 4 months for fingernails and at least 6 months for toenails
   Pediatric: 5 mg/lb/day; *see page* 579 *for dose by weight*
   Grifulvin V *Tab:* 250, 500 mg; *Oral susp:* 125 mg/5 ml (120 ml; alcohol 0.02%)
▷ *griseofulvin, ultramicrosize* (C) 750 mg in a single <u>or</u> divided doses for at least 4 months for fingernails and at least 6 months for toenails
   Pediatric: <2 years: not recommended; ≥2 years: 3.3 mg/lb in a single <u>or</u> divided doses
   Gris-PEG *Tab:* 125, 250 mg
▷ *itraconazole* (C)(G) 200 mg daily x 12 consecutive weeks for toenails; 200 mg bid x 1 week, off 3 weeks, then 200 mg bid x 1 additional week for fingernails
   Pediatric: not recommended
   Sporanox *Cap:* 100 mg; *Soln:* 10 mg/ml (150 ml) (cherry-caramel)
   Pulse Pack: 100 mg caps (7/pck)
▷ *terbinafine* (B)(G) 250 mg daily x 6 weeks for fingernails; 250 mg daily x 12 weeks for toenails
   Pediatric: not recommended
   Lamisil *Tab:* 250 mg

TOPICAL AGENTS

Comment: File and trim nail while nail is free from drug. Remove unattached infected nail as frequently as monthly. For use with mild to moderate onychomycosis of the fingernails and toenails, without lunula involvement due to *Trichophyton rubrum*

immunocompetent patients as part of a comprehensive treatment program. For use on nails and adjacent skin only. Apply evenly to entire onycholytic nail and surrounding 5 mm of skin daily, preferably at HS <u>or</u> 8 hours before washing; apply to nail bed, hyponychium, and under surface of nail plate when it is free of the nail bed; apply over previous coats, then remove with alcohol once per week; treat for up to 48 weeks.

▷ *ciclopirox* (B)
    Pediatric: not established
      Penlac Nail Lacquer *Topical soln (lacquer):* 8% (6.6 ml w. applicator)
▷ *efinaconazole* (C)
    Pediatric: not established
      Jublia *Topical soln:* 5% (10 ml w. brush applicator)
▷ *tavaborole* (C)
    Pediatric: not established
      Kerydin *Topical soln:* 10% (10 ml w. dropper)

OPHTHALMIA NEONATORUM: CHLAMYDIAL

PROPHYLAXIS

▷ *erythromycin* ophthalmic ointment 0.5-1 cm ribbon into lower conjunctival sac of each eye x 1 application
    Ilotycin Ophthalmic Ointment *Ophth oint:* 5 mg/g (1/8 oz)

Comment: The following treatment regimens are published in the **2015 CDC Sexually Transmitted Diseases Treatment Guidelines**. Treatment regimens are presented by generic drug name first, followed by information about brands and dose forms.

RECOMMENDED REGIMENS

Regimen 1

▷ *erythromycin base* 50 mg/kg/day in 4 doses x 14 days

Regimen 2

▷ *erythromycin ethylsuccinate* 50 mg/kg/day in 4 doses x 14 days

DRUG BRANDS AND DOSE FORMS

▷ *erythromycin base* (B)(G)
    Pediatric: <45 kg: 30-50 mg in 2-4 divided doses x 7-10 days; ≥45 kg: same as adult
      Ery-Tab *Tab:* 250, 333, 500 mg ent-coat
      PCE *Tab:* 333, 500 mg

Comment: *erythromycin* may increase INR with concomitant ***warfarin***, as well as increase serum level of ***digoxin***, benzodiazepines and statins.

▷ *erythromycin ethylsuccinate* (B)(G)
    Pediatric: 30-50 mg/kg/day in 4 divided doses x 7 days; may double dose with severe infection; max 100 mg/kg/day for at least 14 days; *see page 574 for dose by weight*
      EryPed *Oral susp:* 200 mg/5 ml (100, 200 ml) (fruit); 400 mg/5 ml (60, 100, 200 ml (banana); *Oral drops:* 200, 400 mg/5 ml (50 ml) (fruit); *Chew tab:* 200 mg wafer (fruit)
      E.E.S. *Oral susp:* 200, 400 mg/5 ml (100 ml) (fruit)

E.E.S. Granules *Oral susp:* 200 mg/5 ml (100, 200 ml) (cherry)
Comment: *erythromycin* may increase INR with concomitant **warfarin**, as well as increase serum level of **digoxin**, benzodiazepines and statins.

 OPHTHALMIA NEONATORUM: GONOCOCCAL

Comment: The following prophylaxis and treatment regimens for gonococcal conjunctivitis is published in the **2015 CDC Sexually Transmitted Diseases Treatment Guidelines**.

Regimen 1

▷ *erythromycin 0.5%* ophthalmic ointment 0.5-1 cm ribbon into lower conjunctival sac of each eye x 1 application
Ilotycin Ophthalmic Ointment *Ophth oint:* 5 mg/g (1/8 oz)

Regimen 2

▷ *ceftriaxone* (B)(G) 25-50 mg/kg IV or IM in a single dose, not to exceed 125 mg
Pediatric: 1 g IM in a single dose
Rocephin *Vial:* 250, 500 mg; 1, 2 g

 OPIOID DEPENDENCE OPIOID WITHDRAWAL SYNDROME

Safety labeling for all immediate-release (IR) opioids has been issued by the FDA. The boxed warning includes serious risks of misuse, abuse, addiction, overdose, and death. The dosing section offers clear steps regarding administration and patient monitoring including initial dose, dose changes, and the abrupt cessation of treatment in physical dependence. Chronic maternal use of opioids during pregnancy can lead to potentially life-threatening neonatal opioid withdrawal. The American Pain Society (APS) has released new evidence-based clinical practice guidelines that include 32 recommendations related to post-op pain management in adults and children.

NARCOTIC ANALGESIC

▷ *methadone* (C) *Narcotic Detoxification:* 15-40 mg daily in decreasing doses not to exceed 21 days; *Narcotic Maintenance:* >21 days; see mfr pkg insert
Pediatric: not established
Dolophine *Tab:* 5, 10 mg; *Dispersible tab:* 40 mg (dissolve in 120 ml orange juice or other citrus drink); *Oral conc:* 5, 10 mg/5 ml; 10 mg/10 ml
Comment: *methadone* maintenance is allowed only by approved providers with strict state and federal regulations.

OPIOID ANTAGONIST

▷ *naltrexone* (C)
Pediatric: not established
ReVia 50 mg daily

Tab: 50 mg
Vivitrol 380 mg IM once monthly; alternate buttocks
Vial: 380 mg

OPIOID PARTIAL AGONIST-ANTAGONIST

Comment: **Belbuca, Butrans, Probuphine, and Subutex** maintenance are allowed only by approved providers with strict state and federal regulations. The drugs are potentiated by CYP3A4 inhibitors (e.g, azole antifungals, macrolides, HIV protease inhibitors) and antagonized by CYP3A4 inducers (monitor for opioid withdrawal). Concomitant NNRTIs (e.g., efavirenz, nevirapine, etravirine, delavirdine) or PIs (e.g., atazanavir with/without ritonavir): monitor. Risk of respiratory or CNS depression with concomitant opioid analgesics, general anesthetics, benzodiazepines, phenothiazines, other tranquilizers, sedative/hypnotics, alcohol, or other CNS depressants. Risk of serotonin syndrome with concomitant SSRIs, SNRIs, TCAs, 5-HT3 receptor antagonists, mirtazapine, trazodone, tramadol, MAO inhibitors.

▷ *buprenorphine* (C)(III)
   Pediatric: <16 years: not established
   Belbuca apply buccal film to inside of cheek; do not chew or swallow; *Opioid naïve:* initially 75 mcg once daily-q 12 hours x at least 4 days; then, increase to 150 mcg q 12 hours; may increase in increments of 150 mcg q 12 hours no sooner than every 4 days; max 900 mcg q 12 hours; see mfr pkg insert for conversion from other opioids; *Severe hepatic impairment or oral mucositis:* reduce initial and titration doses by half
   Buccal film: 75, 150, 300, 450, 600, 750, 900 mcg (60/pck) (peppermint)
   Butrans Transdermal System apply one patch to clean, dry, hairless, intact skin on the upper outer arm, upper chest, upper back, or side of chest every 7 days; rotate sites and do not re-use a site for at least 21 days; *Opioid naïve or oral morphine <30 mg/day or equivalent:* one 5 mcg/hour patch; *Converting from oral morphine equivalents 30-80 mg/day:* taper current opioids for up to 7 days to ≤30 mg/day oral morphine equivalents before starting; then initiate with 10 mcg/hour patch; may use a short-acting analgesic until efficacy is attained; increase dose only after exposure to previous dose x at least 72 hours; max one 20 mcg/hour patch/week; *Conversion from higher opioid doses:* not recommended
   Transdermal patch: 5, 7.5, 10, 15, 20 mcg/hour (4/pck)
   Probuphine initiate when stable on *buprenorphine* ≤8 mg/day; insertion site is the inner side of the upper arm; 4 implants are intended to be in place for 6 months; remove the implants by the end of the 6th month and insert four new implants on the same day in the contralateral arm; if a new implant is not inserted on the same day as removal of a previous implant, maintain the patient on the previous dose of transmucosal *buprenorphine* (i.e., the dose from which the patient was transferred to **Probuphine** treatment).
   Subdermal implant: 74.2 mg of *buprenorphine* (equivalent to 80 mg of *buprenorphine hydrochloride*)
   Comment: Healthcare providers who prescribe, perform insertions and/or perform removals of **Probuphine** must successfully complete a live training program, and demonstrate procedural competency prior to inserting or removing the implants. Further information: visit www.ProbuphineREMS.com or call 1-844-859-6341

Subutex (G) 8 mg in a single dose on day 1; then 16 mg in a single dose on day 2; target dose is 16 mg/day in a single dose; dissolve under tongue; do not chew or swallow whole

    SL tab (lemon-lime) or *SL film (lime):* 2, 8 mg (30/pck)

OPIOID PARTIAL AGONIST-ANTAGONIST/OPIOID ANTAGONIST

Comment: **Bunabail, Suboxone, Sucartonone, Troxyca ER,** and **Zubsolv** maintenance are allowed only by approved providers with strict state and federal regulations.

▷ *buprenorphine/naloxone* (C)(III)

Bunavail administer one buccal film once daily at the same time each day; target dose is 8.4/1.4 once daily; place the side of the **Bunavail** film with the text (BN2, BN4, or BN6) against the inside of the cheek; press and hold the film in place for 5 seconds; maintenance is usually 2.1/0.3 to 12.6/2.1 once daily
Pediatric: <16 years: not recommended; ≥16 years: same as adult

    SL film:

        Bunavail 2.1/0.3 *bup* 2.1 mg/*nal* 0.3 mg (30/carton)

        Bunavail 4.2/0.7 *bup* 4.2 mg/*nal* 0.7 mg (30/carton)

        Bunavail 6.3/1 *bup* 6.3 mg/*nal* 1 mg (30/carton)

Comment: A **Bunavail** 4.2/0.7 mg buccal film provides equivalent ***buprenorphine*** exposure to a **Sucartonone** 8/2 mg sublingual tablet.

Suboxone (G) adjust dose in increments/decrements of 2 mg/0.5 mg or 4 mg/1 mg once daily ***buprenorpnine/naloxone***, based on the patient's daily dose of ***buprenorphine***, to a level that suppresses opioid withdrawal signs and symptoms; *Recommended target dosage:* 16 mg/4 mg as a single daily dose; *Maintenance dose:* generally in the range of 4 mg/1 mg to 24 mg/6 mg per day; higher once daily doses have not been demonstrated to provide any clinical advantage
Pediatric: not established

    SL tab, SL film:

        Suboxone 2/0.5 *bup* 2 mg/*nal* 0.5 mg (lime) (30/bottle)

        Suboxone 8/2 *bup* 8 mg/*nal* 2 mg (lime) (30/bottle)

Sucartonone adjust in 2-4 mg of ***buprenorphine***/day in a single dose; usual range is 4-24 mg/day in a single dose; target dose is 6 mg/day in a single dose; dissolve under tongue; do not chew or swallow whole
Pediatric: <16 years: not recommended; ≥16 years: same as adult

    SL film (lime):

        Sucartonone 2/0.5 *bup* 2 mg/*nal* 0.5 mg (30/pck)

        Sucartonone 4/1 *bup* 4 mg/*nal* 1 mg (30/pck)

        Sucartonone 8/2 *bup* 8 mg/*nal* 2 mg (30/pck)

        Sucartonone 12/3 *bup* 12 mg/*nal* 3 mg (30/pck)

Zubsolv initial induction with buprenorphine sublingual tabs; administer as a single dose once daily; titrate dose in increments of 1.4/0.36 or 2.9/0.72 per day; recommended target dose is 11.4/2.9 per day; usual max 17.2/4.2 per day
Pediatric: <16 years: not recommended; ≥16 years: same as adult

    SL tab:

        Zubsolv 1.4/0.36 *bup* 1.4 mg/*nal* 0.36 mg

        Zubsolv 2.9/0.72 *bup* 2.9 mg/*nal* 0.71 mg

        Zubsolv 5.7/1.4 *bup* 5.7 mg/*nal* 1.4 mg

        Zubsolv 8.6/2.1 *bup* 8.6 mg/*nal* 2.1 mg

> **Zubsolv 11.4/2.9** *bup* 11.4 mg/*nal* 2.9 mg
> **Comment:** One **Subutex 5.7/1.4** SL tab is bioequivalent to one **Sucartonone 8/2** SL film.

➤ *oxycodone/naloxone* (C)(II) *Opioid-naïve and opioid non-tolerant:* initially 10 mg/1.2mg q 12 hours; *Opioid tolerant:* single doses greater than 40 mg/4.8 mg, or a total daily dose greater than 80 mg/9.6 mg are only for use in patients for whom tolerance to an opioid of comparable potency has been established; swallow whole, or sprinkle contents on applesauce and swallow immediately without chewing
Pediatric: <18 years: not recommended
Troxyca ER
    Cap: **Troxyca ER 10/1.2** *oxy 10 mg/nalox 1.2 mg ext-rel*
        Troxyca ER 20/1.2 *oxy 20 mg/nalox 2.4 mg ext-rel*
        Troxyca ER 30/1.2 *oxy 30 mg/nalox 3.6 mg ext-rel*
        Troxyca ER 40/1.2 *oxy 40 mg/nalox 4.8 mg ext-rel*
        Troxyca ER 60/1.2 *oxy 60 mg/nalox 7.2 mg ext-rel*
        Troxyca ER 80/1.2 *oxy 80 mg/nalox 9.6 mg ext-rel*

Comment: Opioid tolerant patients are those taking, for one week or longer, at least 60 mg oral *morphine* per day, 25 mcg transdermal *fentanyl* per hour, 30 mg oral *oxycodone* per day, 8 mg oral *hydromorphone* per day, 25 mg oral *oxymorphone* per day, 60 mg oral *hydrocodone* per day, or an equianalgesic dose of another opioid.

OPIOID-INDUCED CONSTIPATION (OIC)

➤ *lubiprostone* (C) swallow whole; take with food and water; initially 24 mcg bid; *Moderate hepatic impairment (Child Pugh Class B):* 16 mg bid; *Severe hepatic impairment (Child Pugh Class C):* 8 mg bid
Pediatric: not recommended
Amitiza *Cap:* 8, 24 mg

➤ *methylnaltrexone bromide* (C) administer 12 mg SC once daily or once every other day, in the upper arm, abdomen, or thigh; max one dose/24 hrs; discontinue other laxatives; <38 kg-14 kg: 0.15 mg/kg; 38-<62 kg: 8 mg; 62-114 kg: 12 mg; *CrCl <30 mL/min:* reduce dose by half
Pediatric: not established
Relistor *Vial:* 8 mg/0.4 ml; 12 mg/0.6 ml single-use (7/carton); *Prefilled syringes* (7/carton)

➤ *naloxegol* (C) swallow whole; take on an empty stomach; initially 25 mg once daily in the AM; discontinue other laxatives; *CrCl <60 mL/min:* 12.5 mg
Pediatric: not established
Movantik *Tab:* 12.5, 25 mg

OPIOID OVERDOSE

OPIOID ANTAGONISTS

➤ *nalmefene* (B) initially 0.25 mcg/kg IV, IM, or SC, then incremental doses of 0.25 mcg/kg at 2-5 minute intervals; cumulative max 1 mcg/kg; if opioid dependency suspected use 0.1 mg/70 kg initially and then proceed as usual if no response in 2 minutes
Pediatric: not recommended
Revex *Amp:* 100 mcg/1 ml (1 ml); 1 mg/ml (2 ml)

▷ *naloxone* (B)(G) 0.4-2 mg; repeat in 2-3 minutes if no response
  Pediatric: 0.01 mg/kg initially, repeat in 2-3 minutes at 0.1 mg/kg if response inadequate
    Evzio *Prefilled autoinjector:* 0.4 mg/0.4, 2 mg/0.4 ml IM/SC only
    Comment: **Evzio** 2 mg/0.4 ml comes with 2 autoinjectors and one trainer. This strength is indicated for the emergency treatment of known or suspected opioid overdose manifested by CNS depression.
    If the electronic voice instruction system does not operate properly, **Evzio** will still deliver the intended dose of *naloxone* when used according to the printed instructions on the flat surface of the autoinjector label. **Evzio** cannot be administered IV. Due to the short duration of action of naloxone, as compared to opioids which are longer acting, monitoring of the patient is critical as the opioid reversal effects of naloxone may wear off before the effects of the opioid.
    Narcan *Vial/Amp:* 0.4 mg/ml (1 ml), 1 mg/ml (2 ml); *Prefilled syringe:* 0.4 mg/ml (1 ml), 1 mg/ml (2 ml) IV, IM, <u>or</u> SC (parabens-free)
    Narcan Nasal Spray position supine with head tilted back; 1 spray in one nostril; if an additional dose is needed, spray into the opposite nostril
      Nasal spray: 4 mg/0.1 ml, single dose, single use (2 blister pcks, each w a single nasal spray/carton)

OSGOOD-SCHLATTER DISEASE

Acetaminophen for IV Infusion *see Pain page* 306
Oral Prescription NSAIDs *see page* 501
Other Oral Analgesics *see Pain page* 308
Topical/Transdermal NSAIDs *see Pain page* 307
Parenteral Corticosteroids *see page* 511
Oral Corticosteroids *see page* 509
Topical Analgesic and Anesthetic Agents *see page* 499

OSTEOARTHRITIS

Acetaminophen for IV Infusion *see Pain page* 306
Oral Prescription NSAIDs *see page* 501
Other Oral Analgesics *see Pain page* 308
Topical/Transdermal NSAIDs *see Pain page* 307
Parenteral Corticosteroids *see page* 511
Oral Corticosteroids *see page* 509
Topical Analgesic and Anesthetic Agents *see page* 499

TOPICAL ANALGESICS

▷ *capsaicin* (B)(G) apply tid to qid prn to intact skin
  Pediatric: <2 years: not recommended; ≥2 years: same as adult
    Axsain *Crm:* 0.075% (1, 2 oz)
    Capsin *Lotn:* 0.025, 0.075% (59 ml)
    Capzasin-P (OTC) *Crm:* 0.025% (1.5 oz); *Lotn:* 0.025% (2 oz)
    Dolorac *Crm:* 0.025% (28 g)
    Double Cap (OTC) *Crm:* 0.05% (2 oz)
    R-Gel *Gel:* 0.025% (15, 30 g)

Zostrix (OTC) *Crm:* 0.025% (0.7, 1.5, 3 oz)
Zostrix HP (OTC) *Emol crm:* 0.075% (1, 2 oz)
Comment: Provides some relief by 1-2 weeks; optimal benefit may take 4-6 weeks.

ORAL SALICYLATE

▷ *indomethacin* (C) initially 25 mg bid to tid, increase as needed at weekly intervals by
25-50 mg/day; max 200 mg/day
Pediatric: <14 years: usually not recommended; >2 years, if risk warranted: 1-2 mg/
kg/day in divided doses; max 3-4 mg/kg/day (or 150-200 mg/day, whichever is
less); <14 years, ER cap not recommended
  Cap: 25, 50 mg; *Susp:* 25 mg/5 ml (pineapple-coconut, mint) (alcohol 1%);
  Supp: 50 mg; *ER Cap:* 75 mg ext-rel
Comment: *indomethacin* is indicated only for acute painful flares. Administer with
food and/or antacids. Use lowest effective dose for shortest duration.

ORAL NSAIDs

See more Oral NSAIDs page 501

▷ *diclofenac* (C)
Pediatric: <18 years: not recommended
  Zorvolex take on empty stomach; 35 mg tid; *Hepatic impairment:* use lowest dose
  Gelcap: 18, 35 mg
▷ *diclofenac sodium* (C)
Pediatric: <18 years: not recommended
  Voltaren 50 mg bid to qid or 75 mg bid or 25 mg qid with an additional 25 mg
  at HS if necessary
  Tab: 25, 50, 75 mg ent-coat
  Voltaren XR 100 mg once daily; rarely, 100 mg bid may be used
  Tab: 100 mg ext-rel

ORAL NSAIDs PLUS PPI

▷ *esomeprazole/naproxen* (C)(G) 1 tab bid; use lowest effective dose for the shortest
duration swallow whole; take at least 30 minutes before a meal
Pediatric: <18 years: not recommended
  Vimovo *Tab: nap* 375 mg/*eso* 20 mg ext-rel; *nap* 500 mg/*eso* 20 mg ext-rel
  Comment: **Vimovo** is indicated to improve signs/symptoms, and risk of gastric
  ulcer in patients at risk of developing NSAID-associated gastric ulcer.

COX-2 INHIBITORS

Comment: Cox-2 inhibitors are contraindicated with history of asthma, urticaria, and
allergic-type reactions to *aspirin*, other NSAIDs, and sulfonamides, 3rd trimester of
pregnancy, and coronary artery bypass graft (CABG) surgery.
▷ *celecoxib* (C)(G) 100-400 mg daily bid; max 800 mg/day
Pediatric: <18 years: not recommended
  Celebrex *Cap:* 50, 100, 200, 400 mg
▷ *meloxicam* (C)(G) initially 7.5 mg once daily; max 15 mg once daily
Pediatric: <2 years: not recommended; ≥2 years: 0.125 mg/kg; max 7.5 mg once daily
  Mobic *Tab:* 7.5, 15 mg; *Oral susp:* 7.5 mg/5 ml (100 ml) (raspberry)
  Vivlodex *Cap:* 5, 10 mg

INTRA-ARTICULAR INJECTION

▷ **sodium hyaluronate (B)** using strict aseptic technique, administer by intra-articular injection (into the synovial space) once weekly for the prescribed number of weeks (see mfr pkg insert); after preparing the injection site and attaining local analgesia, remove joint synovial fluid or effusion prior to injection
Pediatric: not recommended
    Gelsyn-3 Syringe: 8.4 mg/ml (2 ml) prefilled
    Hyalgan *Vial:* 20 mg (2 ml); Prefilled syringe: 20 mg (2 ml)
    Hylan *Syringe:* 48 mg/6 ml (6 ml) prefilled
    Synvisc One *Syringe:* 46 mg/6 ml (6 ml) prefilled

OSTEOPOROSIS

Comment: Indications for bone density screening include: Postmenopausal women not receiving HRT, maternal history of hip fracture, personal history of fragility fracture, presence of high serum markers of bone resorption, smoker, height >67 inches, weight <125 lb, taking a steroid, GnRH agonist, or antiseizure drug, immobilization, hyperthyroidism, posttransplantation, malabsorption syndrome, hyperparathyroidism, prolactinemia. The mnemonic A̲BONE [A̲ge >65, B̲ulk (weight <140 lbs at menopause), and N̲ever E̲strogens (for more than 6 months)], represent other indications for bone density screening. Foods high in calcium include almonds, broccoli, baked beans, salmon, sardines, buttermilk, turnip greens, collard greens, spinach, pumpkin, rhubarb, and bran. Recommended Daily Calcium Intake: 1-3 years: 700 mg; 4-8 years: 1000 mg; 9-18 years: 1300 mg; 19-50 years: 1000 mg: 51-70 years (males): 1000 mg; ≥51 years (females): 1200 mg; pregnancy or nursing: 1000-1300 mg Recommended Daily Vitamin D Intake: >1 year: 600 IU; 50+ years: 800-1000 IU.

ESTROGEN REPLACEMENT THERAPY

Comment: *estrogen* plus progesterone is indicated for postmenopausal women with an intact uterus. *estrogen* monotherapy is indicated in women without a uterus. The following list is not inclusive; for more estrogen replacement therapies *see **Menopause** page* 264)
▷ **estradiol (X)**
    Alora initially 0.05 mg/day apply patch twice weekly to lower abdomen, upper quadrant of buttocks or outer aspect of hip
        Transdermal patch: 0.025, 0.05, 0.075, 0.1 mg/day (8, 24/pck)
    Climara initially 0.025 mg/day patch once/week to trunk
        Transdermal patch: 0.025, 0.0375, 0.05, 0.075, 0.1 mg/day (4, 8, 24/pck)
    Estrace 1-2 mg daily cyclically (3 weeks on and 1 week off)
        Tab: 0.5, 1, 2*mg (tartrazine)
    Estraderm initially apply one 0.05 mg/day patch twice weekly to trunk
        Transdermal patch: 0.05, 0.1 mg/day (8, 24/pck)
    Menostar apply one patch weekly to lower abdomen, below the waist; avoid the breasts; alternate sites; *Transdermal patch:* 14 mcg/day (4/pck)
    Minivelle initially one 0.0375 mg/day patch twice weekly to trunk area; adjust after one month of therapy
        Transdermal patch: 0.025, 0.0375, 0.05, 0.075, 0.1 mg/day (8/pck)

Vivelle initially one 0.0375 mg/day patch twice weekly to trunk area; use with an oral progestin to prevent endometrial hyperplasia
Transdermal patch: 0.025, 0.0375, 0.05, 0.075, 0.1 mg/day (8, 48/pck)
Vivelle-Dot initially one 0.05 mg/day patch twice weekly to lower abdomen, below the waist; use with an oral progestin to prevent endometrial hyperplasia
Transdermal patch: 0.025, 0.0375, 0.05, 0.075, 0.1 mg/day (8, 24/pck)
▶ *estradiol/levonorgestrel* (X) apply 1 patch weekly to lower abdomen; avoid waistline; alternate sites
Climara Pro *Transdermal patch: estra* 0.045 mg/*levo* 0.015 mg per day (4/pck)
▶ *estradiol/norethindrone* (X) 1 tab daily
Activella (G) *Tab: estra* 1 mg/*noreth* 0.5 mg
FemHRT 1/5 *Tab: estra* 5 mcg/*noreth* 1 mg
▶ *estradiol/norgestimate* (X) one-1mg estradiol tab daily x 3 days, then 1-*estradiol* 1 mg/*norgestimate* 0.09 mg tab once daily x 3 days; repeat this pattern continuously
Ortho-Prefest *Tab: estra* 1 mg/*norgest* 0.09 mg (30/blister pck)
▶ *estrogen, conjugated (equine)* (X)
Premarin 1 tab daily
Tab: 0.3, 0.45, 0.625, 0.9, 1.25, 2.5 mg
▶ *estropipate, piperazine estrone sulfate* (X)(G)
Ogen 0.625-1.25 mg daily cyclically (3 weeks on and 1 week off)
Tab: 0.625, 1.25, 2.5 mg
Ortho-Est 0.75-6 mg daily cyclically (3 weeks on and 1 week off)
Tab: 0.625, 1.25 mg

ESTROGENS, CONJUGATED/ESTROGEN AGONIST-ANTAGONIST COMBINATION

▶ *estrogen, conjugated/bazedoxifene* (X)
Duavee 1 tab daily
Tab: conj estra 0.45 mg/*baze* 20 mg

CALCIUM SUPPLEMENTS

Comment: Take *calcium* supplements after meals to avoid gastric upset. Dosages of calcium over 2000 mg/day have not been shown to have any additional benefit. *calcium* decreases *tetracycline* absorption. *calcium* absorption is decreased by corticosteroids.
▶ *calcitonin-salmon* (C)
Fortical 200 IU intranasally daily; alternate nostrils each day
Nasal spray: 200 IU/actuation (30 doses, 3.7 ml)
Miacalcin Nasal spray 200 IU spray in one nostril once daily; alternate nostrils each day
Nasal spray: 200 IU/actuation (30 doses, 3.7 ml)
Miacalcin Injection 100 units SC <u>or</u> IM every other day
Vial: 200 units/ml (2 ml)
Comment: Supplement diet with calcium (1 g/day) and vitamin D (400 IU/day).
▶ *calcium carbonate* (C)(OTC)(G)
Rolaids chew 2 tabs bid; max 14 tabs/day
Chew tab: 550 mg
Rolaids Extra Strength chew 2 tabs bid; max 8 tabs/day
Chew tab: 1000 mg

Tums chew 2 tabs bid; max 16 tabs/day
  Chew tab: 500 mg
Tums Extra Strength chew 2 tabs bid; max 10 tabs/day
  Chew tab: 750 mg
Tum Sultra chew 2 tabs bid; max 8 tabs/day
  Chew tab: 1000 mg
Os-Cal 500 (OTC) 1-2 tab bid to tid
  Chew tab: elemental calcium carbonate 500 mg
▷ *calcium carbonate/vitamin d* (C)(G)
  Os-Cal 250+D (OTC) 1-2 tab tid
    Tab: elemental calcium carbonate 250 mg/*vit d* 125 IU
  Os-Cal 500+D (OTC) 1-2 tab bid-tid
    Tab: elemental calcium carbonate 500 mg/*vit d* 125 IU
  Viactiv (OTC) 1 tab tid
    Chew tab: elemental calcium 500 mg/*vit d* 100 IU/*vitamin k* 40 mcg
▷ *calcium citrate* (C)(G)
  Citracal (OTC) 1-2 tabs bid
    Tab: elemental calcium citrate 200 mg
▷ *calcium citrate/vitamin d* (C)(G)
  Citracal +D (OTC) 1-2 cplts bid
    Cplt: elemental calcium citrate 315 mg/*vit d* 200 IU
  Citracal 250+D (OTC) 1-2 tabs bid
    Tab: elemental calcium citrate 250 mg/*vit d* 62.3 IU

VITAMIN D ANALOGS

Comment: Concurrent *vitamin D* supplementation is contraindicated for patients
taking *calcitrol* or *doxercalciferol* due to the risk of *vitamin D* toxicity.
▷ *calcitrol* (C) *Predialysis:* initially 0.25 mcg daily; may increase to 0.5 mcg daily; *Dialysis:* initially 0.25 mcg daily; may increase by 0.25 mcg/day at 4-8 week intervals; usual
maintenance 0.5-1 mcg/day; *Hypoparathyroidism:* initially 0.25 mcg q AM; may increase by 0.25 mcg/day at 4- to 8-week intervals; usual maintenance 0.5-2 mcg/day
Pediatric: Predialysis: <3 years: 10-15 ng/kg/day; ≥3 years: initially 0.25 mcg daily;
may increase to 0.5 mcg/day; *Dialysis:* not recommended; *Hypoparathyroidism:*
initially 0.25 mcg daily; may increase by 0.25 mcg/day at 2-4 week intervals; usual
maintenance (1-5 years) 0.25-0.75 mcg/day, (>6 years) 0.5-2 mcg/day
  Rocaltrol *Cap:* 0.25, 0.5 mcg
  Rocaltrol Solution *Soln:* 1 mcg/ml (15 ml, single-use dispensers)
▷ *doxercalciferol* (C) initially 0.25 mcg q AM; may increase by 0.25 mcg/day at 4-8
week intervals; usual maintenance 0.5-2 mcg/day
Pediatric: initially 0.25 mcg daily; may increase by 0.25 mcg; 0.25 mcg/day at 2-4 week
intervals; usual maintenance (1-5 years) 0.25-0.75 mcg/day, (≥6 years) 0.5-2 mcg/day
  Hectorol *Cap:* 0.25, 0.5 mcg

BISPHOSPHONATES (CALCIUM MODIFIERS)

Comment: Biphosphonates should be swallowed whole in the AM with 6-8 oz of
plain water 30 minutes before first meal, beverage, or other medications of the day.
Monitor serum alkaline phosphatase. Contraindications include abnormalities of the
esophagus which delay esophageal emptying such as stricture or achalasia, inability
to stand or sit upright for at least 30 minutes postdose, patients at risk of aspiration,

and hypocalcemia. Co-administration of biphosphonates and *calcium*, antacids, or oral medications containing multivalent cations will interfere with absorption of the bophosphonate. Therefore, instruct patients to wait at least half hour after taking the biphosphonate before taking any other oral medications.

▷ *alendronate (as sodium)* (C) take once weekly, in the AM, 30 minutes before the first food, beverage, or medication of the day; do not lie down (remain upright) for at least 30 minutes and after the first food of the day; *CrCl <35 mL/min:* not recommended with *Pediatric:* not recommended

    Binosto dissolve the effervescent tab in 4 oz (120 ml) of plain, room temperature, water (not mineral or flavored); wait 5 minutes after the effervescence has subsided, then stir for 10 seconds, then drink

        Tab: 70 mg effervescent for buffered solution (4, 12/carton) (strawberry)

    Fosamax (G) swallow tab whole; dosing regimens are the same for men and postmenopausal women; *Prevention:* 5 mg once daily or 35 mg once weekly; *Treatment:* 10 mg once daily or 70 mg once weekly

        Tab: 5, 10, 35, 40, 70 mg

▷ *alendronate/cholecalciferol (vit d3)* (C)(G) take 1 tab once weekly, in the AM, with plain water (not mineral) 30 minutes before the first food, beverage, or medication of the day; do not lie down (remain upright) for at least 30 minutes and after the first food of the day *Pediatric:* not recommended

    Fosamax Plus D

        Tab: **Fosamax Plus D 70/2800:** *alen* 70 mg/*chole* 2800 IU

    Fosamax Plus D 70/5600: *alen* 70 mg/*chole* 5600 IU

▷ *ibandronate (as monosodium monohydrate)* (C)(G)
Pediatric: not recommended

    Boniva take 2.5 mg once daily or 150 mg once monthly on the same day; take in the AM, with plain water (not mineral) 60 minutes before the first food, beverage, or medication of the day; do not lie down (remain upright) for at least 30 minutes and after the first food of the day

        Tab: 2.5, 150 mg

    Boniva Injection administer 3 mg every 3 months by IV bolus over 15-30 seconds; if dose is missed, administer as soon as possible; then every 3 months from the date of the last dose

        Prefilled syringe: 3 mg/3 ml (5 ml)

    Comment: Boniva Injection must be administered by a health care professional.

▷ *risedronate (as sodium)* (C)(G) take in the AM; swallow whole with a full glass of plain water (not mineral); do not lie down (remain upright) for 30 minutes afterward *Pediatric:* not recommended

    Actonel take at least 30 minutes before any food or drink; *Women:* 5 mg once daily or 35 mg once weekly or 75 mg on two consecutive days monthly or 150 mg once monthly; *Men:* 35 mg once weekly

        Tab: 5, 30, 35, 75, 150 mg

    Atelvia 35 mg once weekly immediately after breakfast

        Tab: 35 mg del-rel

▷ *risedronate/calcium* (C) 1 x 5 mg *risedronate* tab weekly plus 1 x 500 mg *calcium* tab on days 2-7 weekly

    Actonel with Calcium *Tab: risedronate* 5 mg and *Tab: calcium* 500 mg (4 *rise-dronate* tabs + 30 *calcium* tabs/pck)

▷ *zoledronic acid* (D)(G)
Pediatric: not recommended

Reclast administer 5 mg via IV infusion over at least 15 minutes mg once a year (for osteoporosis) <u>or</u> once every 2 years (for osteopenia <u>or</u> prophylaxis)
> *Bottle:* 5 mg/100 ml (single-dose)

Comment: **Reclast** is indicated for the treatment of postmenopausal osteoporosis in women who are at high risk for fracture and to increase bone mass in men with primary <u>or</u> hypogonadal osteoporosis who are at high risk for fracture. Administered by a health care professional. Contraindicated in hypocalcemia.

Zometa *Bottle:* 4 mg/5 ml administer 4 mg via IV infusion over at least 15 minutes every 3-4 weeks; optimal duration of treatment not known
> *Vial:* 4 mg/5 ml (single-dose)

Comment: **Zometa** is indicated for the treatment of hypercalcemia of malignancy. The safety and efficacy of **Zometa** in the treatment of hypercalcemia associated with hyperparathyroidism <u>or</u> with other nontumor-related conditions has not been established.

SELECTIVE ESTROGEN RECEPTOR MODULATOR (SERMs)

➤ *raloxifene* (X)(G) 60 mg once daily
Evista *Tab:* 60 mg
Comment: Contraindicated in women who have history of, <u>or</u> current, venous thrombotic event.

HUMAN PARATHYROID HORMONE

➤ *teriparatide* (C) 20 mcg SC daily in the thigh <u>or</u> abdomen; may treat for for up to 2 years
Pediatric: not recommended
Forteo Multidose Pen *Multi-dose pen:* 250 mcg/ml (3 ml)
Comment: **Forteo** is indicated for the treatment of postmenopausal osteoporosis in women who are at high risk for fracture and to increase bone mass in men with primary <u>or</u> hypogonadal osteoporosis who are at high risk for fracture.

BIOENGINEERED REPLICA OF HUMAN PARATHYROID HORMONE

➤ *bioengineered replica of human parathyroid hormone* (C) initially inject mg IM into the thigh once daily; when initiating, decrease dose of active *vitamin D* by 50% if serum *calcium* is above 7.5 mg/dL; monitor serum *calcium* levels every 3 to 7 days after starting <u>or</u> adjusting dose and when adjusting either active *vitamin D* <u>or</u> *calcium* supplements dose
Natpara *Soln for inj:* 25, 50, 75, 100 mcg (2/pkg) multi-dose, dual-chamber glass cartridge containing a sterile powder and diluent
Comment: **Natpara** is indicated as adjunct to *calcium* and *vitamin D* in patients with parathyroidism.

OSTEOCLAST INHIBITOR (RANKL INHIBITOR)

➤ *denosumab* (X) for SC injection 60 mcg SC once every 6 months in the upper arm, abdomen, <u>or</u> upper thigh
Pediatric: not established
Prolia *Vial/Pen:* 60 mg/ml (1 ml) single-dose
Comment: **Prolia** is indicated for the treatment of postmenopausal osteoporosis in women who are at high risk for fracture defined as a history of osteoporotic

fracture, or multiple risk factors for fracture, or patients who have failed or are intolerant to other therapy. Administered by a health care professional. Contraindicated in hypocalcemia.

◯ OTITIS EXTERNA

OTIC ANALGESIC

▷ *antipyrine/benzocaine/zinc acetate dihydrate* (C) fill ear canal with solution; then insert a cotton pluge into meatus; may repeat every 1-2 hours prn
  Pediatric: same as adult
    Otozin *Otic soln:* antipyr 5.4%/*benz* 1%/*zinc*1% per ml (10 ml w. dropper)

OTIC ANTI-INFECTIVE

▷ *chloroxylenol/pramoxine* (C) 4-5 drops tid x 5-10 days
  Pediatric: <1 year: not recommended; 1-12 years: 5 drops bid x 10 days
    PramOtic *Otic drops: chlorox*/*pramox* (5 ml w. dropper)
▷ *finafloxacin* (C) otic 4-5 drops tid x 5-10 days
  Pediatric: <1 year: not recommended; ≥1 year: same as adult
    Xtoro *Otic soln:* 0.3% (5, 8 ml)
▷ *ofloxacin* (C)(G) 10 drops bid x 10 days
  Pediatric: <1 year: not recommended; 1-12 years: 5 drops bid x 10 days
    Floxin Otic *Otic soln:* 0.3% (5, 10 ml w. dropper; 0.25 ml, 5 drop singles, 20/carton)
    Comment: **Floxin Otic** is indicated for adult patients with perforated tympanic membranes and pediatric patients with PE tubes.

OTIC ANTI-INFECTIVE/CORTICOSTEROID COMBINATIONS

▷ *chloroxylenol/pramoxine/hydrocortisone* (C) drops 4 drops tid-qid x 5-10 days
  Pediatric: 3 drops tid-qid x 5-10 days
    Cortane B, Cortane B Aqueous *Otic soln: chlo* 1 mg/*pram* 10 mg/*hydro* 10 mg per ml (10 ml w. dropper)
Comment: **Cortane B Aqueous** may be used to saturate a cotton wick.
▷ *ciprofloxacin/hydrocortisone* (C) susp 3 drops bid x 7 days
  Pediatric: <1 year: not recommended; ≥1 year: same as adult
    Cipro HC Otic *Otic susp: cipro* 0.2%/*hydro* 1% (10 ml w. dropper)
▷ *ciprofloxacin/dexamethasone* (C) 4 drops bid x 7 days
  Pediatric: <6 months: not recommended; ≥6 months: same as adult
    Ciprodex *Otic susp: cipro* 0.3%/*dexa* 1% (7.5 ml)
    Comment: **Ciprodex** is indicated for the treatment of otitis media in pediatric patients with tympanostomy tubes.
▷ *colistin/neomycin/hydrocortisone/thonzonium* (C) 5 drops tid or qid x 5-10 days
  Pediatric: 4 drops tid-qid x 5-10 days
    Coly-Mycin S *Otic susp:* 5, 10 ml
    Cortisporin-TC Otic *Otic susp: colis* 3 mg/*neo* 3.3 mg/*hydro* 10 mg/*thon* 0.5 mg per ml (10 ml w. dropper) (thimerosal)
▷ *polymyxin b/neomycin/hydrocortisone* (C) 4 drops tid-qid; max 10 days
  Pediatric: 3 drops tid-qid; max 10 days

Cortisporin Otic Suspension *Otic susp: poly b* 10,000 u/*neo* 3.5 mg/*hydro* 10 mg per 5 ml (10 ml w. dropper)
Cortisporin Otic Solution *Otic soln: poly b* 10000 u/*neo* 3.5 mg/*hydro* 10 mg per 5 ml (10 ml w. dropper)

OTIC ASTRINGENTS

▷ *acetic acid 2% in aluminum sulfate* (C) 4-6 drops q 2-3 hours
  Pediatric: same as adult
   Domeboro Otic *Otic soln:* 60 ml w. dropper
▷ *acetic acid/propylene glycol/benzethonium chloride/sodium acetate* (C) 3-5 drops q 4-6 hours
  Pediatric: same as adult
   VoSol *Otic soln: acet* 2% (15, 30 ml)
▷ *acetic acid/propylene glycol/hydrocortisone/benzethonium chloride/sod-ium acetate* (C) 3-5 drops q 4-6 hours
  Pediatric: same as adult
   VoSol HC *Otic soln: acet* 2%/*hydro* 1% (10 ml)

OTIC ANESTHETIC/ANALGESIC COMBINATIONS

▷ *antipyrine/benzocaine/glycerine* (C) fill ear canal and insert cotton plug; may repeat q 1-2 hours as needed
  Pediatric: same as adult
   A/B Otic *Otic soln:* 15 ml w. dropper
▷ *benzocaine* (C) 4-5 drops q 1-2 hours
  Pediatric: <1 year: not recommended; ≥1 year: same as adult
   Americaine Otic *Otic soln:* 20% (15 ml w. dropper)
   Benzotic *Otic soln:* 20% (15 ml w. dropper)

SYSTEMIC ANTI-INFECTIVES

Comment: Used for severe disease or with culture.
▷ *amoxicillin/clavulanate* (B)(G) 500 mg tid or 875 mg bid x 10 days
   Augmentin *Tab:* 250, 500, 875 mg; *Chew tab:* 125, 250 mg (lemon-lime); 200, 400 mg (cherry-banana) (phenylalanine); *Oral susp:* 125 mg/5 ml (banana), 250 mg/5 ml (75, 100, 150 ml) (orange); 200, 400 mg/5 ml (50, 75, 100 ml) (orange) (phenylalanine)
     Pediatric: 40-45 mg/kg/day divided tid x 10 days or 90 mg/kg/day divided bid x 10 days *see pages 556-557 for dose by weight*
   Augmentin ES-600 *Oral susp:* 600 mg/5 ml (50, 75, 100, 125, 150, 200 ml) (strawberry cream) (phenylalanine) every 12 hours
     Pediatric: <3 months: not recommended; ≥3 months, <40 kg: 90 mg/kg/day in 2 divided doses; ≥40 kg: not recommended
   Augmentin XR 2 tabs q 12 hours x 10 days
     Pediatric: <16 years: use other forms; ≥16 years: same as adult
     Tab: 1000*mg ext-rel
▷ *cefaclor* (B)(G) 250-500 mg q 8 hours x 7-10 days
  Pediatric: <1 month: not recommended; 20-40 mg/kg bid or q 12 hours x 10 days; max 1 g/day; *see page 558 for dose by weight*

Tab: 500 mg; *Cap:* 250, 500 mg; *Susp:* 125 mg/5 ml (75, 150 ml) (strawberry); 187 mg/5 ml (50, 100 ml) (strawberry); 250 mg/5 ml (75, 150 ml) (strawberry); 375 mg/5 ml (50, 100 ml) (strawberry)

Cefaclor Extended Release
Pediatric: <16 years: ext-rel not recommended; ≥16 years: same as adult
Tab: 375, 500 mg ext-rel

▷ *dicloxacillin* **(B)** 500 mg qid x 7-10 days
Pediatric: 12.5-25 mg/kg/day in 4 divided doses x 7-10 days; *see page 571 for dose by weight*

Dynapen *Cap:* 125, 250, 500 mg; *Oral susp:* 62.5 mg/5 ml (80, 100, 200 ml)

▷ *trimethoprim/sulfamethoxazole* **(C)(G)**
Pediatric: <2 months: not recommended; ≥2 months: 40 mg/kg/day of *sulfamethoxazole* in 2 doses bid x 10 days; *see page 587 for dose by weight*

Bactrim, Septra 2 tabs bid x 10 days
Tab: trim 80 mg/*sulfa* 400 mg*

Bactrim DS, Septra DS 1 tab bid x 10 days
Tab: trim 160 mg/*sulfa* 800 mg*

Bactrim Pediatric Suspension, Septra Pediatric Suspension
Oral susp: trim 40 mg/*sulfa* 200 mg per 5 ml (100 ml) (cherry) (alcohol 0.3%)

Comment: *trimethoprim/sulfamethoxazole* is not recommended in pregnancy or lactation. *CrCl 15-30 mL/min:* reduce dose by 1/2; *CrCl <15 mL/min:* not recommended.

OTITIS MEDIA: ACUTE

OTIC ANALGESIC

▷ *antipyrine/benzocaine/zinc acetate dihydrate* otic **(C)** fill ear canal with solution; then insert cotton plug into meatus; may repeat every 1-2 hours prn
Pediatric: same as adult

Otozin *Otic soln: antipyr* 5.4%/*benz* 1%/*zinc* 1% per ml (10 ml w. dropper)

SYSTEMIC ANTI-INFECTIVES

▷ *amoxicillin* **(B)(G)** 500-875 mg bid or 250-500 mg tid x 10 days
Pediatric: <40 kg (88 lb): 20-40 mg/kg/day in 3 divided doses x 10 days or 25-45 mg/kg/day in 2 divided doses x 10 days; *see page 554 for dose by weight*

Amoxil *Cap:* 250, 500 mg; *Tab:* 875*mg; *Chew tab:* 125, 200, 250, 400 mg (cherry-banana-peppermint) (phenylalanine); *Oral susp:* 125, 250 mg/5 ml (80, 100, 150 ml) (strawberry); 200, 400 mg/5 ml (50, 75, 100 ml) (bubble gum); *Oral drops:* 50 mg/ml (30 ml) (bubble gum)

Moxatag *Tab:* 775 mg ext-rel

Trimox *Tab:* 125, 250 mg; *Cap:* 250, 500 mg; *Oral susp:* 125, 250 mg/5 ml (80, 100, 150 ml) (raspberry-strawberry)

Comment: Consider 80-90 mg/kg/day in 3 divided doses for resistant for cases

▷ *amoxicillin/clavulanate* **(B)(G)** 500 mg tid or 875 mg bid x 10 days

Augmentin *Tab:* 250, 500, 875 mg; *Chew tab:* 125, 250 mg (lemon-lime); 200, 400 mg (cherry-banana) (phenylalanine); *Oral susp:* 125 mg/5 ml (banana), 250 mg/5 ml (75, 100, 150 ml) (orange); 200, 400 mg/5 ml (50, 75, 100 ml) (orange) (phenylalanine)

Pediatric: 40-45 mg/kg/day divided tid x 10 days or 90 mg/kg/day divided bid x 10 days *see pages 556-557 for dose by weight*

Augmentin ES-600 *Oral susp:* 600 mg/5 ml (50, 75, 100, 125, 150, 200 ml) (strawberry cream) (phenylalanine) every 12 hours

Pediatric: <3 months: not recommended; ≥3 months, <40 kg: 90 mg/kg/day in 2 divided doses; ≥40 kg: not recommended

Augmentin XR 2 tabs q 12 hours x 7-10 days

Pediatric: <16 years: use other forms; ≥16 years: same as adult
Tab: 1000*mg ext-rel

➤ *ampicillin* (B) 250-500 mg qid x 10 days
Pediatric: 50-100 mg/kg/day in 4 divided doses x 10 days; *see page 558 for dose by weight*

Omnipen, Principen *Cap:* 250, 500 mg; *Oral susp:* 125, 250 mg/5 ml (100, 150, 200 ml) (fruit)

➤ *azithromycin* (B)(G) 500 mg x 1 dose on day 1, then 250 mg daily on days 2-5 or 500 mg daily x 3 days or **Zmax** 2 g in a single dose
Pediatric: 12 mg/kg/day x 5 days; max 500 mg/day; *see page 559 for dose by weight*

Zithromax *Tab:* 250, 500, 600 mg; *Oral susp:* 100 mg/5 ml (15 ml); 200 mg/5 ml (15, 22.5, 30 ml) (cherry); *Pkt:* 1 g for reconstitution (cherry-banana)

Zithromax Tri-pak *Tab:* 3 x 500 mg tabs/pck

Zithromax Z-pak *Tab:* 6 x 250 mg tabs/pck

Zmax *Oral susp:* 2 g ext-rel for reconstitution (cherry-banana) (148 mg Na$^+$)

➤ *cefaclor* (B)(G) 250-500 mg q 8 hours x 7-10 days
Pediatric: <1 month: not recommended; 20-40 mg/kg bid or q 12 hours x 10 days; max 1 g/day; *see page 560 for dose by weight*
Tab: 500 mg; *Cap:* 250, 500 mg; *Susp:* 125 mg/5 ml (75, 150 ml) (strawberry); 187 mg/5 ml (50, 100 ml) (strawberry); 250 mg/5 ml (75, 150 ml) (strawberry); 375 mg/5 ml (50, 100 ml) (strawberry)

Cefaclor Extended Release

Pediatric: <16 years: ext-rel not recommended
Tab: 375, 500 mg ext-rel

➤ *cefdinir* (B) 300 mg bid or 600 mg daily x 5-10 days
Pediatric: <6 months: not recommended; 6 months-12 years: 14 mg/kg/day in 1-2 divided doses x 10 days; >12 years: same as adult; *see page 562 for dose by weight*

Omnicef *Cap:* 300 mg; *Oral susp:* 125 mg/5 ml (60, 100 ml) (strawberry)

➤ *cefixime* (B)
Pediatric: <6 months: not recommended; 6 months-12 years, <50 kg: 8 mg/kg/day in 1-2 divided doses x 10 days; >12 years, ≥50 kg: same as adult; *see page 563 for dose by weight*

Suprax *Tab:* 400 mg; *Cap:* 400 mg; *Oral susp:* 100, 200 mg/5 ml (50, 75, 100 ml) (strawberry)

➤ *cefpodoxime proxetil* (B) 100 mg bid x 5 days
Pediatric: <2 months: not recommended; 2 months-12 years: 10 mg/kg/day (max 400 mg/dose) or 5 mg/kg/day bid (max 200 mg/dose) x 5 days; >12 years: same as adult; *see page 564 for dose by weight*

Vantin *Tab:* 100, 200 mg; *Oral susp:* 50, 100 mg/5 ml (50, 75, 100 ml) (lemon creme)

➤ *cefprozil* (B) 250-500 mg bid or 500 mg daily x 10 days
Pediatric: <2 years: same as adult; 2-12 years: 7.5 mg/kg bid x 10 days; >12 years: same as adult

see page 565 for dose by weight
> **Cefzil** *Tab:* 250, 500 mg; *Oral susp:* 125, 250 mg/5 ml (50, 75, 100 ml) (bubble gum) (phenylalanine)

▷ *ceftibuten* (B) 400 mg daily x 10 days
Pediatric: 9 mg/kg daily x 10 days; max 400 mg/day; *see page 566 for dose by weight*
> **Cedax** *Cap:* 400 mg; *Oral susp:* 90 mg/5 ml (30, 60, 90, 120 ml); 180 mg/5 ml (30, 60, 120 ml) (cherry)

▷ *ceftriaxone* (B)(G) 1-2 g IM x 1 dose; max 4 g
Pediatric: 50 mg/kg IM x 1 dose
> **Rocephin** *Vial:* 250, 500 mg; 1, 2 g

▷ *cefuroxime axetil* (B)(G) 250-500 mg bid x 10 days
Pediatric: 15 mg/kg bid x 10 days; *see page 567 for dose by weight*
> **Ceftin** *Tab:* 250, 500 mg; *Oral susp:* 125, 250 mg/5 ml (50, 100 ml) (tutti-frutti)

▷ *cephalexin* (B)(G) 250 mg qid x 10 days
Pediatric: 25-50 mg/kg/day in 4 doses x 10 days; *see page 568 for dose by weight*
> **Keflex** *Cap:* 250, 333, 500, 750 mg; *Oral susp:* 125, 250 mg/5 ml (100, 200 ml) (strawberry)

▷ *clarithromycin* (C)(G) 500 mg bid <u>or</u> 500 mg ext-rel daily
Pediatric: <6 months: not recommended; ≥6 months: 7.5 mg/kg divided bid x 7 days; *see page 569 for dose by weight*
> **Biaxin** *Tab:* 250, 500 mg
> **Biaxin Oral Suspension** *Oral susp:* 125, 250 mg/5 ml (50, 100 ml) (fruit-punch)
> **Biaxin XL** *Tab:* 500 mg ext-rel

▷ *erythromycin/sulfisoxazole* (C)(G)
Pediatric: <2 months: not recommended; ≥2 months: 50 mg/kg/day in 3 divided doses x 10 days
> **Eryzole** *Oral susp: eryth* 200 mg/*sulf* 600 mg per 5 ml (100, 150, 200, 250 ml)
> **Pediazole** *Oral susp: eryth* 200 mg/*sulf* 600 mg per 5 ml (100, 150, 200 ml) (strawberry-banana)

Comment: *erythromycin* may increase INR with concomitant *warfarin*, as well as increase serum level of *digoxin*, benzodiazepines and statins. *sulfamethoxazole* is not recommended in pregnancy or lactation. *CrCl 15-30 mL/min*: reduce dose by 1/2; *CrCl <15 mL/min*: not recommended.

▷ *loracarbef* (B) 400 mg bid x 10 days
Pediatric: 30 mg/kg/day in divided bid x 7 days; *see page 581 for dose by weight*
> **Lorabid** *Pulvule:* 200, 400 mg; *Oral susp:* 100 mg/5 ml (50, 100 ml); 200 mg/5 ml (50, 75, 100 ml) (strawberry bubble gum)

▷ *trimethoprim/sulfamethoxazole* (C)(G)
Pediatric: <2 months: not recommended; >2 months: 40 mg/kg/day of *sulfamethoxazole* in divided doses bid x 10 days; *see page 587 for dose by weight*
> **Bactrim, Septra** 2 tabs bid x 10 days
> *Tab: trim* 80 mg/*sulfa* 400 mg*
> **Bactrim DS, Septra DS** 1 tab bid x 10 days
> *Tab: trim* 160 mg/*sulfa* 800 mg*
> **Bactrim Pediatric Suspension, Septra Pediatric Suspension**
> *Oral susp: trim* 40 mg/*sulfa* 200 mg per 5 ml (100 ml) (cherry) (alcohol 0.3%)

Comment: *trimethoprim/sulfamethoxazole* is not recommended in pregnancy <u>or</u> lactation. *CrCl 15-30 mL/min*: reduce dose by 1/2; *CrCl <15 mL/min*: not recommended.

OTIC ANTI-INFECTIVE

▷ *ofloxacin* (C)(G) 10 drops bid x 14 days
   Pediatric: <6 months: not recommended; 6 months-12 years: 5 drops bid x 14
   days; >12 years: same as adult
   Floxin Otic *Otic soln:* 0.3% (5, 10 ml w. dropper)
 Comment: *ofloxacin* may be used with patients with perforated tympanic
membrane <u>or</u> tympanostomy tubes.

Otic Anti-infective/Corticosteroid Combinations

Comment: *neomycin* may cause ototoxicity. Do not use with known <u>or</u> suspected
tympanic membrane rupture.
▷ *chloroxylenol/pramoxine/hydrocortisone* (C) 4 drops tid-qid x 5-10 days
 Pediatric: 3 drops tid-qid x 5-10 days
  Cortane Ear Drops, *Otic drops:* 10 ml
▷ *ciprofloxacin/hydrocortisone* (C) otic susp 3 drops bid x 7 days
 Pediatric: <1 year: not recommended; ≥1 year: same as adult
  Cipro HC *Otic susp:* cipro 0.3%/*dexa* 0.1% (10 ml)
▷ *ciprofloxacin/dexamethasone* (C) otic susp 4 drops bid x 7 days
 Pediatric: <6 months: not recommended; ≥6 months: same as adult
  Ciprodex *Otic susp:* cipro 0.3%/*dexa* 1% (7.5 ml)
  Comment: **Ciprodex** is indicated for the treatment of otitis media in pediatric
  patients with tympanostomy tubes (PE tubes).
▷ *colistin/neomycin/hydrocortisone/thonzonium* (C) 5 drops tid-qid x 5-10 days
 Pediatric: 4 drops tid-qid x 5-10 days
  Coly-Mycin S *Otic susp:* 5, 10 ml
▷ *polymyxin b/neomycin/hydrocortisone* (C)(G) 4 drops tid-qid; max 10 days
 Pediatric: 3 drops tid-qid; max 10 days
  Cortisporin *Otic susp:* 10 ml w. dropper; *Otic soln:* 10 ml w. dropper
  PediOtic *Otic susp:* 7.5 ml w. dropper
▷ *polymyxin B/neomycin/hydrocortisone/surfactant* (C) 4 drops tid-qid
 Pediatric: 3 drops tid-qid; max 10 days
  Cortisporin-TC *Otic susp:* 10 ml w. dropper

OTIC ANESTHETIC/ANALGESIC COMBINATIONS

▷ *antipyrine/benzocaine/glycerine* (C) fill ear canal and insert cotton plug; may repeat
q 1-2 hours as needed
Pediatric: same as adult
  A/B Otic *Otic soln:* antipy 5.4%/*benzo* 1.4% 15 ml w. dropper
▷ *benzocaine* (C)(OTC) 4-5 drops q 1-2 hours
 Pediatric: <1 year: not recommended; ≥1 year: same as adult
  Otic drops: 20% (15 ml dropper-top bottle)
  Americaine Otic *Otic soln:* 15 ml w. dropper
  Benzotic *Otic soln:* 20% (15 ml w. dropper)

 OTITIS MEDIA: SEROUS

Anti-infectives *see* **Otitis Media: Acute** *page* 301
Oral Drugs for Allergy, Cough, and Cold *see page* 535
Oral Corticosteroids *see page* 509

PAGET'S DISEASE: BONE

Comment: Calcium decreases *tetracycline* absorption. **calcium** absorption is decreased by corticosteroids. **calcium** absorption is decreased by foods such as rhubarb, spinach, and bran.

BISPHOSPHONATES (CALCIUM MODIFIERS)

Comment: Biphosphonates should be swallowed whole in the AM with 6-8 oz of plain water 30 minutes before first meal, beverage, <u>or</u> other medications of the day. Monitor serum alkaline phosphatase. Contraindications include abnormalities of the esophagus which delay esophageal emptying such as stricture <u>or</u> achalasia, inability to stand <u>or</u> sit upright for at least 30 minutes post-dose, patients at risk of aspiration, and hypocalcemia. Coadministration of biphosphonates and calcium, antacids, <u>or</u> oral medications containing multivalent cations will interfere with absorption of the bophosphonate. Therefore, instruct patients to wait at least half hour after taking the biphosphonate before taking any other oral medications.

▷ *alendronate (as sodium)* (C) take once weekly, in the AM, 30 minutes before the first food, beverage, <u>or</u> medication of the day; do not lie down (remain upright) for at least 30 minutes and after the first food of the day; not recommended with *CrCl <35 mL/min.*

Pediatric: not recommended

Binosto dissolve the effervescent tab in 4 oz (120 ml) of plain, room temperature, water (not mineral <u>or</u> flavored); wait 5 minutes after the effervescence has subsided, then stir for 10 seconds, then drink

Tab: 70 mg effervescent for buffered solution (4, 12/carton) (strawberry)

Fosamax (G) swallow tab whole; dosing regimens are the same for men and post-menopausal women; *Prevention:* 5 mg once daily <u>or</u> 35 mg once weekly; *Treatment:* 10 mg once daily <u>or</u> 70 mg once weekly

Tab: 5, 10, 35, 40, 70 mg

▷ *alendronate/cholecalciferol (vit d3)* (C)(G) take 1 tab once weekly, in the AM, with plain water (not mineral) 30 minutes before the first food, beverage, <u>or</u> medication of the day; do not lie down (remain upright) for at least 30 minutes and after the first food of the day

Pediatric: not recommended

Fosamax Plus D

Tab: **Fosamax Plus D 70/2800** *alen* 70 mg/*chole* 2800 IU

Fosamax Plus D 70/5600 *alen* 70 mg/*chole* 5600 IU

▷ *ibandronate (as monosodium monohydrate)* (C)(G)

Pediatric: not recommended

Boniva take 2.5 mg once daily <u>or</u> 150 mg once monthly on the same day; take in the AM, with plain water (not mineral) 60 minutes before the first food, beverage, <u>or</u> medication of the day; do not lie down (remain upright) for at least 30 minutes and after the first food of the day

Tab: 2.5, 150 mg

Boniva Injection administer 3 mg every 3 months by IV bolus over 15-30 seconds; if dose is missed, administer as soon as possible, then every 3 months from the date of the last dose

Prefilled syringe: 3 mg/3 ml (5 ml)

Comment: **Boniva Injection** must be administered by a qualified health care professional.

▷ *risedronate (as sodium)* **(C)(G)** take in the AM; swallow whole with a full glass of plain water (not mineral) do not lie down (remain upright) for 30 minutes afterward
Pediatric: not recommended

> **Actonel** take at least 30 minutes before any food or drink; *Women:* 5 mg once daily or 35 mg once weekly or 75 mg on two consecutive days monthly or 150 mg once monthly; *Men:* 35 mg once weekly; *Tab:* 5, 30, 35, 75, 150 mg
> **Atelvia** 35 mg once weekly immediately after breakfast
> *Tab:* 35 mg del-rel

▷ *risedronate/calcium* **(C)** 1 x 5 mg *risedronate* tab weekly and 1 x 500 mg *calcium* tab on days 2-7 weekly

> **Actonel with Calcium** *Tab:* risedronate 5 mg and *Tab:* calcium 500 mg (4 *risedronate* tabs + 30 *calcium* tabs/pck)

▷ *zoledronic acid* **(D)(G)**
Pediatric: not recommended

> **Reclast** administer 5 mg via IV infusion over at least 15 minutes mg once a year (for osteoporosis) or once every 2 years (for osteopenia or prophylaxis)
> *Bottle:* 5 mg/100 ml (single-dose)
> **Comment:** **Reclast** is indicated for the treatment of postmenopausal osteoporosis in women who are at high risk for fracture and to increase bone mass in men with primary or hypogonadal osteoporosis who are at high risk for fracture. Administered by a qualified health care professional. Contraindicated in hypocalcemia.
> **Zometa** administer 4 mg via IV infusion over at least 15 minutes every 3-4 weeks; optimal duration of treatment not known
> *Bottle:* 4 mg/5 ml; *Vial:* 4 mg/5 ml (single-dose)
> **Comment:** **Zometa** is indicated for the treatment of hypercalcemia of malignancy. The safety and efficacy of **Zometa** in the treatment of hypercalcemia associated with hyperparathyroidism or with other nontumor-related conditions has not been established.

 PAIN

Antidepressants *see Depression page* 105
Skeletal Muscle Relaxants *see Muscle Strain page* 273

ACETAMINOPHEN FOR IV INFUSION

▷ *acetaminophen* injectable **(B)** administer by IV infusion over 15 minutes; 1,000 mg q 6 hours prn or 650 mg q 4 hours prn; max 4,000 mg/day
Pediatric: <2 years: not recommended; 2-13 years <50 kg: 15 mg/kg q 6 hours prn or 2.5 mg/kg q 4 hours prn; max 750 mg single-dose; max 75 mg/kg per day; >13 years: same as adult

> **Ofirmev** *Vial:* 10 mg/ml (100 ml) (preservative-free)
> **Comment:** The **Ofirmev** vial is intended for single-use. If any portion is withdrawn from the vial, use within 6 hours. Discard the unused portion. For pediatric patients, withdraw the intended dose and administer via syringe pump. Do not admix **Ofirmev** with any other drugs. **Ofirmev** is physically incompatible with *diazepam* and *chlorpromazine hydrochloride*.

IBUPROFEN FOR IV INFUSION

➤ *ibuprofen* (B) dilute dose in 0.9% NS, D5W, or Lactated Ringers (LR) solution; administer by IV infusion over at least 10 minutes; do not administer via IV bolus or IM; 400-800 mg q 6 hours prn; maximum 3,200 mg/day
Pediatric: <6 months; not recommended; 6 months-<12 years: 10 mg/kg q 4-6 hours prn; max 400 mg/dose; max 40 mg/kg or 2,400 mg/24 hours, whichever is less; 12-17 years: 400 mg q 4-6 hours prn; max 2,400 mg/24 hours
    Caldolor *Vial:* 800 mg/8 ml single-dose
    Comment: Prepare Caldolor dolutiion for IV administration as follows: 100 mg dose: dilute 1 ml of **Caldolor** in at least 100 ml of diluent (IVF); 200 mg dose: dilute 2 ml of **Caldolor** in at least 100 ml of diluent; 400 mg dose: dilute 4 ml of Caldolor in at least 100 ml of diluent; 800 mg dose: dilute 8 ml of **Caldolor** in at least 200 ml of diluent. **Caldolor** is also indicated for management of fever. For adults with fever, 400 mg via IV infusion, followed by 400 mg q 4-6 hours or 100-200 mg q 4 hours prn.

OCULAR PAIN

➤ *difluprednate* (C) apply 1 drop to affected eye qid; for postop ocular pain, begin treatment 24 hours postop and continue x 2 weeks; then bid daily x 1 week; then taper
Pediatric: not recommended
    Durezol *Ophth emul:* 0.05% (5 ml)
    Comment: **Durezol** is an ophthalmic steroid.
➤ *nepafenac* (C) apply 1 drop to affected eye tid; for postop ocular pain, begin treatment 24 hours before surgery and continue day of surgery and for two weeks post-op
Pediatric: <10 years: not recommended; ≥10 years: same as adult
    Nevanac *Ophth susp:* 0.1% (3 ml) (benzalkonium chloride)
    Comment: **Nevanac** is an ophthalmic NSAID.

TOPICAL/TRANSDERMAL NSAIDs

➤ *capsaicin* (B)(G) apply tid-qid prn to intact skin
Pediatric: <2 years: not recommended; ≥2 years: apply sparingly tid-qid prn
    Axsain *Crm:* 0.075% (1, 2 oz)
    Capsin *Lotn:* 0.025, 0.075% (59 ml)
    Capzasin-P (OTC) *Crm:* 0.025% (1.5 oz); *Lotn:* 0.025% (2 oz)
    Dolorac *Crm:* 0.025% (28 g)
    Double Cap (OTC) *Crm:* 0.05% (2 oz)
    R-Gel *Gel:* 0.025% (15, 30 g)
    Zostrix (OTC) *Crm:* 0.025% (0.7, 1.5, 3 oz)
    Zostrix HP (OTC) *Emol crm:* 0.075% (1, 2 oz)
➤ *capsaicin* 8% patch (B) apply up to 4 patches for one 60-minute application to clean dry skin; may prep area with topical anesthetic; wear nonlatex gloves; patches may be cut to size/shape; treatment may be repeated every 3 months; remove with cleansing gel after treatment
Pediatric: <18 years: not recommended
    Qutenza *Patch:* 8% 1640 mcg/cm (179 mg) (1 or 2 patches, each w. 1-50 g tube cleansing gel/carton)

▷ *diclofenac epolamine transdermal patch* (C; D ≥30 wks) apply one patch to affected area bid; remove during bathing; avoid non-intact skin
  Pediatric: not recommended
    Flector Patch *Patch:* 180 mg/patch (30/carton)
▷ *diclofenac sodium* (C; D ≥30 wks)(G)
  Pediatric: not established
    Pennsaid 1.5% in 10 drop increments, dispense and rub into front, side, and back of knee: usually; 40 drops (40 mg) qid
      Topical soln: 1.5% (150 ml)
    Pennsaid 2% apply 2 pump actuations (40 mg) and rub into front, side, and back of knee bid
      Topical soln: 2% (20 mg/pump actuation, 112 g)
    Comment: **Pennsaid** is indicated for the treatment of pain associated with osteoarthritis of the knee.
      Pediatric: not recommended
    Voltaren Gel apply qid; avoid nonintact skin
      Gel: 1% (100 g)
    Comment: *diclofenac* is contraindicated with *aspirin* allergy. As with other NSAIDs, **Voltaren Gel** should be avoided in late pregnancy (≥30 weeks) because it may cause premature closure of the ductus arteriosus.
    Other Prescription NSAIDs *see page* 501

TOPICAL/TRANSDERMAL LIDOCAINE

▷ *lidocaine* transdermal patch (C)(G) apply one patch to affected area for 12 hours (then off for 12 hours); remove during bathing; avoid non-intact skin; do not re-use
  Pediatric: not recommended
    Lidoderm *Patch:* 5% (10 cm x14 cm, 30/carton)

OPIOIDS AND OTHER ORAL ANALGESICS

▷ *butalbital/acetaminophen* (C)(G) 1 tab q 4 hours prn; max 6 tabs/day
  Pediatric: <12 years: not recommended; ≥12 years: same as adult
    Tab: but 50 mg/*acet* 325 mg
    Phrenilin 1-2 tabs q 4 hours prn; max 6 tabs/day
      Tab: but 50 mg/*acet* 325 mg
    Phrenilin Forte 1 tab or cap q 4 hours prn; max 6 caps/day
      Cap: but 50 mg/*acet* 325 mg; *Tab: but* 50 mg/*acet* 325 mg
▷ *butalbital/acetaminophen/caffeine* (C)(G)
  Pediatric: not recommended
    Fioricet 1-2 tabs q 4 hours prn; max 6/day
      Tab: but 50 mg/*acet* 325 mg/*caf* 40 mg
    Zebutal 1 cap q 4 hours prn; max 5/day
      Cap: but 50 mg/*acet* 325 mg/*caf* 40 mg
▷ *butalbital/aspirin/caffeine* (C)(III)(G)
  Pediatric: <12 years: not recommended; ≥12 year: same as adult
    Fiorinal 1-2 tabs or caps q 4 hours prn; max 6 caps/day
      Tab/Cap: but 50 mg/*asa* 325 mg/*caf* 40 mg
▷ *butalbital/aspirin/codeine/caffeine* (C)(III)(G)
  Pediatric: <12 years: not recommended; ≥12 year: same as adult
    Fiorinal with Codeine 1-2 caps q 4 hours prn; max 6 caps/day
      Cap: but 50 mg/*asp* 325 mg/*cod* 30 mg/*caf* 40 mg

➤ *codeine sulfate* (C)(III)(G) 15-60 q 4-6 hours prn; max 60 mg/day
  Tab: 15, 30, 60 mg
➤ *codeine/acetaminophen* (C)(III)(G) 15-60 mg of *codeine* q 4 hours prn; max 360 mg of *codeine*/day
  Pediatric: not recommended
    Tab: **Tylenol #1** *cod* 7.5 mg/*acet* 300 mg (sulfites)
        Tylenol #2 *cod* 15 mg/*acet* 300 mg (sulfites)
        Tylenol #3 *cod* 30 mg/*acet* 300 mg (sulfites)
        Tylenol #4 *cod* 60 mg/*acet* 300 mg (sulfites)
        Tylenol with Codeine Elixir (C)(III)
        Pediatric: 1 mg of *codeine*/kg/dose q 4-6 hours prn; max 60 mg of *codeine*/dose; <3 years: not recommended; 3-6 years: 5 ml tid-qid; 7-12 years: 10 ml tid-qid; >12 years: same as adult
        Elix: cod 12 mg/acet 120 mg per 5 ml (cherry) (alcohol)
➤ *dihydrocodeine/acetaminophen/caffeine* (C)(III)(G)
  Pediatric: not recommended
    Panlor DC 1-2 caps q 4-6 hours prn; max 10 caps/day
      Cap: dihydro 16 mg/acet 325 mg/caf 30 mg
    Panlor SS 1 tab q 4 hours prn; max 5 tabs/day
      Tab: dihydro 32 mg/acet 325 mg/caf 60*mg
➤ *dihydrocodeine/aspirin/caffeine* (D)(III)(G) 1-2 caps q 4 hours prn
  Pediatric: not recommended
    Synalgos-DC
      Cap: dihydro 16 mg/asa 356.4 mg/caf 30 mg
➤ *hydrocodone bitartrate* (C)(II)
  Pediatric: <12 years: not recommended
    Hysingla ER swallow whole; 1 tab once daily at the same time each day
      Tab: 20, 30, 40, 60, 80, 100, 120 mg ext-rel
    Vantrela ER swallow whole; 1 tab once daily at the same time each day
      Tab: 15, 30, 45, 60, 90 mg ext-rel
    Zohydro ER swallow whole; *Opioid naïve:* 10 mg q 12 hours; may increase by 10 mg q 12 hours every 3-7 days; when discontinuing, titrate downward every 2-4 days
      Cap: 10, 15, 20, 30, 40, 50 mg ext-rel
➤ *hydrocodone bitartrate/acetaminophen* (C)(II)(G)
  Pediatric: not recommended
    Hycet 3 tsp (15 ml) q 4-6 hours prn; max 18 tsp/day
      Liq: hydro 7.5 mg/acet 325 mg per 15 ml
    Lorcet 1-2 caps q 4-6 hours prn; max 8 caps/day
      Cap: hydro 5 mg/acet 325 mg
    Lorcet 10/650 1 tab q 4-6 hours prn; max 6 tabs/day
      Tab: hydro 10 mg/acet 325 mg
    Lorcet-HD 1 cap q 4-6 hours prn; max 6 tabs/day
      Cap: hydro 5 mg/acet 325 mg
    Lorcet Plus 1 tab q 4-6 hours prn; max 6 tabs/day
      Tab: hydro 7.5 mg/acet 325 mg
    Lortab 2.5/500 1-2 tabs q 4-6 hours prn; max 8 tabs/day
      Tab: hydro 2.5 mg/acet 325*mg
    Lortab 5/500 1-2 tabs q 4-6 hours prn; max 8 tabs/day
      Tab: hydro 5 mg/acet 325*mg

    Lortab 7.5/500 1 tab q 4-6 hours prn; max 6 tabs/day
      Tab: hydro 7.5 mg/*acet* 325*mg
    Lortab 10/500 1 tab q 4-6 hours prn; max 6 tabs/day
      Tab: hydro 10 mg/*acet* 325*mg
    Lortab Elixir 3 tsp q 4-6 hours prn; max 18 tsp/day
      Liq: hydro 7.5 mg/*acet* 300 mg per 15 ml (tropical fruit punch) (alcohol)
    Maxidone 1 tab q 4-6 hours prn; max 5 tabs/day
      Tab: hydro 10 mg/*acet* 325*mg
    Norco 5/325 1 tab q 4-6 hours prn; max 8 tabs/day
      Tab: hydro 5 mg/*acet* 325*mg
    Norco 7.5/325 1 tab q 4-6 hours prn; max 6 tabs/day
      Tab: hydro 7.5 mg/*acet* 325*mg
    Norco 10/325 1 tab q 4-6 hours prn; max 6 tabs/day
      Tab: hydro 10 mg/*acet* 325*mg
    Vicodin 1-2 tabs q 4-6 hours prn; max 8 tabs/day
      Tab: hydro 5 mg/*acet* 300*mg
    Vicodin ES 1 tab q 4-6 hours prn; max 6 tabs/day
      Tab: hydro 7.5 mg/*acet* 300*mg
    Vicodin HP 1 tab q 4-6 hours prn; max 6 tabs/day
      Tab: hydro 10 mg/*acet* 300*mg
    Xodol 5/300 1-2 tabs q 4-6 hours prn; max 8 caps/day
      Tab: hydro 5 mg/*acet* 300*mg
    Xodol 7.5/300 1 tab q 4-6 hours prn; max 6 caps/day
      Tab: hydro 7.5 mg/*acet* 300*mg
    Xodol 10/300 1 tab q 4-6 hours prn; max 6 caps/day
      Tab: hydro 10 mg/*acet* 300*mg
    Zamicet 10/325 1-2 tabs q 4-6 hours prn; max 8 caps/day
      Liq: hydro 10 mg/*acet* 325 mg per 15 ml
    Zydone 5/400 1-2 tabs q 4-6 hours prn; max 8 caps/day
      Tab: hydro 5 mg/*acet* 400 mg
    Zydone 7.5/400 1 tab q 4-6 hours prn; max 6 caps/day
      Tab: hydro 7.5 mg/*acet* 400 mg
    Zydone 10/400 1 tab q 4-6 hours prn; max 6 caps/day
▶ *hydrocodone/ibuprofen* (C; not for use in 3rd)(II)(G)
  Pediatric: not recommended
    Ibudone 5/200 1 tab q 4-6 hours prn; max 5 tabs/day
      Tab: hydro 5 mg/*ibup* 200 mg
    Ibudone 10/200 1 tab q 4-6 hours prn; max 5 tabs/day
      Tab: hydro 10 mg/*ibup* 200 mg
    Reprexain 1 tab q 4-6 hours prn; max 5 tabs/day
      Tab: hydro 5 mg/*ibup* 200 mg
    Vicoprofen 1 tab q 4-6 hours prn; max 5 tabs/day
      Tab: hydro 7.5 mg/*ibup* 200 mg
▶ *hydromorphone* (C)(II)(G)
  Pediatric: not recommended
    Dilaudid initially 2-4 mg q 4-6 hours prn
      Tab: 2, 4, 8 mg (sulfites)
    Dilaudid Oral Liquid 2.5-10 mg q 3-6 hours prn
      Liq: 5 mg/5 ml (sulfites)
    Dilaudid Rectal Suppository 2.5-10 mg q 6-8 hours prn

       Rectal supp: 3 mg

   Dilaudid Injection initially 1-2 mg SC <u>or</u> IM q 4-6 hours prn
      Amp: 1, 2, 4 mg/ml (1 ml)
   Dilaudid-HP Injection initially 1-2 mg SC <u>or</u> IM q 4-6 hours prn
      Amp: 10 mg/ml (1 ml)
   Exalgo initially 8-64 mg once daily
      Tab: 8, 12, 16, 32 mg ext-rel (sulfites)

▷ *meperidine* **(C; D in 2nd, 3rd)(II)(G)** 50-150 mg q 3-4 hours prn
   Pediatric: 0.5-0.8 mg/lb q 3-4 hours prn; max adult dose
   Demerol *Tab:* 50, 100 mg; *Syr:* 50 mg/5 ml (banana) (alcohol-free)

▷ *meperidine/promethazine* **(C; D in 2nd, 3rd)(II)(G)**
   Pediatric: not recommended
   Mepergan 1-2 tsp q 3-4 hours prn
      Syr: mep 25 mg/*prom* 25 mg per ml
   Mepergan Fortis 1-2 tsp q 4-6 hours prn
      Tab: mep 50 mg/*prom* 25 mg

▷ *methadone* **(C)(II)** 2.5-10 mg PO, SC, <u>or</u> IM q 3-4 hours prn
   Pediatric: not recommended
   Dolophine *Tab:* 5, 10 mg; *Dispersible tab:* 40 mg (dissolve in 120 ml orange juice
   <u>or</u> other citrus drink); *Oral conc:* 5, 10 mg/5 ml; 10 mg/10 ml; *Inj:* 10 mg/ml
Comment: **methadone** maintenance is allowed only by approved treatment
programs with strict state and federal regulations.

▷ *morphine sulfate* **(C)(II)(G)** tabs, usually 15-30 mg q 4 hours prn; solution, usually
10-20 mg q 4 hours prn
   Pediatric: <18 years: not recommended
      Tab: 15*, 30*mg; *Oral soln:* 10 mg/5 ml, 20 mg/5 ml (100, 500 ml), 100 mg/5 ml
      (30, 120 ml)

▷ *morphine sulfate (immed- and sust-rel)* **(C)(II)**
Comment: Dosage dependent upon previous opioid dosage; see mfr pkg insert
for conversion guidelines; not for prn use; swallow whole <u>or</u> sprinkle contents of
caps on applesauce (do not crush, chew, <u>or</u> dissolve). Generic *morphine sulfate* is
available in the following forms: *Tab:* 15*, 30*mg; *Oral soln:* 10, 20 mg/5 ml (100
ml); 100 mg/5 ml (30, 120 ml w. oral syringe)
   Pediatric: <18 years: not recommended
   Arymo ER swallow whole; 1 tab once daily at the same time each day
      Tab: 15, 30, 60 mg ext-rel
   Duramorph administer per anesthesia
      IV/Intrathecal/Epidural: 0.5, 1 mg/ml
   Infumorph administer per anesthesia
      Intrathecal/Epidural: 10, 20 mg/ml
   Kadian (G) 1 cap every 12-24 hours
      Cap: 10, 20, 30, 50, 60, 80, 100, 200 mg sust-rel
   MS Contin (G) 1 tab every 24 hours
      Tab: 15, 30, 60, 100, 200 mg sust-rel
   MSIR 5-30 mg q 4 hours prn
      Tab: 15*, 30*mg; *Cap:* 15, 30 mg
   MSIR Oral Solution 5-30 mg q 4 hours prn
      Oral soln: 10, 20 mg/5 ml (120 ml)
   MSIR Oral Solution Concentrate 5-30 mg q 4 hours prn
      Oral conc: 20 mg/ml (30, 120 ml w. dropper)

Oramorph SR 1 cap every 12-24 hours
Tab: 15, 30, 60, 100 mg sust-rel
Roxanol Oral Solution 10-30 mg q 4 hours prn
Oral soln: 20 mg/ml (1, 4, 8 oz)
Roxanol Rescudose
Oral soln: 10 mg/2.5 ml (25 single-dose)
▷ *morphine sulfate/naltrexone* (C)(II)
Pediatric: <18 years: not recommended
Embeda 1 cap q 12-24 hours
Cap: **Embeda 20/0.8** *morph* 20 mg/*nal* 0.8 mg ext-rel
Embeda 30/1.2 *morph* 30 mg/*nal* 1.2 mg ext-rel
Embeda 50/2 *morph* 50 mg/*nal* 2 mg ext-rel
Embeda 60/2.4 *morph* 60 mg/*nal* 2.4 mg ext-rel
Embeda 80/3.2 *morph* 80 mg/*nal* 3.2 mg ext-rel
Embeda 100/4 *morph* 100 mg/*nal* 4 mg ext-rel
Comment: **Embeda** is not for prn use; for use in opioid-tolerant patients only; swallow whole or sprinkle contents of caps on applesauce (do not crush, chew, or dissolve); do not administer via NG or gastric tube (PEG tube).
▷ *oxycodone* (B)(II)(G) 5-15 mg q 4-6 hours prn
Comment: Concomitant use os CYP3A4 inhibitors may increase opioid effects and CYP3A4 inducers may decrease effects or possibly cause development of an abstinence syndrome (withdrawal symtoms) in patients who are physically *oxycodone* dependent/addicted.
Pediatric: <18 years: not recommended
Oxaydo *Tab:* 5, 7.5 mg
Comment: **Oxaydo** is the first and only immediate-release oral *oxycodone* that discourages intranasal abuse. **Oxaydo** is formulated with sodium lauryl sulfate, an inactive ingredient that may cause nasal burning and throat irritation when snorted and, thus potentially reducing abuse liability. There is no generic equivalent.
Oxecta *Tab:* 5, 7.5 mg
Oxycodone Oral Solution (G) *Oral soln:* 5 mg/5 ml (15, 30 ml)
OxyIR (G) *Cap:* 5 mg
Roxycodone *Tab:* 5, 15*, 30*mg; *Oral soln:* 5 mg/ml
Roxycodone Intensol *Oral soln:* 20 mg/ml
▷ *oxycodone cont-rel* (B)(II)(G) dosage dependent upon previous opioid dosages; see mfr pkg insert: <11 years: not recommended; 11-16 years: must already tolerate minimum opium dose equal to *oxycodone* 20 mg/day x 5 days; >16 year: same as adult
OxyContin dose q 12 hours
Tab: 10, 15, 20, 30, 40, 60, 80 mg cont-rel
OxyFast dose q 6 hours
Oral conc: 20 mg/ml (30 ml w. dropper)
Xtampza ER dose q 12 hours
Pediatric: not recommended
Cap: 10, 15, 20, 30, 40 mg ext-rel
Comment: May open the **Xtampza ER** capsule and sprinkle in water or on soft food.
▷ *oxycodone/acetaminophen* (C)(II)(G)
Comment: Maximum 4 grams acetaminophen per day.
Pediatric: not recommended
Magnacet 2.5/400 1 tab q 6 hours prn; max 10 tabs/day

       Tab: oxy 2.5 mg/*acet* 325 mg
    Magnacet 5/400 1 tab q 6 hours prn; max 10 tabs/day
       Tab: oxy 5 mg/*acet* 325 mg
    Magnacet 7.5/400 1 tab q 6 hours prn; max 8 tabs/day
       Tab: oxy 7.5 mg/*acet* 325 mg
    Magnacet 10/400 1 tab q 6 hours prn; max 6 tabs/day
       Tab: oxy 10 mg/*acet* 325 mg
    Percocet 2.5/325 1 tab q 6 hours prn; max 4 g acet/day
       Tab: oxy 2.5 mg/*acet* 325 mg
    Percocet 5/325 1 tab q 6 hours prn; max 4 g acet/day
       Tab: oxy 5 mg/*acet* 325*mg
    Percocet 7.5/325 1 tab q 6 hours prn; max 4 g acet/day
       Tab: oxy 7.5 mg/*acet* 325 mg
    Percocet 7.5/500 1 tabs q 6 hours prn; max 4 g acet/day
       Tab: oxy 7.5 mg/*acet* 325 mg
    Percocet 10/325 1 tabs q 6 hours prn; max 4 g acet/day
       Tab: oxy 10 mg/*acet* 325 mg
    Percocet 10/650 1 tab q 6 hours prn; max 4 g acet/day
       Tab: oxy 10 mg/*acet* 325 mg
    Roxicet 5/325 1 tab/tsp q 6 hours prn
       Tab: oxy 5 mg/*acet* 325 mg; *Oral soln: oxy* 5 mg/*acet* 325 mg per 5 ml
    Roxicet 5/500 1 caplet q 6 hours prn
       Cplt: oxy 5 mg/*acet* 325 mg
    Roxicet Oral Solution 1 tsp q 6 hours prn
       Oral soln: oxy 5 mg/*acet* 325 mg per 5 ml (alcohol 0.4%)
    Tylox 1 cap q 6 hours prn
       Cap: oxy 5 mg/*acet* 325 mg
    Xartemis XR 2 tabs q 12 hours prn
       Tab: oxy 7.5 mg/*acet* 325 mg
▷ *oxycodone/aspirin* (D)(II)(G)
    Percodan 1 tab q 6 hours prn
       Pediatric: not recommended
       Tab: oxy 4.8355 mg/*asa* 325*mg
    Percodan-Demi 1-2 tabs q 6 hours prn
       Pediatric: 6-12 years: 1/4 tab q 6 hours prn; >12-18 years: 1/2 tab q 6 hours prn
       Tab: oxy 2.25 mg/*oxy tere* 0.19 mg/*asa* 325 mg
▷ *oxycodone/ibuprofen* (C)(II)(G)
    Pediatric: <14 years: not recommended; ≥14 years: same as adult
    Combunox 1 tab q 6 hours prn
       Tab: oxy 5 mg/*ibu* 400*mg
▷ *oxycodone/naloxone* (C)(II) 1 tab q 3-4 hours prn
    Pediatric: not recommended
    Targiniq
       Tab: **Targiniq 10/5** *oxy* 10 mg/*nal* 5 mg
           Targiniq 20/10 *oxy* 20 mg/*nal* 10 mg
           Targiniq 40/20 *oxy* 40 mg/*nal* 20 mg
▷ *oxymorphone* (C)(II)(G)
    Pediatric: <18 years: not recommended
    Numorphan 1 supp q 4-6 hours prn
       Rectal supp: 5 mg; *Vial:* 1 mg/ml (1 ml), *Amp:* 1.5 mg/ml (10 ml);

Comment: Store in refrigerator in original package. 1 mg of **Numorphan** is approximately equivalent in analgesic activity to 10 mg of ***morphine sulfate***.

Opana 1-1 tab q 4-6 hours prn
    Tab: 5, 10 mg
Opana ER 1 tab q 12 hours prn
    Tab: 5, 7.5, 10, 15, 20, 30, 40 mg ext-rel crush-resistant
Opana Injection initially 0.5 mg IV or IM; 1 x 1 mg IM or IV q 4-6 hours prn
    Amp: 1 mg/ml (1 ml) (paraben/sodium dithionite-free)

▷ *pentazocine/aspirin* (D)(IV) 2 cplts tid or qid prn
Pediatric: not recommended
    Talwin Compound *Cplt:* pent 12.5 mg/*asa* 325 mg

▷ *pentazocine/naloxone* (C)(IV) 1 tab q 3-4 hours prn
Pediatric: not recommended
    Talwin NX *Tab:* pent 50 mg/*nal* 0.5*mg

▷ *pentazocine lactate* (C)(IV) 30 mg IM, SC, or IV q 3-4 hours; max 360 mg/day
Pediatric: <1 year: not recommended; >1 year: 0.5 mg/kg IM
    Talwin Injectable *Amp:* pent 30 mg/ml (1, 1.5, 2 ml)

▷ *propoxyphene napsylate/acetaminophen* (C)(IV)(G)
Comment: Max 4 g acetaminophen per day.
Pediatric: not recommended
    Balacet 325 1 tab q 4 hours prn; max 6 tabs/day
    Tab: prop 100 mg/*acet* 325 mg

▷ *tramadol* (C)(IV)(G)
    Rybix ODT initially 100 mg once daily; may increase by 100 mg every 5 days; max 300 mg/day; *CrCl <30 mL/min* or *severe hepatic impairment:* not recommended; *Cirrhosis:* max 50 mg q 12 hours
        Pediatric: <17 years: not recommended
        ODT: 50 mg (mint) (phenylalanine)
    Ryzolt initially 100 mg once daily; may increase by 100 mg every 5 days; max 300 mg/day; *CrCl <30 mL/min* or *severe hepatic impairment:* not recommended
        Pediatric: <16 years: not recommended; ≥16 years: same as adult
        Tab: 100, 200, 300 mg ext-rel
    Ultram 50-100 mg q 4-6 hours prn; max 400 mg/day; *CrCl <30 mL/min:* max 100 mg q 12 hours; *Cirrhosis:* max 50 mg q 12 hours
        Pediatric: <16 years: not recommended; ≥16 year: same as adult
        Tab: 50*mg
    Ultram ER initially 100 mg once daily; may increase by 100 mg every 5 days; max 300 mg/day; *CrCl <30 mL/min* or *severe hepatic impairment:* not recommended
        Pediatric: <18 years: not recommended
        Tab: 100, 200, 300 mg ext-rel

▷ *tramadol/acetaminophen* (C)(IV)(G) 2 tabs q 4-6 hours; max 8 tabs/day; 5 days; *CrCl <30 mL/min:* max 2 tabs q 12 hours; max 4 tabs/day x 5 days
Pediatric: <16 years: not recommended; ≥16 year: same as adult
    Ultracet *Tab:* tram 37.5/*acet* 325 mg

▷ *buprenorphine* (C)(III) change patch every 7 days; do not increase the dose until previous dose has been worn for at least 72 hours; after removal, do not re-use the site for at least 3 weeks; do not expose the patch to heat
Pediatric: <16 years: not recommended; ≥16 years: same as adult
    Butrans Transdermal System
        Transdermal patch: 5, 10, 20 mcg/hour (4/pck)

▶ *fentanyl* transdermal system **(C)(II)** apply to clean, dry, non-irritated, intact, skin; hold in place for 30 seconds; start at lowest dose and titrate upward; *Opioid-naïve*: change patch every 3 days (72 hours)
Pediatric: <18 years or <110 lb: not recommended
    Duragesic *Transdermal patch*: 12, 25, 37.5, 50, 62.5, 75, 87.5, 100 mcg/hour (5/pck)
▶ *fentanyl iontophoretic transdermal system*
    Ionsys is a transdermal patient-controlled device that sticks to the arm or chest; it is activated when the patient pushes the button
    Comment: **Ionsys** is for in-hospital use only and should be discontinued prior to hospital discharge. It is indicated for post-op pain relief.

TRANSMUCOSAL OPIOID

Comment: For chronic severe pain. For management of breakthrough pain in patients with cancer who are already receiving and who are tolerant to opioid therapy. Opioid-tolerant patients are those taking oral *morphine* ≥60 mg/day, transdermal *fentanyl* ≥25 mcg/hr, *oxycodone* ≥30 mg/day, oral *hydromorphone* ≥8 mg/day, or an equianalgesic dose of another opioid, for ≥1 week

ORAL OPIOID PARTIAL AGONIST-ANTAGONIST

▶ *buprenorphine* **(C)**
Pediatric: <16 years: not recommended; ≥16 year: same as adult
    Subutex 8 mg in a single dose on day 1; then 16 mg in a single dose on day 2; target dose is 16 mg/day in a single dose; dissolve under tongue; do not chew or swallow whole
        SL tab (lemon-lime) or *SL film (lime)*: 2, 8 mg (30/pck)
▶ *fentanyl* buccal soluble film **(C)(II)** dissolve 1 film on moistened area inside cheek; initially 200 mcg; no more than 4 doses/day at least 2 hours apart; max 1200 mcg/dose; do not cut film
Pediatric: <18 years: not recommended
    Onsolis *Buccal film*: 200, 400, 600, 800, 1200 mcg (30 films/pck)
▶ *fentanyl citrate* transmucosal unit **(C)(II)(G)** initially one 200 mcg unit placed between cheek and lower gum; move from side to side; suck (not chew); use 6 units before titrating; titrate dose as needed; max 4 units/day
Pediatric: <18 years: not recommended
    Actiq *Unit*: 200, 400, 600, 800, 1200, 1600 mcg (24 units/pck)
    Fentora *Unit*: 100, 200, 400, 600, 800 mcg (24 units/pck)
▶ *fentanyl* sublingual tab **(C)(II)** initially one 100 mcg dose; if inadequate after 30 minutes, may repeat; titrate in increments of 100 mcg; max 2 doses per episode, up to 4 episodes per day; wait at least 2 hours before treating another episode; *Maintenance*: use only one tablet of appropriate strength; do not chew, suck, or swallow tablets; do not convert from other *fentanyl* products on a mcg-per-mcg basis or interchange with other *fentanyl* products
Pediatric: <18 years: not recommended
    Abstral *SL tab*: 100, 200, 300, 400, 600, 800 mcg (32 tabs/pck)
▶ *fentanyl sublingual spray* **(C)(II)**
Pediatric: <18 years: not recommended
    Subsys 100, 200, 400, 600, 800 mcg/S L spray
    Comment: **Subsys** is not bioequivalent with other *fentanyl* products. Do not convert patients from other *fentanyl* products to **Subsys** on a mcg-per-mcg

basis. There are no conversion directions available for patients on any other *fentanyl* products other than **Actiq**. (Note: This includes oral, transdermal, or parenteral formulations of *fentanyl*.)

PARENTERAL OPIOID AGONIST/ANTAGONIST

▷ *nalbuphine* (B)(G) 10 mg/70 kg IM, SC, or IV q 3-6 hours prn
  Pediatric: <18 years: not recommended
    Nubain *Amp:* 10, 20 mg/ml (1 ml) (sulfite-free, parabens-free)
▷ *pentazocine/naloxone* (C)(IV) 1-2 tabs q 3-4 hours prn; max 12 tabs/day
  Pediatric: <12 years: not recommended; ≥12 year: same as adult
    Talwin-NX *Tab: pent* 50 mg/*nal* 0.5*mg

INTRANASAL TRANSMUCOSAL NARCOTIC ANALGESICS

▷ *butorphanol tartrate* nasal spray (C)(IV) initially 1 spray (1 mg) in one nostril and may repeat after 60-90 minutes (*Elderly* 90-120 minutes) in opposite nostril if needed or 1 spray in each nostril and may repeat q 3-4 hours prn
  Pediatric: <18 years: not recommended
    Butorphanol Nasal Spray *Nasal spray:* 1 mg/actuation (10 mg/ml, 2.5 ml)
    Stadol Nasal Spray *Nasal spray:* 1 mg/actuation (10 mg/ml, 2.5 ml)
▷ *fentanyl* nasal spray (C)(II) initially 1 spray (100 mcg) in one nostril and may repeat after 2 hours; when adequate analgesia is achieved, use that dose for subsequent breakthrough episodes
  Titration steps: 100 mcg using 1 x 100 mcg spray; 200 mcg using 2 x 100 mcg spray (1 in each nostril); 400 mcg using 1 x 400 mcg spray; 800 mcg using 2 x 400 mcg (1 in each nostril); max 800 mcg; limit to ≤4 doses per day
  Pediatric: <18 years: not recommended
    Lazanda Nasal Spray *Nasal spray:* 100, 400 mcg/100 mcl (8 sprays/bottle)
    Comment: **Lazanda Nasal Spray** is available by restricted distribution program. Call 855-841-4234 or visit www.LazandaREMS.com to enroll. **Lazanda Nasal Spray** is indicated for the management of breakthrough pain in cancer patients who are already receiving and who are tolerant to opioid therapy for their underlying persistent cancer pain. Patients considered opioid tolerant are those who are taking at least 60 mg of oral morphine/day, 25 mcg of transdermal *fentanyl*/hour, 30 mg oral *oxycodone*/day, 8 mg oral *hydromorphone*/day, 25 mg oral *oxymorphone*/day, or an equianalgesic dose of another opioid for a week or longer. Patients must remain on around-the-clock opioids when using **Lazanda Nasal Spray**. As such, it is contraindicated in the management of acute or post-op pain, including headache/migraine, or dental pain.

INTRATHECAL NARCOTIC ANALGESICS

▷ *ziconotide* intrathecal (IT) infusion (C) initially no more than 2.4 mcg/day (0.1 mcg/hour) and titrate to upward by up to 2.4 mcg/day (0.1 mcg/day at intervals of no more than 2-3 times per week, up to a recommended maximum of 19.2 mcg/day (0.8 mcg/hr) by Day 21; dose increases in increments of less than 2.4 mcg/day (0.1 mcg/hr) and increases in dose less frequently than 2-3 times per week may be used.
  Pediatric: not recommended
    Prialt *Vial:* 25 mcg/ml (20 ml), 100 mcg/ml (1, 2, 5 ml)
    Comment: Patients with a pre-existing history of psychosis should not be treated with *ziconotide*. Contraindications to the use of IT analgesia include conditions

such as the presence of infection at the microinfusion injection site, uncontrolled bleeding diathesis, and spinal canal obstruction that impairs circulation of CSF.

⬤ PANCREATIC ENZYME DEFICIENCY

Comment: Seen in chronic pancreatitis, postpancreatectomy, cystic fibrosis, steatorrhea, post-GI tract bypass surgery, and ductal obstruction from neoplasia. May sprinkle cap; however, do not crush or chew cap or tab. May mix with applesauce or other acidic food; follow with water or juice. Do not let any drug remain in mouth. Take dose just prior to each meal or snack. Base dose on lipase units; adjust per diet and clinical response (i.e., steatorrhea). Pancrelipase products are interchangeable. Contraindicated with pork protein hypersensitivity.

PANCRELIPASE PRODUCTS

▷ *pancreatic enzymes* (C)

Creon 500 units/kg per meal; max 2,500 units/kg per meal or <10,000 units/kg per day or <4,000 units/g fat ingested per day

Pediatric: <12 months: 2,000-4,000 units per 120 ml formula or per breast-feeding (do not mix directly into formula or breast milk; 12 months to 4 years: 1,000 units/kg per meal; max 2,500 units/kg per meal <10,000 units/kg per day; >4 years: same as adult

Cap: **Creon 3000** *lip* 3,000 units/*pro* 9,500 units/*amyl* 15,000 units del-rel
Creon 6000 *lip* 6,000 units/*pro* 19,000 units/*amyl* 30,000 units del-rel
Creon 12000 *lip* 12,000 units/*pro* 38,000 units/amyl 60,000 units del-rel
Creon 24000 *lip* 24,000 units/*prot* 76,000 units/*amyl* 120,000 units del-rel
Creon 36000 *lip* 36,000 units/*pro*114,000 units/*amyl* 180,000 units del-rel

Cotazym 1-3 tabs just prior to each meal or snack

Pediatric: not recommended

Tab: **Cotazym** *lip* 1,000 units/*pro* 12,500 units/*amyl* 12,500 units del-rel
Cotazym-S *lip* 5,000 units/*pro* 20,000 units/*amyl* 20,000 units del-rel

Donnazyme 1-3 caps just prior to each meal or snack

Pediatric: not recommended

Cap: **Donnazyme** *lip* 5,000 units/*pro* 20,000 units/*amyl* 20,000 units del-rel

Ku-Zyme 1-2 caps just prior to each meal or snack

Pediatric: not recommended

Cap: **Ku-Zyme:** *lip* 12,000 units/*pro* 15,000 units/*amyl* 15,000 units del-rel

Kutrase 1-2 caps just prior to each meal or snack

Pediatric: not recommended

Cap: **Kutrase:** *lip* 12,000 units/*pro* 30,000 units/*amyl* 30,000 units del-rel

Pancreaze 2,500 lipase units/kg per meal or <10,000 lipase units/kg per day or <4,000 lipase units/gram fat ingested per day

Pediatric: <12 months: 2,000-4,000 lipase units per 120 ml formula or per breastfeeding; >12 months to <4 years 1,000 lipase units/kg per meal; >4 years: 500 lipase units/kg per meal; max: adult dose

Cap: **Pancreaze 4200** *lip* 4,200 units/*pro* 10,000 units/*amyl* 17,500 units ec-microtabs
Pancreaze 10500 *lip* 10,500 units/*pro* 25,000 units/*amyl* 43,750 units ec microtabs
Pancrease 16800 *lip* 16,800 units/*pro* 40,000 units/*amyl* 70,000 units ec-microtabs

Pancreaze 21000 *lip* 21,000 units/*pro* 37,000 units/*amyl* 61,000 units ec-microtabs

Pertyze *12 months to 4 years and ≥8 kg:* initially 1,000 lipase units/kg per meal; *≥4 years and ≥16 kg:* initially 500 lipase units/kg per meal; *Both:* 2,500 lipase units/kg per meal or <10,000 units/kg per day or <4,000 lipase units/g fat ingested per day

    Cap: **Pertyze 8000** *lip* 8,000 units/*pro* 28,750 units *amyl* 30,250 units del-rel

Pertyze 16000 *lip* 16,000 units/*pro* 57,500 units/*amyl* 65,000 units del-rel

Ultrase 1-3 tabs just prior to each meal or snack

    Pediatric: same as adult

    Cap: **Ultrase** *lip* 4,500 units/*pro* 20,000 units/*amyl* 25,000 units del-rel

        Ultrase MT *lip* 12,000 units/*pro* 39,000 units/*amyl* 39,000 units del-rel

        Ultrase MT 18 *lip* 18,000 units/*pro* 58,500 units/*amyl* 58,500 units del-rel

        Ultrase MT 20 *lip* 20,000 units/*pro* 65,000 units/*amyl* 65,000 units del-rel

Viokace initially 500 lip units/kg per meal; max 2,500 lipase units/kg per meal, or <10,000 lipase units/kg per meal, or <4,000 units/g fat ingested per day

    Pediatric: same as adult

    Tab: **Viokace 8** *lip* 8,000 units/*pro* 30,000 units/*amyl* 30,000 units

        Viokace 16 *lip* 16,000 units/*pro* 60,000 units *amyl* 60,000 units

        Pediatric: not established

Viokace 0440 *lip* 10,440 units/*pro* 39,150 units *amyl* 39,150 units

Viokace 20880 *lip* 20,880 units/*pro* 78,300 units *amyl* 78,300 units

Comment: **Viokace 10440** and **Viokase 20880** should be taken with a daily proton pump inhibitor.

Viokace Powder 1/4 tsp (0.7 g) with meals

Viokace Powder *lip* 16,800 units/*pro* 70,000 units/*amyl* 70,000 units per 1/4 tsp (8 oz)

Zenpep 500 units/kg per meal; max 2,500 units/kg per meal or <10,000 units/kg per day or <4,000 units/g fat ingested per day

    Pediatric: <12 months: 2,000-4,000 units per 120 ml formula or per breast feeding (do not mix directly into formula or breast milk); 12 months-4 years: 1,000 units/kg per meal; max 2,500 units/kg per meal <10,000 units/kg per day; >4 years: same as adult

    Cap: **Zenpep 5000** *lip* 5,000 units/*prot* 17,000 units/*amyl* 27,000 units del-rel

        Zenpep 10000 *lip* 10,000 units/*prot* 34,000 units/*amyl* 55,000 units del-rel

        Zenpep 15000 *lip* 15,000 units/*prot* 51,000 units/*amyl* 82,000 units del-rel

        Zenpep 20000 *lip* 20,000 units/*prot* 68,000 units/*amyl* 109,000 units del-rel

Zymase 1-3 caps just prior to each meal or snack

    Pediatric: not recommended

    Cap: **Zymase** *lip* 12,000 units/*prot* 24,000 units/*amyl* 24,000 units del-rel

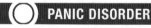

PANIC DISORDER

Comment: If possible when considering a benzodiazepine to treat anxiety, a short-acting benzodiazepines should be used only prn to avert intense anxiety and panic for the least time necessary while a different non-addictive anti-anxiety regimen (e.g., SSRI, SNRI, TCA, buspirone, beta-blocker) is established and effective treatment goals achieved. Co-administration of SSRIs with TCAs requires extreme caution. Concomitant use of MAOIs and SSRIs is absolutely contraindicated. Avoid other serotonergic drugs. A potentially fatal adverse event is *serotonin syndrome*, caused by serotonin excess. Milder symptoms require HCP intervention to avert severe symptoms which can be rapidly fatal without urgent/emergent medical care. Symptoms include restlessness, agitation, confusion, hallucinations, tachycardia, hypertension, dilated pupils, muscle twitching, muscle rigidity, loss of muscle coordination, diaphoresis, diarrhea, headache, shivering, piloerection, hyperpyrexia, cardiac arrhythmias, seizures, loss of consciousness, coma, death. Abrupt withdrawal or interruption of treatment with an antidepressant medication is sometimes associated with an *antidepressant discontinuation syndrome* which may be mediated by gradually tapering the drug over a period of two weeks or longer, depending on the dose strength and length of treatment. Common symptoms of the *serotonin discontinuation syndrome* include flu-like symptoms (nausea, vomiting, diarrhea, headaches, sweating), sleep disturbances (insomnia, nightmares, constant sleepiness), mood disturbances (dysphoria, anxiety, agitation), cognitive disturbances (mental confusion, hyperarousal), sensory and movement disturbances (imbalance, tremors, vertigo, dizziness, electric-shock-like sensations in the brain, often described by sufferers as "brain zaps."

SELECTIVE SEROTONIN REUPTAKE INHIBITORS (SSRIs)

▷ *escitalopram* (C)(G) initially 10 mg daily; may increase to 20 mg daily after 1 week; *Elderly* or *hepatic impairment*: 10 mg once daily
Pediatric: <12 years: not recommended; 12-17 years: initially 10 mg once daily; may increase to 20 mg once daily after 3 weeks
> **Lexapro** *Tab:* 5, 10*, 20*mg
> **Lexapro Oral Solution** *Oral soln:* 1 mg/ml (240 ml) (peppermint) (parabens)

▷ *fluoxetine* (C)(G)
> **Prozac** initially 20 mg daily; may increase after 1 week; doses >20 mg/day should be divided into AM and noon doses; max 80 mg/day
> > *Pediatric:* <7 years: not recommended; 7-17 years: initially 10 mg/day; may increase after 2 weeks to 20 mg/day; range 20-60 mg/day; range for lower weight children 20-30 mg/day
> > *Cap:* 10, 20, 40 mg; *Tab:* 30*, 60*mg; *Oral soln:* 20 mg/5 ml (4 oz) (mint)
> **Prozac Weekly** following daily *fluoxetine* therapy at 20 mg/day for 13 weeks, may initiate **Prozac Weekly** 7 days after the last 20 mg *fluoxetine* dose
> > *Pediatric:* not recommended
> > *Cap:* 90 mg ent-coat del-rel pellets

▷ *paroxetine maleate* (D)(G)
> *Pediatric:* not recommended
> **Paxil** initially 20 mg daily in AM; may increase by 10 mg/day at weekly intervals as needed; max 60 mg/day
> > *Tab:* 10*, 20*, 30, 40 mg
> **Paxil CR** initially 25 mg daily in AM; may increase by 12.5 mg at weekly intervals as needed; max 62.5 mg/day
> > *Tab:* 12.5, 25, 37.5 mg cont-rel ent-coat
> **Paxil Suspension** initially 20 mg daily in AM; may increase by 10 mg/day at weekly intervals as needed; max 60 mg/day
> > *Oral susp:* 10 mg/5 ml (250 ml) (orange)

▷ *sertraline* (C) initially 50 mg daily; increase at 1 week intervals if needed; max 200 mg daily
Pediatric: <6 years: not recommended; 6-12 years: initially 25 mg daily; max 200 mg/day; 13-17 years: initially 50 mg daily; max 200 mg/day
> **Zoloft** *Tab:* 15*, 50*, 100*mg; *Oral conc:* 20 mg per ml (60 ml, dilute just before administering in 4 oz water, ginger ale, lemon-lime soda, lemonade, or orange juice) (alcohol 12%)

SEROTONIN-NOREPINEPHRINE REUPTAKE INHIBITORS (SNRIs)

▷ *desvenlafaxine* (C)(G) swallow whole; initially 50 mg once daily; max 120 mg/day
  Pediatric: not recommended
    Pristiq *Tab:* 50, 100 mg ext-rel
▷ *venlafaxine* (C)
    Effexor initially 75 mg/day in 2-3 doses; may increase at 4 day intervals in
    75 mg increments to 150 mg/day; max 375 mg/day
      Pediatric: <18 years: not recommended
      Tab: 25, 37.5, 50, 75, 100 mg
    Effexor XR initially 75 mg q AM; may start at 37.5 mg x 4-7 days, then
    increase by increments of up to 75 mg/day at intervals of at least 4 days; usual
    max 375 mg/day
      Pediatric: not recommended
      Cap: 37.5, 75, 150 mg ext-rel

TRICYCLIC ANTIDEPRESSANTS (TCAs)

▷ *doxepin* (C)(G)
  Pediatric: not recommended
    Cap: 10, 25, 50, 75, 100, 150 mg; *Oral conc:* 10 mg/ml (4 oz w. dropper)
▷ *imipramine* (C)(G)
  Pediatric: not recommended
    Tofranil initially 75 mg daily (max 200 mg); *Adolescents:* initially 30-40 mg daily
    (max 100 mg/day); if maintenance dose exceeds 75 mg daily, may switch to
    Tofranil PM for divided <u>or</u> bedtime dose
      Tab: 10, 25, 50 mg
    Tofranil PM initially 75 mg daily 1 hour before HS; max 200 mg
      Cap: 75, 100, 125, 150
    Tofranil Injection 50 mg IM; lower dose for adolescents; switch to oral form as
    soon as possible
      Amp: 25 mg/2 ml (2 ml)

1ST GENERATION ANTIHISTAMINE

▷ *hydroxyzine* (C)(G) 50-100 mg qid; max 600 mg/day
  Pediatric: <6 years: 50 mg/day divided qid; ≥6 years: 50-100 mg/day divided qid
    Atarax *Tab:* 10, 25, 50, 100 mg; *Syr:* 10 mg/5 ml (alcohol 0.5%)
    Vistaril *Cap:* 25, 50, 100 mg; *Oral susp:* 25 mg/5 ml (4 oz) (lemon)

AZASPIRONES

▷ *buspirone* (B) initially 7.5 mg bid; may increase by 5 mg/day q 2-3 days; max 60 mg/day
  Pediatric: <6 years: not recommended; 6-17 years: same as adult
    BuSpar *Tab:* 5, 10, 15*, 30* mg

BENZODIAZEPINES

Short Acting

▷ *alprazolam* (D)(IV)(G)
  Pediatric: <18 years: not recommended
    Niravam initially 0.25-0.5 mg tid; may titrate every 3-4 days; max 4 mg/day
      Tab: 0.25*, 0.5*, 1*, 2*mg orally-disint

Xanax initially 0.25-0.5 mg tid; may titrate every 3-4 days; max 4 mg/day
Tab: 0.25*, 0.5*, 1*, 2*mg
Xanax XR initially 0.5-1 mg once daily, preferably in the AM; increase at intervals of at least 3-4 days by up to 1 mg/day. Taper no faster than 0.5 mg every 3 days; max 10 mg/day. When switching from immediate-release *alprazolam*, give total daily dose of immediate-release once daily.
Tab: 0.5, 1, 2, 3 mg ext-rel

▷ *oxazepam* (C)(IV)(G) 10-15 mg tid-qid for moderate symptoms; 15-30 mg tid-qid for severe symptoms
Pediatric: not recommended
Tab: 15 mg; Cap: 10, 15, 30 mg

Intermediate Acting

▷ *lorazepam* (D)(IV)(G) 1-10 mg/day in 2-3 divided doses
Pediatric: not recommended
Ativan *Tab:* 0.5, 1*, 2*mg
Lorazepam Intensol *Oral conc:* 2 mg/ml (30 ml w. graduated dropper)

Long Acting

▷ *chlordiazepoxide* (D)(IV)(G)
Pediatric: <6 years: not recommended; ≥6 years: 5 mg bid-qid; increase to 10 mg bid-tid
Librium 5-10 mg tid-qid for moderate symptoms; 20-25 mg tid-qid for severe symptoms
Cap: 5, 10, 25 mg
Librium Injectable 50-100 mg IM or IV; then 25-50 mg IM tid-qid prn; max 300 mg/day
Inj: 100 mg

▷ *chlordiazepoxide/clidinium* (D)(IV) 1-2 caps tid-qid: max 8 caps/day
Pediatric: not recommended
Librax *Cap: chlor* 5 mg/*clid* 2.5 mg

▷ *clonazepam* (D)(IV)(G) initially 0.25 mg bid; increase to 1 mg/day after 3 days
Pediatric: <18 years: not recommended
Klonopin *Tab:* 0.5*, 1, 2 mg
Klonopin Wafers dissolve in mouth with or without water
Wafer: 0.125, 0.25, 0.5, 1, 2 mg orally-disint

▷ *clorazepate* (D)(IV)(G) 30 mg/day in divided doses; max 60 mg/day
Pediatric: <9 years: not recommended; ≥9 years: same as adult
Tranxene *Tab:* 3.75, 7.5, 15 mg
Tranxene SD do not use for initial therapy
Tab: 22.5 mg ext-rel
Tranxene SD Half Strength do not use for initial therapy
Tab: 11.25 mg ext-rel
Tranxene T-Tab *Tab:* 3.75*, 7.5*, 15*mg

▷ *diazepam* (D)(IV)(G) 2-10 mg bid to qid
Pediatric: not recommended
Diastat *Rectal gel delivery system:* 2.5 mg
Diastat AcuDial *Rectal gel delivery system:* 10, 20 mg
Valium *Tab:* 2*, 5*, 10*mg

Valium Injectable *Vial:* 5 mg/ml (10 ml); *Amp:* 5 mg/ml (2 ml); *Prefilled syringe:* 5 mg/ml (5 ml)
Valium Intensol Oral Solution *Conc oral soln:* 5 mg/ml (30 ml w. dropper) (alcohol 19%)
Valium Oral Solution *Oral soln:* 5 mg/5 ml (500 ml) (wintergreen spice)

PHENOTHIAZINES

▷ *prochlorperazine* (C)(G)
Compazine 5 mg tid-qid
Pediatric: not recommended
Tab: 5 mg; *Syr:* 5 mg/5 ml (4 oz) (fruit); *Rectal supp:* 2.5, 5, 25 mg
Compazine Spansule 15 mg q AM or 10 mg q 12 hours
Pediatric: not recommended
Spansule: 10, 15 mg sust-rel
▷ *trifluoperazine* (C)(G) 1-2 mg bid; max 6 mg/day; max 12 weeks
Pediatric: not recommended
Stelazine *Tab:* 1, 2, 5, 10 mg

 PARKINSON'S DISEASE

Parkinson's Disease-associated Dementia, *see **Dementia** page* 103
Comment: When administering ***carbidopa*** and ***levodopa*** separately, administer each at the same time. Titrate daily dose ratio of 1:10 ***carbidopa*** to ***levodopa***. Max daily ***carbidopa*** 200 mg. Most patients will require ***levodopa*** 400 to 1600 mg/day in divided doses every 4 to 8 hours. After titrating both drugs to the desired effects without intolerable side effects, switch to a ***carbidopa/levodopa*** combination form.

DOPAMINE PRECURSOR

▷ *levodopa* (C)(G)
Tab: 125, 150, 200 mg

DECARBOXYLASE INHIBITOR

▷ *carbidopa* (C)(G)
Lodosyn *Tab:* 25 mg

DOPAMINE RECEPTOR AGONISTS

▷ *amantadine* (C) initially 100 mg bid; may increase after 1-2 weeks by 100 mg/day; max 400 mg/day in divided doses; for extrapyramidal effects, 100 mg bid; max 300 mg/day in divided doses
Symmetrel *Cap:* 100 mg; *Syr:* 50 mg/5 ml (16 oz) (raspberry)
▷ *bromocriptine* (B)(G) initially 1.25 mg bid to 2.5 mg tid with meals; increase as needed every 2-4 weeks by 2.5 mg/day; max 100 mg/day
Parlodel *Tab:* 2.5*mg; *Cap:* 5 mg
▷ *pramipexole* (C)(G) initially 0.125 mg tid; increase at intervals q 5-7 days; max 1.5 mg tid
Mirapex *Tab:* 0.125, 0.25*, 0.5*, 1*, 1.5*mg
▷ *ropinirole* (C) initially 0.25 mg tid for first week; then 0.5 mg tid for second week; then 0.75 mg tid for third week; then 1 mg tid for fourth week; may increase by

1.5 mg/day at 1 week intervals to 9 mg/day; then increase up to 3 mg/day at 1 week intervals; max 24 mg/day

> **Requip** *Tab:* 0.25, 0.5, 1, 2, 4, 5 mg

▷ *rotigotine* transdermal patch (C) apply to clean, dry, intact skin on abdomen, thigh, hip, flank, shoulder, <u>or</u> upper arm; rotate sites and allow 14 days before reusing site; if hairy, shave site at least 3 days before application to site; avoid abrupt cessation; taper by 2 mg/24 hours every other day; *Early stage:* initially 2 mg/24 hour patch once daily; may increase weekly by 2 mg/24 hour if needed; max 6 mg/24 hour once daily; *Advanced stage:* initially 4 mg/24 hour patch once daily; may increase weekly by 2 mg/24 hour if needed; max 8 mg/24 hour once daily

> **Neupro** *Trans patch:* 1 mg/24 hr, 2 mg/24 hr, 3 mg/24 hr, 4 mg/24 hr, 6 mg/24 hr, 8 mg/24 hr (30/carton) (sulfites)

DOPA-DECARBOXYLASE INHIBITORS

Comment: Contraindicated in narrow-angle glaucoma. Use with caution with sympathomimetics and antihypertensive agents.

▷ *carbidopa/levodopa* (C)(G) usually 400-1600 mg *levodopa*/day
Pediatric: <18 years: not established

> **Duopa** *Ent susp: carb* 4.63 mg/*levo* 20 mg single-use cassettes for use w. CADD Legacy 1400 Pump
>
> **Sinemet 10/100** initially 1 tab tid-qid; increase if needed daily <u>or</u> every other day up to qid
>> *Tab: carb* 10 mg/*levo* 100 mg* **Sinemet 25/100** initially 1 tab bid-tid; increase if needed daily <u>or</u> every other day up to qid
>> *Tab: carb* 25 mg/*lev* 100 mg*
>
> **Sinemet 25/250** 1 tab tid-qid
>> *Tab: carb* 25 mg/*lev* 250 mg*
>
> **Sinemet CR 25/100** initially one 25/100 tab bid; allow 3 days between dosage adjustments
>> *Tab: carb* 25 mg/*levo* 100 mg cont-rel
>
> **Sinemet CR 50/200** initially one 50/200 tab bid; allow 3 days between dosage adjustments
>> *Tab: carb* 50 mg/*levo* 200 mg cont-rel*

DOPA-DECARBOXYLASE INHIBITOR/DOPAMINE PRECURSOR/COMT INHIBITOR COMBINATION

▷ *carbidopa/levodopa/entacapone* (C) titrate individually with separate components; then switch to corresponding strength *levodopa* and *carbidopa*; max 8 tabs/day
>> *Tab:* **Stalevo 50**: *carb* 12.5 mg/*levo* 50 mg/*enta* 200 mg
>> **Stalevo 75**: *carb* 12.5 mg/*levo* 75 mg/*enta* 200 mg
>> **Stalevo 100**: *carb* 12.5 mg/*levo* 100 mg/*enta* 200 mg
>> **Stalevo 125**: *carb* 12.5 mg/*levo* 125 mg/*enta* 200 mg
>> **Stalevo 150**: *carb* 12.5 mg/*levo* 150 mg/*enta* 200 mg
>> **Stalevo 200**: *carb* 12.5 mg/*levo* 200 mg/*enta* 200 mg

MONOAMINE OXIDASE INHIBITORS (MAOIS)

▷ *rasagiline* (C)(G) usual maintenance: 0.5-1 mg/day; max: 1 mg/day; initial dose for patients on concomitant *levodopa*: 0.5 mg daily; initial dose for patients not on concomitant *levodopa*: 1 mg daily

Azilect *Tab:* 0.5, 1 mg
Comment: **Azelect** is indicated as monotherapy or as adjunct to *levodopa*. With mild hepatic dysfunction (Child-Pugh 5-6), limit **Azelect** dose to 0.5 mg daily. With moderate to severe hepatic dysfunction (Child-Pugh 7-15), **Azelect** is not recommended. Contraindications include co-administration with *meperidine, methadone, mirtazapine, propoxyphene, tramadol, dextromethorphan, St. John's wort, cyclobenzaprine, methylphenidate, dexmethylphenidate,* or other MAOIs.

▷ *selegiline* (C)(G) 5 mg at breakfast and at lunch; max 10 mg/day
   Tab/Cap: 5 mg
▷ *selegiline* (C)(G) 1.25 mg daily; max 2.5 mg/day
   Zelapar *ODT:* 1.25 mg orally-disint (phenylalanine)

COMT INHIBITORS

▷ *entacapone* (C) 1 tab with each dose of *levodopa* or *carbidopa*; max 8 tabs/day
   Comtan *Tab:* 200 mg
   Comment: **Comtan** is an adjunct to *levodopa/carbidopa* in patients with end-of-dose wearing off.
▷ *tolcapone* (C) 100-200 mg tid; max 600 mg/day
   Tasmar *Tab:* 100, 200 mg
   Comment: Monitor LFTs every 2 weeks. Withdraw **Tasmar** if no substantial improvement in the first 3 weeks of treatment.

CENTRALLY ACTING ANTICHOLINERGICS

▷ *benztropine mesylate* (C) initially 0.5-1 mg q HS, increase if needed; for extrapyrami-dal disorders 1-4 mg once daily-bid; max 6 mg/day
   Cogentin *Tab:* 0.5*, 1*, 2*mg
▷ *biperiden hydrochloride* (C) initially 1 tab tid or qid, then increase as needed; max 8 tabs/day
   Akineton *Tab:* 2 mg
▷ *procyclidine* (C) initially 2.5 mg tid; may increase as needed to 5 mg tid-qid every 3-5 days; max 15 mg/day
   Kemadrin *Tab:* 5 mg
▷ *trihexyphenidyl* (C)(G) initially 1 mg; increase as needed by 2 mg every 3-5 days; max 15 mg/day
   Artane *Tab:* 2*, 5*mg

◯ PARONYCHIA (PERIUNGUAL ABSCESS)

▷ *cephalexin* (B)(G) 500 mg bid x 10 days
   Pediatric: 25-50 mg/day in 2 divided doses x 10 days
   Keflex *Cap:* 250, 333, 500, 750 mg; *Oral susp:* 125, 250 mg/5 ml (100, 200 ml) (strawberry)
▷ *clindamycin* (B)(G) 150-300 mg q 6 hours x 10 days
   Pediatric: 8-16 mg/kg/day in 3-4 divided doses x 10 days
   Cleocin *Cap:* 75 (tartrazine), 150 (tartrazine), 300 mg
   Cleocin Pediatric Granules *Oral susp:* 75 mg/5 ml (100 ml) (cherry)

➤ *dicloxacillin* (B)(G) 500 mg q 6 hours x 10 days
  Pediatric: 12.5-25 mg/kg/day in 4 divided doses x 10 days; *see page* 571 *for dose by weight*
    Dynapen *Cap:* 125, 250, 500 mg; *Oral susp:* 62.5 mg/5 ml (80, 100, 200 ml)
➤ *erythromycin base* (B)(G) 500 mg q 6 hours x 10 days
  Pediatric: <45 kg: 30-50 mg in 2-4 doses x 10 days; ≥45 kg: same as adult
    Ery-Tab *Tab:* 250, 333, 500 mg ent-coat
    PCE *Tab:* 333, 500 mg
  Comment: *erythromycin* may increase INR with concomitant *warfarin*, as well as increase serum level of *digoxin*, benzodiazepines and statins.
➤ *erythromycin ethylsuccinate* (B)(G) 400 mg q 6 hours x 10 days
  Pediatric: 30-50 mg/kg/day in 4 divided doses q 6 hours x 10 days; may double dose with severe infection; max 100 mg/kg/day; *see page* 574 *for dose by weight*
    EryPed *Oral susp:* 200 mg/5 ml (100, 200 ml) (fruit); 400 mg/5 ml (60, 100, 200 ml) (banana); *Oral drops:* 200, 400 mg/5 ml (50 ml) (fruit); *Chew tab:* 200 mg wafer (fruit)
    E.E.S. *Oral susp:* 200, 400 mg/5 ml (100 ml) (fruit)
    E.E.S. Granules *Oral susp:* 200 mg/5 ml (100, 200 ml) (cherry)
    E.E.S. 400 Tablets *Tab:* 400 mg
  Comment: *erythromycin* may increase INR with concomitant *warfarin*, as well as increase serum level of *digoxin*, benzodiazepines and statins.

◯ PEDICULOSIS: PEDICULOSIS HUMANUS CAPITIS (HEAD LICE)/PHTHIRUS (PUBIC LICE)

➤ *ivermectin* (C) thoroughly wet hair; leave on for 10 minutes; then rinse off with water; do not re-treat
  Pediatric: <6 months, <33 lbs: not recommended; ≥6 months, ≥33 lbs: same as adult
    Sklice *Lotn:* 0.5% (4 oz, 117 g, laminate tube)
➤ *lindane* (C)(G) apply, leave on for 4 minutes, then thoroughly wash off
  Pediatric: <2 years: not recommended; ≥2 years: same as adult
    Kwell Shampoo *Shampoo:* 1% (60 ml)
➤ *malathion* (B)(G) thoroughly wet hair; allow to dry naturally; shampoo and rinse after 8-12 hours; use a fine tooth comb to remove lice and nits; if lice persist after 7-9 days, may repeat treatment
  Pediatric: same as adult
    Ovide (OTC) *Lotn:* 59% (2 oz)
➤ *permethrin* (B)(G) apply to washed and towel-dried hair; allow to remain on for 10 minutes, then rinse off; repeat after 7 days if needed
  Pediatric: <2 months: not recommended; ≥2 months: same as adult
    Nix (OTC) *Crm rinse:* 1% (2 oz w. comb)
➤ *pyrethrins with piperonyl butoxide* (C)(G) apply and leave on for 10 minutes, then wash off
    A-200 *Shampoo:* pyr 0.33%/pip but 3%
    Rid Mousse *Shampoo:* pyr 0.33%/pip but 4%
    Rid Shampoo *Shampoo:* pyr 0.33%/pip but 3%
  Comment: To remove nits, soak hair in equal parts white vinegar and water for 15-20 minutes.

⬤ PELVIC INFLAMMATORY DISEASE (PID)

Comment: The following treatment regimens are published in the **2015 CDC Sexually Transmitted Diseases Treatment Guidelines.** Treatment regimens are presented by generic drug name first, followed by information about brands and dose forms. Treat all sexual partners. Because of the high risk for maternal morbidity and preterm delivery, pregnant women who have suspected PID should be hospitalized and treated with parenteral antibiotics. HIV-infected women with PID respond equally well to standard parenteral and antibiotic regimens as HIV-negative women.

OUTPATIENT REGIMENS

Regimen 1

▷ *ceftriaxone* 250 mg IM in a single dose plus
▷ *doxycycline* 100 mg bid x 14 days with or without
▷ *metronidazole* 500 mg PO bid x 14 days

Regimen 2

▷ *cefoxitin* 2 g IM in a single dose plus
▷ *probenecid* 1 g PO in a single dose administered concurrently plus *doxycycline* 100 mg bid x 14 days with or without
▷ *metronidazole* 500 mg PO bid x 14 days

Regimen 3

▷ Other parenteral third-generation cephalosporin (e.g., *ceftizoxime* or *cefotaxime*) in a single dose) plus
▷ *doxycycline* 100 mg bid x 14 days with or without
▷ *metronidazole* 500 mg PO bid x 14 days

DRUG BRANDS AND DOSE FORMS

▷ *cefoxitin* (B)(G)
　　　Mefoxin *Vial:* 1, 2 g
▷ *ceftriaxone* (B)(G)
　　　Rocephin Vials 250, 500 mg: 1, 2 g
▷ *doxycycline* (D)(G)
　　　Actilate *Tab:* 75, 150** mg
　　　Adoxa *Tab:* 50, 75, 100, 150 mg ent-coat
　　　Doryx *Tab:* 50, 75, 100, 150, 200 mg del-rel
　　　Monodox *Cap:* 50, 75, 100 mg
　　　Oracea *Cap:* 40 mg del-rel
　　　Vibramycin *Tab:* 100 mg; *Cap:* 50, 100 mg; *Syr:* 50 mg/5 ml (raspberry-apple) (sulfites); *Oral susp:* 25 mg/5 ml (raspberry)
　　　Vibra-Tab *Tab:* 100 mg film-coat
Comment: *doxycycline* is contraindicated <8 years-of-age, in pregnancy, and lactation (discolors developing tooth enamel). A side effect may be photo-sensitivity (photophobia). Do not give with antacids, calcium supplements, milk or other dairy, or within two hours of taking another drug.

▷ *metronidazole* (not for use in 1st; B in 2nd, 3rd)
    Flagyl *Tab:* 250*, 500*mg
    Flagyl 375 *Cap:* 375 mg
    Flagyl ER *Tab:* 750 mg ext-rel
Comment: Alcohol is contraindicated during treatment with oral *metronidazole* and for 72 hours after therapy due to a possible *disulfiram*-like reaction (nausea, vomiting, flushing, headache).
▷ *probenecid* (B)(G)
    Benemid *Tab:* 500*mg; *Cap:* 500 mg

◯ PEPTIC ULCER DISEASE (PUD)

Helicobacter pylori Eradication Regimens *see page* 180

H₂ ANTAGONISTS

▷ *cimetidine* (B)(G)
Pediatric: <16 years: not recommended; ≥16 years: same as adult
    Tagamet 800 mg bid <u>or</u> 400 mg qid; max 2.4 g/day
        Tab: 300, 400*, 800* mg
    Tagamet HB (OTC) *Prophylaxis:* 1 tab ac; *Treatment:* 1 tab bid
        Tab: 200 mg
    Tagamet HB Oral Suspension (OTC) *Prophylaxis:* 1 tsp ac; *Treatment:* 1 tsp bid
        Oral susp: 200 mg/20 ml (12 oz)
    Tagamet Liquid *Liq:* 300 mg/5 ml (mint-peach) (alcohol 2.8%)
▷ *famotidine* (B)(G) 20 mg bid <u>or</u> 40 mg q HS; *max* 6 weeks
Pediatric: 0.5 mg/kg/day q HS <u>or</u> in 2 divided doses; max 40 mg/day
    Pepcid *Tab:* 20, 40 mg; *Oral susp:* 40 mg/5 ml (50 ml)
    Pepcid AC (OTC) 1 tab ac; max 2 doses/day
        Tab/Rapid dissolving tab: 10 mg
    Pepcid Complete (OTC) 1 tab ac; max 2 doses/day
        Tab: fam 10 mg/$CaCO_2$ 800 mg/*Mg hydroxide* 165 mg
    Pepcid RPD
        Tab: 20, 40 mg rapid-dissolving
▷ *nizatidine* (B)(G) 150 mg bid; max 12 weeks
Pediatric: not recommended
    Axid *Cap:* 150, 300 mg
    Axid AR (OTC) 1 tab ac; max 150 mg/day
        Tab: 75 mg
▷ *ranitidine* (B)(G)
Pediatric: <1 month: not recommended; 1 month-16 years: 2-4 mg/kg/day in 2 divided doses; max 300 mg/day; *Duodenal/Gastric Ulcer:* 2-4 mg/kg/day divided bid; max 300 mg/day; *Erosive Esophagitis:* 5-10 mg/kg/day divided bid; max 300 mg/day; >16 years: same as adult
    Zantac 150 mg bid <u>or</u> 300 mg q HS
        Tab: 150, 300 mg
    Zantac 75 (OTC) 1 tab ac
        Tab: 75 mg
    Zantac EFFERdose dissolve 25 mg tab in 5 ml water; dissolve 150 mg tab in 6-8 oz water

Efferdose: 25, 150 mg effervescent (phenylalanine)
Zantac Syrup *Syr:* 15 mg/ml (peppermint) (alcohol 7.5%)
▷ ***ranitidine bismuth citrate* (C)** 400 mg bid
Pediatric: not recommended
Tritec *Tab:* 400 mg

PROTON PUMP INHIBITORS (PPIs)

Comment: If hepatic impairment, or if patient is Asian, consider reducing the PPI dosage. Research has demonstrated associations between PPI use and fractures of the hip, wrist, and spine, hypomagnesemia, kidney injuries and chronic kidney disease, possible cardiovascular drug interactions, and infections (e.g., Clostridium difficile and pneumonia). Reducing the acidity of the stomach allows bacteria to thrive and spread to other organs like the lungs and intestines. This risk is increased with high dose and chronic use and greatest in the elderly. The most recent class-wide FDA warning cites reports of cutaneous and systemic lupus erythematosis (CLS/SLE) associates with PPIs in patients with both new onset and exacerbation of existing autoimmune disease. PPI treatment should be discontinued and the patient should be referred to a specialist. (http://www.fda.gov/Drugs/DrugSafety/InformationbyDrugClass/ucm213259.htm)
▷ ***dexlansoprazole* (B)(G)** 30-60 mg daily for up to 4 weeks
Pediatric: <18 years: not recommended
Dexilant *Cap:* 30, 60 mg ent-coat del-rel granules; may open and sprinkle on applesauce; do not crush or chew granules
Dexilant SoluTab *Tab:* 30 mg del-rel orally-disint
▷ ***esomeprazole* (B)(OTC)(G)** 20-40 mg daily; max 8 weeks; take 1 hour before food; swallow whole or mix granules with food or juice and take immediately; do not crush or chew granules
Pediatric: <1 year: not recommended; 1-11 years: <20 kg: 10 mg; ≥20 kg: 10-20 mg once daily; 12-17 years: 20-40 mg once daily; max 8 weeks
Nexium *Cap:* 20, 40 mg ent-coat del-rel pellets
Nexium for Oral Suspension *Oral susp:* 10, 20, 40 mg ent-coat del-rel granules/ pkt; mix in 2 tblsp water and drink immediately; 30 pkt/carton
▷ ***lansoprazole* (B)(OTC)(G)** 15-30 mg daily for up to 8 weeks; may repeat course; take before eating
Pediatric: <1 year: not recommended; 1-11, <30 kg: 15 mg once daily; ≥12 years: same as adult
Prevacid *Cap:* 15, 30 mg ent-coat del-rel granules; swallow whole or mix granules with food or juice and take immediately; do not crush or chew granules; follow with water
Prevacid for Oral Suspension *Oral susp:* 15, 30 mg ent-coat del-rel granules/pkt; mix in 2 tblsp water and drink immediately; 30 pkt/carton (strawberry)
Prevacid SoluTab *ODT:* 15, 30 mg (strawberry) (phenylalanine)
Prevacid 24HR 15 mg ent-coat del-rel granules; swallow whole or mix granules with food or juice and take immediately; do not crush or chew granules; follow with water
▷ ***omeprazole* (C)(OTC)(G)** 20-40 mg daily; take before eating; swallow whole or mix granules with applesauce and take immediately; do not crush or chew; follow with water
Pediatric: <1 year: not recommended; 5-<10 kg: 5 mg daily; 10-<20 kg: 10 mg daily; ≥20 kg: same as adult
Prilosec *Cap:* 10, 20, 40 mg ent-coat del-rel granules
Pediatric: <18 years: not recommended

Prilosec OTC *Tab:* 20 mg del-rel (regular, wild berry)
▷ *pantoprazole* (B) initially 40 mg bid
  Pediatric: not recommended
    Protonix (G) *Tab:* 40 mg ent-coat del-rel
    Protonix for Oral Suspension *Oral susp:* 40 mg ent-coat del-rel granules/pkt;
    mix in 1 tsp apple juice for 5 seconds <u>or</u> sprinkle on 1 tsp apple sauce, and
    swallow immediately; do not mix in water <u>or</u> any other liquid <u>or</u> food; take
    approximately 30 minutes prior to a meal; 30 pkt/carton
▷ *rabeprazole* (B)(OTC)(G) initially 20 mg daily; then titrate; may take 100 mg daily in
  divided doses <u>or</u> 60 mg bid
  Pediatric: <12 years: not recommended; ≥12 years: 20 mg once daily; max 8 weeks
    AcipHex *Tab:* 20 mg ent-coat del-rel
    Antacids *see GERD page* 151

OTHER

▷ *glycopyrrolate* (B)(G) initially 1-2 mg bid-tid; *Maintenance:* 1 mg bid; max 8 mg/day
  Pediatric: <12 years: not recommended; ≥12 years: same as adult
    Robinul *Tab:* 1 mg (dye-free)
    Robinul Forte *Tab:* 2 mg (dye-free)
  Comment: *glycopyrrolate* is an anticholinergic adjunct to PUD treatment.
▷ *mepenzolate* (B)(G) 25-50 mg divided qid, with meals and at HS
    Cantil *Tab:* 25 mg
▷ *sucralfate* (B)(G) **Active ulcer:** 1 g qid; *Maintenance:* 1 g bid
    Carafate *Tab:* 1*g; *Oral susp:* 1 g/10 ml (14 oz)

PROPHYLAXIS

▷ *misoprostol* (X) 200 mg qid with food for prevention of NSAID-induced gastric ulcers
    Cytotec *Tab:* 100, 200 mg

PERIPHERAL NEURITIS, DIABETIC NEUROPATHIC PAIN, PERIPHERAL NEUROPATHIC PAIN

▷ **Acetaminophen for IV Infusion** *see Pain page* 306
▷ *acetaminophen* (B)(G) *see Fever page* 143
▷ *aspirin* (D)(G) *see Fever page* 144
  Comment: *aspirin*-containing medications are contraindicated with history of
  allergic-type reaction to *aspirin*, children and adolescents with *Varicella* <u>or</u> other
  viral illness, and 3rd trimester pregnancy.

α₂-DELTA LIGAND

▷ *pregabalin (GABA analog)* (C)(V) initially 150 mg daily divided bid-tid; may titrate
  within one week; max 600 mg divided bid-tid; discontinue over one week
  Pediatric: <18 years: not recommended
    Lyrica *Cap:* 25, 50, 75, 100, 150, 200, 225, 300 mg; *Oral soln:* 20 mg/ml

SEROTONIN AND NOREPINEPHRINE REUPTAKE INHIBITOR (SNRI)

▷ *duloxetine* (C) swallow whole; 30-60 mg once daily; may increase by 30 mg at 1 week
  intervals; usual target 60 mg daily; max 120 mg/day
  Pediatric: not recommended
      Cymbalta *Cap:* 20, 30, 60 mg ent-coat pellets
      Comment: **Cymbalta** is indicated for chronic pain syndromes (e.g., arthritis,
      fibromyalgia, lowback pain).

TOPICAL/TRANSDERMAL NSAIDs

▷ *capsaicin* (B)(G) apply tid-qid prn to intact skin
  Pediatric: <2 years: not recommended; ≥2 years: apply sparingly tid-qid prn
      Axsain *Crm:* 0.075% (1, 2 oz)
      Capsin *Lotn:* 0.025, 0.075% (59 ml)
      Capzasin-P (OTC) *Crm:* 0.025% (1.5 oz); *Lotn:* 0.025% (2 oz)
      Dolorac *Crm:* 0.025% (28 g)
      Double Cap (OTC) *Crm:* 0.05% (2 oz)
      R-Gel *Gel:* 0.025% (15, 30 g)
      Zostrix (OTC) *Crm:* 0.025% (0.7, 1.5, 3 oz)
      Zostrix HP (OTC) *Emol crm:* 0.075% (1, 2 oz)
▷ *capsaicin* 8% patch (B) apply up to 4 patches for one 60-minute application to
  clean dry skin; may prep area with topical anesthetic; wear nonlatex gloves; patches
  may be cut to size/shape; treatment may be repeated every 3 months; remove with
  cleansing gel after treatment
  Pediatric: <18 years: not recommended
      Qutenza *Patch:* 8% 1640 mcg/cm (179 mg) (1 or 2 patches, each w. 1-50 g tube
      cleansing gel/carton)
▷ *diclofenac epolamine transdermal patch* (C) apply one patch to affected area bid;
  remove during bathing; avoid nonintact skin
  Pediatric: not recommended
      Flector Patch *Patch:* 180 mg/patch (30/carton)
▷ *capsaicin* (B)(G) apply tid to qid prn to intact skin
  Pediatric: <2 years: not recommended; ≥2 years: same as adult
      Axsain *Crm:* 0.075% (1, 2 oz)
      Capsin *Lotn:* 0.025, 0.075% (59 ml)
      Capzasin-P (OTC) *Crm:* 0.025% (1.5 oz); *Lotn:* 0.025% (2 oz)
      Dolorac *Crm:* 0.025% (28 g)
      Double Cap (OTC) *Crm:* 0.05% (2 oz)
      R-Gel *Gel:* 0.025% (15, 30 g)
      Zostrix (OTC) *Crm:* 0.025% (0.7, 1.5, 3 oz)
      Zostrix HP (OTC) *Emol crm:* 0.075% (1, 2 oz)
▷ *capsaicin* 8% patch (B) apply up to 4 patches for one 60-minute application to clean
  dry skin; may prep area with topical anesthetic; wear non-latex gloves; patches may
  be cut to size/shape; treatment may be repeated every 3 months; remove with cleansing gel after treatment
  Pediatric: <18 years: not recommended
      Qutenza *Patch:* 8% 1640 mcg/cm (179 mg) (1 or 2 patches w. 1-50 g tube
      cleansing gel/carton)
▷ *lidocaine* 5% patch (B)(G) apply up to 3 patches at one time for up to 12 hours/24-
  hour period (12 hours on/12 hours off); patches may be cut into smaller sizes before
  removal of the release liner; do not re-use

Pediatric: not recommended
    Lidoderm *Patch:* 5% (10x14 cm, 30/carton)

ORAL ANALGESICS

▷ *tramadol* (C)(IV)(G)
    Rybix ODT initially 100 mg once daily; may increase by 100 mg every 5 days; max 300 mg/day; *CrCl <30 mL/min* or *severe hepatic impairment:* not recommended; *Cirrhosis:* max 50 mg q 12 hours
      Pediatric: <17 years: not recommended
      ODT: 50 mg (mint) (phenylalanine)
    Ryzolt initially 100 mg once daily; may increase by 100 mg every; 5 days; max 300 mg/day; *CrCl <30 mL/min* or *severe hepatic impairment:* not recommended
      Pediatric: <16 years: not recommended; ≥16 years: same as adult
      Tab: 100, 200, 300 mg ext-rel
    Ultram 50-100 mg q 4-6 hours prn; max 400 mg/day; *CrCl <30 mL/min:* max 100 mg q 12 hours; *Cirrhosis:* max 50 mg q 12 hours
      Pediatric: <16 years: not recommended; ≥16 years: same as adult
      Tab: 50 mg
    Ultram ER initially 100 mg once daily; may increase by 100 mg every 5 days; max 300 mg/day; *CrCl <30 mL/min* or *severe hepatic impairment:* not recommended
      Pediatric: <18 years: not recommended
      Tab: 100, 200, 300 mg ext-rel
▷ *tramadol/acetaminophen* (C)(IV)(G) 2 tabs q 4-6 hours; max 8 tabs/day; 5 days; *CrCl <30 mL/min:* max 2 tabs q 12 hours; max 4 tabs/day x 5 days
  Pediatric: <16 years: not recommended; ≥16 years: same as adult
    Ultracet *Tab:* tram 37.5/acet 325 mg

MU-OPIOID AGONIST/NOREPINEPHRINE REUPTAKE INHIBITOR

▷ *tapentadol* (C)
  Pediatric: <18 years: not recommended
    Nucynta 50-100 mg q 4-6 hours prn; max 700 mg/day on the first day; 600 mg/day on subsequent days
      Tab: 50, 75, 100 mg
    Nucynta ER *Opioid-naïve:* initially 50 mg q 12 hours, then titrate to optimal dose within therapeutic range; usual therapeutic range 100-250 mg q 12 hours; doses >500 mg not recommended; *Converting from Nucynta:* divide total **Nucynta** daily dose into 2 **Nucynta ER** doses and administer q 12 hours; converting from *oxycodone CR* and other opioids, see mfr recommendations
      Tab: 50, 100, 150, 200, 250 mg ext-rel
    Other Oral Analgesics *see Pain page* 308

PERIPHERAL VASCULAR DISEASE (PVD, ARTERIAL INSUFFICIENCY, INTERMITTENT CLAUDICATION)

ANTIPLATELET THERAPY

▷ *aspirin* (D)(OTC) usually 81 mg once daily; range 75-325 mg once daily
    Ecotrin *Tab/Cap:* 81, 325, 500 mg ent-coat

▷ *cilostazol* (C) 100 mg bid 1/2 hour before or 2 hours after breakfast or dinner; may reduce to 50 mg bid if used with CYP 3A4 (e.g., azole antifungals, macrolides, *diltiazem*, *fluvoxamine*, *fluoxetine*, *nefazodone*, *sertraline*) or CYP 2C19 (e.g., *omeprazole*) inhibitors
  Pletal *Tab:* 50, 100 mg
  Comment: May be used with *aspirin*. Cautious use with other antiplatelet agents and anticoagulants.
▷ *clopidogrel* (B) 75 mg daily
  Plavix *Tab:* 75 mg
▷ *dipyridamole* (B)(G) 25-100 mg tid-qid
  Persantine *Tab:* 25, 50, 75 mg
  Comment: Does not potentiate *warfarin* and may be taken concomitantly. Do not administer *dipyridamole* concomitantly with *aspirin*.
▷ *pentoxifylline* (C) 400 mg tid with food
  PentoPak *Tab:* 400 mg ext-rel
  Trental *Tab:* 400 mg sust-rel
▷ *ticlopidine* (B) 250 mg bid with food
  Ticlid *Tab:* 250 mg
  Comment: Monitor for neutropenia; resolves after discontinuation.
▷ *warfarin* (X) adjust dose to maintain INR in recommended range; *see Anticoagulation Therapy page* 526
  Coumadin *Tab:* 1*, 2*, 2.5*, 5*, 7.5*, 10*mg
  Coumadin for Injection *Vial:* 2 mg/ml (5 mg) pwdr for reconstitution
  Comment: Treatment for over-anticoagulation with *warfarin* is *vitamin K*.

○ PERTUSSIS (WHOOPING COUGH)

Prophylaxis *see Childhood Immunizations page* 478

POSTEXPOSURE PROPHYLAXIS AND TREATMENT

Comment: Antibiotics do not alter the course of illness, but they do prevent transmission. Infected persons should be isolated until after the fifth day of antibiotic treatment.
▷ *azithromycin* (B)(G) 500 mg x 1 dose on day 1, then 250 mg daily on days 2-5 or 500 mg daily x 3 days
  Pediatric: 12 mg/kg/day x 5 days; max 500 mg/day; *see page* 559 *for dose by weight*
    Zithromax *Tab:* 250, 500, 600 mg; *Oral susp:* 100 mg/5 ml (15 ml); 200 mg/5 ml (15, 22.5, 30 ml) (cherry); *Pkt:* 1 g for reconstitution (cherry-banana)
    Zithromax Tri-pak *Tab:* 3 x 500 mg tabs/pck
    Zithromax Z-pak *Tab:* 6 x 250 mg tabs/pck
    Zmax *Oral susp:* 2 g ext-rel for reconstitution (cherry-banana) (148 mg Na$^+$)
  Comment: *azithromycin* is the drug of choice for infants <1 month-of-age.
▷ *clarithromycin* (C)(G) 250 mg bid or 500 mg ext-rel daily x 10 days
  Pediatric: <6 months: not recommended; ≥6 months: 7.5 mg/kg divided bid x 10 days; *see page* 569 *for dose by weight*
    Biaxin *Tab:* 250, 500 mg
    Biaxin Oral Suspension *Oral susp:* 125, 250 mg/5 ml (50, 100 ml) (fruit-punch)
    Biaxin XL *Tab:* 500 mg ext-rel

➤ *erythromycin base* (B)(G) 1 g/day divided qid x 14 days
   Pediatric: 40 mg/kg/day in divided doses x 14 days
      Ery-Tab *Tab:* 250, 333, 500 mg ent-coat
      PCE *Tab:* 333, 500 mg
   Comment: *erythromycin* may increase INR with concomitant *warfarin*, as well as increase serum level of *digoxin*, benzodiazepines and statins.

➤ *erythromycin ethylsuccinate* (B)(G) 1 g/day in 4 divided doses x 14 days
   Pediatric: 40-50 mg/kg/day in 4 divided doses x 7 days; may double dose with severe infection; max 100 mg/kg/day; *see page* 574 *for dose by weight*
      EryPed *Oral susp:* 200 mg/5 ml (100, 200 ml) (fruit); 400 mg/5 ml (60, 100, 200 ml) (banana); *Oral drops:* 200, 400 mg/5 ml (50 ml) (fruit); *Chew tab:* 200 mg wafer (fruit)
      E.E.S. *Oral susp:* 200, 400 mg/5 ml (100 ml) (fruit)
      E.E.S. Granules *Oral susp:* 200 mg/5 ml (100, 200 ml) (cherry)
      E.E.S. 400 Tablets *Tab:* 400 mg
   Comment: *erythromycin* may increase INR with concomitant *warfarin*, as well as increase serum level of *digoxin*, benzodiazepines and statins.

➤ *trimethoprim/sulfamethoxazole* (C)(G)
   Pediatric: <2 months: not recommended; ≥2 months: 40 mg/kg/day of *sulfamethoxazole* in 2 doses bid x 10 days; *see page* 587 *for dose by weight*
      Bactrim, Septra 2 tabs bid x 10 days
         Tab: trim 80 mg/*sulfa* 400 mg*
      Bactrim DS, Septra DS 1 tab bid x 10 days
         Tab: trim 160 mg/*sulfa* 800 mg
      Bactrim Pediatric Suspension, Septra Pediatric Suspension
         Oral susp: trim 40 mg/*sulfa* 200 mg per 5 ml (100 ml) (cherry) (alcohol 0.3%)
   Comment: *trimethoprim/sulfamethoxazole* is <u>not</u> recommended in pregnancy <u>or</u> lactation. *CrCl 15-30 mL/min:* reduce dose by 1/2; *CrCl <15 mL/min:* not recommended.

TREATMENT

Same as Postexposure Prophylaxis

 ## PHARYNGITIS: GONOCOCCAL

Comment: Treat all sexual contacts. Empiric therapy requires concomitant treatment for *Chlamydia*. Post-treatment culture recommended with PMHx history rheumatic fever.

PRIMARY THERAPY

➤ *azithromycin* (B)(G) 1 g x 1 dose
   Pediatric: 12 mg/kg/day x 5 days; max 500 mg/day; *see page* 559 *for dose by weight*
      Zithromax *Tab:* 250, 500, 600 mg; *Oral susp:* 100 mg/5 ml (15 ml); 200 mg/5 ml (15, 22.5, 30 ml) (cherry); *Pkt:* 1 g for reconstitution (cherry-banana)
      Zithromax Tri-pak *Tab:* 3 x 500 mg tabs/pck
      Zithromax Z-pak *Tab:* 6 x 250 mg tabs/pck
      Zmax *Oral susp:* 2 g ext-rel for reconstitution (cherry-banana) (148 mg Na⁺)
   Comment: Per the CDC 2015 STD Treatment Guidelines, *azithromycin* should be used <u>with</u> ceftriaxone 250mg.

▷ *ceftriaxone* (B)(G) 250 mg IM x 1 dose
  Pediatric: <45 kg: 125 mg IM x 1 dose; ≥45 kg: same as adult
      Rocephin *Vial:* 250, 500 mg; 1, 2 g

⃝ PHARYNGITIS: STREPTOCOCCAL

▷ *amoxicillin* (B)(G) 500-875 mg bid or 250-500 mg tid x 10 days
  Pediatric: <40 kg (88 lb): 20-40 mg/kg/day in 3 divided doses x 10 days or 25-45
  mg/kg/day in 2 divided doses x 10 days; ≥40 kg: same as adult; *see page 554 for dose
  by weight*
      Amoxil *Cap:* 250, 500 mg; *Tab:* 875*mg; *Chew tab:* 125, 200, 250, 400 mg (cher-
      ry-banana-peppermint) (phenylalanine); *Oral susp:* 125, 250 mg/5 ml (80, 100,
      150 ml) (strawberry); 200, 400 mg/5 ml (50, 75, 100 ml) (bubble gum); *Oral
      drops:* 50 mg/ml (30 ml) (bubble gum)
      Moxatag *Tab:* 775 mg ext-rel
      Trimox *Tab:* 125, 250 mg; *Cap:* 250, 500 mg; *Oral susp:* 125, 250 mg/5 ml (80,
      100, 150 ml) (raspberry-strawberry)
▷ *amoxicillin/clavulanate* (B)(G) 500 mg tid or 875 mg bid x 10 days
      Augmentin *Tab:* 250, 500, 875 mg; *Chew tab:* 125, 250 mg (lemon-lime); 200,
      400 mg (cherry-banana) (phenylalanine); *Oral susp:* 125 mg/5 ml (banana), 250
      mg/5 ml (75, 100, 150 ml) (orange); 200, 400 mg/5 ml (50, 75, 100 ml) (orange)
      (phenylalanine)
          Pediatric: 40-45 mg/kg/day divided tid x 10 days or 90 mg/kg/day divided
          bid x 10 days *see pages 556-557 for dose by weight*
      Augmentin ES-600 *Oral susp:* 600 mg/5 ml (50, 75, 100, 125, 150, 200 ml)
      (strawberry cream) (phenylalanine) every 12 hours
          Pediatric: <3 months: not recommended; ≥3 months, <40 kg: 90 mg/kg/day
          in 2 divided doses; ≥40 kg: not recommended
      Augmentin XR 2 tabs q 12 hours x 7-10 days
          Pediatric: <16 years: use other forms; ≥16 years: same as adult
          Tab: 1000*mg ext-rel
▷ *azithromycin* (B)(G) 500 mg x 1 dose on day 1, then 250 mg daily on days 2-5 or 500
  mg daily x 3 days
  Pediatric: 12 mg/kg/day x 5 days; max 500 mg/day; *see page 559 for dose by weight*
      Zithromax *Tab:* 250, 500, 600 mg; *Oral susp:* 100 mg/5 ml (15 ml); 200 mg/5 ml
      (15, 22.5, 30 ml) (cherry); *Pkt:* 1 g for reconstitution (cherry-banana)
      Zithromax Tri-pak *Tab:* 3 x 500 mg tabs/pck
      Zithromax Z-pak *Tab:* 6 x 250 mg tabs/pck
      Zmax *Oral susp:* 2 g ext-rel for reconstitution (cherry-banana) (148 mg Na$^+$)
▷ *cefaclor* (B)(G) 250 mg tid or 375 mg bid x 5 days
  Pediatric: <1 month: not recommended; 20-40 mg/kg bid or q 12 hours x 10 days;
  max 1 g/day; *see page 560 for dose by weight*
  Tab: 500 mg; *Cap:* 250, 500 mg; *Susp:* 125 mg/5 ml (75, 150 ml) (strawberry); 187
  mg/5 ml (50, 100 ml) (strawberry); 250 mg/5 ml (75, 150 ml) (strawberry); 375
  mg/5 ml (50, 100 ml) (strawberry)
      Cefaclor Extended Release
          Pediatric: <16 years: ext-rel not recommended; ≥16 years: same as adult
          Tab: 375, 500 mg ext-rel
▷ *cefadroxil* (B) 1 g in 1-2 doses x 10 days
  Pediatric: 30 mg/kg/day in 2 divided doses x 10 days; *see page 561 for dose by weight*

      Duricef *Cap:* 500 mg; *Tab:* 1 g; *Oral susp:* 250 mg/5 ml (100 ml); 500 mg/5 ml (75, 100 ml) (orange-pineapple)

➤ *cefdinir* (B) 300 mg bid x 10 days
Pediatric: <6 months: not recommended; 6 months-12 years: 14 mg/kg/day in 1-2 doses x 10 days; >12 years: same as adult; *see page 562 for dose by weight*
      Omnicef *Cap:* 300 mg; *Oral susp:* 125 mg/5 ml (60, 100 ml) (strawberry)

➤ *cefditoren pivoxil* (B) 200 mg bid x 10 days
Pediatric: not recommended
      Spectracef *Tab:* 200 mg
      Comment: Spectracef is contraindicated with milk protein allergy or carnitine deficiency.

➤ *cefixime* (B) 400 mg daily x 5 days
Pediatric: <6 months: not recommended; 6 months-12 years, <50 kg: 8 mg/kg/day in 1-2 divided doses x 10 days; >12 years, ≥50 kg: same as adult; *see page 563 for dose by weight*
      Suprax *Tab:* 400 mg; *Cap:* 400 mg; *Oral susp:* 100, 200 mg/5 ml (50, 75, 100 ml) (strawberry)

➤ *cefpodoxime proxetil* (B) 100 mg bid x 5-7 days
Pediatric: <2 months: not recommended; 2 months-12 years: 10 mg/kg/day in 2 divided doses x 5-7 days; >12 years: same as adult; *see page 564 for dose by weight*
      Vantin *Tab:* 100, 200 mg; *Oral susp:* 50, 100 mg/5 ml (50, 75, 100 ml) (lemon creme)

➤ *cefprozil* (B) 500 mg daily x 10 days
Pediatric: <2 years: not recommended; 2-12 years: 7.5 mg/kg divided bid x 10 days; >12 years: same as adult; *see page 565 for dose by weight*
      Cefzil *Tab:* 250, 500 mg; *Oral susp:* 125, 250 mg/5 ml (50, 75, 100 ml) (bubble gum) (phenylalanine)

➤ *ceftibuten* (B) 400 mg daily x 5 days
Pediatric: 9 mg/kg daily x 5 days; *see page 566 for dose by weight*
      Cedax *Cap:* 400 mg; *Oral susp:* 90 mg/5 ml (30, 60, 90, 120 ml); 180 mg/5 ml (30, 60, 120 ml) (cherry)

➤ *cefuroxime axetil* (B)(G) 250 mg bid x 10 days
Pediatric: <3 months: not recommended; ≥3 months: 20 mg/kg/day divided bid x 10 days; *see page 567 for dose by weight*
      Ceftin *Tab:* 250, 500 mg; *Oral susp:* 125, 250 mg/5 ml (50, 100 ml) (tutti-frutti)

➤ *cephalexin* (B)(G) 500 mg bid x 10 days
Pediatric: 25-50 mg/kg/day in 2 divided doses x 10 days; *see page 568 for dose by weight*
      Keflex *Cap:* 250, 333, 500, 750 mg; *Oral susp:* 125, 250 mg/5 ml (100, 200 ml) (strawberry)

➤ *clarithromycin* (C)(G) 250 mg bid or 500 mg ext-rel daily x 10 days
Pediatric: <6 months: not recommended; ≥6 months: 7.5 mg/kg divided bid x 10 days; *see page 569 for dose by weight*
      Biaxin *Tab:* 250, 500 mg
      Biaxin Oral Suspension *Oral susp:* 125, 250 mg/5 ml (50, 100 ml) (fruit-punch)
      Biaxin XL *Tab:* 500 mg ext-rel

➤ *dirithromycin* (C)(G) 500 mg daily x 10 days
Pediatric: <12 years: not recommended; ≥12 years: same as adult
      Dynabac *Tab:* 250 mg

➤ *erythromycin base* **(B)(G)** 500 mg qid x 10 days
    Pediatric: <45 kg: 30-50 mg divided bid-qid x 10 days; ≥45 kg: same as adult
        Ery-Tab *Tab:* 250, 333, 500 mg ent-coat
        PCE *Tab:* 333, 500 mg
    Comment: *erythromycin* may increase INR with concomitant *warfarin*, as well as increase serum level of *digoxin*, benzodiazepines and statins.

➤ *erythromycin estolate* **(B)(G)** 250-500 mg qid x 10 days
    Pediatric: 20-50 mg/kg divided q 6 hours x 10 days; *see page 573 for dose by weight*
        Ilosone *Pulvule:* 250 mg; *Tab:* 500 mg; *Liq:* 125, 250 mg/5 ml (100 ml)
    Comment: *erythromycin* may increase INR with concomitant *warfarin*, as well as increase serum level of *digoxin*, benzodiazepines and statins.

➤ *erythromycin ethylsuccinate* **(B)(G)** 400 mg qid or 800 mg bid x 10 days
    Pediatric: 30-50 mg/kg/day in 4 divided doses x 7 days; may double dose with severe infection; max 100 mg/kg/day; *see page 574 for dose by weight*
        EryPed *Oral susp:* 200 mg/5 ml (100, 200 ml) (fruit); 400 mg/5 ml (60, 100, 200 ml) (banana); *Oral drops:* 200, 400 mg/5 ml (50 ml) (fruit); *Chew tab:* 200 mg wafer (fruit)
        E.E.S. *Oral susp:* 200, 400 mg/5 ml (100 ml) (fruit)
        E.E.S. Granules *Oral susp:* 200 mg/5 ml (100, 200 ml) (cherry)
        E.E.S. 400 Tablets *Tab:* 400 mg
    Comment: *erythromycin* may increase INR with concomitant *warfarin*, as well as increase serum level of *digoxin*, benzodiazepines and statins.

➤ *loracarbef* **(B)** 200 mg bid x 5 days
    Pediatric: 15 mg/kg/day in 2 divided doses x 5 days; *see page 581 for dose by weight*
        Lorabid *Pulvule:* 200, 400 mg; *Oral susp:* 100 mg/5 ml (50, 100 ml); 200 mg/5 ml (50, 75, 100 ml) (strawberry bubble gum)

➤ *penicillin G (benzathine)* **(B)(G)** 1.2 million units IM x 1 dose
    Pediatric: <60 lb: 300,000-600,000 units IM x 1 dose; ≥60 lb: 900,000 units x 1 dose
        Bicillin L-A *Cartridge-needle unit:* 600,000 units (1 ml); 1.2 million units (2 ml)

➤ *penicillin G (benzathine and procaine)* **(B)(G)** 2.4 million units IM x 1 dose
    Pediatric: <30 lb: 600,000 units IM x 1 dose; 30-60 lb: 900,000-1.2 million units IM x 1 dose; >60 mg: same as adult
        Bicillin C-R *Cartridge-needle unit:* 600,000 units (1 ml); 1.2 million units; (2 ml); 2.4 million units (4 ml)

➤ *penicillin V potassium* **(B)(G)** 500 mg bid or 250 mg qid x 10 days
    Pediatric: 25-50 mg/kg day in 4 divided doses x 10 days; >12 years: same as adult; *see page 583 for dose by weight*
        Pen-Vee K *Tab:* 250, 500 mg; *Oral soln:* 125 mg/5 ml (100, 200 ml); 250 mg/5 ml (100, 150, 200 ml)
        Veetids *Tab:* 250, 500 mg; *Oral soln:* 125, 250 mg/5 ml (100, 200 ml)

⬤ PHEOCHROMOCYTOMA

ALPHA-BLOCKER

➤ *phenoxybenzamine* **(C)** initially 10 mg bid; increase every other day as needed; usually 20-40 mg bid-tid
    Dibenzyline *Cap:* 10 mg

PINWORM (ENTEROBIUS VERMICULARIS)

Comment: Treatment of all family members is recommended.

ANTHELMINTICS

▷ *albendazole* (C) 400 mg x 1 dose; may repeat in 2-3 weeks if needed; take with a meal
  Pediatric: <20 kg: 200 mg as a single dose; >20kg: same as adult
    Albenza *Tab:* 200 mg
▷ *mebendazole* (C) chew, swallow, <u>or</u> mix with food; 100 mg x 1 dose; may repeat in 3 weeks if needed; take with a meal
  Pediatric: <2 years: not recommended; ≥2 years: same as adult
    Emverm *Chew tab:* 100 mg
    Vermox (G) *Chew tab:* 100 mg
▷ *pyrantel pamoate* (C) 11 mg/kg x 1 dose; max 1 g/dose; may repeat in 2-3 weeks if needed; take with a meal
  Pediatric: 25-37 lb: 1/2 tsp x 1 dose; 38-62 lb: 1 tsp x 1 dose; 63-87 lb: 1 tsp x 1 dose; 88-112 lb: 2 tsp x 1 dose; 113-137 lb: 2 tsp x 1 dose; 138-162 lb: 3 tsp x 1 dose; 163-187 lb: 3 tsp x 1 dose; >187 lb: 4 tsp x 1 dose
    Pin-X (OTC); *Cap:* 180 mg; *Liq:* 50 mg/ml (30 ml); 144 mg/ml (30 ml); *Oral susp:* 50 mg/ml (30 ml)
▷ *thiabendazole* (C) 50 mg/kg x 1 dose after a meal; max 3 g; may repeat in 2-3 weeks if needed; take with a meal
  Pediatric: same as adult
    Mintezol *Chew tab:* 500*mg (orange); *Oral susp:* 500 mg/5 ml (120 ml) (orange)
    Comment: *thiabendazole* should not be used as first-line therapy for pinworms. May impair mental alertness.

PITYRIASIS ALBA

Comment: Pityriasis alba is a chronic skin disorder seen in children with a genetic predisposition to atopic disease. Treatment is directed toward controlling roughness and pruritus. There is no known treatment for the associated skin pigment changes. Pityriasis alba resolves spontaneously and permanently in the 2nd <u>or</u> 3rd decade of life.
    Topical Corticosteroids *see page 506*

COAL TAR PREPARATIONS

▷ *coal tar* (C)
  Pediatric: same as adult
    Scytera (OTC) apply qd-qid; use lowest effective dose
      Foam: 2%
    T/Gel Shampoo Extra Strength (OTC) use every other day; max 4 x/week; massage into affected area for 5 minutes; rinse; repeat
      Shampoo: 1%
    T/Gel Shampoo Original Formula (OTC) use every other day; max 7 x/week; massage into affected area for 5 minutes; rinse; repeat
      Shampoo: 0.5%

> **T/Gel Shampoo Stubborn Itch Control (OTC)** use every other day; max 7 x/ week; massage into affected area for 5 minutes; rinse; repeat
> *Shampoo:* 0.5%

EMOLLIENTS AND OTHER MOISTURIZING AGENTS

see **Dermatitis: Atopic** *page* 110

⃝ PITYRIASIS ROSEA

Topical Corticosteroids *see page* 506
Oral Drugs for Allergy, Cough, and Cold *see page* 535

⃝ PLAGUE (*YERSINIA PESTIS*)

Comment: *Yersinia pestis* is transmitted via the bite of a flea from an infected rodent or the bite, lick, or scratch of an infected cat. Untreated bubonic plague may progress to secondary pneumonic plague, which may be transmitted via contaminated respiratory droplet spread.

▷ *streptomycin* (C)(G) 15mg/kg IM bid x 10 days
Pediatric: same as adult
Amp: 1 g/2.5 ml or 400 mg/ml (2.5 ml)
Comment: For patients with renal impairment, reduce dose of *streptomycin* to 20 mg/kg/day if mild and 8 mg/kg/day q 3 days if advanced). For patients who are pregnant or who have hearing impairment, shorten the course of treatment to 3 days after fever has resolved.

▷ *moxifloxacin* (C)(G) 400 mg daily x 10 days
Pediatric: <18 years: not recommended
Avelox *Tab:* 400 mg; IV soln: 400 mg/250 mg (latex-free, preservative-free)
Comment: *moxifloxacin* is for prophylaxis as well as treatment for pneumonia and septic plague. *moxifloxacin* is contraindicated <18 years of age and during pregnancy and lactation. Risk of tendonitis or tendon rupture, especially 60 years-of-age and older.

▷ *tetracycline* (D)(G) 500 mg qid or 25-50 mg/kg/day divided q 6 hours x 10 days
Comment: *tetracycline* is contraindicated <8 years-of-age, in pregnancy, and lactation (discolors developing tooth enamel). A side effect may be photo-sensitivity (photophobia). Do not give with antacids, calcium supplements, milk or other dairy, or within two hours of taking another drug.

⃝ PNEUMOCYSTIS JIROVECI PNEUMONIA

▷ *atovaquone* (C) take with food; *Treatment:* 750 mg once daily x 21 days; *Prophylaxis:* 1500 mg once daily
Pediatric: see mfr pkg insert
Mepron *Susp:* 750 mg/5 ml (citrus)

▷ *trimethoprim/sulfamethoxazole* (C)(G) *Prophylaxis:* 1 tab 3 x/week; *Treatment:* 1 tab daily x 3 weeks; *Septra* can be given if intolerable to *Bactrim*

Pediatric: <2 months: not recommended; ≥2 months: 40 mg/kg/day of sulfamethoxazole in 2 doses bid x 10 days

> **Bactrim, Septra** 2 tabs bid x 10 days
> > *Tab:* trim 80 mg/sulfa 400 mg*
> **Bactrim DS, Septra DS** 1 tab bid x 10 days
> > *Tab:* trim 160 mg/sulfa 800 mg*
> **Bactrim Pediatric Suspension, Septra Pediatric Suspension**
> > *Oral susp: trim 40 mg/sulfa* 200 mg per 5 ml (100 ml) (cherry) (alcohol 0.3%)

Comment: *trimethoprim/sulfamethoxazole* is not recommended in pregnancy or lactation. *CrCl 15-30 mL/min:* reduce dose by 1/2; *CrCl <15 mL/min:* not recommended

◯ PNEUMONIA: CHLAMYDIAL

RECOMMENDED REGIMEN

▷ *erythromycin base* (B)(G) 500 mg qid hours x 10-14 days
> *Pediatric:* <45 kg: 50 mg in 4 divided doses x 10-14 days; ≥45 kg: same as adult
> > **Ery-Tab** *Tab:* 250, 333, 500 mg ent-coat
> > **PCE** *Tab:* 333, 500 mg

Comment: *erythromycin* may increase INR with concomitant *warfarin*, as well as increase serum level of *digoxin*, benzodiazepines and statins.

▷ *erythromycin ethylsuccinate* (B)(G) 400 mg qid x 10-14 days
> *Pediatric:* <45 kg: 50 mg/kg/day in 4 divided doses x 10-14 days; ≥45 kg: same as adult; *see page 574 for dose by weight*
> > **EryPed** *Oral susp:* 200 mg/5 ml (100, 200 ml) (fruit); 400 mg/5 ml (60, 100, 200 ml) (banana); *Oral drops:* 200, 400 mg/5 ml (50 ml) (fruit); *Chew tab:* 200 mg wafer (fruit)
> > **E.E.S.** *Oral susp:* 200, 400 mg/5 ml (100 ml) (fruit)
> > **E.E.S. Granules** *Oral susp:* 200 mg/5 ml (100, 200 ml) (cherry)
> > **E.E.S. 400 Tablets** *Tab:* 400 mg

Comment: *erythromycin* may increase INR with concomitant *warfarin*, as well as increase serum level of *digoxin*, benzodiazepines and statins.

ALTERNATE REGIMENS

▷ *azithromycin* (B)(G) 500 mg once daily x 10 days
> *Pediatric:* 20 mg/kg per dose once daily x 3 days; max 500 mg/day; *see page 559 for dose by weight*
> > **Zithromax** *Tab:* 250, 500, 600 mg; *Oral susp:* 100 mg/5 ml (15 ml); 200 mg/5 ml (15, 22.5, 30 ml) (cherry); Pkt: 1 g for reconstitution (cherry-banana)
> > **Zithromax Tri-pak** *Tab:* 3 x 500 mg tabs/pck
> > **Zithromax Z-pak** *Tab:* 6 x 250 mg tabs/pck
> > **Zmax** *Oral susp:* 2 g ext-rel for reconstitution (cherry-banana) (148 mg Na⁺)

▷ *levofloxacin* (C) *Uncomplicated:* 500 mg daily x 7 days; *Complicated:* 750 mg daily x 7 days
> *Pediatric:* <18 years: not recommended
> > **Levaquin** *Tab:* 250, 500, 750 mg; *Oral soln:* 25 mg/ml (480 ml) (benzyl alcohol); *Inj conc:* 25 mg/ml for IV infusion after dilution (20, 30 ml single-use vial) (preservative-free); *Premix soln:* 5 mg/ml for IV infusion (50, 100, 150 ml) (preservative-free)

Comment: *levofloxacin* is contraindicated <18 years-of-age, and during pregnancy and lactation. Risk of tendonitis or tendon rupture, especially 60 years-of-age and older. Risk of tendonitis or tendon rupture, especially 60 years-of-age and older.

PNEUMONIA: COMMUNITY ACQUIRED (CAP)/ COMMUNITY ACQUIRED BACTERIAL PNEUMONIA (CABP)

ANTI-INFFECTIVES

Age 3 Months-5 Years

▷ *amoxicillin* (B)(G)
Pediatric: <40 kg (88 lb): 20-40 mg/kg/day in 3 divided doses x 10 days or 25-45 mg/kg/day in 2 divided doses x 10 days; ≥40 kg: same as adult
 Amoxil *Cap:* 250, 500 mg; *Tab:* 875 mg; *Chew tab:* 125, 200, 250, 400 mg (cherry-banana-peppermint) (phenylalanine); *Oral susp:* 125, 250 mg/5 ml (80, 100, 150 ml) (strawberry); 200, 400 mg/5 ml (50, 75, 100 ml) (bubble gum); *Oral drops:* 50 mg/ml (30 ml) (bubble gum)
 Moxatag *Tab:* 775 mg ext-rel
 Trimox *Tab:* 125, 250 mg; *Cap:* 250, 500 mg; *Oral susp:* 125, 250 mg/5 ml (80, 100, 150 ml) (raspberry-strawberry)

▷ *amoxicillin/clavulanate* (B)(G) 500 mg tid or 875 mg bid x 10 days
 Augmentin *Tab:* 250, 500, 875 mg; *Chew tab:* 125, 250 mg (lemon-lime); 200, 400 mg (cherry-banana) (phenylalanine); *Oral susp:* 125 mg/5 ml (banana), 250 mg/5 ml (75, 100, 150 ml) (orange); 200, 400 mg/5 ml (50, 75, 100 ml) (orange) (phenylalanine)
 Pediatric: 40-45 mg/kg/day divided tid x 10 days or 90 mg/kg/day divided bid x 10 days *see pages 556-557 for dose by weight*
 Augmentin ES-600 *Oral susp:* 600 mg/5 ml (50, 75, 100, 125, 150, 200 ml) (strawberry cream) (phenylalanine) every 12 hours
 Pediatric: <3 months: not recommended; ≥3 months, <40 kg: 90 mg/kg/day in 2 divided doses; ≥40 kg: not recommended
 Augmentin XR 2 tabs q 12 hours x 7-10 days
 Pediatric: <16 years: use other forms; ≥16 years: same as adult
 Tab: 1000*mg ext-rel

▷ *azithromycin* (B)(G)
Pediatric: <6 months: not recommended; ≥6 months: 10 mg/kg x 1 dose on day 1, then 5 mg/kg/day on days 2-5; max 500 mg/day; *see page 559 for dose by weight*
 Zithromax *Tab:* 250, 500, 600 mg; *Oral susp:* 100 mg/5 ml (15 ml); 200 mg/5 ml (15, 22.5, 30 ml) (cherry); *Pkt:* 1 g for reconstitution (cherry-banana)
 Zithromax Tri-pak *Tab:* 3 x 500 mg tabs/pck
 Zithromax Z-pak *Tab:* 6 x 250 mg tabs/pck
 Zmax *Oral susp:* 2 g ext-rel for reconstitution (cherry-banana) (148 mg Na⁺)

▷ *cefaclor* (B)(G) 250 mg tid or 375 mg bid x 10 days
Pediatric: <1 month: not recommended; 20-40 mg/kg divided bid or q 12 hours x 10 days; max 1 g/day; *see page 560 for dose by weight*
 Tab: 500 mg; *Cap:* 250, 500 mg; *Susp:* 125 mg/5 ml (75, 150 ml) (strawberry); 187 mg/5 ml (50, 100 ml) (strawberry); 250 mg/5 ml (75, 150 ml) (strawberry); 375 mg/5 ml (50, 100 ml) (strawberry)
 Cefaclor Extended Release

Pediatric: <16 years: ext-rel not recommended; ≥16 years: same as adult
    Tab: 375, 500 mg ext-rel

▷ *ceftriaxone*(B)(G)
Pediatric: 50-75 mg/kg IM in 2 divided doses; max 2 g/day
    Rocephin *Vial:* 250, 500 mg; 1, 2 g

▷ *clarithromycin* (C) 500 mg q 12 hours <u>or</u> 500 mg ext-rel daily x 10 days
Pediatric: <6 months: not recommended; ≥6 months: 7.5 mg/kg divided bid x 7-14
days; *see page 569 for dose by weight*
    Biaxin *Tab:* 250, 500 mg
    Biaxin Oral Suspension *Oral susp:* 125, 250 mg/5 ml (50, 100 ml) (fruit punch)
    Biaxin XL *Tab:* 500 mg ext-rel

▷ *erythromycin base* (B)(G)
Pediatric: <45 kg: 30-50 mg in 2-4 divided doses x 7-10 days; ≥45 kg: same as adult
    Ery-Tab *Tab:* 250, 333, 500 mg ent-coat
    PCE *Tab:* 333, 500 mg

Comment: *erythromycin* may increase INR with concomitant ***warfarin***, as well as
increase serum level of ***digoxin***, benzodiazepines and statins.

▷ *erythromycin estolate* (B)(G)
Pediatric: 30-50 mg/kg/day in divided doses x 10 days; *see page 573 for dose by
weight*
    Ilosone *Pulvule:* 250 mg; *Tab:* 500 mg; *Liq:* 125, 250 mg/5 ml (100 ml)

Comment: *erythromycin* may increase INR with concomitant ***warfarin***, as well as
increase serum level of ***digoxin***, benzodiazepines and statins.

Age 5-18 Years

▷ *amoxicillin* (B)(G) 875 mg bid <u>or</u> 500 mg tid x 10 days
Pediatric: <40 kg (88 lb): 20-40 mg/kg/day in 3 divided doses x 10 days <u>or</u> 25-45
mg/kg/day in 2 divided doses x 10 days; ≥40 kg: same as adult; *see page 554 for dose
by weight*
    Amoxil *Cap:* 250, 500 mg; *Tab:* 875*mg; *Chew tab:* 125, 200, 250, 400 mg (cher-
ry-banana-peppermint) (phenylalanine); *Oral susp:* 125, 250 mg/5 ml (80, 100,
150 ml) (strawberry); 200, 400 mg/5 ml (50, 75, 100 ml) (bubble gum); *Oral
drops:* 50 mg/ml (30 ml) (bubble gum)
    Trimox *Tab:* 125, 250 mg; *Cap:* 250, 500 mg; *Oral susp:* 125, 250 mg/5 ml (80,
100, 150 ml) (raspberry-strawberry)

▷ *amoxicillin/clavulanate* (B)(G) 500 mg tid <u>or</u> 875 mg bid x 10 days
    Augmentin *Tab:* 250, 500, 875 mg; *Chew tab:* 125, 250 mg (lemon-lime); 200,
400 mg (cherry-banana) (phenylalanine); *Oral susp:* 125 mg/5 ml (banana),
250 mg/5 ml (75, 100, 150 ml) (orange); 200, 400 mg/5 ml (50, 75, 100 ml)
(orange) (phenylalanine)
        Pediatric: 40-45 mg/kg/day divided tid x 10 days <u>or</u> 90 mg/kg/day divided
        bid x 10 days *see pages 556-557 for dose by weight*
    Augmentin ES-600 *Oral susp:* 600 mg/5 ml (50, 75, 100, 125, 150, 200 ml)
(strawberry cream) (phenylalanine) every 12 hours
        Pediatric: <3 months: not recommended; ≥3 months, <40 kg: 90 mg/kg/day
        in 2 divided doses; ≥40 kg: not recommended
    Augmentin XR 2 tabs q 12 hours x 7-10 days
        Pediatric: <16 years: use other forms; ≥16 years: same as adult
        Tab: 1000*mg ext-rel

▷ *azithromycin* (B)(G) weight-based or 500 mg x 1 dose on day 1, then 250 mg daily on days 2-5 or 500 mg daily x 3 days or **Zmax** 2 g in a single dose
Pediatric: 10 mg/kg x 1 dose on day 1, then 5 mg/kg/day on days 2-5; max 500 mg/day; *see page 559 for dose by weight*
   Zithromax *Tab:* 250, 500, 600 mg; *Oral susp:* 100 mg/5 ml (15 ml); 200 mg/5 ml (15, 22.5, 30 ml) (cherry); *Pkt:* 1 g for reconstitution (cherry-banana)
   Zithromax Tri-pak *Tab:* 3 x 500 mg tabs/pck
   Zithromax Z-pak *Tab:* 6 x 250 mg tabs/pck
▷ *cefaclor* (B)(G) 250 mg tid or 375 mg bid x 5 days
Pediatric: <1 month: not recommended; 20-40 mg/kg divided bid or q 12 hours x 10 days; max 1 g/day; *see page 560 for dose by weight*
   Tab: 500 mg; *Cap:* 250, 500 mg; *Susp:* 125 mg/5 ml (75, 150 ml) (strawberry); 187 mg/5 ml (50, 100 ml) (strawberry); 250 mg/5 ml (75, 150 ml) (strawberry); 375 mg/5 ml (50, 100 ml) (strawberry)
   Cefaclor Extended Release
      Pediatric: <16 years: ext-rel not recommended; ≥16 years: same as adult
      Tab: 375, 500 mg ext-rel
▷ *cefdinir* (B) 300 mg bid or 600 mg daily x 10 days
Pediatric: <6 months: not recommended; 6 months-12 years: 14 mg/kg/day in a single or 2 divided doses x 10 days; >12 years: same as adult; *see page 562 for dose by weight*
   Omnicef
      Cap: 300 mg; *Oral susp:* 125 mg/5 ml (60, 100 ml) (strawberry)
▷ *cefpodoxime proxetil* (B) 200 mg bid x 14 days
Pediatric: 2 months-2 years: 10 mg/kg/day in 2 doses x 14 days; >12 years: same as adult; *see page 564 for dose by weight*
   Vantin *Tab:* 100, 200 mg; *Oral susp:* 50, 100 mg/5 ml (50, 75, 100 ml) (lemon creme)
▷ *ceftriaxone* (B)
Pediatric: 50-75 mg/kg IM in 2 divided doses; max 2 g/day
   Rocephin *Vial:* 250, 500 mg; 1, 2 g
▷ *clarithromycin* (C) 7.5 mg/kg divided bid x 7-14 days
Pediatric: <6 months: not recommended; ≥6 months: 7.5 mg/kg bid x 7-14 days
   Biaxin *Tab:* 250, 500 mg
   Biaxin Oral Suspension *Oral susp:* 125, 250 mg/5 ml (50, 100 ml) (fruit-punch)
   Biaxin XL *Tab:* 500 mg ext-rel
▷ *dirithromycin* (C)(G) 500 mg daily x 14 days
Pediatric: <12 years: not recommended; ≥12 years: same as adult
   Dynabac *Tab:* 250 mg
▷ *erythromycin base* (B)(G) 500 mg q 6 hours x 10 days
Pediatric: <45 kg: 30-50 mg in 2-4 divided doses x 10 days; ≥45 kg: same as adult
   Ery-Tab *Tab:* 250, 333, 500 mg ent-coat
   PCE *Tab:* 333, 500 mg
   Comment: *erythromycin* may increase INR with concomitant *warfarin*, as well as increase serum level of *digoxin*, benzodiazepines and statins.
▷ *erythromycin estolate* (B) 250 mg q 6 hours x 10 days
Pediatric: 30-50 mg/kg/day in divided doses x 10 days; *see page 573 for dose by weight*
   Ilosone *Pulvule:* 250 mg; *Tab:* 500 mg; *Liq:* 125, 250 mg/5 ml (100 ml)
   Comment: *erythromycin* may increase INR with concomitant *warfarin*, as well as increase serum level of *digoxin*, benzodiazepines and statins.

Age 18-60 Years Without Comorbidity

▷ *amoxicillin* (B)(G) 500-875 mg bid or 250-500 mg tid x 10 days

Amoxil *Cap:* 250, 500 mg; *Tab:* 875*mg; *Chew tab:* 125, 200, 250, 400 mg (cherry-banana-peppermint) (phenylalanine); *Oral susp:* 125, 250 mg/5 ml (80, 100, 150 ml) (strawberry); 200, 400 mg/5 ml (50, 75, 100 ml) (bubble gum); *Oral drops:* 50 mg/ml (30 ml) (bubble gum)

Moxatag *Tab:* 775 mg ext-rel

Trimox *Tab:* 125, 250 mg; *Cap:* 250, 500 mg; *Oral susp:* 125, 250 mg/5 ml (80, 100, 150 ml) (raspberry-strawberry)

▷ *amoxicillin/clavulanate* (B)(G) 500 mg tid or 875 mg bid x 10 days

Augmentin *Tab:* 250, 500, 875 mg; *Chew tab:* 125, 250 mg (lemon-lime); 200, 400 mg (cherry-banana) (phenylalanine); *Oral susp:* 125 mg/5 ml (banana), 250 mg/5 ml (75, 100, 150 ml) (orange); 200, 400 mg/5 ml (50, 75, 100 ml) (orange) (phenylalanine)

    Pediatric: 40-45 mg/kg/day divided tid x 10 days or 90 mg/kg/day divided bid x 10 days *see pages* 556-557 *for dose by weight*

Augmentin ES-600 *Oral susp:* 600 mg/5 ml (50, 75, 100, 125, 150, 200 ml) (strawberry cream) (phenylalanine) every 12 hours

    Pediatric: <3 months: not recommended; ≥3 months, <40 kg: 90 mg/kg/day in 2 divided doses; ≥40 kg: not recommended

Augmentin XR 2 tabs q 12 hours x 7-10 days

    Pediatric: <16 years: use other forms; ≥16 years: same as adult

    Tab: 1000*mg ext-rel

▷ *azithromycin* (B)(G) 500 mg x 1 dose on day 1, then 250 mg daily on days 2-5 or 500 mg daily x 3 days or **Zmax** 2 g in a single dose

Zithromax *Tab:* 250, 500, 600 mg; *Oral susp:* 100 mg/5 ml (15 ml); 200 mg/5 ml (15, 22.5, 30 ml) (cherry); *Pkt:* 1 g for reconstitution (cherry-banana)

Zithromax Tri-pak *Tab:* 3 x 500 mg tabs/pck

Zithromax Z-pak *Tab:* 6 x 250 mg tabs/pck

Zmax *Oral susp:* 2 g ext-rel for reconstitution (cherry-banana) (148 mg Na$^+$)

▷ *cefaclor* (B)(G) 250 mg tid or 375 mg bid x 10 days

Tab: 500 mg; *Cap:* 250, 500 mg; *Susp:* 125 mg/5 ml (75, 150 ml) (strawberry); 187 mg/5 ml (50, 100 ml) (strawberry); 250 mg/5 ml (75, 150 ml) (strawberry); 375 mg/5 ml (50, 100 ml) (strawberry)

Cefaclor Extended Release

    Pediatric: <16 years: ext-rel not recommended; ≥16 years: same as adult

    Tab: 375, 500 mg ext-rel

▷ *cefdinir* (B) 300 mg bid or 600 mg daily x 10 days

Omnicef *Cap:* 300 mg; *Oral susp:* 125 mg/5 ml (60, 100 ml) (strawberry)

▷ *cefpodoxime proxetil* (B) 200 mg bid x 14 days

Vantin *Tab:* 100, 200 mg; *Oral susp:* 50, 100 mg/5 ml (50, 75, 100 ml) (lemon creme)

▷ *ceftaroline fosamil* (B) administer by IV infusion after reconstitution every 12 hours x 5-7 days; *CrCl ≥50 mL/min:* 600 mg; *CrCl >30-<50 mL/min:* 400 mg; *CrCl: >15-<30 mL/min:* 300 mg; ES RD: 200 mg

Teflaro *Vial:* 400, 600 mg

▷ *ceftriaxone* (B)(G) 1-2 g IM daily; max 4 g

Rocephin *Vial:* 250, 500 mg; 1, 2 g

▷ *clarithromycin* (C)(G) 500 mg bid or 500 mg ext-rel daily x 7-14 days

Biaxin *Tab:* 250, 500 mg

Biaxin Oral Suspension *Oral susp:* 125, 250 mg/5 ml (50, 100 ml) (fruit-punch)

Biaxin XL *Tab:* 500 mg ext-rel
▷ *dirithromycin* (C)(G) 500 mg daily x 14 days
    Dynabac *Tab:* 250 mg
▷ *doxycycline* (D)(G) 100 mg bid x 7-14 days
    Actilate *Tab:* 75, 150** mg
    Adoxa *Tab:* 50, 75, 100, 150 mg ent-coat
    Doryx *Tab:* 50, 75, 100, 150, 200 mg del-rel
    Monodox *Cap:* 50, 75, 100 mg
    Oracea *Cap:* 40 mg del-rel
    Vibramycin *Tab:* 100 mg; *Cap:* 50, 100 mg; *Syr:* 50 mg/5 ml (raspberry-apple) (sulfites); *Oral susp:* 25 mg/5 ml (raspberry)
    Vibra-Tab *Tab:* 100 mg film-coat

Comment: *doxycycline* is contraindicated <8 years-of-age, in pregnancy, and lactation (discolors developing tooth enamel). A side effect may be photo-sensitivity (photophobia). Do not give with antacids, calcium supplements, milk or other dairy, or within two hours of taking another drug.

▷ *ertapenem* (B) 1 g daily; *CrCl <30 mL/min:* 500 mg daily x 3-10 days; may switch to an oral antibiotic after 3 days if warranted; *IV infusion:* administer over 30 minutes; *IM injection:* reconstitute with lidocaine only
    Ivanz *Vial:* 1 g pwdr for reconstitution

▷ *erythromycin base* (B)(G) 500 mg q 6 hours x 14-21 days; <45 kg: 30-50 mg in 2-4 doses x 14-21 days; ≥45 kg: same as adult
    Ery-Tab *Tab:* 250, 333, 500 mg ent-coat
    PCE *Tab:* 333, 500 mg

Comment: *erythromycin* may increase INR with concomitant *warfarin*, as well as increase serum level of *digoxin*, benzodiazepines and statins.

▷ *erythromycin estolate* (B) 500 mg q 6 hours x 14-21 days
    Ilosone *Pulvule:* 250 mg; *Tab:* 500 mg; *Liq:* 125, 250 mg/5 ml (100 ml)

Comment: *erythromycin* may increase INR with concomitant *warfarin*, as well as increase serum level of *digoxin*, benzodiazepines and statins.

▷ *gemifloxacin* (C)(G) 320 mg daily x 5-7 days
Pediatric: <18 years: not recommended
    Factive *Tab:* 320* mg

Comment: *gemifloxacin* is contraindicated <18 years-of-age, and during pregnancy and lactation. Risk of tendonitis or tendon rupture, especially 60 years-of-age and older.

▷ *levofloxacin* (C) *Uncomplicated:* 500 mg once daily x 7-14 days; *Complicated:* 750 mg once daily x 7-14 days
Pediatric: <18 years: not recommended
    Levaquin *Tab:* 250, 500, 750 mg; *Oral soln:* 25 mg/ml (480 ml) (benzyl alcohol); *Inj conc:* 25 mg/ml for IV infusion after dilution (20, 30 ml single-use vial) (preservative-free); *Premix soln:* 5 mg/ml for IV infusion (50, 100, 150 ml) (preservative-free)

Comment: *levofloxacin* is contraindicated <18 years-of-age, and during pregnancy and lactation. Risk of tendonitis or tendon rupture, especially 60 years-of-age and older.

▷ *linezolid* (C)(G) 600 mg q 12 hours x 10-14 days
Pediatric: <5 years: 10 mg/kg q 8 hours x 10-14 days; 5-11 years: 10 mg/kg q 12 hours x 10-14 days; >11years: same as adult
    Zyvox *Tab:* 400, 600 mg; *Oral susp:* 100 mg/5 ml (150 ml) (orange) (phenylalanine)

Comment: *linezolid* is indicated to treat susceptible vancomycin-resistant *E. faecium* infections.

▷ *loracarbef* (B) 400 mg bid x 14 days

    Lorabid *Pulvule:* 200, 400 mg; *Oral susp:* 100 mg/5 ml (50, 100 ml); 200 mg/5 ml (50, 75, 100 ml) (strawberry bubble gum)

▷ *moxifloxacin* (C)(G) 400 mg daily x 10 days

    Pediatric: <18 years: recommended

        Avelox *Tab:* 400 mg; IV soln: 400 mg/250 mg (latex-free, preservative-free)

    Comment: *moxifloxacin* is contraindicated <18 years of age and during pregnancy and lactation. Risk of tendonitis or tendon rupture, especially 60 years-of-age and older.

▷ *ofloxacin* (C)(G) 400 mg bid x 10 days

    Pediatric: <18 years: not recommended

        Floxin *Tab:* 200, 300, 400 mg

    Comment: *ofloxacin* is contraindicated <18 years of age and during pregnancy and lactation. Risk of tendonitis or tendon rupture, especially 60 years-of-age and older.

▷ *tedizolid phosphate* (B) administer 200 mg once daily x 6 days, via PO or IV infusion over 1 hour

    Pediatric: <18 years: not established

        Sivextro *Tab:* 200 mg (6/blister pck)

    Comment: Sivextro is indicated for the treatment of adults with community acquired bacterial pneumonia (CABP)

▷ *telithromycin* (C) 2 x 400 mg tabs in a singe dose daily x 7-10 days

        Ketek *Tab:* 300, 400 mg

    Comment: *telithromycin* is contraindicated with PMHx hepatitis or jaundice associated with macrolide use.

▷ *tigecycline* (D)(G) 100 mg once; then 50 mg q 12 hours x 7-14 days; *Severe hepatic impaitment (Child Pugh C):* 100 mg once; then 25 mg q 12 hours

    Pediatric: <18 years: not recommended

        Tygacil *Vial:* 50 mg pwdr for reconstitution and IV infusion (preservative-free)

    Comment: Tygacil is indicated only for the treatment of adults with community acquired bacterial pneumonia (CABP). *tigecycline* is contraindicated <8 years-of-age, in pregnancy, and lactation (discolors developing tooth enamel). A side effect may be photo-sensitivity (photophobia). Do not give with antacids, calcium supplements, milk or other dairy, or within two hours of taking another drug.

Age Over 60 Years or Presence of Comorbidity

Comment: Consider respiratory quinolone for presence of comorbidity

▷ *amoxicillin/clavulanate* (B)(G) 500 mg tid or 875 mg bid x 10 days

    Augmentin *Tab:* 250, 500, 875 mg; *Chew tab:* 125, 250 mg (lemon-lime); 200, 400 mg (cherry-banana) (phenylalanine); *Oral susp:* 125 mg/5 ml (banana), 250 mg/5 ml (75, 100, 150 ml) (orange); 200, 400 mg/5 ml (50, 75, 100 ml) (orange) (phenylalanine)

        Pediatric: 40-45 mg/kg/day divided tid x 10 days or 90 mg/kg/day divided bid x 10 days *see page 556 for dose by weight*

    Augmentin ES-600 *Oral susp:* 600 mg/5 ml (50, 75, 100, 125, 150, 200 ml) (strawberry cream) (phenylalanine) every 12 hours

        Pediatric: <3 months: not recommended; ≥3 months, <40 kg: 90 mg/kg/day in 2 divided doses; ≥40 kg: not recommended

Augmentin XR 2 tabs q 12 hours x 7-10 days
> *Pediatric:* <16 years: use other forms; ≥16 years: same as adult
> *Tab:* 1000*mg ext-rel

▷ *azithromycin* (B)(G) 500 mg x 1 dose on day 1, then 250 mg daily on days 2-5 or 500 mg daily x 3 days or **Zmax** 2 g in a single dose
> **Zithromax** *Tab:* 250, 500, 600 mg; *Oral susp:* 100 mg/5 ml (15 ml); 200 mg/5 ml (15, 22.5, 30 ml) (cherry); *Pkt:* 1 g for reconstitution (cherry-banana)
> **Zithromax Tri-pak** *Tab:* 3 x 500 mg tabs/pck
> **Zithromax Z-pak** *Tab:* 6 x 250 mg tabs/pck
> **Zmax** *Oral susp:* 2 g ext-rel for reconstitution (cherry-banana) (148 mg Na⁺)

▷ *cefaclor* (B)(G) 250 mg tid or 375 mg bid x 7 days
> *Tab:* 500 mg; *Cap:* 250, 500 mg; *Susp:* 125 mg/5 ml (75, 150 ml) (strawberry); 187 mg/5 ml (50, 100 ml) (strawberry); 250 mg/5 ml (75, 150 ml) (strawberry); 375 mg/5 ml (50, 100 ml) (strawberry)
> **Cefaclor Extended Release**
> > *Pediatric:* <16 years: ext-rel not recommended
> > *Tab:* 375, 500 mg ext-rel

▷ *cefdinir* (B) 300 mg bid or 600 mg daily x 10 days
> **Omnicef** *Cap:* 300 mg; *Oral susp:* 125 mg/5 ml (60, 100 ml) (strawberry)

▷ *cefpodoxime proxetil* (B) 200 mg bid x 14 days
> **Vantin** *Tab:* 100, 200 mg; *Oral susp:* 50, 100 mg/5 ml (50, 75, 100 ml) (lemon creme)

▷ *ceftriaxone* (B)(G) 1-2 g IM once daily; max 4 g
> **Rocephin** *Vial:* 250, 500 mg; 1, 2 g

▷ *clarithromycin* (C)(G) 500 mg bid x 7-14 days
> **Biaxin** *Tab:* 250, 500 mg
> **Biaxin Oral Suspension** *Oral susp:* 125, 250 mg/5 ml (50, 100 ml) (fruit-punch)
> **Biaxin XL** *Tab:* 500 mg ext-rel

▷ *dirithromycin* (C)(G) 500 mg daily x 14 days
> **Dynabac** *Tab:* 250 mg

▷ *gemifloxacin* (C)(G) 320 mg daily x 5-7 days
> *Pediatric:* <18 years: not recommended
> > **Factive** *Tab:* 320* mg

Comment: *gemifloxacin* is contraindicated <18 years-of-age, and during pregnancy and lactation. Risk of tendonitis or tendon rupture, especially 60 years-of-age and older.

▷ *levofloxacin* (C)
> *Pediatric:* <18 years: not recommended; *Uncomplicated:* 500 mg daily x 7-14 days; *Complicated:* 750 mg daily x 7-14 days
> > **Levaquin** *Tab:* 250, 500, 750 mg; *Oral soln:* 25 mg/ml (480 ml) (benzyl alcohol); *Inj conc:* 25 mg/ml for IV infusion after dilution (20, 30 ml single-use vial) (preservative-free); *Premix soln:* 5 mg/ml for IV infusion (50, 100, 150 ml) (preservative-free)

Comment: *levofloxacin* is contraindicated <18 years-of-age and during pregnancy and lactation. Risk of tendonitis or tendon rupture, especially 60 years-of-age and older.

▷ *loracarbef* (B) 400 mg bid x 14 days
> **Lorabid** *Pulvule:* 200, 400 mg; *Oral susp:* 100 mg/5 ml (50, 100 ml); 200 mg/5 ml (50, 75, 100 ml) (strawberry bubble gum)

▷ *trimethoprim/sulfamethoxazole* (C)(G)
    Bactrim, Septra 2 tabs bid x 10 days
        Tab: trim 80 mg/*sulfa* 400 mg*
    Bactrim DS, Septra DS 1 tab bid x 10 days
        Tab: trim 160 mg/*sulfa* 800 mg*

Comment: *trimethoprim/sulfamethoxazole* is not recommended in pregnancy or lactation. *CrCl 15-30 mL/min:* reduce dose by 1/2; *CrCl <15 mL/min:* not recommended.

▷ *telithromycin* (C) 2 x 400 mg tabs in a singe dose daily x 7-10 days
    Ketek *Tab:* 300, 400 mg

Comment: *telithromycin* is contraindicated with PMHx hepatitis or jaundice associated with macrolide use.

PNEUMONIA: LEGIONELLA

▷ *ciprofloxacin* (C) 500 mg bid x 14-21 days
    Pediatric: <18 years: not recommended
    Cipro (G) *Tab:* 250, 500, 750 mg; *Oral susp:* 250, 500 mg/5 ml (100 ml) (strawberry)
    Cipro XR *Tab:* 500, 1000 mg ext-rel
    ProQuin XR *Tab:* 500 mg ext-rel

Comment: *ciprofloxacin* is contraindicated <18 years-of-age, and during pregnancy and lactation. Risk of tendonitis or tendon rupture, especially 60 years-of-age and older.

▷ *clarithromycin* (C)(G) 500 mg bid or 500 mg ext-rel daily x 14-21 days
    Biaxin *Tab:* 250, 500 mg
    Biaxin Oral Suspension *Oral susp:* 125, 250 mg/5 ml (50, 100 ml) (fruit-punch)
    Biaxin XL *Tab:* 500 mg ext-rel

▷ *dirithromycin* (C)(G) 500 mg once daily x 14-21 days
    Dynabac *Tab:* 250 mg

▷ *erythromycin base* (B)(G) 500 mg qid x 14-21 days
    Pediatric: <45 kg: 30-50 mg in 2-4 divided doses x 14-21 days; ≥45 kg: same as adult
    Ery-Tab *Tab:* 250, 333, 500 mg ent-coat
    PCE *Tab:* 333, 500 mg

Comment: *erythromycin* may increase INR with concomitant *warfarin*, as well as increase serum level of *digoxin*, benzodiazepines and statins.

▷ *erythromycin estolate* (B)(G) 1-2 g daily in divided doses x 14-21 days
    Pediatric: 30-50 mg/kg/day in divided doses x 14-21 days; *see page* 573 *for dose by weight*
    Ilosone *Pulvule:* 250 mg; *Tab:* 500 mg; *Liq:* 125, 250 mg/5 ml (100 ml)

Comment: *erythromycin* may increase INR with concomitant *warfarin*, as well as increase serum level of *digoxin*, benzodiazepines and statins.

▷ *trimethoprim/sulfamethoxazole* (C)(G)
    Pediatric: <2 months: not recommended; ≥2 months: 40 mg/kg/day of *sulfamethoxazole* in 2 doses bid x 10 days
    Bactrim, Septra 2 tabs bid x 10 days
        Tab: trim 80 mg/*sulfa* 400 mg*
    Bactrim DS, Septra DS 1 tab bid x 10 days
        Tab: trim 160 mg/*sulfa* 800 mg*
    Bactrim Pediatric Suspension, Septra Pediatric Suspension

Oral susp: trim 40 mg/*sulfa* 200 mg per 5 ml (100 ml) (cherry) (alcohol 0.3%)

Comment: *trimethoprim/sulfamethoxazole* is not recommended in pregnancy or lactation. *CrCl 15-30 mL/min:* reduce dose by 1/2; *CrCl <15 mL/min:* not recommended.

⬤ PNEUMONIA: MYCOPLASMA

ANTI-INFECTIVES

▷ *azithromycin* (B)(G) 500 mg x 1 dose on day 1, then 250 mg daily on days 2-5 or 500 mg daily x 3 days or **Zmax** 2 g in a single dose
  Pediatric: 12 mg/kg/day x 5 days; max 500 mg/day; *see page 559 for dose by weight*
      Zithromax *Tab:* 250, 500, 600 mg; *Oral susp:* 100 mg/5 ml (15 ml); 200 mg/5 ml (15, 22.5, 30 ml) (cherry); *Pkt:* 1 g for reconstitution (cherry-banana)
      Zithromax Tri-pak *Tab:* 3 x 500 mg tabs/pck
      Zithromax Z-pak *Tab:* 6 x 250 mg tabs/pck
      Zmax *Oral susp:* 2 g ext-rel for reconstitution (cherry-banana) (148 mg Na⁺)
▷ *clarithromycin* (C)(G) 500 mg bid or 500 mg ext-rel daily x 14-21 days
  Pediatric: <6 months: not recommended; ≥6 months: 7.5 mg/kg bid x 7 days; *see page 569 for dose by weight*
      Biaxin *Tab:* 250, 500 mg
      Biaxin Oral Suspension *Oral susp:* 125, 250 mg/5 ml (50, 100 ml) (fruit-punch)
      Biaxin XL *Tab:* 500 mg ext-rel
▷ *erythromycin base* (B)(G) 500 mg q 6 hours x 14-21 days
  Pediatric: <45 kg: 30-50 mg in 2-4 doses x 14-21 days; ≥45 kg: same as adult
      Ery-Tab *Tab:* 250, 333, 500 mg ent-coat
      PCE *Tab:* 333, 500 mg
  Comment: *erythromycin* may increase INR with concomitant *warfarin*, as well as increase serum level of *digoxin*, benzodiazepines and statins.
▷ *erythromycin ethylsuccinate* (B)(G) 400 mg qid x 14-21 days
  Pediatric: 30-50 mg/kg/day in 4 divided doses x 14-21 days; may double dose with severe infection; max 100 mg/kg/day; *see page 574 for dose by weight*
      EryPed *Oral susp:* 200 mg/5 ml (100, 200 ml) (fruit); 400 mg/5 ml (60, 100, 200 ml) (banana); *Oral drops:* 200, 400 mg/5 ml (50 ml) (fruit); *Chew tab:* 200 mg wafer (fruit)
      E.E.S. *Oral susp:* 200, 400 mg/5 ml (100 ml) (fruit)
      E.E.S. Granules *Oral susp:* 200 mg/5 ml (100, 200 ml) (cherry)
      E.E.S. 400 Tablets *Tab:* 400 mg
  Comment: *erythromycin* may increase INR with concomitant *warfarin*, as well as increase serum level of *digoxin*, benzodiazepines and statins.
▷ *tetracycline* (D)(G) 500 mg qid
  Pediatric: <8 years: not recommended; ≥8 years, <100 lb: 25-50 mg/kg/day in 2-4 divided doses; ≥8 years, ≥100 lb: same as adult; *see page 585 for dose by weight*
      Achromycin V *Cap:* 250, 500 mg
      Sumycin *Tab:* 250, 500 mg; *Cap:* 250, 500 mg; *Oral susp:* 125 mg/5 ml (100, 200 ml) (fruit) (sulfites)
  Comment: *tetracycline* is contraindicated <8 years-of-age, in pregnancy, and lactation (discolors developing tooth enamel). A side effect may be photo-sensitivity (photophobia). Do not give with antacids, calcium supplements, milk or other dairy, or within two hours of taking another drug.

PNEUMONIA: PNEUMOCOCCAL

PROPHYLAXIS

➤ *pneumococcal* vaccine (C) 0.5 ml IM or SC in deltoid x 1 dose
   Pneumovax
   Pediatric: <2 years: not recommended; ≥2 years: same as adult
   Vial: 25 mcg/0.5 ml (0.5 ml single-dose, 10/pck; 2.5 ml)
   Pnu-Imune 23
   Pediatric: <2 years: not recommended; ≥2 years: same as adult
   Vial: 25 mcg/0.5 ml (0.5 ml single-dose, 5/pck; 2.5 ml)
   Prevnar 13 for adults ≥50 years of age
   Pediatric: total 4 doses: 2, 4, 6, and 12-15 months-of-age; may start at 6 weeks
   of age; administer first 3 doses 4-8 weeks apart and the 4th dose at least 2
   months after the 3rd dose
   Vial: 25 mcg/0.5 ml (2.5 ml multi-dose; *Prefilled syringe:* (0.5 ml single-dose
   10/pck)
Comment: Pneumococcal vaccine contains 23 polysaccharide isolates representing
approximately 85-90% of common U.S. isolates. Administer the pneumococcal
vaccine in the anterolateral aspect of the thigh for infants and the deltoid for
toddlers, children, and adults.

TREATMENT

see **CAP/CABP** *page* 340

POLIOMYELITIS

PROPHYLAXIS

➤ *trivalent poliovirus vaccine, inactivated (type 1, 2, and 3)* (C)
   Pediatric: <6 weeks: not recommended; ≥6 weeks: one dose at 2, 4, 6-18 months
   and 4-6 years of age
   Ipol 0.5 ml SC or IM in deltoid area

POLYARTICULAR JUVENILE IDIOPATHIC ARTHRITIS (PJIA)

Acetaminophen for IV Infusion *see Pain page* 306
Oral Prescription NSAIDs *see page* 501
Other Oral Analgesics *see Pain page* 308
Topical/Transdermal NSAIDs *see Pain page* 307
Parenteral Corticosteroids *see page* 511
Oral Corticosteroids *see page* 509
Topical Analgesic and Anesthetic Agents *see page* 499

TOPICAL ANALGESICS

➤ *capsaicin* (B)(G) apply tid or qid prn to intact skin
   Pediatric: <2 years: not recommended; ≥2 years: same as adult

Axsain *Crm:* 0.075% (1, 2 oz)
Capsin *Lotn:* 0.025, 0.075% (59 ml)
Capzasin-P (OTC) *Crm:* 0.025% (1.5 oz); *Lotn:* 0.025% (2 oz)
Dolorac *Crm:* 0.025% (28 g)
Double Cap (OTC) *Crm:* 0.05% (2 oz)
R-Gel *Gel:* 0.025% (15, 30 g)
Zostrix (OTC) *Crm:* 0.025% (0.7, 1.5, 3 oz)
Zostrix HP (OTC) *Emol crm:* 0.075% (1, 2 oz)
Comment: Provides some relief by 1-2 weeks; optimal benefit may take 4-6 weeks.

ORAL SALICYLATES

➤ *indomethacin* (C) initially 25 mg bid <u>or</u> tid, increase as needed at weekly intervals by 25-50 mg/day; max 200 mg/day
Pediatric: <14 years: usually not recommended; >2 years, if risk warranted: 1-2 mg/kg/day in divided doses; max 3-4 mg/kg/day (<u>or</u> 150-200 mg/day, whichever is less; <14 years, ER cap not recommended
Cap: 25, 50 mg; *Susp;* 25 mg/5 ml (pineapple-coconut, mint) (alcohol 1%); *Supp:* 50 mg; *ER Cap:* 75 mg ext-rel
Comment: *indomethacin* is indicated only for acute painful flares. Administer with food <u>and/or</u> antacids. Use lowest effective dose for shortest duration.

➤ *methotrexate* (X) 7.5 mg x 1 dose per week <u>or</u> 2.5 mg x 3 at 12 hour intervals once a week; max 20 mg/week; therapeutic response begins in 3-6 weeks; administer *methotrexate* injection SC only into the abdomen <u>or</u> thigh
Pediatric: <2 years: not recommended; ≥2 years: 10 mg/m^2 once weekly; max 20 mg/m^2
Rasuvo *Autoinjector:* 7.5 mg/0.15 ml, 10 mg/0.20 ml, 12.5 mg/0.25 ml, 15 mg/0.30 ml, 17.5 mg/0.35 ml, 20 mg/0.40 ml, 22.5 mg/0.45 ml, 25 mg/0.50 ml, 27.5 mg/0.55 ml, 30 mg/0.60 ml (solution concentration for SC injection is 50 mg/ml)
Rheumatrex *Tab:* 2.5*mg (5, 7.5, 10, 12.5, 15 mg/week, 4/card unit dose pack)
Trexall *Tab:* 5*, 7.5*, 10*, 15*mg (5, 7.5, 10, 12.5, 15 mg/week, 4/card unit dose pack)
Comment: *methotrexate* (MTX) is contraindicated with immunodeficiency, blood dyscrasias, alcoholism, and chronic liver disease.

POLYCYSTIC OVARIAN SYNDROME (PCOS, STEIN-LEVENTHAL DISEASE)

See **Contraceptives** *page* 486
See **Type 2 Diabetes Mellitus** *page* 431

POLYMYALGIA RHEUMATICA

Comment: Initial treatment is low-dose prednsone at 12-25 mg/day. May attempt a very slow tapering regimen after 2-4 weeks. If relapse occurs, increase the daily dose of corticosteroid to the previous effective dose. Most people with polymyalgia rheumatica need to continue corticosteroid treatment for at least a year. Approximately 30-60% of people will have at least one relapse during corticosteroid tapering. Joint guidelines from the American Academy of Rheumatology (AAR) and the European League

Against Rheumatism (ELAR) suggest using concomitant methotrexate (MTX) along with corticosteroids in some patients. It may be useful early in the course of treatment or later, if the patient relapses or does not respond to corticosteroids. The American Academy of Rheumatology (AAR) recommends the following daily doses for anyone on a chronic oral corticosteroid regimen: Calcium 1,200-1,500 mg/day and vitamin D 800-1,000 IU/day.

Oral Corticosteroids see page 509

For calcium and vitamin D supplementation, see **Hypocalcemia** page 226

▶ *methotrexate* (X) 7.5 mg x 1 dose per week or 2.5 mg x 3 at 12 hour intervals once a week; max 20 mg/week; therapeutic response begins in 3-6 weeks; administer methotrexate injection SC only into the abdomen or thigh

Pediatric: <2 years: not recommended; ≥2 years: 10 mg/m2 once weekly; max 20 mg/m2

> **Rasuvo** *Autoinjector:* 7.5 mg/0.15 ml, 10 mg/0.20 ml, 12.5 mg/0.25 ml, 15 mg/0.30 ml, 17.5 mg/0.35 ml, 20 mg/0.40 ml, 22.5 mg/0.45 ml, 25 mg/0.50 ml, 27.5 mg/0.55 ml, 30 mg/0.60 ml (solution concentration for SC injection is 50 mg/ml)
>
> **Rheumatrex** *Tab:* 2.5*mg (5, 7.5, 10, 12.5, 15 mg/week, 4/card unit dose pack)
>
> **TrexallR** *Tab:* 5*, 7.5*, 10*, 15*mg (5, 7.5, 10, 12.5, 15 mg/week, 4/card unit dose pack)

Comment: *methotrexate* (MTX) is contraindicated with immunodeficiency, blood dyscrasias, alcoholism, and chronic liver disease.

⬤ POSTHERPETIC NEURALGIA

GAMMA AMINOBUTYRIC ACID ANALOG

▶ *gabapentin* (C) *CrCl 30-60 mL/min:* 600-1800 mg; *CrCl <30 mL/min* or *on hemodialysis:* not recommended

Comment: Avoid abrupt cessation of *gabapentin* and *gabapentin enacarbil*. To discontinue, withdraw gradually over 1 week or longer.

Pediatric: <18 years: not recommended

> **Gralise** initially 300 mg on Day 1; then 600 mg on Day 2; then 900 mg on Days 3-6; then 1200 mg on Days 7-10; then 1500 mg on Days 11-14; titrate up to 1800 mg on Day 15; take entire dose once daily with the evening meal; do not crush, split, or chew
>
> *Tab:* 300, 600 mg
>
> **Neurontin** (G) 300mg daily x 1 day, then 300 mg bid x 1 day, then 300 mg tid continuously; max 1,800 mg/day in 3 divided doses; taper over 7 days
>
> *Pediatric:* <3 years: not recommended; 3-12 years: initially 10-15 mg/kg/day in 3 divided doses; max 12 hours between doses; titrate over 3 days; 3-4 years: titrate to 40 mg/kg/day; 5-12 years: titrate to 25-35 mg/kg/day; max 50 mg/kg/day;
>
> *Tab:* 600*, 800* mg; *Cap:* 100, 300, 400 mg; *Oral soln:* 250 mg/5 ml (480 ml) (strawberry-anise) >12 years: same as adult

▶ *gabapentin enacarbil* (C) 600 mg once daily at about 5:00 PM; if dose not taken at recommended time, next dose should be taken the following day; swallow whole; take with food; *CrCl 30-59 mL/min:* 600 mg on Day 1, Day 3, and every day thereafter; *CrCl <30 mL/min:* or on hemodialysis: not recommended

Pediatric: not recommended

> **Horizant** *Tab:* 600 ext-rel

Tricyclic Antidepressants (TCAs)

Comment: Co-administration of SSRIs and TCAs requires extreme caution.

➤ *amitriptyline* (C)(G) initially 75 mg/day in divided doses of 50-100 mg/day q HS; max 300 mg/day
Pediatric: not recommended
Tab: 10, 25, 50, 75, 100, 150 mg

➤ *amoxapine* (C) initially 50 mg bid-tid; after 1 week may increase to 100 mg bid-tid; usual effective dose 200-300 mg/day; if total dose exceeds 300 mg/day, give in divided doses (max 400 mg/day); may give as a single bedtime dose (max 300 mg q HS)
Pediatric: not recommended
Tab: 25, 50, 100, 150 mg

➤ *desipramine* (C)(G) 100-200 mg/day in single or divided doses; max 300 mg/day
Pediatric: not recommended
Norpramin *Tab:* 10, 25, 50, 75, 100, 150 mg

➤ *doxepin* (C)(G) 75 mg/day; max 150 mg/day
Pediatric: not recommended
Cap: 10, 25, 50, 75, 100, 150 mg; Oral conc: 10 mg/ml (4 oz w. dropper)

➤ *imipramine* (C)(G)
Pediatric: not recommended
Tofranil initially 75 mg daily (max 200 mg); adolescents initially 30-40 mg daily (max 100 mg/day); if maintenance dose exceeds 75 mg daily, may switch to
Tofranil PM for divided or bedtime dose
Tab: 10, 25, 50 mg
Tofranil PM initially 75 mg daily 1 hour before HS; max 200 mg
Cap: 75, 100, 125, 150 mg
Tofranil Injection 50 mg IM; lower dose for adolescents; switch to oral form as soon as possible
Amp: 25 mg/2 ml (2 ml)

➤ *nortriptyline* (D)(G) initially 25 mg tid-qid; max 150 mg/day
Pediatric: not recommended
Pamelor *Cap:* 10, 25, 50, 75 mg; Oral soln: 10 mg/5 ml (16 oz)

➤ *protriptyline* (C) initially 5 mg tid; usual dose 15-40 mg/day in 3-4 divided doses; max 60 mg/day
Pediatric: <12 years: not recommended
Vivactyl *Tab:* 5, 10 mg

➤ *trimipramine* (C) initially 75 mg/day in divided doses; max 200 mg/day
Pediatric: not recommended
Surmontil *Cap:* 25, 50, 100 mg

α₂-DELTA LIGAND

➤ *pregabalin (GABA analog)* (C)(V) initially 150 mg daily divided bid-tid and may titrate within one week; max 600 mg divided bid-tid; discontinue over one week
Pediatric: <18 years: not recommended
Lyrica *Cap:* 25, 50, 75, 100, 150, 200, 225, 300 mg; Oral soln: 20 mg/ml

TOPICAL/TRANSDERMAL ANALGESICS

➤ *capsaicin* (B)(G) apply tid-qid prn to intact skin; avoid mucus membranes
Pediatric: <2 years: not recommended; ≥2 years: same as adult

> **Double Cap (OTC)** *Crm:* 0.05% (2 oz)
> **Qutenza** *Patch:* 8% (1-2, both with 50 g tube of cleansing gel)
> **Zostrix (OTC)** *Crm:* 0.025% (0.7, 1.5, 3 oz)
> **Zostrix HP (OTC)** *Emol crm:* 0.075% (1, 2 oz)

Comment: Provides some relief by 1-2 weeks; optimal benefit may take 4-6 weeks.

▷ *diclofenac epolamine* **(C)** apply one patch to affected area bid; remove during bathing; avoid non-intact skin; do not re-use
Pediatric: not recommended

> **Flector Patch** *Patch:* 180 mg/patch (30/carton)

Comment: *diclofenac* is contraindicated with *aspirin* allergy and late pregnancy.

▷ *doxepin* **(B)** cream apply to affected area qid at intervals of at least 3-4 hours; max 8 days
Pediatric: not recommended

> **Prudoxin** *Crm:* 5% (45 g)
> **Zonalon** *Crm:* 5% (30, 45 g)

▷ *tacrolimus* **(C)** apply to affected area bid; continue for 1 week after clearing
Pediatric: <2 years: not recommended; 2-15 years: use 0.03% strength

> **Protopic** *Oint:* 0.03, 0.1% (30, 60 g)

TOPICAL/TRANSDERMAL ANESTHETICS

▷ *lidocaine* cream **(B)**
Pediatric: not recommended

> **LidaMantle** *Crm:* 3% (1, 2 oz)
> **Lidoderm** *Crm:* 3% (85 g)

▷ *lidocaine* lotion **(B)**
Pediatric: not recommended

> **LidaMantle** *Lotn:* 3% (177 ml)

▷ *lidocaine* 5% patch **(B)(G)** apply up to 3 patches at one time for up to 12 hours/24-hour period (12 hours on/12 hours off); patches may be cut into smaller sizes before removal of the release liner; do not re-use
Pediatric: not recommended

> **Lidoderm** *Patch:* 5% (10x14 cm; 30/carton)

▷ *lidocaine/dexamethasone* **(B)**

> **Decadron Phosphate with Xylocaine** *dexa* 4 mg/*lido* 10 mg per ml (5 ml)

▷ *lidocaine/hydrocortisone* **(B)(G)**
Pediatric: not recommended

> **LidaMantle HC** *Crm: lido* 3%/*hydro* 0.5% (1, 3 oz); *Lotn:* (177 ml)
> **Acetaminophen for IV Infusion** *see Pain page* 306

ORAL ANALGESICS

▷ *acetaminophen* **(B)(G)** *see Fever page* 143
▷ *aspirin* **(D)(G)** *see Fever page* 144

Comment: *aspirin*-containing medications are contraindicated with history of allergic-type reaction to *aspirin*, children and adolescents with *Varicella* or other viral illness, and 3rd trimester pregnancy.

▷ *tramadol* **(C)(IV)(G)**

> **Rybix ODT** initially 100 mg once daily; may increase by 100 mg every 5 days; max 300 mg/day; *CrCl <30 mL/min* or *severe hepatic impairment:* not recommended; *Cirrhosis:* max 50 mg q 12 hours

Pediatric: <17 years: not recommended
ODT: 50 mg (mint) (phenylalanine)
Ryzolt initially 100 mg once daily; may increase by 100 mg every 5 days; max 300 mg/day; *CrCl <30 mL/min* or *severe hepatic impairment:* not recommended
Pediatric: <16 years: not recommended; ≥16 years: same as adult
Tab: 100, 200, 300 mg ext-rel
Ultram 50-100 mg q 4-6 hours prn; max 400 mg/day; *CrCl <30 mL/min:* max 100 mg q 12 hours; *Cirrhosis:* max 50 mg q 12 hours
Pediatric: <16 years: not recommended; ≥16 years: same as adult
Tab: 50*mg
Ultram ER initially 100 mg once daily; may increase by 100 mg every 5 days; max 300 mg/day; *CrCl <30 mL/min:* or *severe hepatic impairment:* not recommended
Pediatric: <18 years: not recommended
Tab: 100, 200, 300 mg ext-rel
▷ *tramadol/acetaminophen* **(C)(IV)(G)** 2 tabs q 4-6 hours; max 8 tabs/day; 5 days; *CrCl <30 mL/min:* max 2 tabs q 12 hours; max 4 tabs/day x 5 days
Pediatric: <16 years: not recommended; ≥16 years: same as adult
Ultracet *Tab:* tram 37.5/acet 325 mg
Other Oral Analgesics *see Pain page* 308

TRICYCLIC ANTIDEPRESSANTS (TCAs)

Comment: Co-administration of TCAs with SSRIs requires extreme caution.
▷ *amitriptyline* **(C)(G)** titrate to achieve pain relief; max 300 mg/day
Pediatric: not recommended
Tab: 10, 25, 50, 75, 100, 150 mg
▷ *amoxapine* **(C)** titrate to achieve pain relief; if total dose exceeds 300 mg/day, give in divided doses; max 400 mg/day
Pediatric: not recommended
Tab: 25, 50, 100, 150 mg
▷ *desipramine* **(C)(G)** titrate to achieve pain relief; max 300 mg/day
Pediatric: not recommended
Norpramin *Tab:* 10, 25, 50, 75, 100, 150 mg
▷ *doxepin* **(C)(G)** titrate to achieve pain relief; max 150 mg/day
Pediatric: not recommended
Cap: 10, 25, 50, 75, 100, 150 mg; *Oral conc:* 10 mg/ml (4 oz w. dropper)
▷ *imipramine* **(C)(G)**
Pediatric: not recommended
Tofranil titrate to achieve pain relief; max 200 mg/day; adolescents max 100 mg/day; if maintenance dose exceeds 75 mg/day, may switch to **Tofranil PM** at bedtime
Tab: 10, 25, 50 mg
Tofranil PM titrate to achieve pain relief; initially 75 mg at HS; max 200 mg at HS
Cap: 75, 100, 125, 150 mg
Tofranil Injection 50 mg IM; lower dose for adolescents; switch to oral form as soon as possible
Amp: 25 mg/2 ml (2 ml)
▷ *nortriptyline* **(D)(G)** titrate to achieve pain relief; initially 10-25 mg tid-qid; max 150 mg/day; lower doses for elderly and adolescents
Pediatric: not recommended
Pamelor titrate to achieve pain relief; max 150 mg/day

Cap: 10, 25, 50, 75 mg; *Oral soln:* 10 mg/5 ml (16 oz)

▷ *protriptyline* (C) titrate to achieve pain relief; initially 5 mg tid; max 60 mg/day
  Pediatric: <12 years: not recommended
  Vivactyl *Tab:* 5, 10 mg

▷ *trimipramine* (C) titrate to achieve pain relief; max 200 mg/day
  Pediatric: not recommended
  Surmontil *Cap:* 25, 50, 100 mg

 POST-TRAUMATIC STRESS DISORDER (PTSD)

Comment: No one pharmacological agent has emerged as the best treatment for PTSD. A combination of pharmacological agents (e.g., antidepressants, nonadrenergic agents, antipsychosis drugs) may comprise an individualized treatment plan to successfully manage core symptoms of PTSD as well as associated anxiety, depression, sleep disturbances, and co-occurring psychiatric disorders.

SELECTIVE SEROTONIN REUPTAKE INHIBITORS (SSRIs)

Comment: The FDA has approved two SSRIs for the treatment of PTSD: *paroxetine* and *sertraline*. However, the safety and efficacy of other SSRIs (*fluoxetine, citalopram, escitalopram, fluvoxamine*) have been tested in clinical practice. Co-administration of SSRIs with TCAs requires extreme caution. Concomitant use of MAOIs and SSRIs is absolutely contraindicated. Avoid St. John's wort and other serotonergic agents. A potentially fatal adverse event is *serotonin syndrome*, caused by serotonin excess. Milder symptoms require HCP intervention to avert severe symptoms which can be rapidly fatal without urgent/emergent medical care. Symptoms include restlessness, agitation, confusion, hallucinations, tachycardia, hypertension, dilated pupils, muscle twitching, muscle rigidity, loss of muscle coordination, diaphoresis, diarrhea, headache, shivering, piloerection, hyperpyrexia, cardiac arrhythmias, seizures, loss of consciousness, coma, death. Abrupt withdrawal or interruption of treatment with an antidepressant medication is sometimes associated with an *Antidepressant Discontinuation Syndrome* which may be mediated by gradually tapering the drug over a period of two weeks or longer, depending on the dose strength and length of treatment. Common symptoms of the *serotonin discontinuation Syndrome* include flu-like symptoms (nausea, vomiting, diarrhea, headaches, sweating), sleep disturbances (insomnia, nightmares, constant sleepiness), mood disturbances (dysphoria, anxiety, agitation), cognitive disturbances (mental confusion, hyperarousal), sensory and movement disturbances (imbalance, tremors, vertigo, dizziness, electric-shock-like sensations in the brain, often described by sufferers as "brain zaps."

▷ *paroxetine maleate* (D)(G)
  Pediatric: not recommended
  Paxil initially 20 mg daily in AM; may increase by 10 mg/day at weekly intervals as needed; max 60 mg/day
    Tab: 10*, 20*, 30, 40 mg
  Paxil CR initially 25 mg daily in AM; may increase by 12.5 mg at weekly intervals as needed; max 62.5 mg/day
    Tab: 12.5, 25, 37.5 mg cont-rel ent-coat
  Paxil Suspension initially 20 mg daily in AM; may increase by 10 mg/day at weekly intervals as needed; max 60 mg/day
    Oral susp: 10 mg/5 ml (250 ml; orange)

▷ *sertraline* (C) initially 50 mg daily; increase at 1 week intervals if needed; max 200 mg daily
Pediatric: <6 years: not recommended; 6-12 years: initially 25 mg daily; max 200 mg/day; 13-17 years: initially 50 mg daily; max 200 mg/day
 Zoloft *Tab:* 15*, 50*, 100*mg; *Oral conc:* 20 mg per ml (60 ml [dilute just before administering in 4 oz water, ginger ale, lemon-lime soda, lemonade, or orange juice]) (alcohol 12%)

ATYPICAL ANTIPSYCHOSIS DRUGS

▷ *olanzapine* (C)(G) initially 2.5-5 mg once daily at HS; increase by 5 mg every week to 20 mg at HS; usual maintenance 10-20 mg/day
 Zyprexa *Tab:* 2.5, 5, 7.5, 10, 15, 20 mg
 Zyprexa Zydis *ODT:* 5, 10, 15, 20 mg (phenylalanine)
▷ *quetiapine* (C)(G) initially 25 mg bid; increase total daily dose by 50 mg, as needed and tolerated, to max 300-600 mg/day
 Seroquel *Tab:* 25, 100, 200, 300 mg
 Seroquel XR *Tab:* 50, 150, 200, 300, 400 mg ext-rel
▷ *risperidone* (C)(G) initially 0.5-1 mg bid; titrate to 3 mg bid by the end of the first week; usual maintenance 4-6 mg/day
 Risperdal *Tab:* 0.25, 0.5, 1, 2, 3, 4 mg; *Soln:* 1 mg/ml (30 ml w. pipette); *Consta (Inj):* 25, 37.5, 50 mg
 Risperdal M-Tabs *M-tab:* 0.5, 1, 2, 3, 4 mg orally-disint (phenylalanine)

NONADRENERGIC AGENTS

ALPHA-1 ANTAGONISTS

Comment: *prazosin* is useful in reducing combat-trauma nightmares, normalizing dreams for combat veterans, and mediating other sleep disturbances.
▷ *prazosin* (C)(G) first dose at HS, 1 mg bid-tid; increase dose slowly; usual range 6-15 mg/day in divided doses; max 20-40 mg/day
Pediatric: not recommended
 Minipress *Cap:* 1, 2, 5 mg

CENTRAL ALPHA-2 AGONISTS

Comment: *clonidine* is useful to reduce nightmares, hypervigilance, startle reactions, and outbursts of rage.
▷ *clonidine* (C)
Pediatric: <12 years: not recommended; ≥12 years: same as adult
 Catapres initially 0.1 mg bid; usual range 0.2-0.6 mg/day in divided doses; max 2.4 mg/day *Tab:* 0.1*, 0.2*, 0.3*mg
 Catapres-TTS initially 0.1 mg patch weekly; increase after 1-2 weeks if needed; max 0.6 mg/day
  Patch: 0.1, 0.2 mg/day (12/carton); 0.3 mg/day (4/carton)
 Kapvay (G) initially 0.1 mg bid; usual range 0.2-0.6 mg/day in divided doses; max 2.4 mg/day *Tab:* 0.1, 0.2 mg
 Nexiclon XR initially 0.18 mg (2 ml) suspension or 0.17 mg tab once daily; usual max 0.52 mg (6 ml suspension) once daily
  Tab: 0.17, 0.26 mg ext-rel; *Oral susp:* 0.09 mg/ml ext-rel (4 oz)

BETA-ADRENERGIC BLOCKER (NON-CARDIOSELECTIVE)

Comment: *propranolol* is useful to mediate hyperarousal. For other non-cardioselective beta-adrenergic blockers, *see* **Hypertension**, *page* 208

▶ *propranolol* (C)(G) 40-240 mg daily
  Pediatric: not recommended
    Inderal *Tab:* 10*, 20*, 40*, 60*, 80*mg
    Inderal LA initially 80 mg daily in a single dose; increase q 3-7 days; usual range 120-160 mg/day; max 320 mg/day in a single dose

SEROTONIN AND NOREPINEPHRINE REUPTAKE INHIBITORS (SNRIs)

▶ *desvenlafaxine* (C)(G) swallow whole; initially 50 mg once daily; max 120 mg/day
  Pediatric: not recommended
    Pristiq *Tab:* 50, 100 mg ext-rel
▶ *duloxetine* (C)(G) swallow whole; initially 30 mg once daily x 1 week; then increase to 60 mg once daily; max 120 mg/day
  Pediatric: not recommended
    Cymbalta *Cap:* 20, 30, 40, 60 mg del-rel
▶ *venlafaxine* (C)(G)
    Effexor initially 75 mg/day in 2-3 divided doses; may increase at 4-day intervals in 75 mg increments to 150 mg/day; max 225 mg/day
      Pediatric: <18 years: not recommended
      Tab: 37.5, 75, 150, 225 mg
    Effexor XR initially 75 mg q AM; may start at 37.5 mg daily x 4-7 days, then increase by increments of up to 75 mg/day at intervals of at least 4 days; usual max 375 mg/day
      Pediatric: not recommended
      Tab/Cap: 37.5, 75, 150 mg ext-rel

5HT2/3 RECEPTOR BLOCKERS

▶ *mirtazapine* (C) initially 15 mg q HS; increase at intervals of 1-2 weeks; 1-2 weeks; usual range 15-60 mg/day; max 60 mg/day
  Pediatric: not recommended
    Remeron *Tab:* 15*, 30*, 45*mg
    Remeron SolTab *ODT:* 15, 30, 45 mg (orange) (phenylalanine)

SEROTONIN/ACETYLCHOLINE/NOREPINEPHRINE/DOPAMINE BLOCKER

▶ *trazodone* (C)(G) initially 150 mg/day in divided doses with food; increase by 50 mg/day q 3-4 days; max 400 mg/day in divided doses <u>or</u> 50-400 mg at HS
  Pediatric: <18 years: not recommended
    Oleptro *Tab:* 50, 100*, 150*, 200, 250, 300 mg

TRICYCLIC ANTIDEPRESSANTS (TCAs)

▶ *amitriptyline* (C)(G) 10-20 mg at HS
  Pediatric: not recommended
    Tab: 10, 25, 50, 75, 100, 150 mg
▶ *doxepin* (C)(G) 10-200 mg at HS
  Pediatric: not recommended
    Cap: 10, 25, 50, 75, 100, 150 mg; *Oral conc:* 10 mg/ml (4 oz w. dropper)

➤ *imipramine* (C)(G) 10-200 mg q HS
    Tofranil 100-300 mg at HS <u>or</u> divided bid <u>or</u> tid
        Pediatric: <6 years: not recommended; 6-12 years: initially 25 mg; >12 years:
        50 mg max 2.5 mg/kg/day
        Tab: 10, 25, 50 mg
    Tofranil PM initially 75 mg daily 1 hour before HS; max 200 mg
        Cap: 75, 100, 125, 150 mg
    Tofranil Injection 50 mg IM; lower dose for adolescents; switch to oral form as
    soon as possible
        Amp: 25 mg/2 ml (2 ml)
➤ *nortriptyline* (D)(G) 10-150 mg q HS
    Pediatric: not recommended
        Pamelor *Cap:* 10, 25, 50, 75 mg; *Oral soln:* 10 mg/5 ml

MONOAMINE OXIDASE INHIBITORS (MAOIs)

Comment: Many drug and food interactions with this class of drugs, use cautiously.
MAOIs should be reserved for refractory depression that has not responded to other
classes of antidepressants. Concomitant use of MAOIs and SSRIs is contraindicated.
See mfr pkg insert for drug and food interactions. MAOIs have been used to reduce
recurrent recollections of the trauma, nightmares, flashbacks, numbing, sleep
disturbances, and social withdrawal in PTSD.
➤ *phenelzine* (C)(G) initially 15 mg tid; max 90 mg/day
    Pediatric: <16 years: not recommended; ≥16 years: same as adult
        Nardil
        Tab: 15 mg
➤ *selegiline* (C) initially 10 mg tid; max 60 mg/day
    Pediatric: <12 years: not recommended; ≥12 years: same as adult
        Emsam *Transdermal patch:* 6 mg/24 hrs, 9 mg/24 hrs, 12 mg/24 hrs
        Comment: At the **Emsam** transdermal patch 6 mg/24 hrs dose, the dietary re-
        strictions commonly required when using nonselective MAOIs are not necessary.

⬤ PREGNANCY

see **Appendix Z: Prescription Prenatal Vitamins** *page* 532
Comment: Prenatal vitamins should have at least 400 mcg of folic acid content.
Take one dose once daily. It is recommended that prenatal vitamins be started at
least 3 months prior to conception to improve preconception nutritional status,
and continued throughout pregnancy and the postnatal period, in lactating and
nonlactating women, and throughout the childbearing years.

NAUSEA/VOMITING

➤ *doxyalamine succinate/pyridoxine* (A)(G) do not crush <u>or</u> chew; take on an empty
    stomach with water; initially 2 tabs at HS on day 1; may increase to 1 tab AM and 2
    tabs at HS day 2; may increase to 1 tab AM, 1 tab mid-afternoon, 2 tabs at HS; max
    4 tabs/day
    Diclegis *Tab:* doxyl 10 mg/*pyri* 10 mg del-rel
    Comment: Diclegis is the only FDA-approved drug for the treatment of morning
    sickness. It has not been studied in women with hyperemesis gravidarum.

➤ *promethazine* (C)(G) 12.5-50 mg PO/IM/rectally q 4-6 hours prn
    Phenergan *Tab:* 12.5*, 25*, 50 mg; *Plain syr:* 6.25 mg/5 ml; *Fortis syr:* 25 mg/5 ml; *Rectal supp:* 12.5, 25, 50 mg; *Amp:* 25, 50 mg/ml (1 ml)
➤ *ondansetron* (C)(G) 4-8 mg bid prn
    Zofran *Tab:* 4, 8, 24 mg
    Zofran Injection *Vial:* 2 mg/ml (2 ml single-dose); 2 mg/ml (20 ml multi-dose) for IV or IM administration
    Zofran ODT *ODT:* 4, 8 mg (strawberry) (phenylalanine)
    Zofran Oral Solution *Oral soln:* 4 mg/5 ml (50 ml) (strawberry)
    Zuplenz Oral Soluble Film: 4, 8 mg orally-disint (10/carton) (peppermint)

 # PREMENSTRUAL DYSPHORPHIC DISORDER (PMDD)

Oral Prescription NSAIDs *see page* 501
Other Oral Analgesics *see **Pain** page* 308
Other Oral Contraceptives *see page* 485

ORAL ESTROGEN/PROGESTERONE COMBINATIONS

Comment: **Rajani** (a generic form of **Beyaz**) and **Yaz;** also available in generic Forms (**Gianvi, Ocella, Syeda, Vestura, Yasmin, Zarah**) have an FDA indication for treatment of PMDD in females who choose to use an OCP. Contraindicated with renal and adrenal insufficiency. Monitor k⁺ level during the first cycle if the patient is at risk for hyperkalemia for any reason. If the patient is taking a drug that increase serum potassium (e.g., ACEIs, ARBS, NSAIDs, K⁺ sparing diuretics), the patient is at risk for hyperkalemia.
➤ *ethinyl estradiol/drospirenone* (X)(G) 1 tab once daily x 28 days; repeat cycle; start on first Sunday after menses begins or on first day of next menses
    Yaz *Tab:* ethin estra 20 mcg/*drospir* 3 mg
➤ *ethinyl/estradiol/drospirenone/levomefolate calcium* (X)(G) 1 tab once daily x 28 days; repeat cycle; start on first Sunday after menses begins or on first day of next menses preceded by a negative pregnancy test
    Beyaz *Tab:* ethin estra 20 mcg/*drospir* 3 mg/*levo* 0.451 mg
    Rajani *Tab:* ethin estra 20 mcg/*drospir* 3 mg/*levo* 0.451 mg

DIURETICS

➤ *spironolactone* (D)(G) initially 50-100 mg once daily or in divided doses; titrate at 2-week intervals
Pediatric: not recommended
    Aldactone *Tab:* 25, 50*, 100*mg

ANTIDEPRESSANTS

➤ *fluoxetine* (C)(G)
    Prozac initially 20 mg daily; may increase after 1 week; doses >20 mg/day should be divided into AM and noon doses; max 80 mg/day
        Pediatric: <8 years: not recommended; 8-17 years: initially 10 or 20 mg/day; start lower weight children at 10 mg/day; if starting at 10 mg/day, may increase after 1 week to 20 mg/day
        Tab: 10*mg; *Cap:* 10, 20, 40 mg; *Oral soln:* 20 mg/5 ml (4 oz) (mint)

Prozac Weekly following daily *fluoxetine* therapy at 20 mg/day for 13 weeks, may initiate **Prozac Weekly** 7 days after the last 20 mg *fluoxetine* dose
Pediatric: not recommended
Cap: 90 mg ent-coat del-rel pellets
Sarafem administer daily or 14 days before expected menses and through first full day of menses; initially 20 mg/day; max 80 mg/day
Tab: 10, 15, 20 mg; *Cap:* 20 mg

▷ *paroxetine maleate* (D)(G)
Pediatric: not recommended
Paxil initially 20 mg daily in AM; may increase by 10 mg/day at weekly intervals as needed; max 60 mg/day
Tab: 10*, 20*, 30, 40 mg
Paxil CR initially 25 mg daily in AM; may increase by 12.5 mg at weekly intervals as needed; max 62.5 mg/day; may start 14 days before and continue through day one of menses
Tab: 12.5, 25, 37.5 mg cont-rel ent-coat
Paxil Suspension initially 20 mg daily in AM; may increase by 10 mg/day at weekly intervals as needed; max 60 mg/day
Oral susp: 10 mg/5 ml (250 ml) (orange)

▷ *sertraline* (C)
For 2 weeks prior to onset of menses: initially 50 mg daily x 3; then increase to 100 mg daily for remainder of the cycle; *For full cycle:* initially 50 mg daily; then may increase by 50 mg/day each cycle to max 150 mg/day
Pediatric: not recommended
Zoloft *Tab:* 25*, 50*, 100*mg; *Oral conc:* 20 mg per ml (60 ml) (alcohol 12%); dilute just before administering in 4 oz water, ginger ale, lemon-lime soda, lemonade, or orange juice

▷ *nortriptyline* (D)(G) initially 25 mg tid-qid; max 150 mg/day
Pediatric: not recommended
Pamelor *Cap:* 10, 25, 50, 75 mg; *Oral soln:* 10 mg/5 ml

Contraceptives *see page 485*

CALCIUM SUPPLEMENTS

▷ *calcium* (C) 1200 mg/day
see **Osteoporosis** *page 294*

⬤ PRIMARY IMMUNODEFICIENCY IN ADULTS

▷ *recombinant human hyaluronidase (human normal immunoglobulin)* (C)
HyQvia see mfr pkg insert for dose by weight table and dose schedule table
Vial: 10%; 2.5 g/200 u, 5 g/400 u, 10 g/800 u, 20 g/1600 u, 30 g/2400 u (2 single-use/dual-vial unit (preservative-free)
Comment: HyQvia is an immune globulin with a recombinant human hyaluronidase indicated for the treatment of primary immunodeficiency (PI) in adults. This includes, but is not limited to, common variable immunodeficiency (CVID), X-linked agammaglobulinemia, congenital agammaglobulinemia, Wiskott-Aldrich syndrome, and severe combined immunodeficiencies.
HyQvia contains IgG antibodies, collected from human plasma donated by healthy people. HyQvia is a dual vial unit with one vial of immune globulin

infusion 10% (Human) and one vial of recombinant human hyaluronidase. The hyaluronidase part of **HyQvia** helps more of the immune globulin get absorbed into the body. HyQvia is a ready-for-use sterile, liquid preparation of highly purified, concentrated, broad spectrum IgG antibodies. The distribution of the IgG subclasses is similar to that of normal plasma. Contains 100 mg/ml protein. **HyQvia** is collected only at FDA approved blood establishments and is tested by FDA licensed serological tests for Hepatitis B Surface Antigen (HBsAg), and for antibodies to Human Immunodeficiency Virus (HIV-1/HIV-2) and Hepatitis C Virus (HCV) in accordance with U.S. regulatory requirements. As an additional safety measure, mini-pools of the plasma are tested for the presence of HIV-1 and HCV by FDA licensed Nucleic Acid Testing (NAT). Protect from light. Use within 3 months after removal to room temperature but within the expiration date on the carton and vial labels. Do not return vials to the refrigerator after being stored at room temperature.

 ## PROCTITIS: ACUTE (PROCTOCOLITIS/ENTERITIS)

Comment: The following regimen for the treatment of proctitis, proctocolitis, and enteritis is published in the **2015 CDC Sexually Transmitted Diseases Treatment Guidelines**.

RECOMMENDED REGIMEN

▷ *ceftriaxone* **(B)(G)** 250 mg IM in a single dose
   Rocephin *Vial:* 250, 500 mg; 1, 2 g
       plus
▷ *doxycycline* 100 mg bid x 7 days
   Actilate *Tab:* 75, 150** mg
   Adoxa *Tab:* 50, 75, 100, 150 mg ent-coat
   Doryx *Tab:* 50, 75, 100, 150, 200 mg del-rel
   Monodox *Cap:* 50, 75, 100 mg
   Oracea *Cap:* 40 mg del-rel
   Vibramycin *Tab:* 100 mg; *Cap:* 50, 100 mg; *Syr:* 50 mg/5 ml (raspberry-apple) (sulfites); *Oral susp:* 25 mg/5 ml (raspberry)
   Vibra-Tab *Tab:* 100 mg film-coat

Comment: *doxycycline* is contraindicated <8 years-of-age, in pregnancy, and lactation (discolors developing tooth enamel). A side effect may be photo-sensitivity (photophobia). Do not give with antacids, calcium supplements, milk or other dairy, or within two hours of taking another drug.

 ## PROSTATITIS: ACUTE

ANTI-INFECTIVES

▷ *ciprofloxacin* **(C)** 500 mg bid x 4-6 weeks
   Pediatric: <18 years: not recommended
   Cipro (G) *Tab:* 250, 500, 750 mg; *Oral susp:* 250, 500 mg/5 ml (100 ml) (strawberry)
   Cipro XR *Tab:* 500, 1000 mg ext-rel
   ProQuin XR *Tab:* 500 mg ext-rel

Comment: *ciprofloxacin* is contraindicated <18 years-of-age, and during pregnancy and lactation. Risk of tendonitis or tendon rupture, especially 60 years-of-age and older.

▷ *norfloxacin* (C) 400 mg bid x 28 days
Noroxin *Tab:* 400 mg

Comment: *norfloxacin* is contraindicated <18 years-of-age, and during pregnancy and lactation. Risk of tendonitis or tendon rupture, especially 60 years-of-age and older.

▷ *ofloxacin* (C)(G) 300 mg x bid x 6 weeks
Floxin *Tab:* 200, 300, 400 mg

Comment: *ofloxacin* is contraindicated <18 years-of-age, and during pregnancy and lactation. Risk of tendonitis or tendon rupture, especially 60 years-of-age and older.

▷ *trimethoprim/sulfamethoxazole* (C)(G)
Bactrim, Septra 2 tabs bid x 10 days
Tab: trim 80 mg/*sulfa* 400 mg*
Bactrim DS, Septra DS 1 tab bid x 10 days
Tab: trim 160 mg/*sulfa* 800 mg*
Bactrim Pediatric Suspension, Septra Pediatric Suspension
Oral susp: trim 40 mg/*sulfa* 200 mg per 5 ml (100 ml) (cherry) (alcohol 0.3%)

Comment: *CrCl 15-30 mL/min:* reduce dose by 1/2; *CrCl <15 mL/min:* not recommended

⭕ PROSTATITIS: CHRONIC

ANTI-INFECTIVES

▷ *carbenicillin* (B) 2 tabs qid x 4-12 weeks
Geocillin *Tab:* 382 mg

▷ *ciprofloxacin* (C) 500 mg bid x 3 or more months
Pediatric: <18 years: not recommended
Cipro (G) *Tab:* 250, 500, 750 mg; *Oral susp:* 250, 500 mg/5 ml (100 ml) (strawberry)
Cipro XR *Tab:* 500, 1000 mg ext-rel
ProQuin XR *Tab:* 500 mg ext-rel

Comment: *ciprofloxacin* is contraindicated <18 years-of-age, and during pregnancy and lactation. Risk of tendonitis or tendon rupture, especially 60 years-of-age and older.

▷ *ofloxacin* (C)(G) 300 mg bid x 4-12 weeks
Floxin *Tab:* 200, 300, 400 mg

Comment: *ofloxacin* is contraindicated <18 years-of-age, and during pregnancy and lactation. Risk of tendonitis or tendon rupture, especially 60 years-of-age and older.

▷ *norfloxacin* (C) 400 mg bid x 4-12 weeks
Noroxin *Tab:* 400 mg

Comment: *norfloxacin* contraindicated <18 years-of-age, and during pregnancy and lactation. Risk of tendonitis or tendon rupture, especially 60 years-of-age and older.

▷ *trimethoprim/sulfamethoxazole* (C)(G)
Bactrim, Septra 2 tabs bid x 10 days
Tab: trim 80 mg/*sulfa* 400 mg*
Bactrim DS, Septra DS 1 tab bid x 10 days
Tab: trim 160 mg/*sulfa* 800 mg
Bactrim Pediatric Suspension, Septra Pediatric Suspension 20 ml bid x 10 days

Oral susp: trim 40 mg/*sulfa* 200 mg per 5 ml (100 ml) (cherry) (alcohol 0.3%)
Comment: *CrCl 15-30 mL/min:* reduce dose by 1/2; *CrCl <15 mL/min:* not recommended

SUPPRESSION THERAPY

▷ *trimethoprim/sulfamethoxazole* (C)(G)
  Bactrim, Septra 2 tabs bid x 10 days
   Tab: trim 80 mg/*sulfa* 400 mg*
  Bactrim DS, Septra DS 1 tab bid x 10 days
   Tab: trim 160 mg/*sulfa* 800 mg*
  Bactrim Pediatric Suspension, Septra Pediatric Suspension 20 ml bid x 10 days
   Oral susp: trim 40 mg/*sulfa* 200 mg per 5 ml (100 ml) (cherry) (alcohol 0.3%)
Comment: *CrCl 15-30 mL/min:* reduce dose by 1/2; *CrCl <15 mL/min:* not recommended

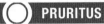

PRURITUS

Oral Drugs for Allergy, Cough, and Cold *see page* 535
Topical Corticosteroids *see page* 506
Parenteral Corticosteroids *see page* 511
Oral Corticosteroids *see page* 509
Eucerin Products (OTC)
Lac-Hydrin Products (OTC)
Lubriderm Products (OTC)
Aveeno Products (OTC)

TOPICAL OIL

▷ *fluocinolone acetamide* 0.01% topical oil (C)
 Pediatric: <6 years: not recommended; ≥6 years: apply sparingly bid for up to 4 weeks
  Derma-Smoothe/FS Topical Oil apply sparingly tid
   Topical oil: 0.01% (4 oz) (peanut oil)

TOPICAL ANALGESICS

▷ *capsaicin* (B)(G) apply tid-qid prn to intact skin
 Pediatric: <2 years: not recommended; ≥2 years: same as adult
  Double Cap (OTC) *Crm:* 0.05% (2 oz)
  Qutenza (B) *Patch:* 8% (1-2, both with 50 g tube of cleansing gel)
  Zostrix (OTC) *Crm:* 0.025% (0.7, 1.5, 3 oz)
  Zostrix HP (OTC) *Emol crm:* 0.075% (1, 2 oz)
Comment: Provides some relief by 1-2 weeks; optimal benefit may take 4-6 weeks.
▷ *doxepin* (B) cream apply to affected area qid at intervals of at least 3-4 hours; max 8 days
 Pediatric: not recommended
  Prudoxin *Crm:* 5% (45 g)
  Zonalon *Crm:* 5% (30, 45 g)
▷ *tacrolimus* (C) apply to affected area bid; continue for 1 week after clearing
 Pediatric: <2 years: not recommended; 2-15 years: use 0.03% strength; apply to affected area bid; continue for 1 week after clearing
  Protopic *Oint:* 0.03, 0.1% (30, 60 g)

PSEUDOBULBAR AFFECT (PBA) DISORDER

Comment: Pseudobulbar affect (PBA), emotional lability, labile affect, or emotional incontinence refers by to a neurologic disorder characterized involuntary crying or uncontrollable episodes of crying and/or laughing, or other emotional displays. PBA occurs secondary to a neurologic disease or brain injury. Brain injury or neurologic diseases such as traumatic brain injury, stroke, Parkinson's disease, multiple sclerosis, and amyotrophic lateral sclerosis (ALS, or Lou Gehrig's disease).

▶ *dextromethorphan/quinidine* (C) 1 cap once daily x 7 days; then starting on day 8, 1 cap bid

    Nuedexta apply bid to lesions and gently rub in completely

      Pediatric: not recommended

      Cap: dextro 20 mg/quini 10 mg

 PSEUDOGOUT

Injectable Acetaminophen *see Pain page* 306
Oral Prescription NSAIDs *see page* 501
Other Oral Analgesics *see Pain page* 308
Topical/Transdermal NSAIDs *see Pain page* 307
Parenteral Corticosteroids *see page* 511
Oral Corticosteroids *see page* 509
Topical Analgesic and Anesthetic Agents *see page* 499

 PSEUDOMEMBRANOUS COLITIS

Comment: Staphylococcal enterocolitis and antibiotic-associated pseudomembranous colitis caused by *C. difficile*.

ANTI-INFECTIVES

▶ *vancomycin* (B, caps; C, susp)(G) 500 mg to 2 g in 3-4 doses x 7-10 days; max 2 g/day
    Pediatric: 40 mg/kg/day in 3-4 doses x 7-10 days; max 2 g/day
▶ *metronidazole* (not for use in 1st; B in 2nd, 3rd)(G) 500 mg tid x 14 days
    Flagyl *Tab:* 250*, 500*mg
    Flagyl 375 *Cap:* 375 mg
    Flagyl ER *Tab:* 750 mg ext-rel

Comment: Alcohol is contraindicated during treatment with oral *metronidazole* and for 72 hours after therapy due to a possible *disulfiram*-like reaction (nausea, vomiting, flushing, headache).

PSITTACOSIS

ANTI-INFECTIVES

▶ *tetracycline* (D)(G) 250 mg qid or 500 mg tid x 7-14 days
    Pediatric: <8 years: not recommended; ≥8 years, <100 lb: 25-50 mg/kg/day in 4 doses x 7-14 days; ≥8 years, ≥100 lb: same as adult

Achromycin V *Cap:* 250, 500 mg
Sumycin *Tab:* 250, 500 mg; *Cap:* 250, 500 mg; *Oral susp:* 125 mg/5 ml (100, 200 ml) (fruit) (sulfites)

Comment: *tetracycline* is contraindicated <8 years-of-age, in pregnancy, and lactation (discolors developing tooth enamel). A side effect may be photo-sensitivity (photophobia). Do not give with antacids or calcium supplements within two hours of another drug.

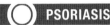

PSORIASIS

Emollients *see* **Dermatitis: Atopic** *page* 110
Topical Corticosteroids *see page* 506

VITAMIN D-3 DERIVATIVES

➤ *calcipotriene* (C)
  Dovonex apply bid to lesions and gently rub in completely
    Pediatric: not recommended
    Crm: 0.005% (30, 120 g)

VITAMIN D-3 DERIVATIVE/CORTICOSTEROID COMBINATIONS

➤ *calcipotriene/betamethasone dipropionate* (C)(G)
  Pediatric: <18 years: not recommended
    Enstilar apply to affected area and gently rub in once daily x up to 4 weeks; limit treatment area to 30% of body surface area; do not occlude; do not use on face, axillae, groin, <u>or</u> atrophic skin; max 100 g/week
      Foam: calci 0.005%/*beta* 0.064% (60 g spray can)
    Taclonex apply to affected area and gently rub in once daily as needed, up to 4 weeks
    Taclonex Ointment apply bid to lesions and gently rub in completely; limit treatment area to 30% of body surface area; do not occlude; do not use on face, axillae, groin, <u>or</u> atrophic skin; max 100 g/week
      Oint: calci 0.005%/*beta* 0.064% (60, 100 g)
    Taclonex Scalp Topical Suspension apply to affected area and gently rub in once daily x 2 weeks <u>or</u> until cleared; max 8 weeks; limit treatment area to 30% of body surface area; do not occlude; do not use on face, axillae, groin, <u>or</u> atrophic skin; max 100 g/week
      Bottle: (30, 60 g; 120 g [2x60 g])
➤ *Calcitrol* (C)
  Vectical apply bid to lesions and gently rub in completely; max weekly dose should not exceed 200 g
    Pediatric: <18 years: not recommended
    Oint: 3 mcg/g (100 g)

IMMUNOSUPPRESSANTS

➤ *alefacept* (B) 7.5 mg IV bolus <u>or</u> 15 mg IM once weekly x 12 weeks; may re-treat x 12 weeks
  Pediatric: not recommended

Amevive *IV dose pack:* 7.5 mg single-use (w. 10 ml sterile water diluents [use 0.6 ml]; 1, 4/pck); *IM dose pack:* 15 mg single-use (w. 10 ml sterile water diluent [use 0.6 ml]; 1, 4/pck)

Comment: CD4+ and T-lymphycyte count should be checked prior to initiating treatment with **alefacept** and then monitored. Treatment should be withheld if CD4+ T-lymphocyte counts are below 250 cells/mcl.

➤ *cyclosporine* (C) 1.25 mg/kg bid; may increase after 4 weeks by 0.5mg/kg/day; then adjust at 2-week intervals; max 4 mg/kg/day; administer with meals
   Pediatric: <18 years: not recommended
      Neoral *Cap:* 25, 100 mg (alcohol)
      Neoral Oral Solution *Oral soln:* 100 mg/ml (50 ml) may dilute in room temperature apple juice <u>or</u> orange juice (alcohol)

ANTIMITOTICS

➤ *anthralin* (C) apply once daily
   Pediatric: not recommended
      Zithranol-RR *Crm:* 1.2% (15, 45 g)

RETINOIDS

➤ *acitretin* (X)(G) 25-50 mg once daily with main meal
   Pediatric: not recommended
      Soriatane *Cap:* 10, 25 mg
➤ *tazarotene* (X)(G) apply once daily at HS
   Pediatric: not recommended
      Avage Cream *Crm:* 0.1% (30 g)
      Tazorac Cream *Crm:* 0.05, 0.1% (15, 30, 60 g)
      Tazorac Gel *Gel:* 0.05, 0.1% (30, 100 g)

COAL TAR PREPARATIONS

➤ *coal tar* (C)(G)
   Pediatric: same as adult
      Scytera (OTC) apply qd-qid; use lowest effective dose
         Foam: 2%
      T/Gel Shampoo Extra Strength (OTC) use every other day; max 4 x/week; massage into affected areas for 5 minutes; rinse; repeat *Shampoo:* 1%
      T/Gel Shampoo Original Formula (OTC) use every other day; max 7 x/week; massage into affected areas for 5 minutes; rinse; repeat *Shampoo:* 0.5%
      T/Gel Shampoo Stubborn Itch Control (OTC) use every other day; max 7 x/week; massage into affected areas for 5 minutes; rinse; repeat *Shampoo:* 0.5%

INTERLEUKIN-17A ANTAGONIST

➤ *secukinumab* (B) inject SC into the upper arm, abdomen, <u>or</u> thigh; rotate sites; administer 300 mg SC (as two separate 150 mg SC injections) at weeks 0, 1, 2, 3, and 4; then 300 mg every 4 weeks; for some patients, 150 mg/dose may be sufficient
   Pediatric: <18 years: not recommended
      Cosentyx *Vial:* 150 mg/ml pwdr for SC inj after reconstitution single-use (preservative-free)
      Comment: **Cosentyx** may be used as monotherapy <u>or</u> in combination with **methotrexate** (MTX).

INTERLEUKIN-12/INTERLEUKIN-23 ANTAGONIST

➤ *ustekinumab* (B) inject SC; rotate sites; <100 kg: 45 mg once; then 4 weeks later; then every 12 weeks; ≥100 kg: 90 mg once; then 4 weeks later; then every 12 weeks
Pediatric: <18 years: not recommended
    Stelara *Vial:* 45 mg/0.5 ml single-use (preservative-free)
    Comment: **Stelara** may be used as monotherapy or in combination with *methotrexate* (MTX).

TUMOR NECROSIS FACTOR (TNF) BLOCKERS

➤ *adalimumab* (B) initially 80 mg SC once followed by 40 mg once every other week starting one week after initial dose; inject into thigh or abdomen; rotate sites
Pediatric: <18 years: not recommended
    Humira *Prefilled syringe:* 20 mg/0.4 ml; 40 mg/0.8 ml single-dose (2/pck; 2, 6/starter pck) (preservative-free)
➤ *etanercept* (B) inject SC into thigh, abdomen, or upper arm; rotate sites; initially 50 mg twice weekly (3-4 days apart) for 3 months; then 50 mg/week maintenance or 25 mg or 50 mg per week for 3 months; then 50 mg/week maintenance
Pediatric: <4 years: not recommended; 4-17 years: Chronic moderate-to-severe plaque psoriasis
    Enbrel *Vial:* 25 mg pwdr for SC injection after reconstitution (4/carton w. supplies) (preservative-free, diluent contains benzyl alcohol); *Prefilled syringe:* 25, 50 mg/ml (preservative-free); *SureClick autoinjector:* 50 mg/ml (preservative-free)
➤ *golimumab* (B) administer SC or IV infusion (in combination with *methotrexate [MTX]*)
Pediatric: <18 years: not established
    Simponi 50 mg SC once monthly; rotate sites
        Prefilled syringe, SmartJect autoinjector: 50 mg/0.5 ml, single-use (preservative-free)
    Simponi Aria 2 mg/kg IV infusion week 0 and week 4; then every 8 weeks thereafter
        Vial: 50 mg/4 ml, single-use, soln for IV infusion after dilution (latex-free, preservative-free)
➤ *infliximab* (B) administer by IV infusion over 2 hours; 5 mg/kg weeks 0, 2, 6; then once every 8 weeks
Pediatric: <6 years: not recommended; ≥6 years: same as adult
    Remicade *Vial:* 100 mg pwdr for reconstitution for IV infusion (20 ml, single-use) (preservative-free)
    Inflectra *Vial:* 100 mg pwdr for reconstitution for IV infusion (20 ml, single-use) (preservative-free)

MOISTURIZING AGENTS

    Aquaphor Healing Ointment (OTC) *Oint:* (1.75, 3.5, 14 oz) (alcohol)
    Eucerin Daily Sun Defense (OTC) *Lotn:* 6 oz (fragrance-free)
    Comment: **Eucerin Daily Sun Defense** is a moisturizer with SPF 15.
    Eucerin Facial Lotion (OTC) *Lotn:* 4 oz
    Eucerin Light Lotion (OTC) *Lotn:* 8 oz
    Eucerin Lotion (OTC) *Lotn:* 8, 16 oz
    Eucerin Original Creme (OTC) *Crm:* 2, 4, 16 oz (alcohol)
    Eucerin Plus Creme *Crm:* 4 oz

Eucerin Plus Lotion (OTC) *Lotn:* 6, 12 oz
Eucerin Protective Lotion (OTC) *Lotn:* 4 oz (alcohol)
Comment: Eucerin Protective Lotion is a moisturizer with SPF 25.
Lac-Hydrin Cream (OTC) *Crm:* 280, 385 g
Lac-Hydrin Lotion (OTC) *Lotn:* 225, 400 g
Lubriderm Dry Skin Scented (OTC) *Lotn:* 6, 10, 16, 32 oz
Lubriderm Dry Skin Unscented (OTC) *Lotn:* 3.3, 6, 10, 16 oz (fragrance-free)
Lubriderm Sensitive Skin Lotion (OTC) *Lotn:* 3.3, 6, 10, 16 oz (lanolin-free)
Lubriderm Dry Skin (OTC) *Lotn (scented):* 2.5, 6, 10, 16 oz;
Lotn (fragrance-free): 1, 2.5, 6, 10, 16 oz
Lubriderm Bath 1-2 capfuls in bath <u>or</u> rub onto wet skin as needed; then rinse
Oil: 8 oz

PSORIATIC ARTHRITIS

Injectable Acetaminophen *see Pain page* 306
Oral Prescription NSAIDs *see page* 501
Other Oral Analgesics *see Pain page* 306
Topical/Transdermal NSAIDs *see Pain page* 307
Parenteral Corticosteroids *see page* 511
Oral Corticosteroids *see page* 509
Topical Analgesic and Anesthetic Agents *see page* 499

TOPICAL ANALGESICS

▷ *capsaicin* (B)(G) apply tid-qid prn to intact skin
  Pediatric: <2 years: not recommended; >2 years: same as adult
      Axsain *Crm:* 0.075% (1, 2 oz)
      Capsin *Lotn:* 0.025, 0.075% (59 ml)
      Capzasin-P (OTC) *Crm:* 0.025% (1.5 oz); *Lotn:* 0.025% (2 oz)
      Dolorac *Crm:* 0.025% (28 g)
      Double Cap (OTC) *Crm:* 0.05% (2 oz)
      R-Gel *Gel:* 0.025% (15, 30 g)
      Zostrix (OTC) *Crm:* 0.025% (0.7, 1.5, 3 oz)
      Zostrix HP (OTC) *Emol crm:* 0.075% (1, 2 oz)
  Comment: Provides some relief by 1-2 weeks; optimal benefit may take 4-6 weeks.
▷ *trolamine salicylate* (NE)
      Mobisyl apply tid-qid
          Crm: 10%
  Comment: Provides some relief by 1-2 weeks; optimal benefit may take 4-6 weeks.
▷ *diclofenac sodium* (C; D ≥30 wks) apply qid prn to intact skin
  Pediatric: not established
      Pennsaid 1.5% in 10 drop increments, dispense and rub into front, side, and
      back of knee: usually; 40 drops (40 mg) qid
          Topical soln: 1.5% (150 ml)
      Pennsaid 2% apply 2 pump actuations (40 mg) and rub into front, side, and
      back of knee bid
          Topical soln: 2% (20 mg/pump actuation, 112 g)
  Comment: Pennsaid is indicated for the treatment of pain associated with
  osteoarthritis of the knee.

Pennsaid 2% apply 2 pump actuations (40 mg) and rub into front, side, and back of knee bid
Topical soln: 2% (20 mg/pump actuation; 112 g)
Voltaren Gel (G) *Gel:* 1% (100 g)

Comment: Contraindicated with ***aspirin*** allergy. As with other NSAIDs, **Voltaren Gel** should be avoided in late pregnancy (≥30 weeks) because it may cause premature closure of the ductus arteriosus.

ORAL SALICYLATE

▷ *indomethacin* (C) initially 25 mg bid-tid, increase as needed at weekly intervals by 25-50 mg/day; max 200 mg/day
Pediatric: <14 years: usually not recommended; >2 years, if risk warranted: 1-2 mg/kg/day in divided doses; max 3-4 mg/kg/day or 150-200 mg/day, whichever is less; <14 years, ER cap not recommended
Cap: 25, 50 mg; *Susp:* 25 mg/5 ml (pineapple-coconut, mint; alcohol 1%); *Supp:* 50 mg; *ER Cap:* 75 mg ext-rel

Comment: *indomethacin* is indicated only for acute painful flares. Administer with food and/or antacids. Use lowest effective dose for shortest duration.

ORAL NSAIDs

See more **Oral NSAIDs** page 511

▷ *diclofenac sodium* (C)
Voltaren 50 mg bid-qid or 75 mg bid or 25 mg qid with an additional 25 mg at HS if necessary
Tab: 25, 50, 75 mg ent-coat
Voltaren XR 100 mg once daily; rarely, 100 mg bid may be used
Tab: 100 mg ext-rel

NSAID PLUS PPI

▷ *esomeprazole/naproxen* (C)(G) 1 tab bid; use lowest effective dose for the shortest duration swallow whole; take at least 30 minutes before a meal
Pediatric: <18 years: not recommended
Vimovo *Tab: nap* 375 mg/*eso* 20 mg ext-rel; *nap* 500 mg/*eso* 20 mg ext-rel
Comment: **Vimovo** is indicated to improve signs/symptoms, and risk of gastric ulcer in patients at risk of developing NSAID-associated gastric ulcer.

COX-2 INHIBITORS

Comment: Cox-2 inhibitors are contraindicated with history of asthma, urticaria, and allergic-type reactions to ***aspirin***, other NSAIDs, and sulfonamides, 3rd trimester of pregnancy, and coronary artery bypass graft (CABG) surgery.

▷ *celecoxib* (C)(G) 50-400 mg once daily-bid; max 800 mg/day
Pediatric: <18 years: not recommended
Celebrex *Cap:* 50, 100, 200, 400 mg

▷ *meloxicam* (C)(G) initially 7.5 mg once daily; max 15 mg once daily
Pediatric: <2 years: not recommended; ≥2 years: 0.125 mg/kg; max 7.5 mg once daily
Mobic *Tab:* 7.5, 15 mg; *Oral susp:* 7.5 mg/5 ml (100 ml) (raspberry)
Vivlodex *Cap:* 5, 10 mg

PHOSPHODIESTERASE 4 (PDE4) INHIBITOR

▶ *apremilast* (C) swallow whole; initial titration over 5 days; maintenance 30 mg bid; *Day 1:* 10 mg in AM; *Day 2:* 10 mg AM and 10 mg PM; *Day 3:* 10 mg AM and 20 mg PM; *Day 4:* 20 mg AM and 20 mg PM; *Day 5:* 20 mg AM and 30 mg PM; *Day 6 and ongoing:* 30 mg AM and 30 mg PM
   Pediatric: <18 years: not established
   Otezla *Tab:* 10, 20, 30 mg; *2-Week Starter Pack*
Comment: Register pregnant patients exposed to by calling 877-311-8972.

INTERLEUKIN-12/INTERLEUKIN-23 ANTAGONIST

▶ *ustekinumab* (B) inject SC; rotate sites; <100 kg: 45 mg once; then 4 weeks later; then every 12 weeks; ≥100 kg: 90 mg once; then 4 weeks later; then every 12 weeks
Pediatric: <18 years: not recommended
   Stelara *Vial:* 45 mg/0.5 ml single-use (preservative-free)
   Comment: **Stelara** may be used as monotherapy or in combination with *methohtrexate* (MTX).

TUMOR NECROSIS FACTOR (TNF) BLOCKERS

▶ *adalimumab* (B) 40 mg SC once every other week; may increase to once weekly without *methotrexate* (MTX); administer in abdomen or thigh; rotate sites; 2-17 years, supervise first dose
Pediatric: <2 years: <10 kg: not recommended; 10-<15 kg: 10 mg every other week; 15-<30 kg: 20 mg every other week; 30 kg: 40 mg every other week
   Humira *Prefilled syringe:* 20 mg/0.4 ml; 40 mg/0.8 ml single-dose (2/pck; 2, 6/ starter pck) (preservative-free)
   Comment: **Humira** may use with *methotrexate* (MTX), DMARDS, corticoids, salicylates, NSAIDs, or analgesics.
▶ *etanercept* (B) 25 mg SC twice weekly (72-96 hours apart) or 50 mg SC weekly; rotate sites
Pediatric: <4 years: not recommended; 4-17 years: 0.4 mg/kg SC twice weekly, 72-96 hours apart (max 25 mg/dose) or 0.8 mg/kg SC weekly (max 50 mg/dose)
   Enbrel *Vial:* 25 mg pwdr for SC injection after reconstitution (4/carton w. supplies) (preservative-free; diluent contains benzyl alcohol); *Prefilled syringe:* 25, 50 mg/ml (preservative-free); *SureClick Autoinjector:* 50 mg/ml (preservative-free)
Comment: *etanercept* reduces pain, morning stiffness, and swelling. May be administered in combination with *methotrexate*. Live vaccines should not be administered concurrently. Do not administer with active infection.
▶ *golimumab* (B) administer SC or IV infusion (in combination with *methotrexate* [MTX])
Pediatric: <18 years: not established
   Simponi 50 mg SC once monthly; rotate sites
      Prefilled syringe, SmartJect autoinjector: 50 mg/0.5 ml, single-use (preservative-free)
   Simponi Aria 2 mg/kg IV infusion week 0 and week 4; then every 8 weeks thereafter
      Vial: 50 mg/4 ml, single-use, soln for IV infusion after dilution (latex-free, preservative-free)

Comment: Corticosteroids, nonbiologic DMARDs, and/or NSAIDs may be continued during treatment with *golimumab*.

▶ *infiximab* (B) administer SC or IV infusion (in combination with *methotrexate* [MTX]) administer by IV infusion over at least 2 hours; 5 mg/kg once weekly at weeks 0, 2, 6, and then every 8 weeks
Pediatric: <18 years: not established
    Remicade *Vial:* 100 mg pwdr for reconstitution and dilution; (preservative-free)

PULMONARY ARTERIAL HYPERTENSION (PAH) (WHO GROUP I)

PROSTACYCLIN RECEPTOR AGONIST

▶ *selexipag* (X) initially 200 mcg bid; increase by 200 mcg bid to highest tolerated dose up to 1600 mcg bid; *Moderate hepatic impairment (Child-Pugh B):* initially 200 mcg once daily; increase by 200 mcg once daily at weekly intervals as tolerated; swallow whole; may take with food to improve tolerability
Pediatric: not established
    Uptravi
        Tab: 200, 400, 600, 800, 1000, 1200, 1400, 1600 mcg; *Titration pck:* 140 x 200 mcg + 60 x 800 mcg)
    Comment: Discontinue **Uptravi** if pulmonary veno-occlusive disease is confirmed or severe hepatic impairment (Child-Pugh C). May be potentiated by concomitant strong CYP2C8 inhibitors (e.g., gemfibrozil); *Nursing mothers:* not recommended. Discontinue breastfeeding or discontinue the drug.

GUANYLATE CYCLASE STIMULATOR

▶ *riociguat* (X) initially 0.5-1 mg tid; titrate every 2 weeks as tolerated (SBP ≥95 and absence of hypotensive symptoms) to highest tolerated dose; max 2.5 mg tid
Pediatric: not recommended
    Adempas
        Tab: 0.5, 1, 1.5, 2, 2.5 mg
    Comment: If **Adempas** is interrupted for ≥3 days, re-titrate. Consider titrating to dosage higher than 2.5 mg tid, if tolerated, in patients who smoke. Consider a starting dose of 0.5 mg tid when initiating **Adempas** in patients receiving strong cytochrome P450 (CYP) and P-glycoprotein/breast cancer resistance protein (P-gp/BCRP) inhibitors such as azole antimycotics (e.g., *ketoconazole*, *itraconazole*) or HIV protease inhibitors (e.g., *ritonavir*). Monitor for signs and symptoms of hypotension with strong CYP and P-gp/BCRP inhibitors. Obtain pregnancy tests prior to initiation and monthly during treatment. **Adempas** has consistently shown to have teratogenic effects when administered to animals. Females can only receive **Adempas** through the Adempas Risk Evaluation and Mitigation Strategy (REMS) Program, a restricted distribution program: **www .AdempasREMS.com** or 855-4 ADEMPAS. It is not known if **Adempas** is present in human milk; however, *riociguat* or its metabolites were present in the milk of rats. Because of the potential for serious adverse reactions in nursing infants from *riociguat*, discontinue nursing or **Adempas**. In placebo-controlled clinical trials, serious bleeding has occurred (including hemoptysis, hematemesis, vaginal hemorrhage, catheter site hemorrhage, subdural

hematoma, and intra-abdominal hemorrhage. Safety and efficacy have not been demonstrated in patients with creatinine clearance <15 mL/min or on dialysis or severe hepatic impairment (Child-Pugh C).

Endothelin Receptor Antagonist, Selective for the Endothelin Type-A (ETA) Receptor

▷ *ambrisentan* (X) 20 mg once daily; at 4-week intervals, either the dose of **Letairis Le-taris** initially 5 mg once daily, with or without or **tadalafil** can be increased, as needed and tolerated, to **Letairis** 10 mg or *tadalafil* 40 mg; do not split, crush, or chew.
Pediatric: not recommended

Letairis
   Tab: 5, 10 mg *film-coat*

Comment: In patients with PAH, plasma ET-1 concentrations are increased as much as 10-fold and correlate with increased mean right atrial pressure and disease severity. ET-1 and ET-1 mRNA concentrations are increased as much as 9-fold in the lung tissue of patients with PAH, primarily in the endothelium of pulmonary arteries. These findings suggest that ET-1 may play a critical role in the pathogenesis and progression of PAH. When taken with *tadalafil*, **Letairis** is indicated to reduce the risk of disease progression and hospitalization, to reduce the risk of hospitalization due to worsening PAH, and to improve exercise tolerance. **Letaris** is contraindicated in idiopathic pulmonary fibrosis (IPF). Exclude pregnancy before the initiation of treatment with **Letairis.** Females of reproductive potential must use acceptable methods of contraception during treatment with **Letairis** and for one month after treatment. Obtain monthly pregnancy tests during treatment and 1 month after discontinuation of treatment. Females can only receive **Letairis** through the **Letairis** Risk Evaluation and Mitigation Strategy (REMS) Program, a restricted distribution program, because of the risk of embryo-fetal toxicity: www.Letairisrems.com or 1-866-664-5327.

PHOSPHODIESTERASE TYPE 5 (PDE5) INHIBITORS, CGMP-SPECIFIC DRUGS

▷ *sildenafil citrate* (B)(G) *Orally:* initially 5 or 20 mg tid, 4-6 hours apart; max 20 mg tid; *IV bolus:* 2.5 mg or 10 mg bolus injection tid, 4-6 hours apart; max 10 mg tid; the dose does not need to be adjusted for body weight.
Pediatric: not recommended

Revatio
   Tab: 20 mg film-coat; *Oral susp:* 10 mg/ml pwdr for reconstitution (1.12 g, 112 ml) (grape) (sorbitol); *Vial:* 10 mg/12.5 ml (0.8 mg/ml)

Comment: A 10 mg IV dose is predicted to provide pharmacological effect equivalent to the 20 mg oral dose. **Revatio** is contraindicated with concomitant nitrate drugs including *nitroglycerin, isosorbide dinitrate,* isosorbide mononitrate, and some recreational drugs such as "poppers." Taking **Revatio** with a nitrate can cause a sudden and serious decrease in blood pressure. **Revatio** is contraindicated with concomitant guanylate cyclase stimulator drugs such as *riociguat* (**Adempas**). Avoid the use of grapefruit products while taking **Revatio.** Stop **Revatio** and get emergency medical help if sudden vision loss. **Revatio** is contraindicated with other phosphodiesterase type 5 (PDE5) Inhibitors, cGMP-specific drugs such as *avanafil* (**Stendra**)*, tadalafil* (**Cialis**) or *vardenafil* (**Levitra**). Caution with history of recent MI, stroke, life-threatening arrhythmia, hypotension, hypertension, cardiac failure, unstable angina, retinitis pigmentosa, CYP3A4 inhibitors (e.g., *cimetidine*, the azoles, *erythromycin*, protease inhibitors (e.g., *ritonavir*), CYP3A4 inducers (e.g., *rifampin, carbamazepine,* *phenytoin, phenobarbital*), alcohol, antihypertensive agents. Side effects include headache, flushing, nasal congestion, rhinitis, dyspepsia, and diarrhea. Use **Revatio** with caution in patients with anatomical deformation of the penis (e.g., angulation, cavernosal fibrosis, or Peyronie's disease) or in patients who have conditions, which may predispose them to priapism (e.g., sickle cell anemia, multiple myeloma, or leukemia). In the event of an erection that persists longer than 4 hours, the patient should seek immediate medical assistance. If priapism (painful erection greater than 6 hours in duration) is not treated immediately, penile tissue damage and permanent loss of potency could result.

▷ *tadalafil* (**B**) 40mg once daily; *CrCl 31-80 mL/min:* initially 20 mg once daily; increase to 40mg once daily if tolerated; *CrCl <30 mL/min:* not recommended; *Mild or moderate hepatic cirrhosis (Child Pugh Class A or B):* initially 20 mg once daily. *Severe hepatic cirrhosis (Child Pugh Class C):* not recommended; *use with ritonavir; Receiving ritonavir for at least 1 week:* initiate **tadalafil** at 20 mg once daily; may increase to 40mg once daily if tolerated; *Already on tadalafil:* stop **tadalafil** at least 24 hours prior to initiating **ritonavir**; resume **tadalafil** at 20 mg once daily after at least 1 week; may increase to 40mg once daily if tolerated
Pediatric: not established
   Adcirca
Comment: Contraindicated with concomitant organic nitrates and guanylate cyclase stimulators (e.g., *riociguat*).

▷ *treprostinil* (**B**) swallow whole; take with food
   Orenitram
      Tab: 0.125, 0.25, 1, 2.5 mg ext-rel
   Comment: **Orenitram** is indicated to improve exercise capacity. It is contraindicated with severe hepatic impairment (Child-Pugh C). **Orenitram** inhibits platelet aggregation and increases the risk of bleeding. Concomitant administration of **Orenitram** with diuretics, antihypertensive agents or other vasodilators increases the risk of symptomatic hypotension.

PYELONEPHRITIS: ACUTE

URINARY TRACT ANALGESIA

▷ *phenazopyridine* (**B**)(**G**) 95-200 mg q 6 hours prn; max 2 days
Pediatric: not recommended
   AZO Standard, Prodium, Uristat (OTC) *Tab:* 95 mg
   AZO Standard Maximum Strength (OTC) *Tab:* 97.5 mg
   Pyridium, Urogesic *Tab:* 100, 200 mg

OUTPATIENT ANTI-INFECTIVE TREATMENT

Comment: Acute pyelonephritis can be treated with a single IM antibiotic administration followed by a PO antibiotic regimen and close follow up. Example: **Rocephin** 1 g IM followed by **Bactrim DS**, *cephalexin*, *ciprofloxacin*, *levofloxacin*, or *loracarbef*.

▷ *cephalexin* (**B**)(**G**) 1-4 g/day in 4 divided doses x 10-14 days
Pediatric: 25-50 mg/kg/day in 4 divided doses x 10-14 days; *see page 568 for dose by weight*
   Keflex *Cap:* 250, 333, 500, 750 mg; *Oral susp:* 125, 250 mg/5 ml (100, 200 ml) (strawberry)

▷ *ciprofloxacin* (C) 500 mg bid or 1000 mg XR once daily x 3-14 days
  Pediatric: <18 years: not recommended
  Cipro (G) *Tab:* 250, 500, 750 mg; *Oral susp:* 250, 500 mg/5 ml (100 ml) (strawberry)
  Cipro XR *Tab:* 500, 1000 mg ext-rel
  ProQuin XR *Tab:* 500 mg ext-rel
  Comment: *ciprofloxacin* is contraindicated <18 years-of-age, and during pregnancy and lactation. Risk of tendonitis or tendon rupture, especially 60 years-of-age and older.
▷ *levofloxacin* (C) *Uncomplicated:* 500 mg once daily x 10 days; *Complicated:* 750 mg once daily x 10 days
  Pediatric: <18 years: not recommended
  Levaquin *Tab:* 250, 500, 750 mg; *Oral soln:* 25 mg/ml (480 ml) (benzyl alcohol); *Inj conc:* 25 mg/ml for IV infusion after dilution for IV infusion (50, 100, 150 ml) (preservative-free)
  Comment: *levofloxacin* is contraindicated <18 years-of-age, and during pregnancy and lactation. Risk of tendonitis or tendon rupture, especially 60 years-of-age and older.
▷ *loracarbef* (B) 400 mg bid x 14 days
  Pediatric: 15 mg/kg/day in 2 divided doses x 14 days; *see page 581 for dose by weight*
  Lorabid *Pulvule:* 200, 400 mg; *Oral susp:* 100 mg/5 ml (50, 100 ml); 200 mg/5 ml (50, 75, 100 ml) (strawberry bubble gum)
▷ *trimethoprim/sulfamethoxazole* (D)(G) bid x 10 days
  Pediatric: <2 months: not recommended; ≥2 months: 40 mg/kg/day of *sulfamethoxazole* in 2 divided doses x 10 days; *see page 587 for dose by weight*
  Bactrim, Septra 2 tabs bid x 10 days
    Tab: trim 80 mg/*sulfa* 400 mg*
  Bactrim DS, Septra DS 1 tab bid x 10 days
    Tab: trim 160 mg/*sulfa* 800 mg*
  Bactrim Pediatric Suspension, Septra Pediatric Suspension
    Oral susp: trim 40 mg/*sulfa* 200 mg per 5 ml (100 ml) (cherry) (alcohol 0.3%)
  Comment: *trimethoprim/sulfamethoxazole* is not recommended in pregnancy or lactation. *CrCl 15-30 mL/min:* reduce dose by 1/2; *CrCl <15 mL/min:* not recommended

 RABIES

PRE-EXPOSURE PROPHYLAXIS

Comment: Postpone pre-exposure prophylaxis during acute febrile illness or infection. Have *epinephrine* 1:1000 readily available.
▷ *rabies immune globulin, human (HRIG)* (C) 3 injections of 1 ml IM each on day 0, 7, and either day 21 or 28; booster doses 1 ml IM every 2 years
  Pediatric: same as adult (except for infants administer in the vastus lateralis muscle)
  Imovax *Vial:* 2.5 u/ml (1 ml, single dose)

POSTEXPOSURE PROPHYLAXIS

Comment: Have *epinephrine* 1:1000 readily available.

▷ *rabies immune globulin, human (HRIG)* (C) 20 IU/kg infiltrated into wound area as much as feasible, then remaining dose administered IM at site remote from vaccine administration
Pediatric: same as adult
BayRab, Imogam Rabies *Vial:* 150 IU/ml (2, 10 ml)
▷ *rabies vaccine, human diploid cell* (C) *Not previously immunized:* administer first dose 1 ml in the deltoid as soon as possible after exposure; then repeat on days 3, 7, 14, 28 or 30, and 90; administer 1st dose with rabies immune globulin; *Previously immunized:* only 2 doses are administered, immediately after exposure and again 3 days later; no rabies immune globulin is needed.
Pediatric: same as adult (except for infants administer in vastus lateralis muscle)
Imovax, RabAvert *Vial:* 2.5 IU/ml (2.5 IU of freeze-dried vaccine w. diluent)

TETANUS PROPHYLAXIS

see **Tetanus** *page* 408 for patients not previously immunized

⬤ RESPIRATORY SYNCYTIAL VIRUS (RSV)

PROPHYLAXIS

▷ *palivizumab* 15 mg/kg IM administered monthly throughout the RSV season
Synagis *Vial:* 100 mg/ml
Treatment see **Bronchiolitis** *page* 58

⬤ RESTLESS LEGS SYNDROME (RLS)

GAMMA AMINOBUTYRIC ACID ANALOGS

▷ *gabapentin* (C)(G) 100 mg once daily x 1 day; then 100 mg bid x 1 day; then 100 mg tid thereafter; max 900 mg tid
Pediatric: not recommended
Gralise (C) initially 300 mg on Day 1; then 600 mg on Day 2; then 900 mg on Days 3-6; then 1200 mg on Days 7-10; then 1500 mg on Days 11-14; titrate up to 1800 mg on Day 15; take entire dose once daily with the evening meal; do not crush, split, or chew
Tab: 300, 600 mg
Neurontin (G) 100 mg daily x 1 day, then 100 mg bid x 1 day, then 100 mg tid continuously; max 900 mg tid
Pediatric: <3 years: not recommended; 3-12 years: initially 10-15 mg/kg/day in 3 divided doses; max 12 hours between doses; titrate over 3 days; 3-4 years: titrate to 40 mg/kg/day; 5-12 years: titrate to 25-35 mg/kg/day; max 50 mg/kg/day;
▷ *gabapentin enacarbil* (C) 600 mg once daily at about 5:00 PM; if dose not taken at recommended time, next dose should be taken the following day; swallow whole; take with food; *CrCl 30-59 mL/min:* 600 mg on Day 1, Day 3, and every day thereafter; *CrCl <30 mL/min* or on hemodialysis: not recommended
Pediatric: not recommended
Horizant *Tab:* 600 ext-rel
Comment: Avoid abrupt cessation of *gabapentin* and *gabapentin enacarbil*. To discontinue, withdraw gradually over 1 week or longer.

DOPAMINE RECEPTOR AGONISTS

▷ *pramipexole dihydrochloride* (C)(G) initially 0.125 mg once daily 2-3 hours before bedtime; may double dose every 4-7 days; max 0.75 mg/day
Pediatric: not recommended
    Mirapex *Tab:* 0.125, 0.25*, 0.5*, 0.75*, 1*, 1.5* mg

▷ *ropinirole* (C) take once daily 1-3 hours prior to bedtime; initially 0.25 mg on days 1 and 2; then 0.5 mg on days 3-7; increase by 0.5 mg/day at 1 week intervals to 3 mg; max 4 mg/day
Pediatric: not recommended
    Requip *Tab:* 0.25, 0.5, 1, 2, 3, 4, 5 mg

▷ *rotigotine* transdermal patch (C) apply to clean, dry, intact skin on abdomen, thigh, hip, flank, shoulder, or upper arm; initially 1mg/24 hour patch once daily; may increase weekly by 1mg/24 hour if needed; max 3mg/24 hour once daily; rotate sites and allow 14 days before reusing site; if hairy, shave site at least 3 days before application to site; avoid abrupt cessation; reduce by 1 mg/24 hour every other day
Pediatric: not recommended
    Neupro *Trans patch:* 1mg/24hrs, 2mg/24hrs, 3mg/24hrs, 4mg/24 hrs, 6mg/24hrs, 8mg/24hrs (30/carton) (sulfites)

◯ RETINITIS: CYTOMEGALOVIRUS (CMV)

Comment: *cidofovir and valganciclovir* are nucleoside analogues and prodrugs of *ganciclovir* indicated for the treatment of AIDS-related *cytomegalovirus* (CMV) retinitis and prevention of CMV disease in adult kidney, heart, and kidney-pancreas transplant patients at high risk, and for prevention of CMV disease in pediatric kidney and heart transplant patients at high risk.

▷ *cidofovir* (C) administer via IV infusion over 1 hour; pre-treat with oral *probenecid* (2 g, 3 hours prior to starting the *cidofovir* infusion and 1 g, 2 and 8 hours after the infusion is ended) and 1 liter of IV NaCl should be infused immediately before each dose of *cidofovir* (a 2nd liter of NaCl should also be infused either during or after each dose of *cidofovir* if a fluid load is tolerable); *Induction:* 5 mg/kg once weekly for 2 consecutive weeks; *Maintenance:* 5 mg/kg once every 2 weeks; reduce to 3 mg/kg if serum Cr increases 0.3-0.4 mg/dL above baseline; discontinue if serum Cr increases to >0.5 mg/dL above baseline or if >3+ proteinuria develops
Pediatric: not recommended
    Vistide *Vial:* 75 mg/ml (5 ml) (preservative-free)

Comment: *cidofovir* is a nucleoside analogue indicated for treatment of AIDS-related *cytomegalovirus* (CMV) retinitis.

▷ *valganciclovir* (C)(G) take with food; *Induction:* 900 mg bid x 21 days; *Maintenance:* 900 mg daily; *CrCl <60 mL/min:* reduce dose (see mfr pkg insert; hemodialysis or CrCl <10 mL/min not recommended (use *ganciclovir*)
Pediatric: <4 months: not recommended; 4 months-16 years: see mfr pkg insert for dosing calculation equation
    Valcyte *Tab:* 450 mg (preservative-free); *Oral pwdr for reconstitution:* 50 mg/ml (tutti-frutti)

◯ RHEUMATOID ARTHRITIS (RA)

Injectable Acetaminophen *see Pain page 306*

TOPICAL ANALGESICS

▷ *capsaicin* (B)(G) apply tid-qid prn to intact skin
Pediatric: <2 years: not recommended; ≥2 years: same as adult
Axsain *Crm:* 0.075% (1, 2 oz)
Capsin *Lotn:* 0.025, 0.075% (59 ml)
Capzasin-P (OTC) *Crm:* 0.025% (1.5 oz); *Lotn:* 0.025% (2 oz)
Dolorac *Crm:* 0.025% (28 g)
Double Cap (OTC) *Crm:* 0.05% (2 oz)
R-Gel *Gel:* 0.025% (15, 30 g)
Zostrix (OTC) *Crm:* 0.025% (0.7, 1.5, 3 oz)
Zostrix HP (OTC) *Emol crm:* 0.075% (1, 2 oz)
▷ *trolamine salicylate* (NE)
Mobisyl apply tid-qid
Crm: 10%
Comment: Provides some relief by 1-2 weeks; optimal benefit may take 4-6 weeks.

ORAL SALICYLATE

▷ *indomethacin* (C) initially 25 mg bid-tid, increase as needed at weekly intervals by 25-50 mg/day; max 200 mg/day
Pediatric: <14 years: usually not recommended; >2 years, if risk warranted: 1-2 mg/kg/day in divided doses; max 3-4 mg/kg/day (or 150-200 mg/day, whichever is less; <14 years, ER cap not recommended
Cap: 25, 50 mg; *Susp:* 25 mg/5 ml (pineapple-coconut, mint; alcohol 1%); *Supp:* 50 mg; *ER Cap:* 75 mg ext-rel
Comment: *indomethacin* is indicated only for acute painful flares. Administer with food and/or antacids. Use lowest effective dose for shortest duration.

NSAID

See more Oral NSAIDs *page* 511

▷ *diclofenac sodium* (C)(G)
Voltaren 50 mg bid-qid or 75 mg bid or 25 mg qid with an additional 25 mg at HS if necessary
Tab: 25, 50, 75 mg ent-coat
Voltaren XR 100 mg once daily; rarely, 100 mg bid may be used
Tab: 100 mg ext-rel

NSAID PLUS PPI

▷ *esomeprazole/naproxen* (C)(G) 1 tab bid; use lowest effective dose for the shortest duration swallow whole; take at least 30 minutes before a meal
Pediatric: <18 years: not recommended
Vimovo *Tab:* nap 375 mg/eso 20 mg ext-rel; *nap* 500 mg/*eso* 20 mg ext-rel

Comment: **Vimovo** is indicated to improve signs/symptoms, and risk of gastric ulcer in patients at risk of developing NSAID-associated gastric ulcer.

COX-2 INHIBITORS

Comment: Cox-2 inhibitors are contraindicated with history of asthma, urticaria, and allergic-type reactions to **aspirin**, other NSAIDs, and sulfonamides, 3rd trimester of pregnancy, and coronary artery bypass graft (CABG) surgery.

▶ *celecoxib* (C)(G) 50-400 mg once daily-bid; max 800 mg/day
   Pediatric: <18 years: not recommended
      Celebrex *Cap:* 50, 100, 200, 400 mg
▶ *meloxicam* (C)(G) initially 7.5 mg once daily; max 15 mg once daily
   Pediatric: <2 years: not recommended; ≥2 years: 0.125 mg/kg; max 7.5 mg once daily
      Mobic *Tab:* 7.5, 15 mg; *Oral susp:* 7.5 mg/5 ml (100 ml) (raspberry)
      Vivlodex *Cap:* 5, 10 mg

JANUS KINASE (JAK) INHIBITOR

▶ *tofacitinib* (C) 5 mg twice daily; reduce to 5 mg once daily for moderate-to-severe renal impairment <u>or</u> moderate hepatic impairment, concomitant potent CYP3A4 inhibitors, <u>or</u> drugs that result in both CYP3A4 and potent CYP2C19 inhibition
   Pediatric: not established
      Xeljanz *Tab:* 5 mg
      Xeljanz XR *Tab:* 11 mg ext-rel

   Comment: **Xeljanz** is indicated for moderate-to-severe RA as monotherapy in patients who have inadequate response <u>or</u> intolerance to **methotrexate** (MTX) <u>and/or</u> in combination with other non-biologic DMARDs.

DISEASE MODIFYING ANTI-RHEUMATIC DRUGS (DMARDs)

Comment: DMARDs are first-line treatment options for RA. DMARDs include penicillamine, gold salts (**auranofin, aurothio-glucose**), immunosuppressants, and **hydroxychloroquine**. The DMARDs reduce ESR, reduce RF, and favorably affect the outcome of RA. Immunosuppressants may require 6 weeks to affect benefits and 6 months for full improvement.

▶ *auranofin (gold salt)* (C) 3 mg bid <u>or</u> 6 mg once daily; if inadequate response after 6 months, increase to 3 mg tid
   Pediatric: not recommended
      Ridaura *Vial:* 100 mg/20 ml
▶ *azathioprine* (D) 1 mg/kg/day in a single <u>or</u> divided doses; may increase by 0.5 mg/kg/day q 4 weeks; max 2.5 mg/kg/day; minimum trial to ascertain effectiveness is 12 weeks
   Pediatric: not recommended
      Azasan *Tab* 75*, 100*mg
      Imuran *Tab* 50*mg
▶ *cyclosporine (immunosuppressant)* (C) 1.25 mg/kg bid; may increase after 4 weeks by 0.5 mg/kg/day; then adjust at 2 week intervals; max 4 mg/kg/day; administer with meals
   Pediatric: not recommended
      Neoral *Cap:* 25, 100 mg (alcohol)

Neoral Oral Solution *Oral soln:* 100 mg/ml (50 ml) may dilute in room temperature apple juice or orange juice (alcohol)

Comment: **Neoral** is indicated for RA unresponsive to *methotrexate* (MTX).

▷ *hydroxychloroquine* (C) 400-600 mg/day
Pediatric: not recommended
    Plaquenil *Tab:* 200 mg

Comment: May require several weeks to achieve beneficial effects. If no improvement in 6 months, discontinue.

▷ *leflunomide* (X)(G) initially 100 mg once daily x 3 days; maintenance dose 20 mg once daily; max 20 mg daily
Pediatric: <18 years: not recommended
    Arava *Tab:* 10, 20, 100 mg
    Comment: **Arava** is contraindicated with breastfeeding.

▷ *methotrexate* (X) 7.5 mg x 1 dose per week or 2.5 mg x 3 at 12 hour intervals once a week; max 20 mg/week; therapeutic response begins in 3-6 weeks; administer *methotrexate* injection SC only into the abdomen or thigh
Pediatric: <2 years: not recommended; ≥2 years: 10 mg/m² once weekly; max 20 mg/m²
    Rasuvo *Autoinjector:* 7.5 mg/0.15 ml, 10 mg/0.20 ml, 12.5 mg/0.25 ml, 15 mg/0.30 ml, 17.5 mg/0.35 ml, 20 mg/0.40 ml, 22.5 mg/0.45 ml, 25 mg/0.50 ml, 27.5 mg/0.55 ml, 30 mg/0.60 ml (solution concentration for SC injection is 50 mg/ml)
    Rheumatrex *Tab:* 2.5*mg (5, 7.5, 10, 12.5, 15 mg/week, 4/card unit-of-use dose pack)
    Trexall *Tab:* 5*, 7.5*, 10*, 15*mg (5, 7.5, 10, 12.5, 15 mg/week, 4/card unit-of-use dose pack)
    Comment: *methotrexate* (MTX) is contraindicated with immunodeficiency, blood dyscrasias, alcoholism, and chronic liver disease.

▷ *penicillamine* (D) 125-250 mg once daily initially; may increase by 125-250 mg/day q 1-3 months; max 1.5 g/day
Pediatric: not recommended
    Cuprimine *Cap:* 125, 250 mg
    Depen *Tab:* 250 mg

▷ *sulfasalazine* (C; D in 2nd, 3rd)(G) initially 0.5 g once daily bid; gradually increase every 4 days; usual maintenance 2-3 g/day in equally divided doses at regular intervals; max 4 g/day
Pediatric: <6 years: not recommended; 6-16 years: initially 1/4 to 1/3 of maintenance dose; increase weekly; maintenance 30-50 mg/kg/day in 2 divided doses at regular intervals; max 2 g/day
    Azulfidine *Tab:* 500 mg
    Azulfidine EN *Tab:* 500 mg ent-coat

TUMOR NECROSIS FACTOR (TNF) BLOCKERS

▷ *adalimumab* (B) 40 mg SC once every other week; may increase to once weekly without *methotrexate* (MTX); administer in abdomen or thigh; rotate sites; 2-17 years, supervise first dose
Pediatric: <2 years, <10 kg: not recommended; 10-<15 kg: 10 mg every other week; 15-<30 kg: 20 mg every other week; ≥30 kg: 40 mg every other week

Humira *Prefilled syringe:* 20 mg/0.4 ml; 40 mg/0.8 ml single-dose (2/pck; 2, 6/ starter pck) (preservative-free)

Comment: **Humira** may use with *methotrexate* (MTX), DMARDs, corticosteroids, salicylates, NSAIDs, <u>or</u> analgesics.

▷ *certolizumab pegol* **(B)** 400 mg SC on day 1, at week 2, and at week 4; then 200 mg every other week; rotate sites

Pediatric: not recommended

Cimzia *Vial:* 200 mg single-dose w. supplies (2/pck, 2, 6/starter pck); *Prefilled syringe:* 200 mg single-dose w. supplies (2/pck, 2, 6/starter pck) (preservative-free)

▷ *etanercept* **(B)** 25 mg SC twice weekly, 72-96 hours apart <u>or</u> 50 mg SC weekly; rotate sites

Pediatric: <4 years: not recommended; 4-17 years: 0.4 mg/kg SC twice weekly, 72-96 hours apart (max 25 mg/dose) <u>or</u> 0.8 mg/kg SC weekly (max 50 mg/dose)

Enbrel *Vial:* 25 mg pwdr for SC injection after reconstitution (4/carton w. supplies) (preservative-free; diluent contains benzyl alco hol); *Prefilled syringe:* 50 mg/ml (preservative-free); *SureClick autoinjector:* 50 mg/ml (preservative-free)

Comment: *etanercept* reduces pain, morning stiffness, and swelling. May be administered in combination with *methotrexate*. Live vaccines should not be administered concurrently. Do not administer with active infection.

▷ *golimumab* **(B)** administer SC <u>or</u> IV infusion (in combination with *methotrexate* [MTX])

Pediatric: <18 years: not established

Simponi 50 mg SC once monthly; rotate sites

Prefilled syringe, SmartJect autoinjector: 50 mg/0.5 ml, single-use (preservative-free)

Simponi Aria 2 mg/kg IV infusion week 0 and week 4; then every 8 weeks thereafter

Vial: 50 mg/4 ml, single-use, soln for IV infusion after dilution (latex-free, preservative-free)

Comment: corticosteroids, non-biologic DMARDs, <u>and/or</u> NSAIDs may be continued during treatment with *golimumab*.

▷ *infiximab* **(B)** administer SC <u>or</u> IV infusion (in combination with *methotrexate* [MTX]) administer by IV infusion over at least 2 hours; 3 mg/kg once weekly at weeks 0, 2, 6, and then every 8 weeks; may increase to 10 mg/kg <u>or</u> *administer* every 4 weeks

Pediatric: <18 years: not established

Remicade *Vial:* 100 mg pwdr for reconstitution and dilution; (preservative-free)

Comment: Use *infliximab* concomitantly with *methotrexate* when there has been insufficient response to *methotrexate* alone.

Interleukin-1 Receptor Antagonist

▷ *anakinra (interleukin-1 receptor antagonist)* **(B)** 100 mg SC once daily; discard any unused portion

Pediatric: not recommended

Kineret *Prefilled syringe:* 100 mg/single-dose syringe (7, 28/pk) (preservative-free)

Interleukin-6 Receptor Antagonist

▷ *tocilizumab* **(B)** administer as an IV infusion over 60 minutes once every 4 weeks; initially 4 mg/kg; may increase to 8 mg/kg based on clinical response

Pediatric: not recommended
    Actemra *Vial:* 80 mg/4 ml, 200 mg/10 ml, 400 mg/20 ml for IV infusion after dilution

Selective Costimulation Modulator

▷ *abatacept* (C) administer as an IV infusion over 30 minutes at weeks 0, 2, and 4; then every 4 weeks thereafter; <60 kg, administer 500 mg/ dose; 60-100 kg, administer 750 mg/dose; >100 kg, administer 1 g/dose; 60-100 kg, administer 750 mg/dose; >100 kg, administer 1 g/dose
Pediatric: <6 years: not recommended; 6-17 years: administer as an IV infusion over 30 minutes at weeks 0, 2, and 4; then every 4 weeks thereafter; <75 kg, administer 10 mg/kg; same as adult (max 1 g)
    Orencia *Vial:* 250 mg pwdr for IV infusion after reconstitution (silicone-free) (preservative-free); *Prefilled syringe:* 125 mg/ml soln for SC injection (preservative-free); *ClickJect Autoinjector:* 125 mg/ml soln for SC injection

CD20 ANTIBODY

▷ *rituximab* (C) administer corticosteroid 30 minutes prior to each infusion; concomitant *methotrexate* therapy, administer a 1000 mg IV infusion at 0 and 2 weeks; then every 24 weeks <u>or</u> based on response, but not sooner than every 16 weeks.
Pediatric: <6 years: not recommended; >6 years: same as adult
    Rituxan *Vial:* 10 mg/ml (10, 50 ml) (preservative-free)

INTRA-ARTICULAR INJECTION

▷ *sodium hyaluronate* 20 mg as intra-articular injection weekly x 5 weeks
Pediatric: not recommended
    Hyalgan *Prefilled syringe:* 20 mg/2 ml
    Comment: Remove joint effusion and inject with *lidocaine* if possible before injecting **Hyalgan**.

 ## RHINITIS/SINUSITIS: ALLERGIC

Oral Prescription Drugs for the Management of Allergy, Cough, and Cold Symptoms
see page 535
Parenteral Corticosteroids *see page* 511
Oral Corticosteroids *see page* 509

ALLERGEN EXTRACTS

Comment: Allergen extracts (**Grastek, Oralair, Ragwitek**) are not for immediate relief of allergic symptoms. Contraindicated with severe, unstable, and uncontrolled asthma, history of eosinophilic esophagitis, and severe local <u>or</u> systemic reaction. First dose under supervision HCP and observe ≥30 minutes. Subsequent doses may be taken at home.
▷ *short ragweed pollen allergen extract* (C) one SL tab once daily
Pediatric: <18 years: not established
    Ragwitek *SL tab: Amerosia artemisiifolia 12 amb a 1-unit* (30, 90/blister pck)

Comment: Initiate **Ragwitek** at least 12 weeks before onset of ragweed pollen season and continue throughout season.

▷ *sweet vernal, orchard, perennial rye, timothy, Kentucky blue grass mixed pollen allergen extract* (C) 300 IR once daily
  Pediatric: <10 years: not established; 10-17 years: Day 1: 100 IR; Day 2: 200 IR; Day 3 and thereafter: 300 IR once daily
  Oralair *SL tab:* 100, 300 IR (index of reactivity) (30/blister pck)
  Comment: **Oralair** is indicated for grass pollen-induced allergic rhinitis with or without conjunctivitis confirmed by positive skin test. Initiate **Orlair** at least 4 months before onset of grass pollen season and continue throughout season.

▷ *timothy grass pollen allergen extract* (C) one SL tab once daily
  Pediatric: <5 years: not established; ≥5 years: same as adult
  Grastek *SL tab:* 2800 bioequivalent allergy units (BAUS) (30/blister pck)
  Comment: **Grastek** is indicated for grass pollen-induced allergic rhinitis with or without conjunctivitis confirmed by positive skin test. Initiate **Grastek** at least 12 weeks before onset of grass pollen season and continue throughout season.

NASAL DECONGESTANT

▷ *tetrahydrozoline* (C)
  Tyzine 2-4 drops or 3-4 sprays in each nostril q 3-8 hours prn
    Pediatric: <6 years: not recommended; ≥6 years: same as adult
    Nasal spray: 0.1% (15 ml); *Nasal drops:* 0.1% (30 ml)
  Tyzine Pediatric Nasal Drops 2-3 sprays or drops in each nostril q 3-6 hours prn
    Nasal drops: 0.05% (15 ml)

LEUKOTRIENE RECEPTOR ANTAGONISTS

Comment: For prophylaxis and chronic treatment only. Not for primary (rescue) treatment of acute asthma attack.

▷ *montelukast* (B)(G) 10 mg once daily in the PM; for EIB, take at least 2 hours before exercise; max 1 dose/day
  Pediatric: <12 months: not recommended; 12-23 months: one 4 mg granule pkt daily; 2-5 years: one 4 mg chew tab or granule pkt daily; 6-14 years: one 5 mg chew tab daily daily; >15 years: same as adult
  Singulair *Tab:* 10 mg
  Singulair Chewable *Chew tab:* 4, 5 mg (cherry, phenylalanine)
  Singulair Oral Granules: 4 mg/pkt; take within 15 minutes of opening pkt; may mix with applesauce, carrots, rice, or ice cream

▷ *zafirlukast* (B)(G) 20 mg bid, 1 hour ac or 2 hours pc
  Pediatric: <7 years: not recommended; 7-11 years: 10 mg bid 1 hour ac or 2 hours pc; >11 years: same as adult
  Accolate *Tab:* 10, 20 mg

▷ *zileuton* (C) 1 tab qid
  Pediatric: <12 years: not recommended; ≥12 years: same as adult
  Zyflo *Tab:* 600 mg

NASAL CORTICOSTEROIDS

▷ *beclomethasone dipropionate* (C)
  Beconase 1 spray in each nostril bid-qid

Pediatric: <6 years: not recommended; 6-12 years: 1 spray in each nostril tid; >12 years: same as adult
Nasal spray: 42 mcg/actuation (6.7 g, 80 sprays; 16.8 g, 200 sprays)

Beconase AQ 1-2 sprays in each nostril bid
Pediatric: <6: not recommended; ≥6 years: same as adult
Nasal spray: 42 mcg/actuation (25 g, 180 sprays)

Beconase Inhalation Aerosol 1-2 sprays in each nostril bid to qid
Pediatric: <6: not recommended; 6-12 years: 1 spray in each nostril tid; >12 years: same as adult
Nasal spray: 42 mcg/actuation (6.7 g, 80 sprays; 16.8 g, 200 sprays)

Vancenase AQ 1-2 sprays in each nostril bid
Pediatric: <6 years: not recommended; ≥6 years: same as adult
Nasal spray: 84 mcg/actuation (25 g, 200 sprays)

Vancenase AQ DS 1-2 sprays in each nostril once daily
Pediatric: <6 years: not recommended; ≥6 years: same as adult
Nasal spray: 84, 168 mcg/actuation (19 g, 120 sprays)

Vancenase Pockethaler 1 spray in each nostril bid <u>or</u> qid
Pediatric: <6: not recommended; ≥6 years: 1 spray in each nostril tid
Pockethaler: 42 mcg/actuation (7 g, 200 sprays)

QNASL Nasal Aerosol 2 sprays, 80 mcg/spray, in each nostril once daily
Pediatric: <12 years: 2 sprays, 40 mcg/spray, in each nostril once daily; ≥12 years: same as adult
Nasal spray: 40 mcg/actuation (4.9 g, 60 sprays); 80 mcg/actuation (8.7 g, 120 sprays)

▷ *budesonide* (C)
Rhinocort initially 2 sprays in each nostril bid in the AM and PM, <u>or</u> 4 sprays in each nostril in the AM; max 4 sprays each nostril/day; use lowest effective dose
Pediatric: <6 years: not recommended; >6 years: same as adult
Nasal spray: 32 mcg/actuation (7 g, 200 sprays)

Rhinocort Aqua Nasal Spray initially 1 spray in each nostril once daily; max 4 sprays in each nostril once daily
Pediatric: <6 years: not recommended; ≥6-12 years: initially 1 spray in each nostril once daily; max 2 sprays in each nostril once daily
Nasal spray: 32 mcg/actuation (10 ml, 60 sprays)

▷ *ciclesonide* (C)
Pediatric: <6 years: not recommended; ≥6 years: same as adult
Omnaris 2 sprays in each nostril once daily
Nasal spray: 50 mcg/actuation (12.5 g, 120 sprays)
Zetonna 1-2 sprays in each nostril once daily
Nasal spray: 37 mcg/actuation (6.1 g, 60 sprays) (HFA)

▷ *dexamethasone* (C) 2 sprays in each nostril bid-tid; max 12 sprays/day; maintain at lowest effective dose
Pediatric: <6 years: not recommended; ≥6-12 years: 1-2 sprays in each nostril bid; max 8 sprays/day; maintain at lowest effective dose; >12 years: same as adult
Dexacort Turbinaire *Nasal spray:* 84 mcg/actuation (12.6 g, 170 sprays)

▷ *fluticasone furoate* (C) 2 sprays in each nostril once daily; may reduce to 1 spray each nostril once daily

Pediatric: <2 years: not recommended; ≥2-11 years: 1 spray in each nostril once daily; ≥12 years: same as adult
> **Veramyst** *Nasal spray:* 27.5 mcg/actuation (10 g, 120 sprays) (alcohol-free)
▷ *fluticasone propionate* (C)(OTC)(G) initially 2 sprays in each nostril once daily or 1 spray bid; maintenance 1 spray once daily
Pediatric: <4 years: not recommended; >4 years: initially 1 spray in each nostril once daily; may increase to 2 sprays in each nostril once daily; maintenance 1 spray in each nostril once daily; max 2 sprays in each nostril/day
> **Flonase** *Nasal spray:* 50 mcg/actuation (16 g, 120 sprays)
▷ *flunisolide* (C) 2 sprays in each nostril bid; may increase to 2 sprays in each nostril tid; max 8 sprays/nostril/day
Pediatric: <6 years: not recommended; 6-14 years: initially 1 spray in each nostril tid or 2 sprays in each nostril bid; max 4 sprays/nostril/day; >14 years: same as adult
> **Nasalide** *Nasal spray:* 25 mcg/actuation (25 ml, 200 sprays)
> **Nasarel** *Nasal spray:* 25 mcg/actuation (25 ml, 200 sprays)
▷ *mometasone furoate* (C)(G) 2 sprays in each nostril once daily
Pediatric: <2 years: not recommended; 2-11 years: 1 spray in each nostril once daily; max 2 sprays in each nostril once daily; >11 years: same as adult
> **Nasonex** *Nasal spray:* 50 mcg/actuation (17 g, 120 sprays)
▷ *olopatadine* (C) 2 sprays in each nostril bid
Pediatric: <6 years: not recommended; 6-11 years: 1 spray each nostril bid; >11 years: same as adult
> **Patanase** *Nasal spray:* 0.6%; 665 mcg/actuation (30.5 g, 240 sprays) (benzalkonium chloride)
▷ *triamcinolone acetonide* (C)(G) initially 2 sprays in each nostril once daily; max 4 sprays in each nostril once daily or 2 sprays in each nostril bid or 1 spray in each nostril qid; maintain at lowest effective dose
Pediatric: <6 years: not recommended; ≥6 years: 1 spray in each nostril once daily; max 2 sprays in each nostril once daily
> **Nasacort Allergy 24HR (OTC)** *Nasal spray:* 55 mcg/actuation (10 g, 120 sprays)
> **Tri-Nasal** *Nasal spray:* 50 mcg/actuation (15 ml, 120 sprays)

NASAL MAST CELL STABILIZERS

▷ *cromolyn sodium* (B)(OTC) 1 spray in each nostril tid-qid; max 6 sprays in each nostril/day
Pediatric: <2 years: not recommended; ≥2 years: same as adult
> **Children's NasalCrom, NasalCrom** *Nasal spray:* 5.2 mg/spray (13 ml, 100 sprays; 26 ml, 200 sprays)
Comment: Begin 1-2 weeks before exposure to known allergen. May take 2-4 weeks to achieve maximum effect.

NASAL ANTIHISTAMINES

▷ *azelastine* (C) 1 spray in each nostril bid
Pediatric: <5 years: not recommended; ≥5-12 years: 1 spray in each nostril once daily bid; >12 years: same as adult
> **Astelin Ready Spray** 2 sprays in each nostril bid
> *Nasal spray:* 137 mcg/actuation (30 ml, 200sprays) (benzalkonium chloride)
> **Astepro 0.15% Nasal Spray** 1 or 2 sprays each nostril once daily bid

Pediatric: not recommended
Nasal spray: 205.5 mcg/actuation (17 ml, 106 sprays; 30 ml, 200 sprays) (benzalkonium chloride)

NASAL ANTIHISTAMINE/CORTICOSTEROID COMBINATION

▷ *azelastine/fluticasone* (C) 1 spray in each nostril bid
   Pediatric: <6 years: not recommended; ≥6 years: same as adult
     Dymista *Nasal spray:* azel 137 mcg/*flutic* 50 mcg per actuation (23 g, 120 sprays) (benzalkonium chloride)

NASAL ANTICHOLINERGICS

▷ *ipratropium bromide* (B)(G)
     Atrovent Nasal Spray 0.03% 2 sprays in each nostril bid-tid
       Pediatric: <6 years: not recommended; ≥6 years: same as adult
       Nasal spray: 21 mcg/actuation (30 ml, 345 sprays)
     Atrovent Nasal Spray 0.06% 2 sprays in each nostril tid-qid; max 5-7 days
       Pediatric: <5 years: not recommended; ≥5-11 years: 2 sprays in each nostril tid; >11 years: same as adult
       Nasal spray: 42 mcg/actuation (15 ml, 165 sprays)
   Comment: Avoid use with narrow-angle glaucoma, prostate hyperplasia, and bladder neck obstruction.

⦿ RHINITIS MEDICAMENTOSA

Comment: The nasal/oral regimen selected should be instituted with concurrent weaning from the nasal decongestant.
Oral Prescription Drugs for the Management of Allergy, Cough, and Cold Symptoms *see page 535*
Nasal Corticosteroids *see Allergic Rhinitis page 382*
Oral Corticosteroids *see page 509*
Parenteral Corticosteroids *see page 511*

NASAL ANTICHOLINERGICS

▷ *ipratropium bromide* (B)(G)
     Atrovent Nasal Spray 0.03% stop nasal decongestant; 2 sprays in each nostril bid-tid with progressive weaning as tolerated
       Pediatric: <6 years: not recommended; ≥6 years: same as adult
       Nasal spray: 21 mcg/actuation (30 ml, 345 sprays)
     Atrovent Nasal Spray 0.06% stop nasal decongestant; 2 sprays in each nostril tid-qid with progressive weaning as tolerated
       Pediatric: <5 years: not recommended; ≥5-11 years: 2 sprays in each nostril tid; ≥11 years: same as adult
       Nasal spray: 42 mcg/actuation (15 ml, 165 sprays)
   Comment: Avoid use with narrow-angle glaucoma, prostate hyperplasia, and bladder neck obstruction

NASAL ANTIHISTAMINE

▷ *azelastine* (C) 2 sprays in each nostril bid
  Pediatric: <5 years: not recommended; ≥5-12 years: 1 spray in each nostril bid
    Astelin Ready Spray
      Nasal spray: 137 mcg/actuation (30 ml, 200 sprays)

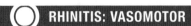

RHINITIS: VASOMOTOR

NASAL ANTICHOLINERGICS

▷ *ipratropium bromide* (B)(G)
    Atrovent Nasal Spray 0.03% stop nasal decongestant; 2 sprays in each nostril
    bid-tid with progressive weaning as tolerated
      Pediatric: <6 years: not recommended; ≥6 years: same as adult
      Nasal spray: 21 mcg/actuation (30 ml, 345 sprays)
    Atrovent Nasal Spray 0.06% stop nasal decongestant; 2 sprays in each nostril
    tid-qid with progressive weaning as tolerated
      Pediatric: <5 years: not recommended; ≥5-11 years: 2 sprays in each nostril
      tid; >11 years: same as adult
      Nasal spray: 42 mcg/actuation (15 ml, 165 sprays)
Comment: Avoid use with narrow-angle glaucoma, prostate hyperplasia, and bladder
neck obstruction

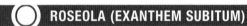

ROSEOLA (EXANTHEM SUBITUM)

  Antipyretics *see Fever page* 143

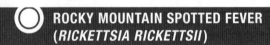

ROCKY MOUNTAIN SPOTTED FEVER (*RICKETTSIA RICKETTSII*)

ANTI-INFECTIVES

▷ *doxycycline* (D)(G) 200 mg on first day; then 100 mg bid x 7-10 days
  Pediatric: <8 years: not recommended; ≥8 years, <100 lb: 2-2.5 mg/kg q 12 hours x
  7-10 days; ≥8 years, >100 lb: same as adult
    Actilate *Tab:* 75, 150**mg
    Adoxa *Tab:* 50, 75, 100, 150 mg ent-coat
    Doryx *Tab:* 50, 75, 100, 150, 200 mg del-rel
    Monodox *Cap:* 50, 75, 100 mg
    Oracea *Cap:* 40 mg del-rel
    Vibramycin *Tab:* 100 mg; *Cap:* 50, 100 mg; *Syr:* 50 mg/5 ml (raspberry-apple)
    (sulfites); *Oral susp:* 25 mg/5 ml (raspberry)
    Vibra-Tab *Tab:* 100 mg film-coat
  Comment: *doxycycline* contraindicated <8 years-of-age, in pregnancy, and lactation
  (discolors developing tooth enamel). A side effect may be photo-sensitivity
  (photophobia). Do not give with antacids, calcium supplements, milk or other
  dairy, or within two hours of taking another drug.

▶ *tetracycline* (D)(G) 500 mg q 6 hours x 7-10 days
Pediatric: <8 years: not recommended; ≥8 years, <100 lb: 10 mg/kg/day q 6 hours x
7-10 days; ≥8 years, >100 lb: same as adult
   Achromycin V *Cap:* 250, 500 mg
   Sumycin *Tab:* 250, 500 mg; *Cap:* 250, 500 mg; *Oral susp:* 125 mg/5 ml (100, 200
   ml) (fruit) (sulfites)
Comment: *tetracycline* is contraindicated <8 years-of-age, in pregnancy, and
lactation (discolors developing tooth enamel). A side effect may be photo-sensitivity
(photophobia). Do not give with antacids, calcium supplements, milk or other dairy,
or within two hours of taking another drug.

 ROTAVIRUS GASTROENTERITIS

PROPHYLAXIS

Comment: **RotaTeq** targets the most common strains of rotavirus (G1, G2, G3, G4),
which are responsible for more than 90% of rotavirus disease in the United States.
▶ *rotavirus vaccine, live* not recommended for adults
Pediatric: <6 weeks or >32 weeks: not recommended; >6 weeks and <32 weeks:
administer 1st dose at 6-12 weeks of age; administer 2nd and 3rd doses at 4-10-
week intervals for a total of 3 doses; if an incomplete dose is administered, do
not administer a replacement dose, but continue with the remaining doses in the
recommended series
   RotaTeq *Oral susp:* 2 ml single-use tube (fetal bovine serum [trace], preservative-
   free, thimerosal-free)

 ROUNDWORM (ASCARIASIS)

ANTHELMINTICS

▶ *albendazole* (C) 400 mg once daily x 7 days; take with a meal
Pediatric: <2 years: 200 mg once daily x 3 days; may repeat in 3 weeks; ≥2-12 years:
400 mg once daily x 3 days; may repeat in 3 weeks
   Albenza *Tab:* 200 mg
▶ *mebendazole* (C) chew, swallow, or mix with food; 100 mg bid x 3 days; may repeat
in 3 weeks if needed; take with a meal
Pediatric: <2 years: not recommended; ≥2 years: same as adult
   Emverm *Chew tab:* 100 mg
   Vermox (G) *Chew tab:* 100 mg
▶ *pyrantel pamoate* (C) 11 mg/kg once daily x 3 days; max 1 g/dose; take with a meal
Pediatric: 25-37 lb: 1/2 tsp x 1 dose; 38-62 lb: 1 tsp x 1 dose; 63-87 lb: 1 tsp x 1 dose;
88-112 lb: 2 tsp x 1 dose; 113-137 lb: 2 tsp x 1 dose; 138-162 lb: 3 tsp x 1 dose; 163-
187 lb: 3 tsp x 1 dose; >187 lb: 4 tsp x 1 dose
   Pin-X (OTC) *Cap:* 180 mg; *Liq:* 50 mg/ml (30 ml); 144 mg/ml (30 ml); *Oral
   susp:* 50 mg/ml (30 ml)
▶ *thiabendazole* (C) 25 mg/kg bid x 7 days; max 1.5 g/dose; max 3000 mg/day; take
with a meal
Pediatric: same as adult
   Mintezol *Chew tab:* 500*mg (orange); *Oral susp:* 500 mg/5 ml (120 ml) (orange)
   Comment: *thiabendazole* is not for prophylaxis. May impair mental alertness.

RUBELLA (GERMAN MEASLES)

PROPHYLAXIS

▷ *rubella virus, live, attenuated/neomycin* vaccine (C)
  Pediatric: <12 months: not recommended (if vaccinated <12 months, revaccinate at
  12 months); ≥12 months: 25 mcg SC
  Meruvax II 25 mcg SC
▷ *measles, mumps, rubella, live, attenuated, neomycin vaccine* (C)
  MMR II 25 mcg SC (preservative-free)
Comment: Contraindications: hypersensitivity to *neomycin* or eggs, primary or
acquired immune deficiency, immunosuppressant therapy, bone marrow or lymphatic
malignancy, and pregnancy (within 3 months following vaccination).
  *see **Childhood Immunizations** page* 478

TREATMENT

▷ *immune globulin* (Ig) 0.25 ml/kg IM (0.5 mg/kg in immunocompromised children)
*Antipyretics see **Fever** page 143*

 RUBEOLA (RED MEASLES)

PROPHYLAXIS

▷ *measles, mumps, rubella, live, attenuated, neomycin vaccine* (C)
  MMR II 25 mcg SC (preservative-free)
  Comment: Contraindications: hypersensitivity to *neomycin* or eggs, primary
  or acquired immune deficiency, immunosuppressant therapy, bone marrow or
  lymphatic malignancy, and pregnancy (within 3 months following vaccination).
  *see **Childhood Immunizations** page 478*

TREATMENT

▷ *immune globulin* (Ig) 0.25 ml/kg IM (0.5 mg/kg in immunocompromised
  children)
  *Antipyretics see **Fever** page 143*

SALMONELLOSIS

▷ *ciprofloxacin* (C) 500 mg bid x 3-5 days
  Pediatric: <18 years: not recommended
  Cipro (G) *Tab:* 250, 500, 750 mg; *Oral susp:* 250, 500 mg/5 ml (100 ml) (strawberry)
  Cipro XR *Tab:* 500, 1000 mg ext-rel
  ProQuin XR *Tab:* 500 mg ext-rel
Comment: *ciprofloxacin* is contraindicated <18 years-of-age, and during pregnancy
and lactation. Risk of tendonitis or tendon rupture, especially 60 years-of-age and
older.

> *trimethoprim/sulfamethoxazole* (D)(G)
  Pediatric: <2 months: not recommended; ≥2 months: 40 mg/kg/day of *sulfamethox-azole* in 2 divided doses bid x 10 days; *see page 587 for dose by weight*
    Bactrim, Septra 2 tabs bid x 10 days
      Tab: trim 80 mg/*sulfa* 400 mg*
    Bactrim DS, Septra DS 1 tab bid x 10 days
      Tab: trim 160 mg/*sulfa* 800 mg*
    Bactrim Pediatric Suspension, Septra Pediatric Suspension
      Oral susp: trim 40 mg/*sulfa* 200 mg per 5 ml (100 ml) (cherry) (alcohol 0.3%)
  Comment: *trimethoprim/sulfamethoxazole* is not recommended in pregnancy
  or lactation. *CrCl 15-30 mL/min:* reduce dose by 1/2; *CrCl <15 mL/min:* not recommended

SCABIES (*SARCOPTES SCABIEI*)

Comment: This section presents treatment regimens for scabies infestation published in the **2015 CDC Sexually Transmitted Diseases Treatment Guidelines**, as well as other available treatments.

RECOMMENDED REGIMEN

> *permethrin* (B)(G) massage into skin from head to soles of feet; leave on x 8-14 hours, then rinse off
  Pediatric: <2 months: not recommended; ≥2 months: same as adult
    Acticin, Elimite *Crm:* 5% (60 g)

ALTERNATIVE REGIMEN

> *lindane* (B)(G) 1 oz of lotion or 30 g of cream apply to all skin surfaces from neck down to the soles of the feet; leave on x 8 hours, then wash off thoroughly; may repeat if needed in 14 days
  Pediatric: <2 months: not recommended; ≥2 months: same as adult
    Kwell *Lotn:* 1% (60, 473 ml); *Crm:* 1% (60 g); *Shampoo:* 1% (60, 473 ml)

OTHER TOPICAL TREATMENTS

> *crotamiton* (C) massage into skin from chin down; repeat in 24 hours
  Pediatric: not recommended
    Eurax *Lotn:* 10% (60 g); *Crm:* 10% (60 g)

SCARLET FEVER (SCARLATINA)

Comment: Microorganism responsible for scarlet fever is Group A beta-hemolytic *Streptococcus* (GABHS). Strep cultures and screens will be positive.
> *azithromycin* (B) 500 mg x 1 dose on day 1, then 250 mg once daily on days 2-5 or 500 mg once daily x 3 days
  Pediatric: 12 mg/kg/day x 5 days; max 500 mg/day; *see page 559 for dose by weight*
    Zithromax *Tab:* 250, 500, 600 mg; *Oral susp:* 100 mg/5 ml (15 ml); 200 mg/5 ml (15, 22.5, 30 ml) (cherry); *Pkt:* 1 g for reconstitution (cherry-banana)
    Zithromax Tri-pak *Tab:* 3 x 500 mg tabs/pck

Zithromax Z-pak *Tab:* 6 x 250 mg tabs/pck
Zmax *Oral susp:* 2 g ext-rel for reconstitution (cherry-banana) (148 mg Na⁺)
▷ *cefadroxil* (B)
  Pediatric: 15-30 mg/kg/day in 2 divided doses x 10 days; *see page* 561 *for dose by weight*
    Duricef *Cap:* 500 mg; *Tab:* 1 g; *Oral susp:* 250 mg/5 ml (100 ml); 500 mg/5 ml (75, 100 ml) (orange-pineapple)
▷ *cephalexin* (B)(G)
  Pediatric: 25-50 mg/kg/day in 2 divided doses x 10 days; *see page* 568 *for dose by weight*
    Keflex *Cap:* 250, 333, 500, 750 mg; *Oral susp:* 125, 250 mg/5 ml (100, 200 ml) (strawberry)
▷ *clarithromycin* (C)(G) 250 mg bid *or* 500 mg ext-rel once daily x 10 days
    Pediatric: <6 months: not recommended; ≥6 months: 7.5 mg/kg bid x 10 days; *see page* 569 *for dose by weight*
    Biaxin *Tab:* 250, 500 mg
    Biaxin Oral Suspension *Oral susp:* 125, 250 mg/5 ml (50, 100 ml) (fruit punch)
    Biaxin XL *Tab:* 500 mg ext-rel
▷ *clindamycin* (B)(G) 150-300 mg q 6 hours x 10 days
    Pediatric: 8-16 mg/kg/day in 3-4 divided doses x 10 days
    Cleocin *Cap:* 75 (tartrazine), 150 (tartrazine), 300 mg
    Cleocin Pediatric Granules *Oral susp:* 75 mg/5 ml (100 ml) (cherry)
▷ *erythromycin estolate* (B)(G) 250 mg q 6 hours x 10 days
    Pediatric: 20-50 mg/kg q 6 hours x 10 days; *see page* 573 *for dose by weight*
    Ilosone *Pulvule:* 250 mg; *Tab:* 500 mg; *Liq:* 125, 250 mg/5 ml (100 ml)
    Comment: *erythromycin* may increase INR with concomitant *warfarin*, as well as increase serum level of *digoxin*, benzodiazepines and statins.
▷ *erythromycin ethylsuccinate* (B)(G) 400 mg qid *or* 800 mg bid x 10 days
    Pediatric: 30-50 mg/kg/day in 4 divided doses x 10 days; may double dose with severe infection; max 100 mg/kg/day; *see page* 574 *for dose by weight*
    EryPed *Oral susp:* 200 mg/5 ml (100, 200 ml) (fruit); 400 mg/5 ml (60, 100, 200 ml) (banana); *Oral drops:* 200, 400 mg/5 ml (50 ml) (fruit); *Chew tab:* 200 mg wafer (fruit)
    E.E.S. *Oral susp:* 200, 400 mg/5 ml (100 ml) (fruit)
    E.E.S. Granules *Oral susp:* 200 mg/5 ml (100, 200 ml) (cherry)
    E.E.S. 400 Tablets *Tab:* 400 mg
Comment: *erythromycin* may increase INR with concomitant *warfarin*, as well as increase serum level of *digoxin*, benzodiazepines and statins.
▷ *penicillin G (benzathine and procaine)* (B)(G) 2.4 million units IM x 1 dose
    Pediatric: <30 lb: 600,000 units IM x 1 dose; 30-60 lb: 900,000-1.2 million units IM x 1 dose
    Bicillin C-R Cartridge-needle unit: 600,000 units (1 ml); 1.2 million units; (2 ml); 2.4 million units (4 ml)
▷ *penicillin V potassium* (B) 250 mg tid x 10 days
    Pediatric: 25-50 mg/kg day in 4 divided doses x 10 days; ≥12 years: same as adult; *see page* 583 *for dose by weight*
    Pen-Vee K *Tab:* 250, 500 mg; *Oral soln:* 125 mg/5 ml (100, 200 ml); 250 mg/5 ml (100, 150, 200 ml)

SEIZURE DISORDER

Status Epilepticus *see Status Epilepticus page* 402
Anticonvulsant Drugs *see page* 520

SEXUAL ASSAULT (STD/STI/VD EXPOSURE)

Comment: The following treatment regimens for victims of sexual assault are
published in the **2015 CDC Sexually Transmitted Diseases Treatment Guidelines.**

RECOMMENDED PROPHYLAXIS REGIMEN

▷ *ceftriaxone* 250 mg IM in a single dose plus *metronidazole* 2 g in a single dose plus
azithromycin 1 g in a single dose

ALTERNATE PROPHYLAXIS REGIMENS

Regimen 1

▷ *ceftriaxone* 250 mg IM in a single dose plus *metronidazole* 2 g in a single dose plus
doxycycline 100 mg bid x 7 days

Regimen 2

▷ *cefixime* 400 mg in a single dose plus *metronidazole* 2 g in a single dose plus *azith-romycin* 1 g in a single dose

Regimen 3

▷ *cefixime* 400 mg in a single dose plus *metronidazole* 2 g in a single dose plus *doxycy-cline* 100 mg bid x 7 days

Regimen 4

▷ *azithromycin* (B) 1 g as a single dose plus *metronidazole* 2 g in a single dose

DRUG BRANDS AND DOSE FORMS

▷ *azithromycin* (B)
   Zithromax *Tab:* 250, 500, 600 mg; *Oral susp:* 100 mg/5 ml (15 ml); 200 mg/5 ml
   (15, 22.5, 30 ml) (cherry); *Pkt:* 1 g for reconstitution (cherry-banana)
   Zithromax Tri-pak *Tab:* 3 x 500 mg tabs/pck
   Zithromax Z-pak *Tab:* 6 x 250 mg tabs/pck
   Zmax *Oral susp:* 2 g ext-rel for reconstitution (cherry-banana) (148 mg Na⁺)
▷ *cefixime* (B)
   Suprax *Tab:* 400 mg; *Cap:* 400 mg; *Oral susp:* 100, 200 mg/5 ml (50, 75, 100 ml)
   (strawberry)
▷ *ceftriaxone* (B)(G)
   Rocephin *Vial:* 250, 500 mg; 1, 2 g
▷ *doxycycline* (D)(G)
   Actilate *Tab:* 75, 150**mg
   Adoxa *Tab:* 50, 75, 100, 150 mg ent-coat
   Doryx *Tab:* 50, 75, 100, 150, 200 mg del-rel
   Monodox *Cap:* 50, 75, 100 mg
   Oracea *Cap:* 40 mg del-rel

Vibramycin *Tab:* 100 mg; *Cap:* 50, 100 mg; *Syr:* 50 mg/5 ml (raspberry-apple) (sulfites); *Oral susp:* 25 mg/5 ml (raspberry)
Vibra-Tab *Tab:* 100 mg film-coat

Comment: *Doxycycline* is contraindicated <8 years-of-age, in pregnancy, and lactation (discolors developing tooth enamel). A side effect may be photosensitivity (photophobia). Do not give with antacids, calcium supplements, milk or other dairy, or within two hours of taking another drug.

▷ *metronidazole* **(not for use in 1st; B in 2nd, 3rd)(G)**
Flagyl *Tab:* 250*, 500*mg
Flagyl 375 *Cap:* 375 mg
Flagyl ER *Tab:* 750 mg ext-rel

Comment: Alcohol is contraindicated during treatment with oral *metronidazole* and for 72 hours after therapy due to a possible *disulfiram*-like reaction (nausea, vomiting, flushing, headache).

 SHIGELLOSIS

ANTI-INFECTIVES

▷ *azithromycin* **(B)** 500 mg x 1 dose on day 1, then 250 mg once daily on days 2-5 or 500 mg once daily x 3 days or **Zmax** 2 g in a single dose
Pediatric: <6 months: not recommended; >6 months: 10 mg/kg x 1 dose on day 1; then 5 mg/kg/day on days 2-5; max 500 mg/day; *see page 559 for dose by weight*
Zithromax *Tab:* 250, 500, 600 mg; *Oral susp:* 100 mg/5 ml (15 ml); 200 mg/5 ml (15, 22.5, 30 ml) (cherry); *Pkt:* 1 g for reconstitution (cherry-banana)
Zithromax Tri-pak *Tab:* 3 x 500 mg tabs/pck
Zithromax Z-pak *Tab:* 6 x 250 mg tabs/pck
Zmax *Oral susp:* 2 g ext-rel for reconstitution (cherry-banana) (148 mg Na$^+$)

▷ *ciprofloxacin* **(C)** 500 mg bid x 3 days
Pediatric: <18 years: not recommended
Cipro (G) *Tab:* 250, 500, 750 mg; *Oral susp:* 250, 500 mg/5 ml (100 ml) (strawberry)
Cipro XR *Tab:* 500, 1000 mg ext-rel
ProQuin XR *Tab:* 500 mg ext-rel

Comment: *ciprofloxacin* is contraindicated <18 years-of-age, and during pregnancy and lactation. Risk of tendonitis or tendon rupture, especially 60 years-of-age and older.

▷ *ofloxacin* **(C)(G)** 400 mg bid x 3 days
Pediatric: <18 years: not recommended
Floxin *Tab:* 200, 300, 400 mg

Comment: *ofloxacin* is contraindicated <18 years-of-age, and during pregnancy and lactation. Risk of tendonitis or tendon rupture, especially 60 years-of-age and older.

▷ *tetracycline* **(D)(G)** 250-500 mg qid x 5 days
Pediatric: <8 years: not recommended; ≥8 years, <100 lb: 25-50 mg/kg/day in 4 divided doses x 5 days; ≥8 years, >100 lb: same as adult; *see page 585 for dose by weight*
Achromycin V *Cap:* 250, 500 mg
Sumycin *Tab:* 250, 500 mg; *Cap:* 250, 500 mg; *Oral susp:* 125 mg/5 ml (100, 200 ml) (fruit) (sulfites)

Comment: *tetracycline* is contraindicated <8 years-of-age, in pregnancy, and lactation (discolors developing tooth enamel). A side effect may be photo-sensitivity (photophobia). Do not give with antacids, calcium supplements, milk or other dairy, or within two hours of taking another drug.

▷ *trimethoprim/sulfamethoxazole* (D)(G)
　　Bactrim, Septra 2 tabs bid x 10 days
　　　Tab: trim 80 mg/*sulfa* 400 mg*
　　Bactrim DS, Septra DS 1 tab bid x 10 days
　　　Tab: trim 160 mg/*sulfa* 800 mg*
　　Bactrim Pediatric Suspension, Septra Pediatric Suspension 20 ml bid x 10 days
　　　Oral susp: trim 40 mg/*sulfa* 200 mg per 5 ml (100 ml) (cherry) (alcohol 0.3%)
　　Comment: *trimethoprim/sulfamethoxazole* is not recommended in pregnancy or lactation. *CrCl 15-30 mL/min:* reduce dose by 1/2; *CrCl <15 mL/min:* not recommended

SINUSITIS/RHINOSINUSITIS: ACUTE BACTERIAL (ABRS)

ANTI-INFECTIVES

▷ *amoxicillin* (B)(G) 500-875 mg bid or 250-500 mg tid x 10 days
Pediatric: <40 kg (88 lb): 20-40 mg/kg/day in 3 divided doses x 10 days or 25-45 mg/kg/day in 2 divided doses x 10 days; *see page 554 for dose by weight*
　　Amoxil *Cap:* 250, 500 mg; *Tab:* 875*mg; *Chew tab:* 125, 200, 250, 400 mg (cherry-banana-peppermint) (phenylalanine); *Oral susp:* 125, 250 mg/5 ml (80, 100, 150 ml) (strawberry); 200, 400 mg/5 ml (50, 75, 100 ml) (bubble gum); *Oral drops:* 50 mg/ml (30 ml) (bubble gum)
　　Moxatag *Tab:* 775 mg ext-rel
　　Trimox *Tab:* 125, 250 mg; *Cap:* 250, 500 mg; *Oral susp:* 125, 250 mg/5 ml (80, 100, 150 ml) (raspberry-strawberry)
▷ *amoxicillin/clavulanate* (B)(G) 500 mg tid or 875 mg bid x 10 days
　　Augmentin *Tab:* 250, 500, 875 mg; *Chew tab:* 125, 250 mg (lemon-lime); 200, 400 mg (cherry-banana) (phenylalanine); *Oral susp:* 125 mg/5 ml (banana), 250 mg/5 ml (75, 100, 150 ml) (orange); 200, 400 mg/5 ml (50, 75, 100 ml) (orange) (phenylalanine)
　　　Pediatric: 40-45 mg/kg/day divided tid x 10 days or 90 mg/kg/day divided bid x 10 days *see pages 556-557 for dose by weight*
　　Augmentin ES-600 *Oral susp:* 600 mg/5 ml (50, 75, 100, 125, 150, 200 ml) (strawberry cream) (phenylalanine) every 12 hours
　　　Pediatric: <3 months: not recommended; ≥3 months, <40 kg: 90 mg/kg/day in 2 divided doses; ≥40 kg: not recommended
　　Augmentin XR 2 tabs q 12 hours x 7-10 days
　　　Pediatric: <16 years: use other forms; ≥16 years: same as adult
　　　Tab: 1000*mg ext-rel
▷ *cefaclor* (B)(G) 250-500 mg q 8 hours x 10 days; max 2 g/day
Pediatric: <1 month: not recommended; 20-40 mg/kg bid or q 12 hours x 10 days; max 1 g/day; *see page 560 for dose by weight*
Tab: 500 mg; *Cap:* 250, 500 mg; *Susp:* 125 mg/5 ml (75, 150 ml) (strawberry); 187 mg/5 ml (50, 100 ml) (strawberry); 250 mg/5 ml (75, 150 ml) (strawberry); 375 mg/5 ml (50, 100 ml) (strawberry)
Pediatric: <16 years: ext-rel not recommended; ≥16 years: same as adult
　　Cefaclor Extended Release *Tab:* 375, 500 mg ext-rel

➤ *cefdinir* (B) 300 mg bid or 600 mg once daily x 10 days
Pediatric: <6 months: not recommended; 6 months-12 years: 14 mg/kg/day in a single or 2 divided doses x 10 days; 12 years: same as adult; *see page 562 for dose by weight*
   Omnicef *Cap:* 300 mg; *Oral susp:* 125 mg/5 ml (60, 100 ml) (strawberry)
➤ *cefixime* (B) 400 mg once daily x 10 days
Pediatric: <6 months: not recommended; 6 months-12 years, <50 kg: 8 mg/kg/day in 1-2 divided doses x 10 days; >12 years, >50 kg: same as adult; *see page 563 for dose by weight*
   Suprax *Tab:* 400 mg; *Cap:* 400 mg; *Oral susp:* 100, 200 mg/5 ml (50, 75, 100 ml) (strawberry)
➤ *cefpodoxime proxetil* 200 mg bid x 10 days
Pediatric: <2 months: not recommended; 2 months-12 years: 10 mg/kg/day (max 400 mg/dose) or 5 mg/kg/day bid (max 200 mg/dose) x 10 days; *see page 564 for dose by weight*
   Vantin *Tab:* 100, 200 mg; *Oral susp:* 50, 100 mg/5 ml (50, 75, 100 mg) (lemon creme)
➤ *cefprozil* (B) 250-500 mg bid x 10 days
Pediatric: <6 months: not recommended; 6 months-12 years: *Mild:* 7.5 mg/kg bid x 10 days; *Moderate/Severe:* 15 mg/kg q 12 hours x 10 days; >12 years: same as adult; *see page 565 for dose by weight*
   Cefzil *Tab:* 250, 500 mg; *Oral susp:* 125, 250 mg/5 ml (50, 75, 100 ml) (bubble gum) (phenylalanine)
➤ *ceftibuten* (B) 400 mg once daily x 10 days
Pediatric: 9 mg/kg once daily x 10 days; max 400 mg/day; *see page 566 for dose by weight*
   Cedax *Cap:* 400 mg; *Oral susp:* 90 mg/5 ml (30, 60, 90, 120 ml); 180 mg/5 ml (30, 60, 120 ml) (cherry)
➤ *cefuroxime axetil* (B)(G) 250 mg bid x 10 days
Pediatric: <3 months: not recommended; 3 months-12 years: 20-30 mg/kg/day in 2 divided doses x 10 days; >12 years: same as adult; *see page 567 for dose by weight*
   Ceftin *Tab:* 250, 500 mg; *Oral susp:* 125, 250 mg/5 ml (50, 100 ml) (tutti-frutti)
➤ *ciprofloxacin* (C) 500 mg bid x 10 days
Pediatric: <18 years: not recommended
   Cipro (G) *Tab:* 250, 500, 750 mg; *Oral susp:* 250, 500 mg/5 ml (100 ml) (strawberry)
   Cipro XR *Tab:* 500, 1000 mg ext-rel
   ProQuin XR *Tab:* 500 mg ext-rel
   Comment: *ciprofloxacin* is contraindicated <18 years-of-age, and during pregnancy and lactation. Risk of tendonitis or tendon rupture, especially 60 years-of-age and older.
➤ *clarithromycin* (C)(G) 500 mg bid or 1000 mg ext-rel once daily x 10 days
Pediatric: <6 months: not recommended; ≥6 months: 7.5 mg/kg bid x 10 days; *see page 569 for dose by weight*
   Biaxin *Tab:* 250, 500 mg
   Biaxin Oral Suspension *Oral susp:* 125, 250 mg/5 ml (50, 100 ml) (fruit punch)
   Biaxin XL *Tab:* 500 mg ext-rel
➤ *levofloxacin* (C) *Uncomplicated:* 500 mg once daily x 10-14 days; *Complicated:* 750 mg once daily x 10-14 days
Pediatric: <18 years: not recommended

Levaquin *Tab:* 250, 500, 750 mg; *Oral soln:* 25 mg/ml (480 ml) (benzyl alcohol); *Inj conc:* 25 mg/ml for IV infusion after dilution (20, 30 ml single-use vial) (preservative-free); *Premix soln:* 5 mg/ml for IV infusion (50, 100, 150 ml) (preservative-free)

Comment: *levofloxacin* is contraindicated <18 years-of-age, and during pregnancy and lactation. Risk of tendonitis or tendon rupture, especially 60 years-of-age and older.

▷ *loracarbef* (B) 400 mg bid x 10 days
Pediatric: 15 mg/kg/day in 2 divided doses x 10 days; *see page 581 for dose by weight*

Lorabid *Pulvule:* 200, 400 mg; *Oral susp:* 100 mg/5 ml (50, 100 ml); 200 mg/5 ml (50, 75, 100 ml) (strawberry bubble gum)

▷ *moxifloxacin* (C)(G) 400 mg once daily x 10 days
Pediatric: <18 years: not recommended

Avelox *Tab:* 400 mg

Comment: *moxifloxacin* is contraindicated <18 years of age, and during pregnancy and lactation. Risk of tendonitis or tendon rupture, especially 60 years-of-age and older.

▷ *trimethoprim/sulfamethoxazole* (D)(G)
Pediatric: <2 months: not recommended; ≥2 months: 40 mg/kg/day of *sulfamethoxazole* in 2 divided doses bid x 10 days; *see page 587 for dose by weight*

Bactrim, Septra 2 tabs bid x 10 days
Tab: trim 80 mg/*sulfa* 400 mg*

Bactrim DS, Septra DS 1 tab bid x 10 days
Tab: trim 160 mg/*sulfa* 800 mg*

Bactrim Pediatric Suspension, Septra Pediatric Suspension
Oral susp: trim 40 mg/*sulfa* 200 mg per 5 ml (100 ml) (cherry) (alcohol 0.3%)

Comment: *trimethoprim/sulfamethoxazole* is not recommended in pregnancy or lactation. *CrCl 15-30 mL/min:* reduce dose by 1/2; *CrCl <15 mL/min:* not recommended

⬤ SJOGRENS, SYNDROME (CHRONIC DRY MOUTH)

CHOLINERGIC/MUSCARINIC AGONIST COMBINATION

▷ *cevimeline* (C)(G) 30 mg tid
Evoxac *Cap:* 30 mg

Comment: *cevimeline* is contraindicated in acute iritis, narrow angle glaucoma, and uncontrolled asthma.

▷ *pilocarpine* (C)(G) 5 mg qid or 7.5 mg tid
Salagen *Tab:* 5, 7.5 mg

ORAL ENZYME RINSE

▷ *xylitol/solazyme/selectobac* (NE) swish 5 ml for 30 seconds bid-tid
Orazyme Dry Mouth Rinse *Oral soln:* 1.5, 16 oz

SKIN: CALLOUSED

KERATOLYTICS

▷ *salicylic acid* (C)(OTC) apply lotion, cream or gel to affected area once daily-bid;
apply patch to affected area and leave on x 48 hours with max 5 applications/14 days
Pediatric: <12 years: not recommended; ≥12 years: same as adult
▷ *urea* (C)
Pediatric: <12 years: not recommended; ≥12 years: same as adult
Carmol 40 apply to affected area with applicator stick provided once daily-tid;
smooth over until cream is absorbed; protect surrounding tissue; may cover
with adhesive bandage or gauze secured with adhesive tape
Crm/Gel: 40% (30 g)
Keratol 40 apply to affected area with applicator stick provided once daily-tid;
smooth over until cream is absorbed; protect surrounding tissue; may cover
with adhesive bandage or gauze secured with adhesive tape
Crm: 40% (1, 3, 7 oz); *Gel:* 40% (15 ml); *Lotn:* 40% (8 oz)
Comment: The moisturizing effect of **Carmol 40** and **Keratol 40** is enhanced by
applying while the skin is still moist (after washing or bathing).

SKIN INFECTION: BACTERIAL (CARBUNCLE, FOLLICULITIS, FURUNCLE)

Comment: Abscesses usually require surgical incision and drainage.

ANTIBACTERIAL SKIN CLEANSERS

Dial soap (OTC) bid
Lever 2000 Antibacterial soap (OTC) bid
▷ *hexachlorophene* (C)
pHisoHex dispense 5 ml into wet hand, work up into lather; then apply to area
to be cleansed; rinse thoroughly
Liq clnsr: 5, 16 oz

TOPICAL ANTI-INFECTIVES

▷ *mupirocin* (B)(G) apply to lesions bid
Pediatric: same as adult
Bactroban *Oint:* 2% (22 g); *Crm:* 2% (15, 30 g)
Centany *Oint:* 2% (15, 30 g)
▷ *polymyxin B/neomycin* (C) oint apply once daily-tid
Neosporin (OTC) *Oint:* 15 g

ORAL ANTI-INFECTIVES

▷ *amoxicillin* (B)(G) 500-875 mg bid or 250-500 mg tid x 10 days
Pediatric: <40 kg (88 lb): 20-40 mg/kg/day in 3 divided doses x 10 days or
25-45 mg/kg/day in 2 divided doses x 10 days; *see page 554 for dose by weight*

Amoxil *Cap:* 250, 500 mg; *Tab:* 875*mg; *Chew tab:* 125, 200, 250, 400 mg (cherry-banana-peppermint) (phenylalanine); *Oral susp:* 125, 250 mg/5 ml (80, 100, 150 ml) (strawberry); 200, 400 mg/5 ml (50, 75, 100 ml) (bubble gum); *Oral drops:* 50 mg/ml (30 ml) (bubble gum)

Moxatag *Tab:* 775 mg ext-rel

Trimox *Tab:* 125, 250 mg; *Cap:* 250, 500 mg; *Oral susp:* 125, 250 mg/5 ml (80, 100, 150 ml) (raspberry-strawberry)

➤ *azithromycin* **(B)** 500 mg x 1 dose on day 1, then 250 mg once daily on days 2-5 or 500 mg once daily x 3 days or **Zmax** 2 g in a single dose

Pediatric: 12 mg/kg/day x 5 days; max 500 mg/day; *see page 559 for dose by weight*

Zithromax *Tab:* 250, 500, 600 mg; *Oral susp:* 100 mg/5 ml (15 ml); 200 mg/5 ml (15, 22.5, 30 ml) (cherry); *Pkt:* 1 g for reconstitution (cherry-banana)

Zithromax Tri-pak *Tab:* 3 x 500 mg tabs/pck

Zithromax Z-pak *Tab:* 6 x 250 mg tabs/pck

Zmax *Oral susp:* 2 g ext-rel for reconstitution (cherry-banana) (148 mg Na⁺)

➤ *cefaclor* **(B)(G)** 250-500 mg q 8 hours x 10 days; max 2 g/day

Pediatric: <1 month: not recommended; 20-40 mg/kg bid or q 12 hours x 10 days; max 1 g/day; *see page 560 for dose by weight*

Tab: 500 mg; *Cap:* 250, 500 mg; *Susp:* 125 mg/5 ml (75, 150 ml) (strawberry); 187 mg/5 ml (50, 100 ml) (strawberry); 250 mg/5 ml (75, 150 ml) (strawberry); 375 mg/5 ml (50, 100 ml) (strawberry)

Cefaclor Extended Release

Pediatric: <16 years: ext-rel not recommended

Tab: 375, 500 mg ext-rel

➤ *cefadroxil* **(B)** 1-2 g in a single or 2 divided doses x 10 days

Pediatric: 15-30 mg/kg/day in 2 divided doses x 10 days; *see page 561 for dose by weight*

Duricef *Cap:* 500 mg; *Tab:* 1 g; *Oral susp:* 250 mg/5 ml (100 ml); 500 mg/5 ml (75, 100 ml) (orange-pineapple)

➤ *cefdinir* **(B)** 300 mg bid x 10 days

Pediatric: <6 months: not recommended; 6 months-12 years: 14 mg/kg/day in 1-2 divided doses x 10 days; *see page 562 for dose by weight*

Omnicef *Cap:* 300 mg; *Oral susp:* 125 mg/5 ml (60, 100 ml) (strawberry)

➤ *cefditoren pivoxil* **(B)** 200 mg bid x 10 days

Pediatric: not recommended

Spectracef *Tab:* 200 mg

Comment: Contraindicated with milk protein allergy or carnitine deficiency.

➤ *cefpodoxime* **(B)** *proxetil* 400 mg bid x 7-14 days

Pediatric: <2 months: not recommended; 2 months-12 years: 10 mg/kg/day (max 400 mg/dose) or 5 mg/kg/day bid (max 200 mg/dose) x 7-14 days; *see page 564 for dose by weight*

Vantin *Tab:* 100, 200 mg; *Oral susp:* 50, 100 mg/5 ml (50, 75, 100 ml) (lemon creme)

➤ *cefprozil* **(B)** 250-500 mg bid or 500 mg once daily x 10 days

Pediatric: 2-12 years: 7.5 mg/kg bid x 10 days; >12 years: same as adult; *see page 565 for dose by weight*

Cefzil *Tab:* 250, 500 mg; *Oral susp:* 125, 250 mg/5 ml (50, 75, 100 ml) (bubble gum) (phenylalanine)

➤ *ceftriaxone* **(B)(G)** 1-2 g IM once daily; max 4 g/day

Rocephin

Pediatric: 50-75 mg/kg IM in 1-2 divided doses; max 2 g/day
Vial: 250, 500 mg; 1, 2 g

▷ *cefuroxime axetil* (B)(G) 250-500 mg bid x 10 days
Pediatric: <3 months: not recommended; 3 months-12 years: 20-30 mg/kg/day
in 2 divided doses x 10 days; >12 years: same as adult; *see page 567 for dose by
weight*
   Ceftin *Tab:* 250, 500 mg; *Oral susp:* 125, 250 mg/5 ml (50, 100 ml) (tutti-frutti)

▷ *cephalexin* (B)(G) 500 mg bid x 10 days
Pediatric: 25-50 mg/kg/day in 4 divided doses x 10 days; *see page 568 for dose by
weight*
   Keflex *Cap:* 250, 333, 500, 750 mg; *Oral susp:* 125, 250 mg/5 ml (100, 200 ml)
   (strawberry)

▷ *clarithromycin* (C)(G) 250-500 mg bid <u>or</u> 500-1000 mg ext-rel once daily x 7-14 days
Pediatric: <6 months: not recommended; >6 months: 7.5 mg/kg bid x 7-14 days; *see
page 569 for dose by weight*
   Biaxin *Tab:* 250, 500 mg
   Biaxin Oral Suspension *Oral susp:* 125, 250 mg/5 ml (50, 100 ml) (fruit punch)
   Biaxin XL *Tab:* 500 mg ext-rel

▷ *dicloxacillin* (B) 500 mg qid x 10 days
Pediatric: 12.5-25 mg/kg/day in 4 divided doses x 10 days; *see page 571 for dose by
weight*
   Dynapen *Cap:* 125, 250, 500 mg; *Oral susp:* 62.5 mg/5 ml (80, 100, 200 ml)

▷ *dirithromycin* (C)(G) 500 mg once daily x 5-7 days
Pediatric: <12 years: not recommended; ≥12 years: same as adult
   Dynabac *Tab:* 250 mg

▷ *doxycycline* (D)(G) 100mg bid x 9 days
Pediatric: <8 years: not recommended; ≥8 years, <100 lb: 1 mg/lb in a single dose
once daily x 9 days x 9 days; ≥8 years, >100 lb: same as adult; *see page 572 for dose
by weight*
   Actilate *Tab:* 75, 150**mg
   Adoxa *Tab:* 50, 75, 100, 150 mg ent-coat
   Doryx *Tab:* 50, 75, 100, 150, 200 mg del-rel
   Monodox *Cap:* 50, 75, 100 mg
   Oracea *Cap:* 40 mg del-rel
   Vibramycin *Tab:* 100 mg; *Cap:* 50, 100 mg; *Syr:* 50 mg/5 ml (raspberry-apple)
   (sulfites); *Oral susp:* 25 mg/5 ml (raspberry)
   Vibra-Tab *Tab:* 100 mg film-coat

Comment: **Doxycycline** is contraindicated <8 years-of-age, in pregnancy, and
lactation (discolors developing tooth enamel). A side effect may be photo-
sensitivity (photophobia). Do not give with antacids, calcium supplements, milk or
other dairy, or within two hours of taking another drug.

▷ *erythromycin base* (B)(G) 250-500 mg tid x 10 days
Pediatric: 30-50 mg/kg/day in 2-4 divided doses x 10 days
   Ery-Tab *Tab:* 250, 333, 500 mg ent-coat
   PCE *Tab:* 333, 500 mg

Comment: **erythromycin** may increase INR with concomitant **warfarin**, as well as
increase serum level of **digoxin**, benzodiazepines and statins.

▷ *erythromycin estolate* (B)(G) 250-500 mg q 6 hours x 10 days
Pediatric: 20-50 mg/kg q 6 hours x 10 days; *see page 573 for dose by weight*
   Ilosone *Pulvule:* 250 mg; *Tab:* 500 mg; *Liq:* 125, 250 mg/5 ml (100 ml)

Comment: *erythromycin* may increase INR with concomitant *warfarin*, as well as increase serum level of *digoxin*, benzodiazepines and statins.

▷ *erythromycin ethylsuccinate* (B)(G) 400 mg qid x 10 days
Pediatric: 30-50 mg/kg/day in 4 divided doses x 10 days; may double dose with severe infection; max 100 mg/kg/day; *see page 574 for dose by weight*

> **EryPed** *Oral susp:* 200 mg/5 ml (100, 200 ml) (fruit); 400 mg/5 ml (60, 100, 200 ml) (banana); *Oral drops:* 200, 400 mg/5 ml (50 ml) (fruit); *Chew tab:* 200 mg wafer (fruit)
> **E.E.S.** *Oral susp:* 200, 400 mg/5 ml (100 ml) (fruit)
> **E.E.S. Granules** *Oral susp:* 200 mg/5 ml (100, 200 ml) (cherry)
> **E.E.S. 400 Tablets** *Tab:* 400 mg

Comment: *erythromycin* may increase INR with concomitant *warfarin*, as well as increase serum level of *digoxin*, benzodiazepines and statins.

▷ *gemifloxacin* (C)(G) 320 mg once daily x 5-7 days
Pediatric: <18 years: not recommended

> **Factive** *Tab:* 320*mg

Comment: *gemifloxacin* is contraindicated <18 years-of-age, and during pregnancy and lactation. Risk of tendonitis or tendon rupture, especially 60 years-of-age and older.

▷ *levofloxacin* (C) *Uncomplicated:* 500 mg once daily x 7-10 days; *Complicated:* 750 mg once daily x 7-10 days
Pediatric: <18 years: not recommended

> **Levaquin** *Tab:* 250, 500, 750 mg; *Oral soln:* 25 mg/ml (480 ml) (benzyl alcohol); *Inj conc:* 25 mg/ml for IV infusion after dilution (20, 30 ml single-use vial) (preservative-free); *Premix soln:* 5 mg/ml for IV infusion (50, 100, 150 ml) (preservative-free)

Comment: *levofloxacin* is contraindicated <18 years-of-age, and during pregnancy and lactation. Risk of tendonitis or tendon rupture, especially 60 years-of-age and older.

▷ *linezolid* (C)(G) 400-600 mg q 12 hours x 10-14 days
Pediatric: <5 years: 10 mg/kg q 8 hours x 10-14 days; 5-11 years: 10 mg/kg q 12 hours x 10-14 days; >11 years: same as adult

> **Zyvox** *Tab:* 400, 600 mg; *Oral susp:* 100 mg/5 ml (150 ml) (orange) (phenylalanine)

Comment: *linezolid* is indicated to treat susceptible vancomycin-resistant *E. faecium* infections.

▷ *loracarbef* (B) 200 mg bid x 7 days
Pediatric: 15 mg/kg/day in 2 divided doses x 7 days; *see page 581 for dose by weight*

> **Lorabid** *Pulvule:* 200, 400 mg; *Oral susp:* 100 mg/5 ml (50, 100 ml); 200 mg/5 ml (50, 75, 100 ml) (strawberry bubble gum)

▷ *minocycline* (D)(G) 200 mg on first day; then 100 mg q 12 hours x 9 more days
Pediatric: <8 years: not recommended; ≥8 years, <100 lb: 2 mg/lb on first day in 2 divided doses, followed by 1 mg/lb q 12 hours x 9 more days; ≥8 years, >100 lb: same as adult

> **Dynacin** *Cap:* 50, 100 mg
> **Minocin** *Cap:* 50, 75, 100 mg; *Oral susp:* 50 mg/5 ml (60 ml) (custard) (sulfites, alcohol 5%)

Comment: *minocycline* is contraindicated <8 years-of-age, in pregnancy, and lactation (discolors developing tooth enamel). A side effect may be photosensitivity (photophobia). Do not give with antacids, calcium supplements, milk or other dairy, or within two hours of taking another drug.

▷ *moxifloxacin* (C)(G) 400 mg once daily x 10 days
  Pediatric: <18 years: not recommended
    Avelox *Tab:* 400 mg
  Comment: *moxifloxacin* is contraindicated <18 years-of-age, and during pregnancy and lactation. Risk of tendonitis or tendon rupture, especially 60 years-of-age and older.
▷ *ofloxacin* (C)(G) 400 mg bid x 10 days
  Pediatric: <18 years: not recommended
    Floxin *Tab:* 200, 300, 400 mg
  Comment: *ofloxacin* is contraindicated <18 years-of-age, and during pregnancy and lactation. Risk of tendonitis or tendon rupture, especially 60 years-of-age and older.
▷ *tetracycline* (D)(G) 500 mg qid x 10 days
  Pediatric: <8 years: not recommended; ≥8 years, <100 lb: 25-50 mg/kg/day in 4 divided doses x 10 days; ≥8 years, >100 lb: same as adult; *see page 585 for dose by weight*
    Achromycin V *Cap:* 250, 500 mg
    Sumycin *Tab:* 250, 500 mg; *Cap:* 250, 500 mg; *Oral susp:* 125 mg/5 ml (100, 200 ml) (fruit) (sulfites)
  Comment: *tetracycline* is contraindicated <8 years-of-age, in pregnancy, and lactation (discolors developing tooth enamel). A side effect may be photo-sensitivity (photophobia). Do not give with antacids, calcium supplements, milk or other dairy, or within two hours of taking another drug.

SLEEP APNEA (HYPOPNEA SYNDROME)

ANTI-NARCOLEPTIC AGENTS

▷ *armodafinil* (C)(IV)(G) *OSAHS:* 150-250 mg once daily in the AM; *SWSD:* 150 mg 1 hour before starting shift; reduce dose with severe hepatic impairment
  Pediatric: <17 years: not recommended
    Nuvigil *Tab:* 50, 150, 200, 250 mg
▷ *modafinil* (C)(IV) 100-200 mg q AM; max 400 mg/day
  Pediatric: <16 years: not recommended; ≥16 years: same as adult
    Provigil *Tab:* 100, 200*mg
  Comment: *modafinil* promotes wakefulness in patients with excessive sleepiness due to obstructive sleep apnea/hypopnea syndrome.

SLEEPINESS: EXCESSIVE/SHIFT WORK SLEEP DISORDER (SWSD)

ANTI-NARCOLEPTIC AGENT

▷ *armodafinil* (C)(IV)(G) *OSAHS:* 150-250 mg once daily in the AM; *SWSD:* 150 mg 1 hour before starting shift; reduce dose with severe hepatic impairment
  Pediatric: <17 years: not recommended
    Nuvigil *Tab:* 50, 150, 200, 250 mg

▷ *modafinil* (C)(IV) 100-200 mg q AM; max 400 mg/day
Pediatric: <16 years: not recommended; ≥16 years: same as adult
Provigil *Tab:* 100, 200*mg
Comment: **Provigil** promotes wakefulness in patients with narcolepsy, shift work sleep disorder, and excessive sleepiness due to obstructive sleep apnea/hypopnea syndrome.

SMALLPOX (VARIOLA MAJOR)

PROPHYLAXIS

▷ *vaccina virus* vaccine *(dried, calf lymph type)* (C)
Pediatric: <12 months: not recommended; 12 months-18 years, non-emergency: not recommended
DRYvax
Kit: vial dried smallpox vaccine (1), 0.25 ml diluent in syringe (1), vented needle (1), 100 individually wrapped bifurcated needles (5 needles/strip, 20 strips) (polymyxin B sulfate, dihydrostreptomycin sulfate, chlortetracycline HCL, neomycin sulfate, glycerin, phenol)
Comment: **DRYvax** is a dried live vaccine with approximately 100 million *Infectious vaccina* viruses (pock-forming units [pfu] per ml). Contact with immunosuppressed individuals should be avoided until the scab has separated from the skin (2 to 3 weeks) and/or a protective occlusive dressing covers the inoculation site. Scarification only. Do not inject IV, IM, or SC. Revaccination is recommended every 10 years.

SPRAIN

Comment: RICE: Rest; Ice; Compression; Elevation.
Injectable Acetaminophen *see Pain page* 306
Oral Prescription NSAIDs *see Pain page* 501
Other Oral Analgesics *see Pain page* 308
Topical/Transdermal NSAIDs *see Pain page* 307
Parenteral Corticosteroids *see page* 511
Oral Corticosteroids *see page* 509
Topical Analgesic and Anesthetic Agents *see page* 499

STATUS ASTHMATICUS

Inhaled Beta-Agonists (Bronchodilators) *see Asthma page* 32
Oral Beta-Agonists (Bronchodilators) *see Asthma page* 35
Inhaled Anticholinergics *see Asthma page* 29
Inhaled Anticholinergic/Beta-Agonist Combination *see Asthma page* 33
Methylxanthines *see Asthma page* 36
Parenteral Corticosteroids *see page* 511
Oral Corticosteroids *see page* 509

EPINEPHRINE

▷ *epinephrine* (C)(G) 0.3-0.5 mg (0.3-0.5 ml of a 1:1000 soln) SC q 20-30 minutes as needed up to 3 doses
Pediatric: <2 years: 0.05-0.1 ml; 2-6 years: 0.1 ml; 6-12 years: 0.2 ml; All: q 20-30 minutes as needed up to 3 doses; >12 years: same as adult

ANAPHYLAXIS EMERGENCY TREATMENT KITS

▷ *epinephrine* (C) 0.3 ml IM <u>or</u> SC in thigh; may repeat if needed
Pediatric: 0.01 mg/kg SC <u>or</u> IM in thigh; may repeat if needed; <15 kg: not recommended; 15-30 kg: 0.15 mg; >30 kg: same as adult
    AdrenaClick *Auto-injector:* 0.15, 0.3 mg (1 mg/ml; 2/carton) (sulfites)
    Auvi-Q *Auto-injector:* 0.15, 0.3 mg (1 mg/ml; 2/carton w. 1 nonactive training device) (sulfites)
    EpiPen *Autoinjector 0.3 mg* (*epi* 1:1000, 0.3 ml (2/carton) (sulfites)
    EpiPen Jr *Autoinjector 0.15 mg* (*epi* 1:2000, 0.3 ml (2/carton) (sulfites)
    Twinject *Autoinjector: 0.15, 0.3 mg* (epi 1:1000, 2/carton) (sulfites)
▷ *epinephrine/chlorpheniramine* (C) epinephrine 0.3 ml SC <u>or</u> IM <u>plus</u> 4 tabs *chlorpheniramine* by mouth
Pediatric: infants-2 years: 0.05-0.1 ml SC <u>or</u> IM; 2-6 years: 0.15 ml SC <u>or</u> IM <u>plus</u> 1 tab *chlor;* 6-12 years: 0.2 ml SC <u>or</u> IM <u>plus</u> 2 tabs *chlor;* >12 years: same as adult
    Ana-Kit: 0.3 ml syringes of *epi* 1:1000 (2/carton) for self-injection <u>plus</u> *chlor* 2 mg chewable tabs x 4

⬤ STATUS EPILEPTICUS

Anticonvulsant Drugs *see page* 520
▷ *diazepam* injectable (D)(IV) initially 5-10 mg IV in large vein; may repeat q 10-15 minutes; max 30 mg; may repeat in 2-4 hours if needed; do not dilute; may give IM if IV not accessible
Pediatric: 1 month-5 years: 0.2-0.5 mg IV q 2-5 minutes; max 5 mg; >5 years: 1 mg IV q 2-5 minutes; max 10 mg; may repeat in 2-4 hours if needed
    Diastat *Rectal gel delivery system:* 2.5 mg
    Diastat AcuDial *Rectal gel delivery system:* 10, 20 mg
    Valium Injectable *Vial:* 5 mg/ml (10 ml); *Amp:* 5 mg/ml (2 ml); *Prefilled syringe:* 5 mg/ml (5 ml)
    Valium Intensol Oral Solution *Conc oral soln:* 5 mg/ml (30 ml w. dropper) (alcohol 19%)
    Valium Oral Solution *Oral soln:* 5 mg/5 ml (500 ml) (wintergreen-spice)
▷ *lorazepam* injectable (D)(IV) 4 mg IV over 2 minutes (dilute first); may repeat in 10-15 minutes; may give IM if needed (undiluted)
Pediatric: <18 years: not recommended
    Ativan Injectable *Vial:* 2 mg/ml (1, 10 ml); *Tubex:* 2 mg/ml (0.5 ml); *Cartridge:* 2, 4 mg/ml (1 ml)
▷ *phenytoin (injectable)* (D)(G) 10-15 mg/kg IV, not to exceed 50 mg/minute; follow with 100 mg orally <u>or</u> IV q 6-8 hours; do not dilute in IV fluid
Pediatric: 15-20 mg/kg IV, not to exceed 1-2 mg/kg/minute
    Dilantin *Vial:* 50 mg/ml (2, 5 ml); *Amp:* 50 mg/ml (2 ml)
Comment: Monitor *phenytoin* serum levels. Therapeutic serum level: 10-20 g/ml. Side effects include gingival hyperplasia.

◯ STYE (HORDEOLUM)

OPHTHALMIC ANTI-INFECTIVES

➤ *erythromycin* ophthalmic ointment (B) 1 cm up to 6 times/day
  Pediatric: same as adult
  Ilotycin Ophthalmic Ointment *Ophth oint:* 5 mg/g (1/8 oz)
➤ *erythromycin* ophthalmic solution (B) initially 1-2 drops q 1-2 hours; may then in-
  crease dose interval
  Pediatric: same as adult
  Isopto Cetamide Ophthalmic Solution *Ophth soln:* 15% (15 ml)
➤ *gentamicin* ophthalmic ointment (C) 1 cm bid-tid
  Pediatric: same as adult
  Garamycin Ophthalmic Ointment *Ophth oint:* 3 mg/g (3.5 g)
  Genoptic Ophthalmic Ointment *Ophth oint:* 3 mg/g (3.5 g)
  Gentacidin Ophthalmic Ointment *Ophth oint:* 3 mg/g (3.5 g)
➤ *polymyxin B/bacitracin* ophthalmic ointment (C) apply 1/2 inch q 3-4 hours
  Pediatric: same as adult
  Polysporin *Ophth oint:* *poly* 10,000 U/*bac* 500 units per g (3.75 g)
➤ *polymyxin B/bacitracin/neomycin* ophthalmic ointment (C)(G) apply 1/2 inch q 3-4
  hours
  Pediatric: same as adult
  Neosporin Ophthalmic Ointment *Ophth oint:* *poly* B 10,000 U/*bac* 400 U/
  neo 3.5 mg/g (3.75 g)
➤ *polymyxin B/neomycin/gramicidin* ophthalmic solution (C) 1-2 drops 2-3 times q
  1 hour; then 1-2 drops bid-qid x 7-10 days
  Pediatric: same as adult
  Neosporin Ophthalmic Solution
  Ophth soln: *poly* 10,000 U/*neo* 1.75 mg/gram 0.025 mg/ml (10 ml)
➤ *sodium sulfacetamide* ophthalmic solution and ointment (C)
  Bleph-10 Ophthalmic Solution 2 drops q 4 hour x 7-14 days
    Pediatric: <2 years: not recommended; ≥2 years: 1-2 drops q 2-3 hours
    during the day
    Ophth soln: 10% (2.5, 5, 15 ml; benzalkonium chloride)
  Bleph-10 Ophthalmic Ointment apply 1/2 inch qid and HS
    Pediatric: <2 years: not recommended; ≥2 years: apply 1/4-1/3 inch qid and HS
    Ophth oint: 10% (3.5 g) (phenylmercuric acetate)

◯ SUNBURN

➤ *prednisone* (C)(G) 10 mg qid x 4-6 days if severe and extensive
➤ *silver sulfadiazine* (C)(G) apply topically to burn once daily-bid
  Pediatric: not recommended
  Silvadene *Crm:* 1% (20, 50, 85, 400, 1000 g jar; 20 g tube)

◯ SYPHILIS (*TREPONEMA PALLIDUM*)

Comment: The following treatment regimens for *T. pallidum* are published in the 2015
CDC Sexually Transmitted Diseases Treatment Guidelines. Treat all sexual contacts.

Consider testing for other STDs. *Penicillin G*, administered parenterally, is the preferred drug for treating all stages of syphilis. The preparation used (i.e., benzathine, aqueous procaine, or aqueous crystalline), the dosage, and the length of treatment depend on the stage and clinical manifestations of the disease. Combinations of *benzathine penicillin, procaine penicillin,* and oral penicillin preparations are not appropriate (e.g., **Bicillin C-R**). All women should be screened serologically for syphilis early in pregnancy. There are no proven alternatives to penicillin for the treatment of syphilis during pregnancy. Pregnant patients who are allergic to penicillin should be desensitized and treated with *penicillin*. Sexual transmission of *T. pallidum* is thought to occur only when mucotaneous syphilis at any stage should be evaluated clinically and serologically and treated with a recommended regimen according to CDC guidelines.

PRIMARY, SECONDARY, AND EARLY LATENT (<1 YEAR) SYPHILIS

Regimen 1

▷ *penicillin G (benzathine)* 2.4 million units IM in a single dose

LATE LATENT, LATENT SYPHILIS OF UNKNOWN DURATION, AND TERTIARY SYPHILIS

Regimen 1

▷ *penicillin G (benzathine)* 7.2 million units total administered in 3 divided doses of 2.4 million units each IM at 1 week intervals

REGIMEN: ADULT, NEUROSYPHILIS

Regimen 1

▷ *aqueous crystalline penicillin G* 18-24 million units per day, administered as 3-4 million units IV every 4 hours or continuous IV infusion, for 10-14 days

ALTERNATIVE REGIMEN: ADULT, NEUROSYPHILIS

Regimen 1

▷ *penicillin G (procaine)* 2.4 million units IM once daily x 10-14 days plus *probenecid* 500 mg qid x 10-14 days

PRIMARY AND SECONDARY SYPHILIS IN HIV-INFECTED PERSONS

Regimen 1

▷ *penicillin G (benzathine)* 2.4 million units IM in a single dose

LATENT SYPHILIS AMONG HIV-INFECTED PERSONS

Comment: Treatment is the same as for HIV-negative persons.

CONGENITAL SYPHILIS

Regimen 1

▷ *aqueous crystalline penicillin G* 100,000-150,000 units/kg/day, administered as 50,000 units IV every 12 hours during the first 7 days of life and every 8 hours thereafter for a total of 10 days

ALTERNATE REGIMEN

Regimen 1

▷ *penicillin G (benzathine)* 50,000 units/kg IM in a single dose

Regimen 2

▷ *penicillin G (procaine)* 50,000 units/kg/dose IM, administered in a single daily dose x 10 days

OLDER INFANTS AND CHILDREN

Regimen 1

▷ *aqueous crystalline penicillin G* 200,000-300,000 units/kg/day, administered as 50,000 units IV every 12 hours during the first 7 days of life and every 4-6 hours thereafter for a total of 10 days

DRUG BRANDS AND DOSE FORMS

▷ *aqueous crystalline penicillin G* (B)(G)
▷ *penicillin G (benzathine)* (B)(G)
   Bicillin L-A *Cartridge-needle unit:* 600,000 million units (1 ml); 1.2 million units (2 ml); 2.4 million units (4 ml)
▷ *penicillin G (procaine)* (B)(G)
   Bicillin C-R Cartridge-needle unit: 600,000 units (1 ml); 1.2 mill- ion units; (2 ml); 2.4 million units (4 ml)
▷ *probenecid* (B)(G)
   Benemid *Tab:* 500*mg; *Cap:* 500 mg

⬤ TAPEWORM (CESTODE)

▷ *albendazole* (C)(G) <2 years: 200 mg once daily x 3 days; may repeat in 3 weeks; ≥2-12 years: 400 mg once daily x 3 days; may repeat in 3 weeks; ≥12 years: 400 mg bid x 7 days; take after a meal
   Albenza *Tab:* 200 mg
   Comment: *albendazole* is a broad-spectrum benzimidazole carbamate anthelmintic.
▷ *praziquantel* (B) <4 years: not established; ≥4 years: 5-10 mg/kg as a single dose
   Biltricide *Tab:* 600 mg film-coat (scored for half or quarter dose)
   Comment: Therapeutically effective levels of **Biltricide** may not be achieved when administered concomitantly with strong P450 inducers, such as *rifampin.* Females should not breastfeed on the day of **Biltricide** treatment and during the subsequent 72 hours. Use caution with hepatosplenic patients who have moderate to severe liver impairment (Child-Pugh class B and C).
▷ *nitazoxanide* (B) <12 months: not recommended; ≥12 months: treat q 12 hours x 3 days; <11 years: [suspension]12-47 months: 5 ml; 4-11 years: 10 ml; ≥11 years: [tab/suspension] 500 mg
   Alinia *Tab:* 500 mg; *Oral susp:* 100 mg/5 ml (60 ml)

TEMPORAL ARTERITIS

Parenteral Corticosteroids *see page* 511
Oral Corticosteroids *see page* 509

 TEMPOROMANDIBULAR JOINT (TMJ) DISORDER

Injectable Acetaminophen *see* **Pain** *page* 306
Oral Prescription NSAIDs *see page* 501
Other Oral Analgesics see **Pain** *page* 308
Topical/Transdermal NSAIDs *see* **Pain** *page* 307
Parenteral Corticosteroids *see page* 511
Oral Corticosteroids *see page* 509
Topical Analgesic and Anesthetic Agents *see page* 499

 TESTOSTERONE DEFICIENCY, HYPOTESTOSTERONEMIA, HYPOGONADISM

Comment: *testosterone* is contraindicated in male breast cancer and prostate cancer. *testosterone* replacement therapy is indicated in males with primary hypogonadism (congenital or acquired due to cryptorchidism, bilateral torsion, orchitis, vanishing testis syndrome, or orchidectomy), or hypogonadotropic hypogonadism (congenital or acquired), and delayed puberty not secondary to a pathological disorder (x-ray of the hand and wrist to determine bone age should be obtained every 6 months to assess the effect of treatment on the epiphyseal centers).

ORAL ANDROGENS

▷ *fluoxymesterone* (X)(III) *Hypogonadism:* 5-20 mg once daily; *Delayed puberty:* use low dose and limit duration to 4-6 months
Pediatric: use by specialist only
Halotestin *Tab:* 2*, 5*, 10*mg (tartrazine)

▷ *methyltestosterone* (X)(III) usually 10-50 mg once daily; for delayed puberty, use low dose and limit duration to 4-6 months
Android *Cap:* 10 mg
Methitest *Tab:* 10*mg
Testred *Cap:* 10 mg

▷ *testosterone* (X)(III) 30 mg q 12 hours to gum region, just above the incisor tooth on either side of the mouth; hold system in place for 30 seconds; rotate sites with each application
Striant *Buccal tab:* 30 mg (6 blister pks; 10 buccal systems/blister pck)
Comment: Serum total *testosterone* concentrations may be checked 4 to 12 weeks after initiating treatment with **Striant**. To capture the maximum serum concentration, an early morning sample (just prior to applying the AM dose) is recommended.

TOPICAL ANDROGENS

Comment: Wash hands after application. Allow solution to dry before it touches clothing. Do not wash site for at least 2 hours after application. Pregnant and nursing women, and children, must avoid skin contact with application sites on men. If there is contact, wash the area as soon as possible with soap and water.

▷ *testosterone* (X)(III)
Pediatric: <18 years: not recommended

AndroGel 1% initially apply 5 g once daily in the AM to clean, dry, intact skin of the shoulders, upper arms, <u>and/or</u> abdomen; do not apply to scrotum; may increase to 7.5 g/day and then to 10 g/day if needed

Gel: 2.5, 5 g (30 pkts); 75 g (60 metered 1.25 g doses)

AndroGel 1.62% initially apply 2.5 g (2 pump actuations) once daily in the AM to clean, dry, intact skin of the shoulders and upper arms intact skin of the upper arms; do not apply to abdomen <u>or</u> genitals; may adjust dose between 1 and 4 pump actuations based on the pre-dose morning serum testosterone concentration at approximately 14 and 28 days after starting treatment <u>or</u> adjusting dose

Gel: 2.25 mg pump actuation (75 g, 60 metered 1.25 g doses)

Axiron apply to clean dry intact skin of the axillae; do not apply to the scrotum, penis, abdomen, shoulders, <u>or</u> upper arms; initially apply 60 mg (30 mg/axilla) once daily in the AM; adjust dose based on serum testosterone concentration 2 to 8 hours after applying and at least 14 days after starting therapy <u>or</u> following dose adjustment; may increase dose in 30 mg increments if serum testosterone <300 ng/dL up to 120 mg; reduce dose to 30 mg if levels >1050 ng/dL; discontinue if serum testosterone remains at >1050 ng/dL

Soln: 30 mg/1.5 ml pump actuation (90 ml; 60 metered actuations) (alcohol, latex-free)

Fortesta (G) initially 40 mg of testosterone (4 pump actuations) applied to the thighs once daily in the AM; may adjust between 10 mg minimum and 70 mg maximum.

Gel: 10 mg/0.5 g pump actuation (120 actuations)

Comment: The **Fortesta** dose should be based on the serum *testosterone* concentration 2 hours after applying **Fortesta** and at approximately 14 days and 35 days after starting treatment <u>or</u> following dose adjustment. Dose adjustment criteria: ≤500 ng/dL, increase daily dose by 10 mg; 500-≤1250 ng/dL, no change; 1250-≤2500 ng/dL, decrease daily dose by 10 mg; ≥2500 ng/dL, decrease daily dose by 20 mg.

Gel: 10 mg (0.5 g)/pump actuation (60 g; 120 metered dose actuations) (ethanol)

Testim (G) initially apply 5 g once daily in the AM to clean, dry, intact skin of the shoulders <u>and/or</u> upper arms; do not apply to the genitals <u>or</u> abdomen; may increase to 10 g after 2 weeks

Gel: 1%, clear, hydroalcoholic (5 mg/5 g, 5 g single-use tube)

Vogelxo Gel (G) 1% initially apply 5 g once daily in the AM to clean, dry, intact skin of the shoulders, upper arms, <u>and/or</u> abdomen; do not apply to scrotum; may increase to 7.5 g/day and then to 10 g/day if needed

Gel: 5 g/pkt (30 pkts); 5 g/tube (30 tubes); metered dose pumps (2 x 75 g, 1.25 g actuation)

INTRANASAL ANDROGENS

▷ *testosterone (nasal gel)* (X)(III) initially one pump actuation each nostril (33 mg) 3x/day, at least 6-8 hours apart, at the same times each day max: 6 pump actuation/day
Pediatric: <18 years: not established

Natesto

Gel: 5.5 mg/actuation, metered dose pump (11 g, 60 actuations)

TRANSDERMAL ANDROGEN

▷ *testosterone* (X)(III)
 Androderm initially apply 4 mg nightly at approximately 10 PM to clean, dry
 area of the arm, back, or upper buttocks; leave on x 24 hours; may increase
 to 7.5 mg or decrease to 2.5 mg based on confirmed AM serum testosterone
 concentrations
   Pediatric: <15 years: not recommended
   Transdermal patch: 2, 4 mg/24hr

TETANUS (*CLOSTRIDIUM TETANI*)

PROPHYLAXIS

see **Childhood Immunizations** *page* 578

POSTEXPOSURE PROPHYLAXIS IN PREVIOUSLY NONIMMUNIZED PERSONS

▷ *tetanus immune globulin, human* (C) 250 mg deep IM in a single dose
 Pediatric: >7 years: same as adult
  BayTET, Hyper-TET
    Vial: 250 units single dose; *Prefilled syringe:* 250 units
▷ *tetanus toxoid* vaccine (C) 0.5 ml IM x 3 dose series
    Vial: 5 Lf units/0.5 ml (0.5, 5 ml); *Prefilled syringe:* 5 Lf units/0.5 ml (0.5 ml)
Comment: Dose of **BayTET/HyperTET** S/D is calculated as 4 units/kg. However,
it may be advisable to administer the entire contents of the syringe of **BayTET/
HyperTET** S/D (250 units) regardless of the child's size, since theoretically the
same amount of toxin will be produced in the child's body by the infecting tetanus
organism as it will in an adult's body. At the same time but in a different extremity
and with a different syringe, administer Diphtheria and Tetanus Toxoids and Pertussis
Vaccine Adsorbed (DTP) or Diphtheria and Tetanus Toxoids Adsorbed (For Pediatric
Use) (DT), if pertussis vaccine is contraindicated, should be administered per mfr
pkg insert. Tetanus immune globulin may interact with live viral vaccines such as
measles, mumps, rubella, and polio. It is also unknown if **BayTET/HyperTET** can
cause fetal harm when administered to a pregnant woman or can affect reproduction
capacity. The single injection of tetanus toxoid only initiates the series for producing
active immunity in the recipient. Impress upon the patient the need for further
toxoid injections in 1 month and 1 year, otherwise the active immunization series
is incomplete. If a contraindication to using tetanus toxoid-containing preparations
exists for a person who has not completed a primary series of tetanus toxoid
immunization, and that person has a wound that is neither clean nor minor, only
passive immunization should be given using tetanus immune globulin.

THREADWORM (*STRONGYLOIDIDES STERCORALIS*)

ANTHELMINTICS

▷ *albendazole* (C) 400 mg bid x 7 days; take with a meal
 Pediatric: <2 years: 200 mg once daily x 3 days; may repeat in 3 weeks; ≥2-12 years:
 400 mg once daily x 3 days; may repeat in 3 weeks; >12 years: same as adult

Albenza *Tab:* 200 mg
▶ *ivermectin* (C) take with water; 200 mcg/kg as a single dose; may re-treat in 3 weeks
Pediatric: <15 kg: not recommended; ≥15 kg: same as adult
Stromectol *Tab:* 3, 6*mg
▶ *mebendazole* (C) chew, swallow, or mix with food; 100 mg bid x 3 days; may repeat
in 3 weeks if needed; take with a meal
Pediatric: <2 years: not recommended; ≥2 years: same as adult
Emverm *Chew tab:* 100 mg
Vermox (G) *Chew tab:* 100 mg
▶ *pyrantel pamoate* (C) 11 mg/kg x 1 dose; max 1 g/dose; take with a meal
Pediatric: 25-37 lb: 1/2 tsp x 1 dose; 38-62 lb: 1 tsp x 1 dose; 63-87 lb: 1 tsp x 1 dose;
88-112 lb: 2 tsp x 1 dose; 113-137 lb: 2 tsp x 1 dose; 138-162 lb: 3 tsp x 1 dose; 163-
187 lb: 3 tsp x 1 dose; >187 lb: 4 tsp x 1 dose
Pin-X (OTC) *Cap:* 180 mg; *Liq:* 50 mg/ml (30 ml); 144 mg/ml (30 ml); *Oral
susp:* 50 mg/ml (30 ml)
▶ *thiabendazole* (C) 25 mg/kg dosed bid x 7 days; max 1.5 g/dose; take with meals
Pediatric: same as adult; <30 lb: consult mfr pkg insert; >30 lb: 25 mg/kg/dose bid
with meals; 30-50 lb: 250 mg bid with meals; >50 lb: 10 mg/lb/dose bid with meals;
max 3g/day Mintezol *Chew tab:* 500*mg (orange); *Oral susp:* 500 mg/5 ml (120 ml)
(orange)
Comment: *thiabendazole* is not for prophylaxis. May impair mental alertness.

 TINEA CAPITIS

Comment: Tinea capitis must be treated with an oral anti-fungal.

FOR SEVERE KERION PRURITUS

▶ *prednisone* (C) 1 mg/kg/day for 7-14 days
see **Oral Corticosteroids** *page 509*

SYSTEMIC ANTI-FUNGALS

▶ *griseofulvin, microsize* (C)(G) 500 mg once daily x 4-6 weeks or longer; max 1 g/day
Pediatric: <30 lb: 5 mg/lb/day; 30-50 lb: 125-250 mg/day; >50 lb: 250-500 mg/day;
5 mg/lb/day x 4-6 weeks or longer; *see page 579 for dose by weight*
Grifulvin V *Tab:* 250, 500 mg; *Oral susp:* 125 mg/5 ml (120 ml; alcohol 0.02%)
▶ *griseofulvin, ultramicrosize* (C)(G) 375 mg/day in a single or divided doses x 4-6
weeks or longer
Pediatric: <2 years: not recommended; ≥2 years: 3.3 mg/lb/day in a single or divided
doses x 4-6 weeks or longer
Gris-PEG *Tab:* 125, 250 mg
Comment: *griseofulvin* should be taken with fatty foods (e.g., milk, ice cream).
Liver enzymes should be monitored.
▶ *ketoconazole* (C)(G) initially 200 mg once daily; max 400 mg/day x 4 weeks
Pediatric: <2 years: not recommended; ≥2 years: 3.3-6.6 mg/kg once daily x 4 weeks
Nizoral *Tab:* 200 mg
Comment: Caution with *ketoconazole* due to concerns about potential for
hepatotoxicity.

TINEA CORPORIS (RINGWORM)

TOPICAL ANTI-FUNGALS

▷ *butenafine* (C)(G) apply bid x 1 week or once daily x 4 weeks
  Pediatric: <12 years: not recommended; ≥12 years: same as adult
    Lotrimin Ultra (OTC) *Crm:* 1% (12, 24 g)
    Mentax *Crm:* 1% (15, 30 g)
  Comment: *butenafine* is a benzylamine, not an azole. Fungicidal activity continues
  for at least 5 weeks after last application.

▷ *ciclopirox* (B)
    Loprox Cream apply bid; max 4 weeks
      Pediatric: <10 years: not recommended; ≥10 years: same as adult
      Crm: 0.77% (15, 30, 90 g)
    Loprox Lotion apply bid; max 4 weeks
      Pediatric: <10 years: not recommended; ≥10 years: same as adult
      Lotn: 0.77% (30, 60 ml)
    Loprox Gel apply bid; max 4 weeks
      Pediatric: <16 years: not recommended
      Gel: 0.77% (30, 45 g)

▷ *clotrimazole* (B)(G) apply to affected area bid x 7 days
  Pediatric: same as adult
    Lotrimin *Crm:* 1% (15, 30, 45 g)
    Lotrimin AF (OTC) *Crm:* 1% (12 g); *Lotn:* 1% (10 ml); *Soln:* 1% (10 ml)

▷ *econazole* (C) apply once daily x 14 days
  Pediatric: same as adult
    Spectazole *Crm:* 1% (15, 30, 85 g)

▷ *ketoconazole* (C) apply once daily x 14 days
  Pediatric: not recommended
    Nizoral Cream *Crm:* 2% (15, 30, 60 g)

▷ *miconazole* 2% (C) apply once daily-bid x 2 weeks
  Pediatric: same as adult
    Lotrimin AF Spray Liquid (OTC) *Spray liq:* 2% (113 g) (alcohol 17%)
    Lotrimin AF Spray Powder (OTC) *Spray pwdr:* 2% (90 g) (alcohol 10%)
    Monistat-Derm *Crm:* 2% (1, 3 oz); *Spray liq:* 2% (3.5 oz); *Spray pwdr:* 2% (3 oz)

▷ *naftifine* (B)(G)
  Pediatric: not recommended
    Naftin Cream apply once daily x 14 days
      Crm: 1% (15, 30, 60 g)
    Naftin Gel apply bid x 14 days
      Gel: 1% (20, 40, 60 g)

▷ *oxiconazole nitrate* (B)(G) apply once daily-bid x 2 weeks
  Pediatric: same as adult
    Oxistat *Crm:* 1% (15, 30, 60 g); *Lotn:* 1% (30 ml)

▷ *sulconazole* (C) apply once daily-bid x 3 weeks
  Pediatric: not recommended
    Exelderm *Crm:* 1% (15, 30, 60 g); *Lotn:* 1% (30 mg)

▷ *terbinafine* (B)(G)
  Pediatric: <12 years: not recommended

Lamisil Cream (OTC) apply to affected and surrounding area once daily-bid x
1-4 weeks until significantly improved
   Crm: 1% (15, 30 g)
Lamisil AT Cream (OTC) apply to affected and surrounding area once daily-bid
x 1-4 weeks until significantly improved
   Crm: **1% (15, 30 g)**
Lamisil Solution (OTC) apply to affected and surrounding area once daily x 1 week
   Soln: 1% (30 ml spray bottle)

TOPICAL ANTIFUNGAL/STEROID COMBINATION

▷ *clotrimazole/betamethasone* (C)(G) apply bid x 2 weeks; max 4 weeks
   Pediatric: <12 years: not recommended; >12 years: same as adult
      Lotrisone *Crm:* clotrim 1 mg/*beta* 0.5 mg (15, 45 g); *Lotn:* clotrim 1 mg/*beta* 0.5
      mg (30 ml)

SYSTEMIC ANTIFUNGALS

▷ *griseofulvin, microsize* (C)(G) 500 mg/day x 2-4 weeks; max 1 g/day
   Pediatric: <30 lb: 5 mg/lb/day; 30-50 lb: 125-250 mg/day; >50 lb: 250-500 mg/day;
   see page 579 for dose by weight
      Grifulvin V *Tab:* 250, 500 mg; *Oral susp:* 125 mg/5 ml (120 ml) (alcohol 0.02%)
▷ *griseofulvin, ultramicrosize* (C)(G) 375 mg/day in a single or divided doses x 2-4
   weeks
   Pediatric: <2 years: not recommended; ≥2 years: 3.3 mg/lb/day in a single or divided
   doses
      Gris-PEG *Tab:* 125, 250
   Comment: *griseofulvin* should be taken with fatty foods (e.g., milk, ice cream).
   Liver enzymes should be monitored.
▷ *ketoconazole* (C) initially 200 mg once daily; max 400 mg/day x 4 weeks
   Pediatric: <2 years: not recommended; >2 years: 3.3-6.6 mg/kg/day x 4 weeks
      Nizoral *Tab:* 200 mg
   Comment: Caution with *ketoconazole* due to concerns about potential for
   hepatotoxicity.

⬤ TINEA CRURIS (JOCK ITCH)

TOPICAL ANTIFUNGALS

▷ *butenafine* (B)(G) apply bid x 1 week or once daily x 4 weeks
   Pediatric: <12 years: not recommended; ≥12 years: same as adult
      Lotrimin Ultra (C)(OTC) *Crm:* 1% (12, 24 g)
      Mentax *Crm:* 1% (15, 30 g)
   Comment: *butenafine* is a benzylamine, not an azole. Fungicidal activity continues
   for at least 5 weeks after last application.
▷ *ciclopirox* (B)
      Loprox Cream apply bid; max 4 weeks
         Pediatric: <10 years: not recommended; ≥10 years: same as adult
         Crm: 0.77% (15, 30, 90 g)
      Loprox Lotion apply bid; max 4 weeks
         Pediatric: <10 years: not recommended; ≥10 years: same as adult

Lotn: 0.77% (30, 60 ml)
Loprox Gel apply bid; max 4 weeks
Pediatric: <16 years: not recommended; ≥16 years: same as adult
Gel: 0.77% (30, 45 g)

▷ *clotrimazole* (B)(G) apply to affected area bid x 7 days
Pediatric: same as adult
Lotrimin *Crm:* 1% (15, 30, 45 g)
Lotrimin AF (OTC) *Crm:* 1% (12 g); *Lotn:* 1% (10 ml); *Soln:* 1% (10 ml)

▷ *econazole* (C) apply once daily x 2 weeks
Pediatric: same as adult
Spectazole *Crm:* 1% (15, 30, 85 g)

▷ *ketoconazole* (C)(G) apply bid x 4 weeks
Pediatric: not recommended
Nizoral Cream *Crm:* 2% (15, 30, 60 g)

▷ *miconazole* 2% (C)(G) apply once daily-bid x 2 weeks
Pediatric: same as adult
Lotrimin AF Spray Liquid (OTC) *Spray liq:* 2% (113 g) (alcohol 17%)
Lotrimin AF Spray Powder (OTC) *Spray pwdr:* 2% (90 g) (alcohol 10%)
Monistat-Derm *Crm:* 2% (1, 3 oz); *Spray liq:* 2% (3.5 oz); *Spray pwdr:* 2% (3 oz)

▷ *naftifine* (B)(G)
Pediatric: not recommended
Naftin Cream apply once daily x 2 weeks
Crm: 1% (15, 30, 60 g)
Naftin Gel apply bid x 2 weeks
Gel: 1% (20, 40, 60 g)

▷ *oxiconazole nitrate* (B)(G) apply once daily-bid x 2 weeks
Pediatric: same as adult
Oxistat *Crm:* 1% (15, 30, 60 g); *Lotn:* 1% (30 ml)

▷ *sulconazole* (C) apply once daily-bid x 3 weeks
Pediatric: not recommended
Exelderm *Crm:* 1% (15, 30, 60 g); *Lotn:* 1% (30 mg)

▷ *terbinafine* (B)(G)
Pediatric: <12 years: not recommended; ≥12 years: same as adult
Lamisil Cream (OTC) apply bid x 1-4 weeks
Crm: 1% (15, 30 g)
Lamisil AT Cream (OTC) apply to affected and surrounding area once daily-bid
x 1-4 weeks until significantly improved
Crm: 1% (15, 30 g)
Lamisil Solution (OTC) apply to affected and surrounding area once daily x 1 week
Soln: 1% (30 ml spray bottle)

▷ *tolnaftate* (C)(OTC)(G) apply sparingly bid x 2-4 weeks
Pediatric: <2 years: not recommended; ≥2 years: same as adult
Tinactin *Crm:* 1% (15, 30 g); *Pwdr:* 1% (45, 90 g); *Soln:* 1% (10 ml); *Aerosol liq:* 1% (4 oz); *Aerosol pwdr:* 1% (3.5, 5 oz)

▷ *undecylenate acid* (NE) apply bid x 4 weeks
Pediatric: same as adult
Desenex (OTC) *Pwdr:* 25% (1.5, 3 oz); *Spray pwdr:* 25% (2.7 oz); *Oint:* 25% (0.5, 1 oz)

TOPICAL ANTIFUNGAL/ANTI-INFLAMMATORY AGENTS

▷ *clotrimazole/betamethasone* (C)(G) apply bid x 4 weeks; max 4 weeks

Pediatric: <12 years: not recommended; ≥12 years: same as adult
Crm: clotrim 10 mg/*beta* 0.5 mg (15, 45 g); *Lotn: clotrim* 10 mg/*beta* 0.5 mg (30 ml)

SYSTEMIC ANTIFUNGALS

▷ *griseofulvin, microsize* (C)(G) 1 g once daily x 2 weeks
   Pediatric: <30 lb: 5 mg/lb/day; 30-50 lb: 125-250 mg/day; >50 lb: 250-500 mg/day;
   5 mg/lb/day x 4-6 weeks <u>or</u> longer; *see page 579 for dose by weight*
      Grifulvin V *Tab:* 250, 500 mg; *Oral susp:* 125 mg/5 ml (120 ml) (alcohol 0.02%)
▷ *griseofulvin, ultramicrosize* (C) 375 mg/day in a single <u>or</u> divided doses x 2 weeks
   Pediatric: <2 years: not recommended; ≥2 years: 3.3 mg/lb/day in a single <u>or</u> divided doses
      Gris-PEG *Tab:* 125, 250 mg
Comment: *griseofulvin* should be taken with fatty foods (e.g., milk, ice cream). Liver
enzymes should be monitored.
▷ *ketoconazole* (C) initially 200 mg once daily; max 400 mg once daily x 4 weeks
   Pediatric: <2 years: not recommended; ≥2 years: 3.3-6.6 mg/kg/day
      Nizoral *Tab:* 200 mg
   Comment: Caution with *ketoconazole* due to concerns about potential for
   hepatotoxicity.

 TINEA PEDIS (ATHLETE'S FOOT)

TOPICAL ANTIFUNGALS

▷ *butenafine* (B)(G) apply bid x 1 week <u>or</u> once daily x 4 weeks
   Pediatric: <12 years: not recommended; ≥12 years: same as adult
      Lotrimin Ultra (C)(OTC) *Crm:* 1% (12, 24 g)
      Mentax *Crm:* 1% (15, 30 g)
   Comment: *butenafine* is a benzylamine, not an azole. Fungicidal activity continues
   for at least 5 weeks after last application.
▷ *Burrows solution* (NE) wet dressings
▷ *ciclopirox* (B)
      Loprox Cream apply bid; max 4 weeks
         Pediatric: <10 years: not recommended; ≥10 years: same as adult
         Crm: 0.77% (15, 30, 90 g)
      Loprox Lotion apply bid; max 4 weeks
         Pediatric: <10 years: not recommended; ≥10 years: same as adult
         Lotn: 0.77% (30, 60 ml)
      Loprox Gel apply bid; max 4 weeks
         Pediatric: <16 years: not recommended; ≥16 years: same as adult
         Gel: 0.77% (30, 45 g)
▷ *clotrimazole* (C)(G) apply bid to affected area x 4 weeks
   Pediatric: same as adult
      Desenex *Crm:* 1% (0.5 oz)
      Lotrimin *Crm:* 1% (15, 30, 45, 90 g); *Lotn:* 1% (30 ml); *Soln:* 1% (10, 30 ml)
      Lotrimin AF (OTC) *Crm:* 1% (15, 30, 45, 90 g); *Lotn:* 1% (20 ml); *Soln:* 1%
      (20 ml)
▷ *econazole* (C) apply once daily x 4 weeks
   Pediatric: same as adult
      Spectazole *Crm:* 1% (15, 30, 85 g)

▷ *ketoconazole* (C) apply once daily x 6 weeks
  Pediatric: not recommended
    Nizoral Cream *Crm:* 2% (15, 30, 60 g)
▷ *miconazole 2%* (C)(G) apply bid x 4 weeks
  Pediatric: same as adult
    Lotrimin AF Spray Liquid (OTC) *Spray liq:* 2% (113 g) (alcohol 17%)
    Lotrimin AF Spray Powder (OTC) *Spray pwdr:* 2% (90 g; alcohol 10%)
    Monistat-Derm *Crm:* 2% (1, 3 oz); *Spray liq:* 2% (3.5 oz); *Spray pwdr:* 2% (3 oz)
▷ *naftifine* (B)(G)
  Pediatric: not recommended
    Naftin Cream apply once daily x 4 weeks
      Crm: 1% (15, 30, 60 g)
    Naftin Gel apply bid x 4 weeks
      Gel: 1% (20, 40, 60 g)
▷ *oxiconazole nitrate* (B)(G) apply once daily-bid x 4 weeks
  Pediatric: same as adult
    Oxistat *Crm:* 1% (15, 30, 60 g); *Lotn:* 1% (30 ml)
▷ *sertaconazole* (C) apply once daily-bid x 4 weeks
  Pediatric: <12 years: not recommended; ≥12 years: same as adult
    Ertaczo *Crm:* 2% (15, 30 g)
▷ *sulconazole* (C) apply once daily-bid x 4 weeks
  Pediatric: not recommended
    Exelderm *Crm:* 1% (15, 30, 60 g); *Lotn:* 1% (30 mg)
▷ *terbinafine* (B)(G)
  Pediatric: <12 years: not recommended; ≥12 years: same as adult
    Lamisil Cream (OTC) apply bid x 1-4 weeks
      Crm: 1% (15, 30 g)
    Lamisil AT Cream (OTC) apply to affected and surrounding area once daily-bid
    x 1-4 weeks until significantly improved
      Crm: 1% (15, 30 g)
    Lamisil Solution (OTC) apply to affected and surrounding area bid x 1 week
      Soln: 1% (30 ml spray bottle)
▷ *tolnaftate* (C)(OTC)(G) apply sparingly bid x 2-4 weeks
  Pediatric: <2 years: not recommended; ≥2 years: same as adult
    Tinactin *Crm:* 1% (15, 30 g); *Pwdr:* 1% (45, 90 g); *Soln:* 1% (10 ml); *Aerosol liq:*
    1% (4 oz); *Aerosol pwdr:* 1% (3.5, 5 oz)

TOPICAL ANTIFUNGAL/ANTI-INFLAMMATORY COMBINATION

▷ *clotrimazole/betamethasone* (C)(G) apply bid x 4 weeks; max 4 weeks
  Pediatric: <12 years: not recommended; ≥12 years: same as adult
    Lotrisone *Crm: clotrim* 1 mg/*beta* 0.5 mg (15, 45 g); *Lotn: clotrim* 1 mg/*beta* 0.5
    mg (30 ml)

SYSTEMIC ANTIFUNGALS

▷ *griseofulvin, microsize* (C)(G) 1 g once daily x 4-8 weeks
  Pediatric: <30 lb: 5 mg/lb/day; 30-50 lb: 125-250 mg/day; >50 lb: 250-500 mg/day;
  5 mg/lb/day x 4-6 weeks <u>or</u> longer; *see page 579 for dose by weight*
    Grifulvin V *Tab:* 250, 500 mg; *Oral susp:* 125 mg/5 ml (120 ml) (alcohol 0.02%)

➤ *griseofulvin, ultramicrosize* (C) 750 mg/day in a single or divided doses x 4-6 weeks
　Pediatric: <2 years: not recommended; ≥2 years: 3.3 mg/lb/day in a single or divided doses
　　Gris-PEG *Tab:* 125, 250
　Comment: *griseofulvin* should be taken with fatty foods (e.g., milk, ice cream). Liver enzymes should be monitored.
➤ *ketoconazole* (C) initially 200 mg once daily; max 400 mg/day x 4 weeks
　Pediatric: <2 years: not recommended; ≥2 years: 3.3-6.6 mg/kg once daily x 4 weeks
　　Nizoral *Tab:* 200 mg
　Comment: Caution with *ketoconazole* due to concerns about potential for hepatotoxicity.

⬤ TINEA VERSICOLOR

Comment: Resolution may take 3-6 months.

TOPICAL ANTIFUNGALS

➤ *butenafine* (G) apply once daily x 2 weeks
　Pediatric: <12 years: not recommended; ≥12 years: same as adult
　　Lotrimin Ultra (C)(OTC) *Crm:* 1% (12, 24 g)
　　Mentax (B) *Crm:* 1% (15, 30 g)
　Comment: *butenafine* is a benzylamine, not an azole. Fungicidal activity continues for at least 5 weeks after last application.
➤ *ciclopirox* (B)
　　Loprox Cream apply bid; max 4 weeks
　　　Pediatric: <10 years: not recommended; ≥10 years: same as adult
　　　Crm: 0.77% (15, 30, 90 g)
　　Loprox Lotion apply bid; max 4 weeks
　　　Pediatric: <10 years: not recommended; ≥10 years: same as adult
　　　Lotn: 0.77% (30, 60 ml)
　　Loprox Gel apply bid; max 4 weeks
　　　Pediatric: <16 years: not recommended; ≥16 years: same as adult
　　　Gel: 0.77% (30, 45 g)
➤ *clotrimazole* (B)(G) apply bid x 7 days
　Pediatric: same as adult
　　Lotrimin *Crm:* 1% (15, 30, 45 g)
　　Lotrimin AF (OTC) *Crm:* 1% (12 g); *Lotn:* 1% (10 ml); *Soln:* 1% (10 ml)
➤ *econazole* (C) apply once daily x 2 weeks
　Pediatric: same as adult
　　Spectazole *Crm:* 1% (15, 30, 85 g)
➤ *miconazole* 2% (C)(G) apply once daily x 2 weeks
　Pediatric: same as adult
　　Lotrimin AF Spray Liquid (OTC) *Spray liq:* 2% (113 g) (alcohol 17%)
　　Lotrimin AF Spray Powder (OTC) *Spray pwdr:* 2% (90 g) alcohol 10%)
　　Monistat-Derm *Crm:* 2% (1, 3 oz); *Spray liq:* 2% (3.5 oz); *Spray pwdr: 2% (3 oz)*
➤ *ketoconazole* (C)(G)
　Pediatric: not recommended

Nizoral Cream apply once daily x 2 weeks
  Crm: 2% (15, 30, 60 g)
Nizoral Shampoo lather into area and leave on 5 minutes x 1 application
  Shampoo: 2% (4 oz)
▷ *oxiconazole nitrate* (B)(G) apply once daily x 2 weeks
  Pediatric: same as adult
    Oxistat *Crm:* 1% (15, 30, 60 g); *Lotn:* 1% (30 ml)
▷ *selenium sulfide* shampoo (C)(G) apply after shower, allow to dry, leave on overnight; then scrub off vigorously in AM; repeat in 1 week and again q 3 months until resolution occurs
  Pediatric: same as adult
    Selsun Blue *Shampoo:* 1% (120, 210, 240, 330 ml); 2.5% (120 ml)
▷ *sulconazole* (C) apply once daily-bid x 3 weeks
  Pediatric: not recommended
    Exelderm *Crm:* 1% (15, 30, 60 g); *Lotn:* 1% (30 mg)
▷ *terbinafine* (B) apply bid to affected and surrounding area x 1 week
  Pediatric: <12 years: not recommended; ≥12 years: same as adult
    Lamisil Solution (OTC) *Soln:* 1% (30 ml spray bottle)

ORAL ANTI-FUNGALS

▷ *ketoconazole* (C) initially 200 mg once daily; max 400 mg/day x 4 weeks
  Pediatric: <2 years: not recommended; ≥2 years: 3.3-6.6 mg/kg once daily x 4 weeks
    Nizoral *Tab:* 200 mg

TOBACCO DEPENDENCE/NICOTINE WITHDRAWAL SYNDROME

NON-NICOTINE PRODUCTS

Alpha₄-Beta₂ Nicotinic Acetylcholine Receptor Partial Agonist

▷ *varenicline* (C)
  Pediatric: <18 years: not recommended
    Chantix set target quit date; begin therapy 1 week prior to target quit date; take after eating with a full glass of water; initially 0.5 mg once daily for 3 days; then 0.5 mg bid x 4 days; then 1 mg bid; treat x 12 weeks; may continue treatment for 12 more weeks
      Tab: 0.5, 1 mg; *Starting Month Pak:* 0.5 mg x 11 tabs + 1 mg x 42 tabs; *Continuing Month Pak:* 1 mg x 56 tabs
  Comment: Caution with **Chantix** due to potential risk for anxiety or suicidal ideation.

AMINOKETONES

▷ *bupropion HBr* (C)(G)
  Pediatric: <18 years: not recommended
    Aplenzin initially 100 mg bid for at least 3 days; may increase to 375 <u>or</u> 400 mg/day after several weeks; then after at least 3 more days, 450 mg in 4 divided doses; max 450 mg/day, 174 mg/single dose

Tab: 174, 348, 522 mg
▷ *bupropion HCl* (B)(G)
  Pediatric: <18 years: not recommended
    Wellbutrin initially 100 mg bid for at least 3 days; may increase to 375 or 400
    mg/day after several weeks; then after at least 3 more days, 450 mg in 4 divided
    doses; max 450 mg/day, 150 mg/single dose
      Tab: 75, 100 mg
    Wellbutrin SR initially 150 mg in AM for at least 3 days; may increase to 150
    mg bid if well tolerated; usual dose 300 mg/day; max 400 mg/day
      Tab: 100, 150 mg sust-rel
    Wellbutrin XL initially 150 mg in AM for at least 3 days; increase to 150 mg bid
    if well tolerated; usual dose 300 mg/day; max 400 mg/day
      Tab: 150, 300 mg sust-rel
    Zyban 150 mg once daily x 3 days; then 150 mg bid x 7-12 weeks; max 300 mg/day
      Pediatric: <18 years: not recommended
      Tab: 150 mg sust-rel
Comment: Contraindications to *bupropion* include seizure disorder, eating
disorder, concurrent MAOI and alcohol use. Smoking should be discontinued after
the 7th day of therapy with *bupropion*. Avoid bedtime dose.

TRANSDERMAL NICOTINE SYSTEMS (D)

    Habitrol (OTC) initially one 21 mg/24 hour patch/day x 4-6 weeks; then one
    14 mg/24 hour patch/day x 2-4 weeks; then one 7 mg/24 hour patch/day x 2-4
    weeks; then discontinue
      Pediatric: not recommended
      Transdermal patch: 7, 14, 21 mg/24 hour
    Nicoderm CQ (OTC) initially one 21 mg/24 hour patch/day x 6 weeks, then
    one 14 mg/24 hour patch/day x 2 weeks; then one 7 mg/24 hour patch/day x 2
    weeks
      Pediatric: not recommended
      Transdermal patch: 7, 14, 21 mg/24 hour
    Comment: Nicoderm CQ is available as a clear patch.
    Nicotrol Step-down Patch (OTC) 1 patch/day x 6 weeks
      Pediatric: not recommended
      Transdermal patch: 5, 10, 15 mg/16 hour (7/pck)
    Nicotrol Transdermal (OTC) 1 patch/day x 6 weeks
      Pediatric: not recommended
      Transdermal patch: 15 mg/16 hour (7/pck)
    Prostep initially one 22 mg/24 hour patch/day x 4-8 weeks; then discontinue or
    one 11 mg/24 hour patch/day x 2-4 additional weeks
      Pediatric: not recommended
      Transdermal patch: 11, 22 mg/24 hour (7/pck)

NICOTINE GUM

▷ *nicotine polacrilex* (D) chew one piece of gum slowly and intermittently over 30
minutes q 1-2 hours x 6 weeks; then q 2-4 hours x 3 weeks; then q 4-8 hours x 3
weeks; max 24 pieces/day; 2 mg if smoked <25 cigarettes/day; 4 mg if smoked >24
cigarettes/day
  Pediatric: not recommended

Nicorette (OTC) *Gum squares:* 2, 4 mg (108 piece starter kit and 48 piece refill) (orange, mint, or original, sugar-free)

NICOTINE LOZENGE

▷ *nicotine polacrilex* **(X)(OTC)(G)** dissolve over 20-30 minutes; minimize swallowing; do not eat or drink for 15 min before and during use; Use 2 mg lozenge if first cigarette smoked >30 minutes after waking; Use 4 mg lozenge if first cigarette smoked within 30 min of waking; 1 lozenge q 1-2 hours (at lest 9/day) x 6 weeks; then q 2-4 hours x 3 weeks; then q 4-8 hours x 3 weeks; then stop; max 5 lozenges/6 hours and 20 lozenges/day
Pediatric: <18 years: not recommended
    Commit Lozenge *Loz:* 2, 4 mg (72/pck) (phenylalanine)
    Nicorette Mini Lozenge (G) *Loz:* 2, 4 mg (72/pck) (mint; phenylalanine)

NICOTINE INHALATION PRODUCTS

▷ *nicotine* 0.5 mg aqueous nasal spray **(D)**
Pediatric: not recommended
    Nicotrol NS 1-2 doses/hour nasally; max 5 doses/hour or 40 doses/day; usual max 3 months
      Nasal spray: 0.5 mg/spray; 10 mg/ml (10 ml, 200 doses)
▷ *nicotine* 10 mg inhalation system **(D)**
Pediatric: not recommended
    Nicotrol Inhaler individualize therapy; at least 6 cartridges/day x 3-6 weeks; max 16 cartridges/day x first 12 weeks; then reduce gradually over 12 more weeks
      Inhaler: 10 mg/cartridge, 4 mg delivered (42 cartridge/pck) (menthol)
Comment: Nicotrol Inhaler is a smoking replacement; to be used with decreasing frequency. Smoking should be discontinued before starting therapy. Side effects include cough, nausea, mouth, or throat irritation. This system delivers nicotine, but no tars or carcinogens. Each cartridge lasts about 20 minutes with frequent continuous puffing and provides nicotine equivalent to 2 cigarettes.

◯ TONSILLITIS: ACUTE

▷ *amoxicillin* **(B)(G)** 500-875 mg bid or 250-500 mg tid x 10 days
Pediatric: <40 kg (88 lb): 20-40 mg/kg/day in 3 divided doses x 10 days or 25-45 mg/kg/day in 2 divided doses x 10 days; *see page 554 for dose by weight*
    Amoxil *Cap:* 250, 500 mg; *Tab:* 875*mg; *Chew tab:* 125, 200, 250, 400 mg (cherry-banana-peppermint) (phenylalanine); *Oral susp:* 125, 250 mg/5 ml (80, 100, 150 ml) (strawberry); 200, 400 mg/5 ml (50, 75, 100 ml) (bubble gum); *Oral drops:* 50 mg/ml (30 ml) (bubble gum)
    Moxatag *Tab:* 775 mg ext-rel
    Trimox *Tab:* 125, 250 mg; *Cap:* 250, 500 mg; *Oral susp:* 125, 250 mg/5 ml (80, 100, 150 ml) (raspberry-strawberry)
▷ *azithromycin* **(B)** 500 mg x 1 dose on day 1, then 250 mg once daily on days 2-5 or 500 mg once daily x 3 days or **Zmax** 2 g in a single dose
Pediatric: 12 mg/kg/day x 5 days; max 500 mg/day; *see page 559 for dose by weight*
    Zithromax *Tab:* 250, 500, 600 mg; *Oral susp:* 100 mg/5 ml (15 ml); 200 mg/5 ml (15, 22.5, 30 ml) (cherry); *Pkt:* 1 g for reconstitution (cherry-banana)

Zithromax Tri-pak *Tab:* 3 x 500 mg tabs/pck
Zithromax Z-pak *Tab:* 6 x 250 mg tabs/pck
Zmax *Oral susp:* 2 g ext-rel for reconstitution (cherry-banana) (148 mg Na⁺)

▷ *cefaclor* (B)(G) 250-500 mg q 8 hours x 10 days; max 2 g/day
Pediatric: <1 month: not recommended; 20-40 mg/kg bid or q 12 hours x 10 days; max 1 g/day; *see page 560 for dose by weight*
Tab: 500 mg; *Cap:* 250, 500 mg; *Susp:* 125 mg/5 ml (75, 150 ml) (strawberry); 187 mg/5 ml (50, 100 ml) (strawberry); 250 mg/5 ml (75, 150 ml) (strawberry); 375 mg/5 ml (50, 100 ml) (strawberry)
    Pediatric: <16 years: ext-rel not recommended; ≥16 years; same as adult
    Cefaclor Extended Release *Tab:* 375, 500 mg ext-rel

▷ *cefadroxil* (B) 1 g once daily or divided bid x 10 days
Pediatric: 30 mg/kg/day in 2 divided doses/day x 10 days; *see page 561 for dose by weight*
    Duricef *Cap:* 500 mg; *Tab:* 1 g; *Oral susp:* 250 mg/5 ml (100 ml); 500 mg/5 ml (75, 100 ml) (orange-pineapple)

▷ *cefdinir* (B) 300 mg bid x 5-10 days or 600 mg once daily x 10 days
Pediatric: <6 months: not recommended; 6 months-12 years: 14 mg/kg/day in a single or 2 divided doses x 10 days; >12 years: same as adult; *see page 562 for dose by weight*
    Omnicef *Cap:* 300 mg; *Oral susp:* 125 mg/5 ml (60, 100 ml) (strawberry)

▷ *cefditoren pivoxil* (B) 200 mg bid x 10 days
Pediatric: <12 years: not recommended
    Spectracef *Tab:* 200 mg
Comment: Contraindicated with milk protein allergy or carnitine deficiency.

▷ *ceftibuten* (B) 200 mg once daily x 10 days
Pediatric: 9 mg/kg once daily x 10 days; max 400 mg/day; *see page 566 for dose by weight*
    Cedax *Cap:* 400 mg; *Oral susp:* 90 mg/5 ml (30, 60, 90, 120 ml); 180 mg/5 ml (30, 60, 120 ml) (cherry)

▷ *cefixime* (B) 400 mg once daily x 10 days
Pediatric: <6 months: not recommended; 6 months-12 years, <50 kg: 8 mg/kg/day in a single or 2 divided doses x 10 days; >12 years, >50 kg: same as adult; *see page 563 for dose by weight*
    Suprax *Tab:* 400 mg; *Cap:* 400 mg; *Oral susp:* 100, 200 mg/5 ml (50, 75, 100 ml) (strawberry)

▷ *cefpodoxime proxetil* (B) 200 mg bid x 5-7 days
Pediatric: <2 months: not recommended; 2 months-12 years: 10 mg/kg/day (max 400 mg/dose) or 5 mg/kg/day bid (max 200 mg/dose) x 5-7 days; *see page 564 for dose by weight*
    Vantin *Tab:* 100, 200 mg; *Oral susp:* 50, 100 mg/5 ml (50, 75, 100 mg) (lemon creme)

▷ *cefprozil* (B) 500 mg once daily x 10 days
Pediatric: 2-12 years: 7.5 mg/kg bid x 10 days; >12 years: same as adult; *see page 565 for dose by weight*
    Cefzil *Tab:* 250, 500 mg; *Oral susp:* 125, 250 mg/5 ml (50, 75, 100 ml) (bubble gum) (phenylalanine)

▷ *cephalexin* (B)(G) 250 mg tid x 10 days
Pediatric: 25-50 mg/kg/day in 4 divided doses x 10 days; *see page 568 for dose by weight*
    Keflex *Cap:* 250, 333, 500, 750 mg; *Oral susp:* 125, 250 mg/5 ml (100, 200 ml) (strawberry)

▷ *clarithromycin* (C)(G) 250 mg bid <u>or</u> 500 mg ext-rel once daily 10 days
   Pediatric: <6 months: not recommended; ≥6 months: 7.5 mg/kg bid x 10 days; *see page* 569 *for dose by weight*
      Biaxin *Tab:* 250, 500 mg
      Biaxin Oral Suspension *Oral susp:* 125, 250 mg/5 ml (50, 100 ml) (fruit punch)
      Biaxin XL *Tab:* 500 mg ext-rel
▷ *dirithromycin* (C)(G) 500 mg once daily x 10 days
   Pediatric: <12 years: not recommended; ≥12 years: same as adult
      Dynabac *Tab:* 250 mg
▷ *erythromycin base* (B)(G) 300-400 mg tid x 10 days
   Pediatric: 30-50 mg/kg/day in 2-4 divided doses x 10 days
      Ery-Tab *Tab:* 250, 333, 500 mg ent-coat
      PCE *Tab:* 333, 500 mg
   Comment: *erythromycin* may increase INR with concomitant *warfarin*, as well as increase serum level of *digoxin*, benzodiazepines and statins.
▷ *erythromycin ethylsuccinate* (B)(G) 400 mg qid x 7 days
   Pediatric: 30-50 mg/kg/day in 4 divided doses x 7 days; may double dose with severe infection; max 100 mg/kg/day; *see page* 574 *for dose by weight*
      EryPed *Oral susp:* 200 mg/5 ml (100, 200 ml) (fruit); 400 mg/5 ml (60, 100, 200 ml) (banana); *Oral drops:* 200, 400 mg/5 ml (50 ml) (fruit); *Chew tab:* 200 mg wafer (fruit)
      E.E.S. *Oral susp:* 200, 400 mg/5 ml (100 ml) (fruit)
      E.E.S. Granules *Oral susp:* 200 mg/5 ml (100, 200 ml) (cherry)
      E.E.S. 400 Tablets *Tab:* 400 mg
   Comment: *erythromycin* may increase INR with concomitant *warfarin*, as well as increase serum level of *digoxin*, benzodiazepines and statins.
▷ *loracarbef* (B) 200 mg bid x 10 days
   Pediatric: 15 mg/kg/day in 2 divided doses x 10 days; *see page* 581 *for dose by weight*
      Lorabid *Pulvule:* 200, 400 mg; *Oral susp:* 100 mg/5 ml (50, 100 ml); 200 mg/5 ml (50, 75, 100 ml) (strawberry bubble gum)
▷ *penicillin V potassium* (B)(G) 250 mg tid x 10 days
   Pediatric: 25-50 mg/kg day in 4 divided doses x 10 days; ≥12 years: same as adult; *see page* 583 *for dose by weight*
      Pen-Vee K *Tab:* 250, 500 mg; *Oral soln:* 125 mg/5 ml (100, 200 ml); 250 mg/5 ml (100, 150, 200 ml)

 TRICHINOSIS (*TRICHINELLA SPIRALIS*)

Comment: Trichinosis is caused by eating raw <u>or</u> undercooked pork or wild game infected with the larvae of a parasitic worm, *Trichinella spiralis*. The initial symptoms are abdominal discomfort, nausea, vomiting, diarrhea, fatigue, and fever beginning one to two days following ingestion. These parasites then invade other organs (e.g., muscles) causing muscle aches, itching, fever, chills, and joint pains that begins about two to eight weeks after ingestion. The treatment is oral anthelmintics which may cause abdominal pain, diarrhea, and (rarely) hypersensitivity reactions, convulsions, neutropenia, agranulocytosis, and hepatitis.

ANTHELMINTICS

▷ *albendazole* (C) 400 mg as bid x 15 days; take with a meal

Pediatric: <2 years: 200 mg once daily x 3 days; may repeat in 3 weeks; 2-12 years: 400 mg once daily x 3 days; may repeat in 3 weeks; >12 years: same as adult

    Albenza *Tab:* 200 mg

▶ *mebendazole* (C) chew, swallow, or mix with food; 200-400 mg tid x 3 days; then 400-500 mg tid x 10 days; take with a meal

Pediatric: <2 years: not recommended; ≥2 years: same as adult

    Emverm *Chew tab:* 100 mg

    Vermox (G) *Chew tab:* 100 mg

▶ *pyrantel pamoate* (C) 11 mg/kg x 1 dose; max 1 g/dose; take with a meal

Pediatric: 25-37 lb: 1/2 tsp x 1 dose; 38-62 lb: 1 tsp x 1 dose; 63-87 lb: 1 tsp x 1 dose; 88-112 lb: 2 tsp x 1 dose; 113-137 lb: 2 tsp x 1 dose; 138-162 lb: 3 tsp x 1 dose; 163-187 lb: 3 tsp x 1 dose; >187 lb: 4 tsp x 1 dose

    Pin-X (OTC) *Cap:* 180 mg; *Liq:* 50 mg/ml (30 ml); 144 mg/ml (30 ml); *Oral susp:* 50 mg/ml (30 ml)

▶ *thiabendazole* (C) 25 mg/kg bid x 7 days; max 1.5 g/dose; take with a meal

Pediatric: same as adult; <30 lb: consult mfr pkg insert; ≥30 lb: 25 mg/kg in 2 divided doses/day with meals; 30-50 lbs: 250 mg bid with meals; >50 lb: 10 mg/lb/dose bid with meals; max 3g/day

    Mintezol *Chew tab:* 500*mg (orange); *Oral susp:* 500 mg/5 ml (120 ml) (orange)

Comment: *thiabendazole* is not for prophylaxis. May impair mental alertness.

TRICHOMONIASIS (*TRICHOMONAS VAGINALIS*)

Comment: The following treatment regimens for *Trichomoniasis* are published in the **2015 CDC Sexually Transmitted Diseases Treatment Guidelines**. Treat all sexual contacts. A multi-dose treatment regimen should be considered in HIV-positive women.

RECOMMENDED REGIMENS (NON-PREGNANT)

Regimen 1

▶ *metronidazole* 2 g once in a single dose

Regimen 2

▶ *tinidazole* 2 g once in a single dose

RECOMMENDED ALTERNATE REGIMEN

Regimen 1

▶ *metronidazole* 500 mg bid x 7 days

DRUG BRANDS AND DOSE FORMS

▶ *metronidazole* (not for use in 1st; B in 2nd, 3rd)(G)

    Flagyl *Tab:* 250*, 500*mg

    Flagyl 375 *Cap:* 375 mg

    Flagyl ER *Tab:* 750 mg ext-rel

Comment: Alcohol is contraindicated during treatment with oral *metronidazole* and for 72 hours after therapy due to a possible *disulfiram*-like reaction (nausea, vomiting, flushing, headache).

▷ *tinidazole* (not for use in 1st; B in 2nd, 3rd)
Tindamax *Tab:* 250*, 500*mg
Comment: Alcohol is contraindicated during treatment with oral *tinidazole* and for 72 hours after therapy due to a possible *disulfiram*-like reaction (nausea, vomiting, flushing, headache).

RECOMMENDED REGIMENS: PREGNANCY/LACTATION

Comment: All pregnant women should be considered for treatment. Women can be treated with 2 g *metronidazole* in a single dose at any stage of pregnancy. Lactating women who are administered *metronidazole* should be instructed to interrupt breastfeeding for 12-24 hours after receiving the 2 g dose of *metronidazole*.

TRIGEMINAL NEURALGIA (TIC DOULOUREUX)

▷ *baclofen* (C)(G) initially 5-10 mg tid with food; usual dose 10-80 mg/day
Pediatric: not recommended
Lioresal *Tab:* 10*, 20*mg
Tab: 10, 20 mg
Comment: Potential for seizures or hallucinations on abrupt withdrawal of *baclofen*.
▷ *carbamazepine* (C)
Carbatrol initially 200 mg bid; may increase weekly as needed by 200 mg/day; usual maintenance 800 mg-1.2 g/day
Pediatric: <12 years: max <35 mg/kg/day; use ext-rel form above 400 mg/day; 12-15 years: max 1 g/day in 2 divided doses; >15 years: usual maintenance 1.2 g/day in 2 divided doses
Cap: 200, 300 mg ext-rel
Tegretol (G) initially 100 mg bid or 1/2 tsp susp qid; may increase dose by 100 mg q 12 hours or by 1/2 tsp susp q 6 hours; usual maintenance 400-800 mg/day; max 1200 mg/day
Pediatric: <6 years: initially 10-20 mg/kg/day in 2 divided doses; increase weekly as needed in 3-4 divided doses; max 35 mg/kg/day in 3-4 divided doses; ≥6 years: initially 100 mg bid; increase weekly as needed by 100 mg/day in 3-4 divided doses; max 1 g/day in 3-4 divided doses
Tab: 200*mg; *Chew tab:* 100*mg; *Oral susp:* 100 mg/5 ml (450 ml) (citrus-vanilla)
Tegretol XR (G) initially 200 mg bid; may increase weekly by 200 mg/day in 2 divided doses
Pediatric: <6 years: use other forms; ≥6 years: initially 100 mg bid; may increase weekly by 100 mg/day in 2 divided doses; max 1 g/day
Tab: 100, 200, 400 mg ext-rel
▷ *clonazepam* (D)(IV)(G) initially 0.25 mg bid; increase to 1 mg/day after 3 days
Pediatric: <10 years, <30 kg: initially 0.1-0.3 mg/kg/day; may increase up to 0.05 mg/kg/day bid-tid; usual maintenance 0.1-0.2 mg/kg/day tid
Klonopin *Tab:* 0.5*, 1, 2 mg
Klonopin Wafers dissolve in mouth with or without water
Wafer: 0.125, 0.25, 0.5, 1, 2 mg orally-disint
▷ *divalproex sodium* (D) initially 250 mg bid; gradually increase to max 1000 mg/day if needed
Pediatric: <10 years: not recommended; ≥10 years: same as adult

Depakene *Cap:* 250 mg; *Syr:* 250 mg/5 ml
Depakote *Tab:* 125, 250 mg
Depakote ER *Tab:* 250, 500 mg ext-rel
Depakote Sprinkle *Cap:* 125 mg
▷ *phenytoin* (D) 400 mg/day in divided doses
Dilantin *Cap:* 30, 100 mg; *Oral susp:* 125 mg/5 ml (8 oz); *Infatab:* 50 mg
Comment: Monitor *phenytoin* serum levels. Therapeutic serum level: 10-20 g/ml.
Side effects include gingival hyperplasia.
▷ *valproic acid* (D) initially 15 mg/kg/day; may increase weekly by 5-10 mg/kg/day;
max 60 mg/kg/day <u>or</u> 250 mg/day
Depakene *Cap:* 250 mg; *Syr:* 250 mg/5 ml

TRICYCLIC ANTIDEPRESSANTS (TCAs)

Comment: Co-administration of TCAs with SSRIs requires extreme caution.
▷ *amitriptyline* (C)(G) titrate to achieve pain relief; max 300 mg/day
Pediatric: not recommended
Tab: 10, 25, 50, 75, 100, 150 mg
▷ *amoxapine* (C) titrate to achieve pain relief; if total dose exceeds 300 mg/day, give
in divided doses; max 400 mg/day
Pediatric: not recommended
Tab: 25, 50, 100, 150 mg
▷ *desipramine* (C)(G) titrate to achieve pain relief; max 300 mg/day
Pediatric: not recommended
Norpramin *Tab:* 10, 25, 50, 75, 100, 150 mg
▷ *doxepin* (C)(G) titrate to achieve pain relief; max 150 mg/day
Pediatric: not recommended
Cap: 10, 25, 50, 75, 100, 150 mg; *Oral conc:* 10 mg/ml (4 oz w. dropper)
▷ *imipramine* (C)(G)
Pediatric: not recommended
Tofranil titrate to achieve pain relief; max 200 mg/day; adolescents max 100
mg/day; if maintenance dose exceeds 75 mg/day, may switch to **Tofranil PM** at
bedtime
Tab: 10, 25, 50 mg
Tofranil PM titrate to achieve pain relief; initially 75 mg at HS; max 200 mg at HS
Cap: 75, 100, 125, 150 mg
Tofranil Injection 50 mg IM; lower dose for adolescents; switch to oral form as
soon as possible
Amp: 25 mg/2 ml (2 ml)
▷ *nortriptyline* (D)(G) titrate to achieve pain relief; initially 10-25 mg tid-qid; max
150 mg/day; lower doses for elderly and adolescents
Pediatric: not recommended
Pamelor titrate to achieve pain relief; max 150 mg/day
Cap: 10, 25, 50, 75 mg; *Oral soln:* 10 mg/5 ml (16 oz)
▷ *protriptyline* (C) titrate to achieve pain relief; initially 5 mg tid; max 60 mg/day
Pediatric: <12 years: not recommended
Vivactyl *Tab:* 5, 10 mg
▷ *trimipramine* (C) titrate to achieve pain relief; max 200 mg/day
Pediatric: not recommended
Surmontil *Cap:* 25, 50, 100 mg

**PULMONARY TUBERCULOSIS (TB)
(*MYCOBACTERIUM TUBERCULOSIS*)**

SCREENING

▷ *purified protein derivative (PPD)* **(C)** 0.1 ml intradermally; examine inoculation site
for induration at 48 to 72 hours.
Pediatric: same as adult
   Aplisol, Tubersol *Soln:* 5 US units/0.1 ml (1, 5 ml)

ANTI-TUBERCULAR AGENTS

Comment: Avoid *streptomycin* in pregnancy. *pyridoxine* (*vitamin B-6*) 25 mg once
daily x 6 months should be administered concomitantly with *INH* for prevention of
side effects. *rifapentine* produces red-orange discoloration of body tissues and body
fluids and may stain contact lenses.
▷ *bedaquiline* **(B)(G)**
   Sirturo *Tab:* 100 mg
   Comment: *bedaquiline* is a diarylquinoline antimycobacterial ATP synthase for the
   treatment of pulmonary multi-drug resistant TB (MDR-TB).
▷ *ethambutol (EMB)* **(B)(G)**
   Myambutol *Tab:* 100, 400*mg
▷ *isoniazid (INH)* **(C)** *Tab:* 300*mg
▷ *pyrazinamide (PZA)* **(C)** *Tab:* 500*mg
▷ *rifampin (RIF)* **(C)(G)**
   Rifadin, Rimactane *Cap:* 150, 300 mg
▷ *rifapentine* **(C)**
   Priftin *Tab:* 150 mg (24, 32 ct pck)
   Comment: The 32-count packs of **Priftin** are intended for patients with active
   tuberculosis infection (TB). The 24-count packs are are intended for patients
   with latent tuberculosis infection (LTBI) who are at high risk for progression to
   tuberculosis disease. **Priftin** for active TB is indicated for patients ≥12 years-of-age.
   Priftin for LTBI is indicated for patients ≥2 years-of-age.
▷ *rilipivirine* **(C)** *Tab:* 25 mg
   Rifabutin *Cap:* 150 mg
▷ *streptomycin (SM)* **(C)(G)** *Amp:* 1 g/2.5 ml <u>or</u> 400 mg/ml (2.5 ml)

COMBINATION AGENTS

▷ *rifampin/isoniazid* **(C)**
   Rifamate *Cap:* rif 300 mg/iso 150 mg
▷ *rifampin/isoniazid/pyrazinamide* **(C)**
   Rifater *Tab:* rif 120 mg/iso 50 mg/pyr 300 mg

PROPHYLAXIS AFTER EXPOSURE TO TUBERCULOSIS, WITH NEGATIVE PPD

▷ *isoniazid* **(C)** 300 mg once daily in a single dose x at least 6 months
Pediatric: 10-20 mg/kg/day x 9 months

PROPHYLAXIS AFTER EXPOSURE, WITH NEW PPD CONVERSION

▷ *isoniazid* **(C)** 300 mg once daily in a single dose x 12 months

Pediatric: 10-20 mg/kg/day x 9 months
Tab: 100, 300*mg; *Syr:* 50 mg/5 ml; *Inj:* 100 mg/ml
▷ *rifampin* (C) 600 mg once daily + *isoniazid* (C) 300 mg once daily x 4 months
Pediatric: rifampin (C) 10-20 mg/kg + *isoniazid* (C) 10-20 mg/kg once daily x 4 months
▷ *rifapentine* (C) 600 mg once weekly + *isoniazid* (C) 300 mg once weekly x 12 weeks
Pediatric: ≤12 years: Treat x 12 weeks; 10-14 kg: *rifapentine* (C) 300 mg once weekly + *isoniazid* (C) 25 mg/kg (max 900 mg) once weekly; 14.1-25 kg: *rifapentine* (C) 450 mg once weekly + *isoniazid* (C) 25 mg/kg (max 900 mg) once weekly; 25.1-32 kg: *rifapentine* (C) 600 mg once weekly + *isoniazid* (C) 25 mg/kg (max 900 mg) once weekly; 32.1-50 kg: *rifapentine* (C) 750 mg once weekly + *isoniazid* (C) 25 mg/kg (max 900 mg) once weekly; >50 kg: *rifapentine* (C) 900 mg once weekly + *isoniazid* (C) 25 mg/kg (max 900 mg) once weekly; >12 years: same as adult

ADULT TREATMENT REGIMENS (>12 YEARS)

Regimen 1

▷ *rifampin* (C) 600 mg + *isoniazid* (C) 300 mg + *pyrazinamide* (C) 2 g + *ethambutol* (C) 15-25 mg/kg or *streptomycin* (C) 1 g once daily x 8 weeks; then *isoniazid* (C) 300 mg + *rifampin* (C) 600 mg once daily x 16 weeks or *isoniazid* 900 mg + *rifampin* (C) 600 mg 2-3 times/week x 16 weeks

Regimen 2

▷ *rifampin* 600 mg + *isoniazid* 300 mg + *pyrazinamide* 2 g + *ethambutol* 15-25 mg/kg or *streptomycin* 1 g once daily x 2 weeks; then *rifampin* 600 mg + *isoniazid* 900 mg + *pyrazinamide* 4 g + *ethambutol* 50 mg/kg or *streptomycin* 1.5 g 2 times/week x 6 weeks; then *isoniazid* 300 mg + *rifampin* 600 mg once daily x 16 weeks or 2 times/week x 16 weeks *rifampin* 600 mg once daily x 16 weeks or 2 times/week x 16 weeks

Regimen 3

▷ *rifampin* 600 mg + *isoniazid* 900 mg + *pyrazinamide* 3 g + *ethambutol* 25-30 mg/kg or *streptomycin* 1.5 g 3 times/week x 6 months

Regimen 4 (for smear and culture negative for pulmonary TB in adult)

▷ Options 1, 2, or 3 x 8 weeks; then *isoniazid* 300 mg + *rifampin* 600 mg once daily x 16 weeks; then *rifampin* 600 mg + *isoniazid* 300 mg + *pyrazinamide* 2 g + *ethambutol* 15-25 mg/kg or *streptomycin* 1 g once daily x 8 weeks or 2-3 times/week x 8 weeks

Regimen 5 (for smear and culture negative for pulmonary TB in adult)

▷ *rifanpentine* 600 mg twice weekly x 2 months (at least 72 hours between doses) + once daily *isoniazid* 300 mg, *ethambutol* 15-25 mg/kg + *pyrazinamide* 2 g; then *rifanpentine* 600 mg once weekly x 4 months + once daily *isoniazid* 300 mg + another appropriate anti-tuberculosis agent for susceptible organisms

Regimen 6 (when pyrazinamide is contraindicated)

▷ *rifampin* 600 mg + *isoniazid* 300 mg + *ethambutol* 15-25 mg/kg + *streptomycin* 1 g once daily x 4-8 weeks; then *isoniazid* 300 mg + *rifampin* 600 mg once daily x 24 weeks or 2 x/week x 24 weeks

PEDIATRIC TREATMENT REGIMENS

Regimen 1

▷ *rifampin* 10-20 mg/kg + *isoniazid* 10-20 mg/kg + *pyrazinamide* 15-20 mg/kg + *ethambutol* 15-25 mg/kg or *streptomycin* 20-40 mg/kg once daily x 8 weeks; then *isoniazid* 10-20 mg/kg + *rifampin* 10-20 mg/kg once daily x 16 weeks or *isoniazid* 20-40 mg/kg + *rifampin* 10-20 mg/kg 2-3 times/week x 16 weeks

Regimen 2

▷ *rifampin* 10-20 mg/kg + *isoniazid* 10-20 mg/kg + *pyrazinamide* 15-30 mg/kg + *ethambutol* 15-25 mg/kg or *streptomycin* 20-40 mg/kg once daily x 2 weeks; then *rifampin* 10-20 mg/kg + *isoniazid* 20-40 mg/kg + *pyrazinamide* 50-70 mg/kg + *ethambutol* 50 mg/kg or *streptomycin* 25-30 mg/kg 2 times/week x 6 weeks; then *isoniazid* 10-20 mg/kg + *rifampin* 10-20 mg/kg once daily x 16 weeks or *rifampin* 10-20 mg/kg + *isoniazid* 20-40 mg/kg 2 times/week x 16 weeks

Regimen 3

▷ *rifampin* 10-20 mg/kg + *isoniazid* 20-40 mg/kg + *pyrazinamide* 50-70 mg/kg + *ethambutol* 25-30 mg/kg or *streptomycin* 25-30 mg/kg 3 times/week x 6 months

Regimen 4 (when pyrazinamide is contraindicated)

▷ *rifampin* 10-20 mg/kg + *isoniazid* 10-20 mg/kg + *ethambutol* 15-25 mg/kg + *streptomycin* 20-40 mg/kg once daily x 4-8 weeks; then *isoniazid* 10-20 mg/kg + *rifampin* 10-20 mg/kg once daily x 24 weeks or *rifampin* 10-20 mg/kg + *isoniazid* 20-40 mg/kg 2 x/week x 24 weeks

◯ TYPE 1 DIABETES MELLITUS

Comment: Target glycosylated hemoglobin (HbA1c) is <7%. Addition of daily ACE-I and/or ARB therapy is strongly recommended for renal protection. Insulin may be indicated in the management of Type 2 diabetes with or without concomitant oral anti-diabetic agents.

TREATMENT FOR ACUTE HYPOGLYCEMIA

▷ *glucagon (recombinant)* (B) administer SC, IM, or IV; if patient does not respond in 15 minutes, may administer a single dose or 2 divided doses; <20 kg: 0.5 mg or 20-30 mg/kg; ≥20 kg: 1 mg
Pediatric: same as adult

INHALED INSULIN

Rapid-Acting Inhalation Powder Insulin

▷ *insulin human (inhaled)* (C) one inhaler may be used for up to 15 days, then discard; dose at meal times as follows: *Insulin naïve:* initially 4 units at each meal; adjust according to blood glucose monitoring
Conversion from SC to inhaled mealtime insulin:
SC 1-4 units: inhal 4 units
SC 5-8 units: inhal 8 units

SC 9-12 units: inhal 12 units
SC 13-16 units: inhal 16 units
SC 17-20 units: inhal 20 units
SC 21-24 units: inhal 24 units
Pediatric: <18 years: not established

Afrezza Inhalation Powder administer at the beginning of the meal; *Mealtime insulin naïve:* initially 4 units at each meal; *Using SC prandial insulin:* convert dose to **Afrezza** using a conversion table (see mfr pkg insert); *Using SC pre-mixed:* divide 1/2 of total daily injected pre-mixed insulin equally among 3 meals of the day; administer 1/2 total injected pre-mixed dose as once daily injected basal insulin dose

Inhal: 4, 8, 12 unit single-inhalation color-coded cartridges (30, 60, 90/pkg w. 2 disposable inhalers)

Comment: **Afrezza** is not a substitute for long-acting insulin. **Afrezza** must be used in combination with long-acting insulin in patients with T1DM. **Afrezza** is not recommended for the treatment of diabetic ketoacidosis. **Afrezza** is contraindicated with chronic lung disease because of the risk of acute bronchospasm. The use of **Afrezza** is not recommended in patients who smoke <u>or</u> who have recently stopped smoking. Each card contains 5 blister strips with 3 cartridges each (total 15 cartridges). The doses are color-coded. **Afrezza** is contraindicated with chronic respiratory disease (e.g., asthma, COPD) and patients prone to episodes of hypoglycaemia.

INJECTABLE INSULINS

Rapid-Acting Insulins

▷ *insulin aspart (recombinant)* **(B)** onset <15 minutes; peak 1-3 hours; duration 3-5 hours; administer 5-10 minutes prior to a meal; SC <u>or</u> infusion pump <u>or</u> IV infusion
Pediatric: <3 years: not recommended; ≥3 years: same as adult
NovoLog *Vial:* 100 U/ml (10 ml); *PenFill cartridge:* 100 U/ml (3 ml, 5/pk) (zinc, m-cresol)

▷ *insulin glulisine (rDNA origin)* **(C)** onset <15 minutes; peak 1 hour; duration 2-4 hours; administer up to 15 minutes before, <u>or</u> within 20 minutes after starting a meal; use with an intermediate <u>or</u> long-acting insulin; SC only; may administer via insulin pump; do not dilute <u>or</u> mix with other insulin in pump
Pediatric: <4 years: not recommended; ≥4 years: same as adult
Apidra *Vial:* 100 U/ml (10 ml); *Cartridge:* 100 U/ml (3 ml, 5/pck; m-cresol)

▷ *insulin lispro (recombinant)* **(B)** onset <15 minutes; peak 1 hour; duration 3.5-4.5 hours; administer up to 15 minutes before, <u>or</u> immediately after, a meal; SC <u>or</u> IV infusion pump only
Pediatric: <3 years: not recommended; ≥3 years: same as adult
Humalog
Vial: 100 U/ml (10 ml); *Prefilled disposable KwikPen:* 100 U/ml (3 ml, 5/pck) (zinc, m-cresol); *HumaPen Memoir* and *HumaPen Luxura* HD inj device for *Humulog cartridges* (100 U/ml, 3 ml 5/pck) (zinc, m-cresol)

▷ *insulin regular* **(B)**
Humulin R U-100 *(human, recombinant)* **(OTC)** onset 30 minutes; peak 2-4 hours; duration up to 6-8 hours; SC <u>or</u> IV <u>or</u> IM
Vial: 100 U/ml (10 ml)
Humulin R U-500 *(human, recombinant)* onset 30 minutes; peak 1.75-4 hours; duration up to 24 hours; SC only; for in-hospital use only

Vial: 500 U/ml (20 ml); *KwikPen:* 3 ml (2, 5/carton)

Comment: Humulin R U-500 formulation is 5 times more concentrated than standard U-100 concentration, indicated for adults and children who require ≥200 units of insulin/day, allowing patients to inject 80% less liquid to receive the desired dose. Recommend using U-500 syringe (BD, Eli Lilly). The U-500 syringe (0.5 ml, 6 mm x 31 gauge) is marked in 5 unit increments and allows for dosing up to 250 units.

Iletin II Regular *(pork)* **(OTC)** onset 30 minutes; peak 2-4 hours; duration 6-8 hours; SC, IV or IM

Vial: 100 U/ml (10 ml)

Novolin R *(human)* **(OTC)** onset 30 minutes; peak 2.5-5 hours; duration 8 hours; SC, IV, or IM

Vial: 100 U/ml (10 ml); *PenFill cartridge:* 100 U/ml (1.5 ml, 5/pck); *Prefilled syringe:* 100 U/ml (1.5 ml, 5/pck)

▷ *pramlintide* (*amylin analogue/amylinomimetic*) **(C)** administer immediately before major meals (≥250 kcal or ≥30 g carbohydrates); initially 15 mcg; titrate in 15 mcg increments for 3 days if no significant nausea occurs; if nausea occurs at 45 or 60 mcg, reduce to 30 mcg; if not tolerated, consider discontinuing therapy; *Maintenance:* 60 mcg (30 mcg *only* if 60 mcg not tolerated)

Symlin *Vial:* 0.6 mg/ml (5 ml) (m-cresol, mannitol)

Comment: Symlin is indicated as adjunct to mealtime insulin with or without a sulfonylurea and/or **metformin** when blood glucose control is suboptimal despite optimal insulin therapy. Do not mix with insulin. When initiating **Symlin**, reduce preprandial short/rapid-acting insulin dose by 50% and monitor pre- and post-prandial and bedtime blood glucose. Do not use in patients with poor compliance, HgbA1c is >9%, recurrent hypoglycemia requiring assistance in the previous 6 months, or if taking a prokinetic drug. With Type 2 DM, initial therapy is 60 mcg/dose and max is 120 mcg/dose.

RAPID-ACTING AND INTERMEDIATE-ACTING INSULIN

Insulin Aspart Protamine Suspension/Insulin Aspart Combinations

▷ *insulin aspart protamine suspension 70%/insulin aspart 30%* (*recombinant*) **(B)** onset 15 min; peak 2.4 hours; duration up to 24 hours; SC only
Pediatric: not recommended

NovoLog Mix 70/30 (OTC) *Vial:* 100 U/ml (10 ml)

NovoLog Mix 70/30 FlexPen (OTC) *Prefilled disposable pen:* 100 U/ml (3 ml, 5/pck); *PenFill cartridge:* 100 U/ml (3 ml, 5/pck)

LONG-ACTING INSULINS

▷ *insulin detemir (human)* **(B)** administer SC once daily with evening meal or at HS as a basal insulin; may administer twice daily (AM/PM); administer in the deltoid, abdomen, or thigh; onset 1-2 hours; peak 6-8 hours; duration 24 hours; switching from another basal insulin, dose should be the same on a unit-to-unit basis; may need more *insulin detemir* when switching from **NPH**; *Type 1:* starting dose 1/3 of total daily insulin requirements; rapid-acting or short-acting, pre-meal insulin should be used to satisfy the remainder of daily insulin requirements; *Type 2 (inadequately controlled on oral antidiabetic agents):* initially 10 units or 0.1-0.2 units/kg, once daily in the evening or divided twice daily (AM/PM); do not add-mix or dilute *insulin detemir* with other insulins.

Pediatric: <2 years: not recommended; ≥2 years: same as adult
Levemir *Vial:* 100 U/ml (10 ml); *FlexPen:* 100 U/ml (3 ml, 5/pck; (zinc, m-cresol)
Comment: Do not mix or dilute ***insulin detemir*** with other insulins.
▷ *insulin glargine (recombinant)* (C)
    Basaglar administer SC once daily, at the same time each day, as a basal insulin in the deltoid, abdomen, or thigh; onset 1-1.5 hours, no pronounced peak, duration 20-24 hours; *T1DM (adults and children >6 years-of-age):* initially 1/3 of total daily insulin dose; administer the remainder of the total dose as short- or rapid-acting pre-prandial insulin; *T2DM (adults only):* initially 2 units/kilogram or up to 10 units once daily; *Switching from once daily insulin glargine 300 units/ml (i.e., **Toujeo**) to 100 units/ml:* initially 80% of the insulin glargine 300 units/ml; *Switching from twice daily NPH:* initially 80% of the total daily NPH dose; do not add-mix or dilute ***insulin glargine*** with other insulins.
    Pediatric: <6 years: not established; ≥6 years: individualize and adjust as needed
        Prefilled KwikPen (disposable), 100 U/ml (3 ml)
    Lantus administer SC once daily at the same time each day as a basal insulin; onset 1-1.5 hours, no pronounced peak, duration 20-24 hours; initial average starting dose 10 units for insulin-naïve patients; *Switching from once daily NPH or Ultralente insulin:* initial dose of ***insulin glargine*** should be on a unit-for-unit basis; *Switching from twice daily NPH insulin:* start at 20% lower than the total daily ***NPH*** dose
        Pediatric: <6 years: not recommended; ≥6 years: same as adult
        Vial: 100 U/ml (10 ml); *Cartridge:* 100 U/ml (3 ml, for use in the *OptiPen One Insulin Delivery Device*) (5/carton) (m-cresol); *SoloStar pen (disposable):* 100 U/ml (3 ml) (5/carton)
    Toujeo administer SC once daily at the same time each day as a basal insulin; in the upper arm, abdomen, or thigh; onset of action 6 hours; duration 20-24 hours; *T2DM, insulin naïve:* initially 0.2 units/kg; titrate every 3-4 days; *T1DM, insulin naïve:* initially 1/3-1/2 total daily insulin dose; remainder as short-acting insulin divided between each meal; *Switch from once daily long- or intermediate-acting insulin:* on a unit-for-unit basis; *Switching from **Lantus:*** a higher daily dose is expected; *Switching from twice daily NPH:* reduce initial dose by 20% of total daily NPH dose
        Pediatric: <18 years: not established
        Soln for SC injection: 300 units/ml prefilled disposable SoloStar Pen (1.5 ml, 3-5/carton)
▷ *insulin isophane suspension (NPH)* (B)
    Humulin N *(human, recombinant)* (OTC) onset 1-2 hours; peak 6-12 hours; duration 18-24 hours; SC only
        Vial: 100 U/ml (10 ml); *Prefilled disposable pen:* 100 U/ml (3 ml, 5/pck)
    Novolin N *(recombinant)* (OTC) onset 1.5 hours; peak 4-12 hours; duration 24 hours; SC only
        Vial: 100 U/ml (10 ml); *PenFill cartridge:* 1.5 ml (5/pck); *KwikPens:* 1.5 ml (5/pck)
    Iletin II NPH *(pork)* (OTC) onset 1-2 hours; peak 6-12 hours; duration 18-26 hours; SC only
        Vial: 100 U/ml (10 ml)
▷ *insulin zinc suspension (lente)* (B)
    Pediatric: <18 years: not recommended
    Humulin L *(human)* (OTC) onset 1-3 hours; peak 6-12 hours; duration 18-24 hours; SC only
        Vial: 100 U/ml (10 ml)

Iletin II Lente *(pork)* (OTC) onset 1-3 hours; peak 6-12 hours; duration 18-26 hours; SC only
>   *Vial:* 100 U/ml (10 ml)
Novolin L *(human)* (OTC) onset 2.5 hours; peak 7-15 hours; duration 22 hours; SC only
>   *Vial:* 100 U/ml (10 ml)

Ultra Long-Acting Insulin

▷ *insulin deglutec (insulin analog)* (C) administer by SC injection once daily at any time of day, with or without food, into the upper arm, abdomen, or thigh; titrate every 3-4 days; *Insulin naïve with type 1 diabetes:* initially 1/3-1/2 of total daily insulin dose, usually 0.2-0.4 units/kg; administer the remainder of the total dose as short-acting insulin divided between each daily meal; *Insulin naive with type 2 diabetes:* initially 10 units once daily; adjust dose of concomitant oral antidiabetic agent; *Already on insulin (type 1 or type 2):* initiate at same unit dose as total daily long- or intermediate-acting insulin unit dose
Pediatric: <1 year: not established; ≥1 year: same as adult
>   Tresiba FlexTouch *Pen:* 100 U/ml (3 ml, 5 pens/carton), 200 U/ml (3 ml, 3 pens/carton) (zinc, m-cresol)

Comment: Tresiba U-200 FlexTouch is the only long-acting insulin in a 160-unit pen allowing up to 160 units in a single injection. The U-200 dose counter always shows the desired dose (i.e., no conversion from U/100 to U-200 is required)
▷ *insulin extended zinc suspension (Ultralente) (human)* (B) onset 4-6 hours; peak 8-20 hours; duration 24-48 hours; SC only
Pediatric: <18 years: not recommended
>   Humulin U (OTC) *Vial:* 100 U/ml (10 ml)

Insulin Lispro Protamine/Insulin Lispro Combinations

▷ *insulin lispro protamine75%/insulin lispro 25%* (B)
Pediatric: <18 years: not recommended
>   Humalog Mix 75/25 *(human)* onset 15 minutes; peak 30 minutes to 1 hour; duration 24 hours; SC only
>   *Vial:* 100 U/ml (10 ml); *Prefilled disposable KwikPen:* 100 U/ml (3 ml, 5/pck) (zinc, m-cresol); *HumaPen Memoir* and *HumaPen Luxura* HD inj device for *Humalog cartridges* (100 U/ml, 3 ml, 5/pck) (zinc, m-cresol)
▷ *insulin lispro protamine 50%/insulin lispro 50%* (B)
Pediatric: <18 years: not recommended
>   Humalog Mix 50/50 *(recombinant)* (B) onset 15 minutes; peak 2.3 hours; range 1-5 hours; SC only
>   *Vial:* 100 U/ml (10 ml); *Prefilled disposable KwikPen:* 100 U/ml (3 ml, 5/pck) (zinc, m-cresol); *HumaPen Memoir* and *Huma-Pen Luxura* HD inj device for *Humalog cartridges* (100 U/ml, 3 ml, 5/pck) (zinc, m-cresol)

Insulin Isophane Suspension (NPH)/Insulin Regular Combinations

▷ *NPH 70%/regular 30%* (B)
Pediatric: same as adult
>   Humulin 70/30 *(human, recombinant)* (OTC) onset 30 minutes; peak 2-12 hours; duration up to 24 hours; SC only
>   *Vial:* 100 U/ml (10 ml)

Novolin 70/30 *(recombinant)* **(OTC)** onset 30 minutes; peak 2-12 hours; duration up to 24 hours; SC only
> *Vial:* 100 U/ml (10 ml)

▷ *NPH 50%/regular 50% (B)*
> *Pediatric:* <18 years: not recommended
> Humulin 50/50 *(human)* **(OTC)** onset 30 minutes; peak 3-5 hours; duration up to 24 hours; SC only
> > *Vial:* 100 U/ml (10 ml)

Insulin Lispro Protamine/Insulin Lispro Combinations

▷ *insulin lispro protamine 75%/insulin lispro 25% (B)*
> *Pediatric:* <18 years: not recommended
> Humalog Mix 75/25 *(recombinant)* onset 15 minutes; peak 30-90 minutes; duration 24 hours; SC only
> > *Vial:* 100 U/ml (10 ml); *Prefilled disposable KwikPen:* 100 U/ml (3 ml, 5/pck) (zinc, m-cresol); *HumaPen Memoir* and *Huma-Pen Luxura* HD inj device for *Humalog cartridges* (100 U/ml, 3 ml 5/pck) (zinc, m-cresol)

▷ *insulin lispro protamine 50%/insulin lispro 50% (B)*
> *Pediatric:* <18 years: not recommended
> Humalog Mix 50/50 *(recombinant)* onset 15 minutes; peak 1 hour; duration up to 16 hours; SC only
> > *Vial:* 100 U/ml (10 ml); *Prefilled disposable KwikPen:* 100 U/ml (3 ml, 5/pck) (zinc, m-cresol); *HumaPen Memoir* and *HumaPen LUXURA* HD inj device for *Humalog cartridges* (100 U/ml, 3 ml 5/pck) (zinc, m-cresol); U/ml (3 ml, 5/pck) (zinc, m-cresol); *HumaPen Memoir* and *HumaPen LUXURA* HD inj device for *Humalog cartridges* (100 U/ml, 3 ml 5/pck) (zinc, m-cresol); (100 U/ml, 3 ml 5/pck (zinc, m-cresol)

Basal Insulin/GLP-1 RA Combinations

▷ *insulin degludec (insulin analog)/liraglutide* **(C)** for treatment of type 2 diabetes only in adults inadequately controlled on <50 units of basal insulin daily or ≤1.8 mg of *liraglutide* daily; administer by SC injection once daily, with or without food, into the upper arm, abdomen, or thigh; titrate every 3-4 days
> *Pediatric:* <18 years: not recommended
> *Xultophy Prefilled pen:* 100/3.6 U/ml (3 ml, 5 pens/carton)

▷ *insulin glargine (insulin analog)/lixisenatide* **(C)** for treatment of type 2 diabetes only in adults inadequately controlled on <60 units of basal insulin daily or lixisenatide; administer by SC injection once daily, with or without food, into the upper arm, abdomen, or thigh; titrate every 3-4 days
> *Pediatric:* <18 years: not recommended
> *Soliqua Prefilled pen:* 100/33 U/ml (3 ml, 5 pens/carton) covering 15-60 mg *insulin glargine* 100 units/ml and 15-20 mcg of *lixisenatide (m-cresol)*

◯ TYPE 2 DIABETES MELLITUS

Comment: Normal fasting glucose is <100 mg/dL. Impaired glucose tolerance is a risk factor for type 2 diabetes and a marker for cardiovascular disease risk; it occurs early in the natural history of these two diseases. Impaired fasting glucose is >100 mg/dL and <125 mg/dL. Impaired glucose tolerance is OGTT, 2 hour post-load 75 g glucose >140 mg/dL and <200 mg/dL. Target pre-prandial glucose is 80 mg/dL to 120 mg/dL. Target bedtime glucose is 100mg/dL to 140 mg/dL. Target glycosylated hemoglobin (HbA1c) is <7.0%. Addition of daily ACE-I and/or ARB therapy is strongly recommended for renal protection. Consider diabetes screening at age 25 years for persons in high-risk groups (non-Caucasian, positive family history for DM, obesity). Hypertension and hyperlipidemia are common comorbid conditions. Macrovascular complications include cerebral vascular disease, coronary artery disease, and peripheral vascular disease. Microvascular complications include retinopathy, nephropathy, neuropathy, and cardiomyopathy. Oral hypoglycemics are contraindicated in pregnancy.

Insulins *see Type 1 Diabetes Mellitus page* 426

TREATMENT FOR ACUTE HYPOGLYCEMIA

▷ *glucagon (recombinant)* (B) administer SC, IM, or IV; if patient does not respond in 15 minutes, may administer a single or 2 divided doses
Adults and Children: <20 kg: 0.5 mg or 20-30 mg/kg; >20 kg: 1 mg

SULFONYLUREAS

Comment: Sulfonylureas are secretagogues (i.e., stimulate pancreatic insulin secretion); therefore, the patient taking a sulfonylurea should be alerted to the risk for hypoglycemia. Action is dependent on functioning beta cells in the pancreatic islets.

1st Generation Sulfonylureas

▷ *chlorpropamide* (C)(G) initially 250 mg/day with breakfast; max 750 mg
Pediatric: not recommended
    Diabinese *Tab:* 100*, 250*mg
▷ *tolazamide* (C)(G) initially 100-250 mg/day with breakfast; increase by 100-250 mg/day at weekly intervals; maintenance 100 mg 1 g/day; max 1 g/day
Pediatric: not recommended
    Tolinase *Tab:* 100, 250, 500 mg
▷ *tolbutamide* (C) initially 1-2 g in divided doses; max 2 g/day
Pediatric: not recommended
    Tab: 500 mg

2nd Generation Sulfonylureas

▷ *glimepiride* (C) initially 1-2 mg once daily with breakfast; after reaching dose of 2 mg, increase by 2 mg at 1-2 week intervals as needed; usual maintenance 1-4 mg once daily; max 8 mg/day
Pediatric: not recommended
    Amaryl *Tab:* 1*, 2*, 4*mg
▷ *glipizide* (C)(G)
Pediatric: not recommended
    Glucotrol initially 5 mg before breakfast; increase by 2.5-5 mg every few days if needed; max 15 mg/day; max 40 mg/day in divided doses
      Tab: 5*, 10* mg
    Glucotrol XL initially 5 mg with breakfast; usual range 5-10 mg/day; max 20 mg/day
      Tab: 2.5, 5, 10 mg ext-rel

▷ *glyburide* (C)(G) initially 2.5-5 mg/day with breakfast; increase by 2.5 mg at weekly intervals; maintenance 1.25-20 mg/day in a single or 2 divided doses; max 20 mg/day
Pediatric: not recommended
    DiaBeta, Micronase *Tab:* 1.25*, 2.5*, 5*mg

▷ *glyburide, micronized* (B)
Pediatric: not recommended
    Glynase PresTab initially 1.5-3 mg/day with breakfast; increase by 1.5 mg at weekly intervals if needed; usual maintenance 0.75-12 mg/day in single or divided doses; max 12 mg/day
        Tab: 1.5*, 3*, 6*mg

ALPHA-GLUCOSIDASE INHIBITORS

Comment: Alpha-glucosidase inhibitors block the enzyme that breaks down carbo-hydrates in the small intestine, delaying digestion and absorption of complex carbo-hydrates, and lowering peak post-prandial glycemic concentrations. Use as monotherapy or in combination with a sulfonylurea. Contraindicated in inflammatory bowel disease, colon ulceration, and intestinal obstruction. Side effects include flatulence, diarrhea, and abdominal pain.

▷ *acarbose* (B) initially 25 mg tid ac, increase at 4-8 week intervals; or initially 25 mg once daily, increase gradually to 25 mg tid; usual range 50-100 mg tid; max 100 mg tid
Pediatric: not recommended
    Precose *Tab:* 25, 50, 100 mg

▷ *miglitol* (B) initially 25 mg tid at the start of each main meal, titrated to 50 mg tid at the start of each main meal; max 100 mg tid
Pediatric: not recommended
    Glyset *Tab:* 25, 50, 100 mg

BIGUANIDE

Comment: The biguanides decrease gluconeogenesis by the liver in the presence of insulin. Action is dependent on the presence of circulating insulin. Lower hepatic glucose production leads to lower overnight, fasting, and pre-prandial plasma glucose levels. Common side effects include GI distress, nausea, vomiting, bloating, and flatulence which usually eventually resolve. May be used as monotherapy (in adults only) or with a sulfonylurea or insulin.

▷ *metformin* (B)(G) take with meals
Comment: *metformin* is contraindicated with renal impairment, metabolic acidosis, ketoacidosis. Suspend *metformin*, prior to, and for 48 hours after, surgery or receiving IV iodinated contrast agents.
    Fortamet initially 1000 mg once daily; may increase by 500 mg/day at 1 week intervals; max 2.5 g/day
        Pediatric: <17 years: not recommended
        Tab: 500, 1000 mg ext-rel
    Glucophage initially 500 mg bid; may increase by 500 mg/day at 1 week intervals; max 1 g bid or 2.5 g in 3 divided doses; or initially 850 mg once daily in AM; may increase by 850 mg/day in divided doses at 2 week intervals; max 2000 mg/day; take with meals

Pediatric: <10 years: not recommended; ≥10-16 years: use only as monotherapy; dose same as adult
Tab: 500, 850, 1000*mg

Glucophage XR initially 500 mg by mouth every evening; may increase by 500 mg/day at 1 week intervals; max 2 g/day
Pediatric: <10 years: not recommended; ≥10-16 years: use immediate release form; >16 years: same as adult
Tab: 500, 750 mg ext-rel

Glumetza ER (G) initially 1000 mg once daily; may increase by 500 mg/day at week intervals; max 2 g/day
Pediatric: <18 years: not recommended
Tab: 500, 1000 mg ext-rel

Riomet XR initially 500 mg once daily; may increase by 500 mg/day at 1 week intervals; max 2 g/day in divided doses; take with meals
Pediatric: <10 years: not recommended; ≥10 years: monotherapy only
Oral soln: 500 mg/ml (4 oz; cherry)

MEGLITINIDES

Comment: Meglitinides are secretagogues (i.e., stimulate pancreatic insulin secretion) in response to a meal. Action is dependent on functioning beta cells in the pancreatic islets. Use as monotherapy or in combination with *metformin*.

➤ *nateglinide* (C) 60-120 mg tid ac 1-30 minutes prior to start of the meal
Pediatric: not recommended
Starlix *Tab:* 60, 120 mg

➤ *repaglinide* (C)(G) initially 0.5 mg with 2-4 meals/day; take 30 minutes ac; titrate by doubling dose at intervals of at least 1 week; range 0.5-4 mg with 2-4 meals/day; max 16 mg/day
Pediatric: not recommended
Prandin *Tab:* 0.5, 1, 2 mg

THIAZOLIDINEDIONES (TZDs)

Comment: The TZDs decrease hepatic gluconeogenesis and reduce insulin resistance (i.e., increase glucose uptake and utilization by the muscles). Liver function tests are indicated before initiating these drugs. Do not start if ALT more than 3 times greater than normal. Recheck ALT monthly for the first six months of therapy; then every two months for the remainder of the first year and periodically thereafter. Liver function tests should be obtained at the first symptoms suggestive of hepatic dysfunction (nausea, vomiting, fatigue, dark urine, anorexia, abdominal pain).

➤ *pioglitazone* (C)(G) initially 15-30 mg once daily; max 45 mg/day as a monotherapy; usual max 30 mg/day in combination with *metformin*, insulin, or a sulfonylurea
Pediatric: <18 years: not recommended
Actos *Tab:* 15, 30, 45 mg

➤ *rosiglitazone* (C)(G) initially 4 mg/day in a single or 2 divided doses; may increase after 8-12 weeks; max 8 mg/day as a monotherapy or combination therapy with *metformin* or a sulfonylurea; not for use with *insulin*
Pediatric: <18 years: not recommended
Avandia *Tab:* 2, 4, 8 mg

DIPEPTIDYL PEPTIDASE-4 (DPP-4) INHIBITOR/THIAZOLIDINEDIONE COMBINATION

Comment: The FDA has reported that alogliptin-containing drugs may increase the risk of heart failure, especially in patients who already have cardiovascular or renal disease. The drug Oseni (*alogliptin/pioglitazone*) is in this risk group.

▷ *alogliptin/pioglitazone* (C) take 1 dose once daily with first meal of the day; max: *rosiglitazone* 8 mg and max *glimepiride* per day; Same precautions as *alogliptin* and *pioglitazone*

Pediatric: <18 years: not recommended

    Oseni

       Tab: **Oseni 12.5/15:** *alo* 12.5 mg/*pio* 15 mg;
             Oseni 12.5/30: *alo* 12.5 mg/*pio* 30 mg
             Oseni 12.5/45: *alo* 12.5 mg/*pio* 45 mg
             Oseni 25/15: *alo* 25/*pio* 15 mg
             Oseni 25/30: *alo* 25/*pio* 30 mg
             Oseni 25/45: *alo* 25 mg/*pio* 45 mg

2ND GENERATION SULFONYLUREA/BIGUANIDE COMBINATIONS

Comment: *Metaglip* and *Glucovance* are combination secretagogues (sulfonylureas) and insulin sensitizers (biguanides). *Sulfonylurea:* Action is dependent on functioning beta cells in the pancreatic islets; patient should be alerted to the risk for hypoglycemia. Common side effects of the biguanide include GI distress, nausea, vomiting, bloating, and flatulence which usually eventually resolve. Take with food. *metformin* is contraindicated with renal impairment, metabolic acidosis, ketoacidosis. Suspend *metformin*, prior to, and for 48 hours after, surgery or receiving IV iodinated contrast agents.

▷ *glipizide/metformin* (C) take with meals; *Primary therapy:* 2.5/250 once daily or if FBS is 280-320 mg/dL, may start at 2.5/250 bid; may increase by 1 tab/day every 2 weeks; max 10/2000 per day in 2 divided doses; *Second Line Therapy:* 2.5/500 or 5/500 bid; may increase by up to 5/500 every 2 weeks; max: 20/2000 per day; Same precautions as *glipizide* and *metformin*

Pediatric: not recommended

    Metaglip

       Tab: **Metaglip 2.5/250:** *glip* 2.5 mg/*met* 250 mg
             Metaglip 2.5/500: *glip* 2.5 mg/*met* 500 mg
             Metaglip 5/500: *glip* 5 mg/*met* 500 mg

▷ *glyburide/metformin* (B) take with meals; *Primary therapy (initial therapy if HgbA1c <9.0%):* initially 1.25/250 once daily; max *glyburide* 20 mg and *metformin* 2000 mg per day; *Primary therapy (initial therapy if HbA1c >9.0% or FBS >200):* initially 1.25/250 bid; max *glyburide* 20 mg and *metformin* 2000 mg per day; *Second line therapy (initial therapy if HbA1c >7.0%):* initially 2.5/500 or 5/500 bid; max *glyburide* 20 mg and *metformin* 2000 mg per day; *Previously treated with a sulfonylurea and metformin:* dose to approximate total daily doses of *glyburide* and *metformin* already being taken; max: *glyburide* 20 mg and *metformin* 2000 mg per day; Same precautions as *glyburide* and *metformin*

Pediatric: not recommended

    Glucovance

       Tab: **Glucovance 1.25/250:** *glyb* 1.25 mg/*met* 250 mg
             Glucovance 2.5/500: *glyb* 2.5 mg/*met* 500 mg

Glucovance 5/500: *glyb* 5 mg/*met* 500 mg

Comment: *metformin* is contraindicated with renal impairment, metabolic acidosis, ketoacidosis. Suspend *metformin*, prior to, and for 48 hours after, surgery or receiving IV iodinated contrast agents.

THIAZOLIDINEDIONE/BIGUANIDE COMBINATION

▶ *pioglitazone/metformin* (C) take in divided doses with meals; *Previously on metformin alone:* initially 15mg/500mg or 15mg/850 mg once or twice daily; *Previously on pioglitazone alone:* initially 15mg/500mg bid; *Previously on pioglitazone and metformin:* switch on a mg/mg basis; may increase after 8-12 weeks; max: *pioglitazone* 45 mg and *metformin* 2000 mg per day; Same precautions as *pioglitazone* and *metformin*
Pediatric: not recommended

    Actoplus Met, Actoplis Met R (G)
      Tab: **Actoplus Met 15/500:** *pio* 15 mg/*met* 500 mg
           Actoplus Met 15/850: *pio* 15 mg/*met* 850 mg
           Actoplus Met XR 15/1000: *pio* 15 mg/*met* 1000 mg
           Actoplus Met XR 30/1000: *pio* 30 mg/*met* 1000 mg

Comment: *metformin* is contraindicated with renal impairment, metabolic acidosis, ketoacidosis. Suspend *metformin*, prior to, and for 48 hours after, surgery or receiving IV iodinated contrast agents.

▶ *rosiglitazone/metformin* (C) take in divided doses with meals; *Previously on metformin alone:* add *rosiglitazone* 4 mg/day; may increase after 8-12 weeks; *Previously on rosiglitazone alone:* add *metformin* 1000 mg/day; may increase after 1-2 weeks; *Previously on rosiglitazone and metformin:* switch on a mg/mg basis; may increase *rosiglitazone* by 4 mg and/or *metformin* by 500 mg per day; max: *rosiglitazone* 8 mg and *metformin* 2000 mg per day; Same precautions as *rosiglitazone* and *metformin*
Pediatric: not recommended

    Avandamet
      Tab: **Avandamet 2/500:** *rosi* 2 mg/*met* 500 mg
           Avandamet 2/1000: *rosi* 2 mg/*met* 1000 mg
           Avandamet 4/500: *rosi* 4 mg/*met* 500 mg
           Avandamet 4/1000: *rosi* 4 mg/*met* 1000 mg

Comment: *rosiglitazone* has been withdrawn from retail pharmacies. In order to enroll and receive *rosiglitazone*, healthcare providers and patients must enroll in the *Avandia-Rosiglitazone Medicines Access Program.* The program limits the use of *rosiglitazone* to patients already being treated successfully, and those whose blood sugar cannot be controlled with other antidiabetic medicines. *metformin* is contraindicated with renal impairment, metabolic acidosis, ketoacidosis. Suspend *metformin*, prior to, and for 48 hours after, surgery or receiving IV iodinated contrast agents.

THIAZOLIDINEDIONE/SULFONYLUREA COMBINATIONS

▶ *pioglitazone/glimepiride* (C) take 1 dose daily with first meal of the day; *Previously on sulfonylurea alone:* initially 30mg/2mg; *Previously on pioglitazone and glimepiride:* switch on a mg/mg basis; max: *pioglitazone* 30 mg and *glimepiride* 4 mg per day; Same precautions as *pioglitazone* and *glimepiride*
Pediatric: <18 years: not recommended

Duetact
> *Tab:* **Duetact 30/2:** *pio* 30 mg/*glim* 2 mg
> **Duetact 304:** *pio* 30 mg/*glim* 4 mg

▶ *rosiglitazone/glimepiride* (C) take 1 dose daily with first meal of the day; max: *rosiglitazone* 8 mg and *glimepiride* 4 mg per day; Same precautions as *rosiglitazone* and *glimepiride*
Pediatric: <18 years: not recommended
Avandaryl
> *Tab:* **Avandaryl 4/1:** *rosi* 4 mg/*glim* 1 mg
> **Avandaryl 4/2:** *rosi* 4 mg/*glim* 2 mg
> **Avandaryl 4/4:** *rosi* 4 mg/*glim* 4 mg
> **Avandaryl 8/2:** *rosi* 8 mg/*glim* 2 mg
> **Avandaryl 8/4:** *rosi* 8 mg/*glim* 4 mg

GLUCAGON-LIKE PEPTIDE-1 (GLP-1) RECEPTOR AGONISTS

Comment: GLP-1 receptor agonists act as an agonist at the GLP-1 receptors. They have a longer half-life than the native protein allowing them to be dosed once daily. They increase intracellular cAMP resulting in *insulin* release in the presence of increased serum concentration, decrease *glucagon* secretion, and delay gastric emptying, thus, reducing fasting, premeal, and post-prandial glucose throughout the day. GLP-1 receptor agonists are not a substitute for *insulin*, not for treatment of DKA, and not for post-prandial administration.

▶ *albiglutide* (C) administer by SC injection into the upper arm, abdomen, or thigh once daily; initially 30 mg once weekly on the same day; may increase to max 50 mg once weekly
Pediatric: <18 years: not established
Tanzeum *Prefilled pen/syringe:* 30, 50 mg/pen pwdr for injection after reconstitution (4/pck) (preservative-free)

▶ *dulaglutide* (C) administer by SC injection into the upper arm, abdomen, or thigh once daily; initially 0.6 mg/day for 1 week; then 1.2 mg/day; may increase to max 1.8 mg/day; if more than 3 days since last dose, restart at 0.6 mg/day and titrate as before
Pediatric: <18 years: not established
Trulicity *Prefilled pen/syringe:* 0.75, 1.5 mg/0.5 ml single-dose (4/pck)

▶ *exenatide* (C) administer by SC injection into the upper arm, abdomen, or thigh
Pediatric: not recommended
Bydureon administer 2 mg weekly (every 7 days); inject immediately after mixing; if changing from **Byetta**, discontinue and start *Vial:* 2 mg pwdr for reconstitution (1 vial pwdr and 1 syringe prefilled w. diluents, vial connector, and needles, 4/pck)
Byetta inject within 60 minutes before AM and PM meals; initially 5 mcg/dose; may increase to 10 mcg/dose after one month
Prefilled pen: 250 mcg/ml (5, 10 mcg/dose; 60 doses, needles not included) (m-cresol, mannitol)

▶ *liraglutide* (C) administer by SC injection into the upper arm, abdomen, or thigh once daily; initially 0.6 mg/day for 1 week; then 1.2 mg/day; may increase to 1.8 mg/day
Pediatric: <18 years: not recommended
Victoza *Prefilled pen:* 6 mg/ml (3 ml; needles not included)

▶ *lixisenatide* (C) administer SC in the upper arm, abdomen, or thigh once daily; initially 10 mcg SC x 14 days; maintenance: 20 mcg beginning on day 15; administer within one hour of the first meal of the day and the same meal of the day

Pediatric: <18 years: not established

Adlyxin Soln for SC inj; *Starter Pen:* 50 mcg/ml (14 doses of 10 mcg; 3 ml); *Maintenance Pen:* 100 mcg/ml (14 doses of 20 mcg); *Starter Pack:* 1 prefilled starter pen and 1 prefilled maintenance pen; *Maintenance Pack:* 2 prefilled maintenance pens

Comment: **Adlyxin** is indicated as an adjunct to diet and exercise for T2DM. Not indicated for treatment of T1DM. Do not use with **Victoza**, **Saxenda**, other GLP-1 receptor agonists, or insulin. Contraindicated with gastroparesis and GFR <15 mL/min. Poorly controlled diabetes in pregnancy increases the maternal risk for diabetic ketoacidosis, pre-eclampsia, spontaneous abortions, preterm delivery, stillbirth and delivery complications. Poorly controlled diabetes increases the fetal risk for major birth defects, still birth, and macrosomia related morbidity. **Adlyxin** should be used during pregnancy only if the potential benefit justifies the potential risk to the fetus. Estimated background risk of major birth defects and miscarriage in clinically recognized pregnancies is 2-4% and 15-20%, respectively.

SODIUM-GLUCOSE CO-TRANSPORTER 2 (SGLT2) INHIBITORS

Comment: SGLT2 inhibitors block the SGLT2 protein involved in 90% of glucose reabsorption in the proximal renal tubule, resulting in increased renal glucose excretion (typically >2000 mg/dL), and lower blood glucose levels (low risk of hypoglycemia), modest weight loss, and mild reduction in blood pressure (probably due to sodium loss). These agents probably also increase insulin sensitivity, decrease gluconeogenesis, and improve *insulin* release from pancreatic beta cells. SGLT2 inhibitors are contraindicated in T1DM, and are decreased or contraindicated with decreased GFR, increased SCr, renal failure, ESRD, renal dialysis, metabolic acidosis, or diabetic ketoacidosis. The most commen side effects are UTI, female genital mycotic infection, and increased urination. These effects may be managed with adequate hydration and genital hygiene. The SGLT2 inhibitors are not recommended in nursing women. There is potential for a hypersensitivity reaction to include angioedema and anaphylaxis. Caution with SGLT2 use due to reports of increased risk of treatment-emergent bone fractures.

➤ *canagliflozin* (C) take one tab before the first meal of the day; initially 100 mg; may titrate up to max 300 mg once daily; *GFR <45 mL/min:* do not initiate
Pediatric: <18 years: not established

Invokana *Tab:* 100, 300 mg

Comment: **Invokana** is contraindicated with GFR <45 *mL/min;* If GFR 45-≤60 *mL/min,* max 100 mg once daily or consider other antihyperglycemic

➤ *dapagliflozin* (C) take one tab before the first meal of the day; initially 5 mg; may increase to max 10 mg once daily
Pediatric: <18 years: not established

Farxiga *Tab:* 5, 10 mg

Comment: **Farxiga** is contraindicated with GFR <60 mL/min.

➤ *empagliflozin* (C) take one tab before the first meal of the day; initially 10 mg; may increase to max 25 mg once daily
Pediatric: <18 years: not established

Jardiance *Tab:* 10, 25 mg

Comment: **Jardiance** is contraindicated with GFR <45 mL/min.

SODIUM-GLUCOSE CO-TRANSPORTER 2 (SGLT2) INHIBITOR/BIGUANIDE COMBINATIONS

Comment: Caution with **SGLT2** use due to reports of increased risk of treatment-emergent bone fractures. *metformin* is contraindicated with renal impairment, metabolic acidosis, ketoacidosis. Suspend *metformin*, prior to, and for 48 hours after, surgery or receiving IV iodinated contrast agents.

▷ *canagliflozin/metformin* (C) take 1 dose twice daily with meals; max daily dose 300/2000; *GFR 45-≤60 mL/min: canagliflozin* max 100 mg once daily or consider other antihyperglycemic; *GFR <45 mL/min:* do not initiate
Pediatric: <18 years: not established
   Invokamet
      Tab: **Invokamet 50/500:** *cana* 50 mg/*met* 500 mg
            Invokamet 50/1000: *cana* 50 mg/*met* 1000 mg
            Invokamet 150/500: *cana* 150 mg/*met* 500 mg
            Invokamet 150/1000: *cana* 150 mg/*met* 1000 mg

▷ *dapagliflozin/metformin* (C) swall whole; do not crush or chew; take once daily first meal of the day; max daily dose 10/2000
Pediatric: <18 years: not established
   Xigduo XR
      Tab: **Xigduo XR 5/500:** *dapa* 5 mg/*met* 500 mg ext-rel
            Xigduo XR 5/1000: *dapa* 5 mg/*met* 1000 mg ext-rel
            Xigduo XR 10/500: *dapa* 10 mg/*met* 500 mg ext-rel
            Xigduo XR 10/1000: *dapa* 10 mg/*met* 1000 mg ext-rel
   Comment: **Xigduo** is contraindicated with GFR <60 mL/min, SCr >1.5 (men), or SCr >1.4 (women)

▷ *empagliflozin/metforman* (C) take 1 dose twice daily with meals; max daily dose 25/2000
Pediatric: <18 years: not established
   Synjardy
      Tab: **Synjardy 5/500:** *empa* 5 mg/*met* 500 mg
            Synjardy 5/1000: *empa* 5 mg/*met* 1000 mg
            Synjardy 12.5/500: *empa* 12.5 mg/*met* 500 mg
            Synjardy 12.5/1000: *empa* 12.5 mg/*met* 1000 mg
   Synjardy XR
      Tab: **Synjardy XR 5/1000:** *empa* 5 mg/*met* 1000 mg
            Synjardy XR 12.5/1000: *empa* 12.5 mg/*met* 1000 mg
            Synjardy XR 10/1000: *empa* 10 mg/*met* 1000 mg
            Synjardy XR 25/1000: *empa* 25 mg/*met* 1000 mg
   Comment: **Synjardy** is contraindicated with *GFR <45 mL/min, SCr >1.5* (men), or *SCr >1.4* (women).

SODIUM-GLUCOSE CO-TRANSPORTER 2 (SGLT2) INHIBITOR/DIPEPTIDYL PEPTIDASE-4 (DPP-4) INHIBITOR COMBINATION

Comment: Caution with **SGLT2** use due to reports of increased risk of treatment-emergent bone fractures.

▷ *empagliflozin/linagliptin* (C) initially 10/5 once daily with the first meal of the day; max daily dose 25/5
Pediatric: <18 years: not established

Glyxambi
> *Tab:* **Glyxambi 10/5:** *empa* 10 mg/*lina* 5 mg
> **Glyxambi 25/5:** *empa* 25 mg/*lina* 5 mg
Comment: **Glyxambi** is contraindicated with GFR <45 mL/min.

DIPEPTIDYL PEPTIDASE-4 (DPP-4) INHIBITOR

Comment: DPP-4 is an enzyme that degrades incretin hormones glucagon-like peptide-1 (GLP-1) and glucose-dependent insulinotropic polypeptide (GIP). Thus, DPP-4 inhibitors increase the concentration of active incretin hormones, stimulating the release of **insulin** in a glucose-dependent manner and decreasing the levels of circulating **glucagon**. The FDA has reported that saxagliptin- and alogliptin-containing drugs may increase the risk of heart failure, especially in patients who already have cardiovascular or renal disease. Drugs in this risk group include Nesina (alogliptin) and Onglyza (saxagliptin)

▷ *algogliptin* (B) take twice daily with meals; max 25 mg/day
   Pediatric: <18 years: not recommended
      Nesina *Tab:* 6.25, 12.5, 25 mg
▷ *linagliptin* (B) 5 mg once daily
   Pediatric: <18 years: not recommended
      Tradjenta *Tab:* 5 mg
▷ *saxagliptin* (B) 2.5-5 mg once daily
   Pediatric: <18 years: not recommended
      Onglyza *Tab:* 2.5, 5 mg
▷ *sitagliptin* (B) as monotherapy or as combination therapy with metfor- min or a TZD
   Pediatric: <18 years: not recommended
      Januvia 25-100 mg once daily
         Tab: 25, 50, 100 mg

DIPEPTIDYL PEPTIDASE-4 (DPP-4) INHIBITOR/BIGUANIDE COMBINATIONS

Comment: DPP-4 inhibitor/**metformin** combinations are contraindicated with renal impairment (men: SCr ≥1.5 mg/dL; women: SCr ≥1.4 mg/dL) or abnormal CrCl, metabolic acidosis, ketoacidosis, or history of angioedema. Suspend **metformin**, prior to, and for 48 hours after, surgery or receiving IV iodinated contrast agents. Avoid in the elderly, malnourished, dehydrated, or with clinical or lab evidence of hepatic disease. For other DPP-4 and/or **metformin** precautions, see mfr pkg insert. The FDA has reported that **saxagliptin**- and **alogliptin**-containing drugs may increase the risk of heart failure, especially in patients who already have cardiovascular or renal disease. These drugs include: **Onglyza** (*saxagliptin*), **Kombiglyze XR** (*saxagliptin/metformin*), **Nesina** (*alogliptin*), **Kazano** (*alogliptin/metformin*), and **Oseni** (*alogliptin/pioglitazone*).

▷ *alogliptin/metformin* (B) take twice daily with meals; max *algogliptin* 25 mg/day, max *metformin* 2000 mg/day
   Pediatric: <18 years: not recommended
      Kazano
         Tab: **Kazano 12.5/500:** *algo* 12.5 mg/*met* 500 mg
            Kazano 2.5/1000: *algo* 12.5 mg/*met* 1000 mg
▷ *linagliptin/metformin* (B)
   Pediatric: <18 years: not recommended
      Jentadueto take twice daily with meals; max *linagliptin* 5 mg/day, max *metformin* 2000 mg/day
         Tab: **Jentadueto 2.5/500:** *lina* 2.5 mg/*met* 500 mg film-coat

Jentadueto 2.5/850: *lina* 2.5 mg/*met* 850 mg film-coat
Jentadueto 2.5/1000: *lina* 2.5 mg/*met* 1000 mg film-coat
Jentadueto XR *Currently not treated with* **metformin**: initiate **Jentadueto XR 5/1000** once daily; *Already treated with* **metformin**: initiate **Jentadueto XR** 5 mg *linagliptin* total daily dose and a similar total daily dose of **metformin** once daily; *Already treated with* **linagliptin and metformin** or *Jentadueto*: switch to **Jentadueto XR** containing 5 mg of *linagliptin* total daily dose and a similar total daily dose of **metformin** once daily; max *linagliptin 5 mg* and **metformin** *2000 mg*; take as a single dose once daily; take with food; do not crush or chew *eGFR <30 mL/min*: contraindicated; *eGFR 30-45 mL/min*: not recommended
 Tab: **Jentadueto 2.5/1000**: *lina* 2.5 mg/*met* 1000 mg film-coat ext-rel
 Jentadueto 5/1000: *lina* 5 mg/*met* 1000 mg film-coat ext-rel
▷ *saxagliptin/metformin* (B) take once daily with meals; max *saxagliptin* 5 mg/day, max *metformin* 2000 mg/day; do not crush or chew
Pediatric: <18 years: not recommended
 Kombiglyze XR
  Tab: **Kombiglyze XR 5/500**: *saxa* 5 mg/*met* 500 mg
  Kombiglyze XR 2.5/1000: *saxa* 2.5 mg/*met* 1000 mg
  Kombiglyze XR 5/1000: *saxa* 5 mg/*met* 1000 mg
Comment: The FDA has reported that *saxagliptin*-containing drugs may increase the risk of heart failure, especially in patients who already have cardiovascular or renal disease. The drug Kombiglyze XR (*saxagliptin/metformin*) is in this risk group. *metformin* is contraindicated with renal impairment, metabolic acidosis, ketoacidosis. Suspend *metformin*, prior to, and for 48 hours after, surgery or receiving IV iodinated contrast agents.
▷ *sitagliptin/metformin* (B) take twice daily with meals; max *sitagliptin* 100 mg/day, max *metformin* 2000 mg/day
Pediatric: <18 years: not recommended
 Janumet
  Tab: **Janumet 50/500**: *sita* 50 mg/*met* 500 mg
  Janumet 50/1000: *sita* 50 mg/*met* 1000 mg
 Janumet XR
  Tab: **Janumet XR 50/500**: *sita* 50 mg/*met* 500 mg ext-rel
  Janumet XR 50/1000: *sita* 50 mg/*met* 1000 mg ext-rel
  Janumet XR 100/1000: *sita* 100 mg/*met* 1000 mg ext-rel
Comment: *metformin* is contraindicated with renal impairment, metabolic acidosis, ketoacidosis. Suspend *metformin*, prior to, and for 48 hours after, surgery or receiving IV iodinated contrast agents.

MEGLITINIDE/BIGUANIDE COMBINATION

▷ *repaglinide/metformin* (C)(G) take in 2-3 divided doses within 30 minutes before food; max 4/1000 per meal and 10/2000 per day
Pediatric: not recommended
 Prandimet
  Tab: **Prandimet 1/500**: *repa* 1 mg/*met* 500 mg
  Prandimet 2/500: *repa* 2 mg/*met* 500 mg
Comment: *metformin* is contraindicated with renal impairment, metabolic acidosis, ketoacidosis. Suspend *metformin*, prior to, and for 48 hours after, surgery or receiving IV iodinated contrast agents.

DIPEPTIDYL PEPTIDASE-4 (DPP-4) INHIBITOR/HMG-COA REDUCTASE INHIBITOR COMBINATION

▷ *sitagliptin/simvastatin* (B) take once daily in the PM; swallow whole; adjust dose if needed after 4 weeks; *Concomitant* **verapamil** or **diltiazem**: max 100/10 once daily; *Concomitant* **amiodarone, amlodipine,** or **ranolazine**: max 100/20 once daily; *Homogenous familial hypercholesterolemia:* max 100/40 once daily; *Chinese patients taking lipid-modifying doses (>1 g/day niacin) of niacin-containing products:* caution with 100/40 dose; increase risk of myopathy
Pediatric: <18 years: not recommended
    Juvisync
        Tab: **Juvisync 100/10**: *sita* 100 mg/*simva* 10 mg
              Juvisync 100/20: *sita* 100 mg/*simva* 20 mg
              Juvisync 100/40: *sita* 100 mg/*simva* 40 mg

DOPAMINE RECEPTOR AGONIST

▷ *bromocriptine mesylate* (B) take with food in the morning within 2 hours of waking; initially 0.8 mg once daily; may increase by 0.8 mg/week; max 4.8 mg/week; *Severe psychotic disorders:* not recommended
Pediatric: not recommended
    Cycloset *Tab:* 0.8 mg
    Comment: **Cycloset** is an adjunct to diet and exercise to improve glycemic control. Contraindicated with syncopal migraines, nursing mothers, and other ergot-related drugs.

Bile Acid Sequestrant

▷ *colesevelam* (B) *Monotherapy:* 3 tabs bid or 6 tabs once daily or one **1.875 g pkt bid** or one 3.75 g pkt once daily
Pediatric: not recommended
    WelChol *Tab:* 625 mg; *Pwdr for oral susp:* 1.875 g pwdr pkts (60/carton); 3.75 g pwdr pkts (30/carton) (citrus; phenylalanine)
    Comment: *colesevelam* (WelChol) is indicated as an adjunctive therapy to improve glycemic control in adults with type 2 diabetes. It can be added to **metformin**, sulfonylureas, or **insulin** alone or in combination with other antidiabetic agents

⬤ TYPHOID FEVER (*SALMONELLA TYPHI*)

PRE-EXPOSURE PROPHYLAXIS

▷ *typhoid* vaccine, oral, live, attenuated strain
    Vivotif Berna 1 cap every other day, 1 hour before a meal, with a lukewarm (not > body temperature) or cold drink for a total of 4 doses; do not crush or chew; complete therapy at least 1 week prior to expected exposure; re-immunization recommended every 5 years if repeated exposure
        Pediatric: <6 years: not recommended; ≥6 years: same as adult
        Cap: ent-coat
▷ *typhoid Vi polysaccharide* vaccine (C)
    Typhim Vi 0.5 ml IM in deltoid; re-immunization recommended every 2 years if repeated exposure

Pediatric: <2 years: not recommended; ≥2 years: same as adult
Vial: 20, 50 dose; *Prefilled syringe:* 0.5 ml

Comment: Febrile illness may require delaying administration of the vaccine; have *epinephrine* 1:1000 readily available.

TREATMENT

▷ *azithromycin* (B) 8-10 mg/kg/day; *Mild Illness:* treat x 7 days; *Severe Illness:* treat x 14 days
Pediatric: 8-10 mg/kg/day; max 500 mg/day; *Mild Illness:* treat x 7 days; *Severe Illness:* treat x 14 days; *see page 559 for dose by weight*
Zithromax *Tab:* 250, 500, 600 mg; *Oral susp:* 100 mg/5 ml (15 ml); 200 mg/5 ml (15, 22.5, 30 ml) (cherry); *Pkt:* 1 g for reconstitution (cherry-banana)
Zithromax Tri-pak *Tab:* 3 x 500 mg tabs/pck
Zithromax Z-pak *Tab:* 6 x 250 mg tabs/pck
Zmax *Oral susp:* 2 g ext-rel for reconstitution (cherry-banana) (148 mg Na+)

▷ *cefixime* (B) *Mild Illness:* 15-20 mg/kg/day x 7-14 days; *Severe Illness:* 20 mg/kg/day x 10-14 days
Pediatric: <6 months: not recommended; 6 months-12 years, <50 kg: *Mild Illness:* 15-20 mg/kg/day x 7-14 days; *Severe Illness:* 20 mg/kg/day x 10-14 >50 kg: same as adult; *see page 563 for dose by weight*
Suprax *Tab:* 400 mg; *Cap:* 400 mg; *Oral susp:* 100, 200 mg/5 ml (50, 75, 100 ml) (strawberry)

▷ *ciprofloxacin* (C) 15 mg/kg/day; *Mild Illness:* treat x 5-7 days; *Severe Illness:* treat x 10-14 days
Pediatric: <18 years: not recommended
Cipro (G) *Tab:* 250, 500, 750 mg; *Oral susp:* 250, 500 mg/5 ml (100 ml) (strawberry)
Cipro XR *Tab:* 500, 1000 mg ext-rel
ProQuin XR *Tab:* 500 mg ext-rel

Comment: *ciprofloxacin* is contraindicated <18 years-of-age, and during pregnancy and lactation. Risk of tendonitis or tendon rupture, especially 60 years-of-age and older.

▷ *ofloxacin* (C) 15 mg/kg/day; *Mild Illness:* treat x 5-7 days; *Severe Illness:* treat x 10-14 days
Pediatric: <18 years: not recommended
Pediatric: <18 years: not recommended
Floxin *Tab:* 200, 300, 400 mg

Comment: *ofloxacin* is contraindicated <18 years-of-age, and during pregnancy and lactation. Risk of tendonitis or tendon rupture, especially 60 years-of-age and older.

▷ *cefotaxime* 80 mg/kg/day IM/IV x 10-14 days; max 2 g/day
Pediatrics: 80 mg/kg/day IM/IV x 10-14 days; max 2 g/day
Claforan *Vial:* 500 mg; 1, 2 g

▷ *ceftriaxone* (B)(G) 75 mg/kg/day IM/IV x 10-14 days; max 2 g/day
Pediatrics: 75 mg/kg/day IM/IV x 10-14 days; max 2 g/day
Rocephin *Vial:* 250, 500 mg; 1, 2 g

▷ *trimethoprim/sulfamethoxazole* (D)(G) 8-40 mg/kg/day x 14 days
Pediatric: <2 months: not recommended; ≥2 months: 8-40 mg/kg/day of *sulfamethoxazole* in 2 divided doses bid x 10 days; *see page 587 for dose by weight*
Bactrim, Septra 2 tabs bid x 10 days
Tab: trim 80 mg/*sulfa* 400 mg*

Bactrim DS, Septra DS 1 tab bid x 10 days
Tab: trim 160 mg/*sulfa* 800 mg*
Bactrim Pediatric Suspension, Septra Pediatric Suspension 20 ml bid x 10 days
Oral susp: trim 40 mg/*sulfa* 200 mg per 5 ml (100 ml) (cherry) (alcohol 0.3%)
Comment: **trimethoprim/sulfamethoxazole** is not recommended in pregnancy
or lactation. *CrCl 15-30 mL/min:* reduce dose by 1/2; *CrCl <15 mL/min:* not
recommended

ULCER: DIABETIC, NEUROPATHIC (LOWER EXTREMITY) ULCER: VENOUS INSUFFICIENCY (LOWER EXTREMITY)

NUTRITIONAL SUPPLEMENT

▷ *L-methylfolate calcium (as metafolin)/pyridoxyl 5-phosphate/methylcobalamin* (NE)
take 1 cap daily
Pediatric: not recommended
Metanx *Cap: metafo* 3 mg/*pyrid* 35 mg/*methyl* 2 mg (gluten-free, yeast-free,
lactose-free)
Comment: **Metanx** is indicated as adjunct treatment of endothelial dysfunction
and/or hyperhomocysteinemia in patients who have lower extremity ulceration.

DEBRIDING/CAPILLARY STIMULANT AGENT

▷ *trypsin/balsam peru/castor oil* (NE) apply at least twice daily; may cover with a wet
bandage
Granulex *Aerosol liq: tryp* 0.12 mg/*bal peru* 87 mg/*cast* 788 mg per 0.82 ml

GROWTH FACTOR

▷ *becaplermin* (C) apply once daily with a cotton swab or tongue depressor; then cover
with saline moistened gauze dressing; rinse after 12 hours; then re-cover with a clean
saline dressing
Regranex *Gel:* 0.01% (2, 7.5, 15 g) (parabens)
Comment: Store in refrigerator; do not freeze. Not for use in wounds that close by
primary intention.

ULCER: DECUBITUS/PRESSURE

DEBRIDING/CAPILLARY STIMULANT AGENT

Granulex (*trypsin* 0.1 mg/*balsam peru* 72.5 mg/castor oil 650 mg per 0.82 ml)
apply at least twice daily; may cover with a wet bandage
Aerosol liq: (2, 4 oz)

GROWTH FACTOR

▷ *becaplermin* (C) apply once daily with a cotton swab or tongue depressor; then cover
with saline moistened gauze dressing; rinse after 12 hours; then recover with a clean
saline dressing
Regranex *Gel:* 0.01% (2, 7.5, 15 g) (parabens)

Comment: Store in refrigerator; do not freeze. Not for use in wounds that close by primary intention.

 ULCERATIVE COLITIS

Comment: Standard treatment regimen is anti-infective, anti-spasmodic, and bowel rest; progressing to clear liquids; then to high fiber.

Parenteral Corticosteroids *see page* 511

Oral Corticosteroids *see page* 509

▷ *budesonide micronized* (C)(G) 9 mg once daily in the AM for up to 8 weeks; may repeat an 8-week course; *Maintenance of remission:* 6 mg once daily for up yo 3 months; taper other systemic steroids when transferring to *bunesonide*

Pediatric: not recommended

    Entocort EC *Cap:* 3 mg ent-coat granules

    Uceris *Tab:* 9 mg ext-rel

RECTAL CORTICOSTEROIDS

▷ *hydrocortisone* rectal (C)

Pediatric: not recommended

    Anusol-HC Suppositories 1 supp rectally 3 times daily <u>or</u> 2 supp rectally twice daily for 2 weeks; max 8 weeks

      Rectal supp: 25 mg (12, 24/pck)

    Cortenema 1 enema q HS x 21 days <u>or</u> until symptoms controlled

      Enema: 100 mg/60 ml (1, 7/pck)

    Cortifoam 1 applicator full once daily-bid x 2-3 weeks and every 2nd day thereafter until symptoms are controlled

      Aerosol: 80 mg/applicator (14 application/container)

    Proctocort 1 supp rectally in AM and PM x 2 weeks; for more severe cases, may increase to 1 supp rectally 3 times daily <u>or</u> 2 supp rectally twice daily; max 4-8 weeks

      Rectal supp: 30 mg (12, 24/pck)

Comment: Use *hydrocortisone* foam as adjunctive therapy in the distal portion of the rectum when *hydrocortisone* enemas cannot be retained.

RECTAL CORTICOSTEROID/ANESTHETIC

Hydrocortisone/Pramoxine

    Proctofoam HC apply to anal/rectal area 3-4 times daily; max 4-8 weeks

      Rectal foam: hydrocort 1%/*pram* 1% (10 g w. applicator)

SALICYLATES

▷ *balsalazide disodium* (B)

    Colazal 2.25 g 3 times daily x 8 weeks; max 12 weeks; swallow whole <u>or</u> sprinkle contents into apple sauce

      Pediatric: <5 years: not recommended; ≥5 years: 2.25 g 3 times daily <u>or</u> 750 mg once daily x 8 weeks; swallow whole <u>or</u> sprinkle contents into apple sauce

      Cap: 750 mg

Comment: *balsalazide* 6.75 g provides 2.4 g of *mesalazine* to the colon.

Giazo take 3 tabs bid; max 8 weeks
Tab: 1.1 g (sodium 126 mg/tab) film-coat
➤ *mesalamine* (B)
Pediatric: not recommended
Apriso take 1.5 g once daily in the AM for maintenance of remission
Cap: 0.375 g ext-rel (phenylalanine 0.56 mg/cap)
Asacol HD 1600 mg tid x 6 weeks; maintenance 1.6 g/day in divided doses;
swallow whole; do not crush <u>or</u> chew
Tab: 800 mg del-rel
Canasa 1 g qid for up to 8 weeks
Rectal supp: 1 g del-rel (30, 42/pck)
Delzicol 800 mg tid x 6 weeks; maintenance once daily for up to 8 weeks;
Maintenance: 1.6 g/day in 2-4 divided doses once daily; swallow whole; do not
crush <u>or</u> chew
Cap: 400 mg del-rel
Lialda 2.4-4.8 g once daily for up to 8 weeks; maintenance 2.4 g once daily;
swallow whole; do not crush <u>or</u> chew
Tab: 1.2 g del-rel
Pentasa 1 g qid for up to 8 weeks
Cap: 250, 500 mg cont-rel
Rowasa Suppository 1 supp rectally bid x 3-6 weeks; retain for 1-3 hours <u>or</u> longer
Rectal supp: 500 mg (12, 24/pck)
Sulfite-Free Rowasa Rectal Suspension 4 g rectally by enema q HS; retain for 8
hours x 3-6 weeks
Enema: 4 g/60 ml (7, 14, 28/pck; kit, 7, 14, 28/pck w. wipes)
➤ *olsalazine* (C) 1 g/day in 2 divided doses
Dipentum *Cap:* 250 mg
➤ *sulfasalazine* (B; D in 2nd, 3rd)(G)
Pediatric: <2 years: not recommended; 2-16 years: initially 40-60 mg/kg/day in 3
to 6 divided doses; max 30 mg/kg/day in 4 divided doses; max 2 g/day; >16 years:
same as adult
Azulfidine initially 1-2 g/day; increase to 3-4 g/day in divided doses pc until
clinical symptoms controlled; maintenance 2 g/day; max 4 g/day
Tab: 500*mg
Azulfidine EN-Tabs initially 500 mg in the PM x 7 days; then 500 mg bid x 7 days;
then 500 mg in the AM and 1 g in the PM x 7 days; then 1 g bid; max 4 g/day
Tab: 500 mg ent-coat

TUMOR NECROSIS FACTOR (TNF) BLOCKER

➤ *adalimumab* (B) initially 180 mg SC (as 4 injections in 1 day <u>or</u> divided over 2 days)
on week 0; then 80 mg at week 2; start 40 mg every other week maintenance at week
4; only continue if evidence of clinical remission by 8 weeks; administer in abdomen
<u>or</u> thigh; rotate sites
Pediatric: <18 years not recommended
Humira *Prefilled syringe:* 20 mg/0.4 ml; 40 mg/0.8 ml single-dose (2/pck; 2, 6/
starter pck) (preservative-free)
➤ *infliximab* (B) administer by IV infusion over 2 hours; 5 mg/kg weeks 0, 2, 6; then
once every 8 weeks
Pediatric: <6 years: not recommended; ≥6 years: same as adult
Vial: 100 mg pwdr for reconstitution for IV infusion (preservative-free)

▷ *vedolizumab* (B) administer by IV infusion over 30 minutes; 300 mg at weeks 0, 2, 6; then once every 8 weeks
Pediatric: not established
   Entyvio
      Vial: 300 mg (20 ml) single dose, pwdr for IV infusion after reconstitution (preservative-free)

ANTI-DIARRHEAL AGENTS

▷ *difenoxin/atropine* (C) 2 tabs; then 1 tab after each loose stool <u>or</u> 1 tab q 3-4 hours; max 8 tabs/day x 2 days
   Motofen *Tab: dif* 1 mg/*atro* 0.025 mg
▷ *diphenoxylate/atropine* (C)(G) 2 tabs <u>or</u> 10 ml qid
   Lomotil *Tab: diphen* 2.5 mg/*atro* 0.025 mg; *Liq: diphen* 2.5 mg/*atro* 0.025 mg/5 ml (2 oz w. dropper)
▷ *loperamide* (B)(G)
   Imodium (OTC) 4 mg initially; then 2 mg after each loose stool; max 16 mg/day
      Cap: 2 mg
   Imodium A-D (OTC) 4 mg initially; then 2 mg after each loose stool; usual max 8 mg/day x 2 days
      Cplt: 2 mg; *Liq:* 1 mg/5 ml (2, 4 oz)
   Imodium Advanced (OTC) 2 tabs chewed after first loose stool; then 1 after the next loose stool; max 4 tabs/day
      Chew tab: loperamide 2 mg/simethicone 125 mg

 URETHRITIS: NONGONOCOCCAL (NGU)

Comment: The following treatment regimens for NGU are published in the **2015 CDC Sexually Transmitted Diseases Treatment Guidelines**. Treatment regimens are for adults only; consult a specialist for treatment of patients less than 18 years-of-age. Treatment regimens are presented by generic drug name first, followed by information about brands and dose forms. All persons who have confirmed <u>or</u> suspected urethritis should be tested for gonorrhea and chlamydia. Men treated for NGU should be instructed to abstain from sexual intercourse for 7 days after a single-dose regimen <u>or</u> until completion of a 7-day regimen.

RECOMMENDED REGIMEN: UNCOMPLICATED NGU

▷ *azithromycin* 1 g in a single dose <u>or</u> 100 mg orally bid x 7 days
   plus
▷ *doxycycline* 100 mg bid x 7 days

PERSISTENT/RECURRENT NGU

Men Initially Treated With Azithromycin+Doxycycline

▷ *azithromycin* 1 g PO in a single dose

Men Who Fail a Regimen of Azithromycin

▷ *moxifloxacin* 400 mg PO once daily x 7 days

Heterosexual Men Who Live in Areas Where *T. Vaginalis* is Highly Prevalent

▷ *metronidazole* 2 g PO in a single dose

  or

▷ *tinidazole* 2 g PO in a single dose

ALTERNATIVE REGIMENS

▷ *erythromycin base* 500 mg PO qid x 7 days

  or

▷ *erythromycin ethylsuccinate* 800 mg PO qid x 7 days

  or

▷ *levofloxacin* 500 mg once daily x 7 days

  or

▷ *ofloxacin* 300 mg PO bid x 7 days

DRUG BRANDS AND DOSE FORMS

▷ *azithromycin* (B)
  Zithromax *Tab:* 250, 500, 600 mg; *Oral susp:* 100 mg/5 ml (15 ml); 200 mg/5 ml
  (15, 22.5, 30 ml) (cherry); *Pkt:* 1 g for reconstitution (cherry-banana)
  Zithromax Tri-pak *Tab:* 3 x 500 mg tabs/pck
  Zithromax Z-pak *Tab:* 6 x 250 mg tabs/pck
  Zmax *Oral susp:* 2 g ext-rel for reconstitution (cherry-banana) (148 mg Na⁺)

▷ *doxycycline* (D)(G)
  Actilate *Tab:* 75, 150**mg
  Adoxa *Tab:* 50, 75, 100, 150 mg ent-coat
  Doryx *Tab:* 50, 75, 100, 150, 200 mg del-rel
  Monodox *Cap:* 50, 75, 100 mg
  Oracea *Cap:* 40 mg del-rel
  Vibramycin *Tab:* 100 mg; *Cap:* 50, 100 mg; *Syr:* 50 mg/5 ml (raspberry-apple)
  (sulfites); *Oral susp:* 25 mg/5 ml (raspberry)
  Vibra-Tab *Tab:* 100 mg film-coat
  Comment: *doxycycline* is contraindicated <8 years-of-age, in pregnancy, and
  lactation (discolors developing tooth enamel). A side effect may be photo-
  sensitivity (photophobia). Do not give with antacids, calcium supplements, milk or
  other dairy, or within two hours of taking another drug.

▷ *erythromycin base* (B)
  Ery-Tab *Tab:* 250, 333, 500 mg ent-coat
  PCE *Tab:* 333, 500 mg
  Comment: *erythromycin* may increase INR with concomitant *warfarin*, as well as
  increase serum level of *digoxin*, benzodiazepines and statins.

▷ *erythromycin ethylsuccinate* (B)(G)
  EryPed *Oral susp:* 200 mg/5 ml (100, 200 ml) (fruit); 400 mg/5 ml (60, 100, 200
  ml) (banana); *Oral drops:* 200, 400 mg/5 ml (50 ml) (fruit); *Chew tab:* 200 mg
  wafer (fruit)
  E.E.S. *Oral susp:* 200, 400 mg/5 ml (100 ml) (fruit)
  E.E.S. Granules *Oral susp:* 200 mg/5 ml (100, 200 ml) (cherry)
  E.E.S. 400 Tablets *Tab:* 400 mg

Comment: *erythromycin* may increase INR with concomitant *warfarin*, as well as increase serum level of *digoxin*, benzodiazepines and statins.

➤ *levofloxacin* (C)
    Levaquin *Tab:* 250, 500, 750 mg; *Oral soln:* 25 mg/ml (480 ml) (benzyl alcohol); *Inj conc:* 25 mg/ml for IV infusion after dilution (20, 30 ml single-use vial) (preservative-free); *Premix soln:* 5 mg/ml for IV infusion (50, 100, 150 ml) (preservative-free)

Comment: *levofloxacin* is contraindicated <18 years-of-age, and during pregnancy and lactation. Risk of tendonitis or tendon rupture, especially 60 years-of-age and older.

➤ *metronidazole* (not for use in 1st; B in 2nd, 3rd)(G)
    Flagyl *Tab:* 250*, 500*mg
    Flagyl 375 *Cap:* 375 mg
    Flagyl ER *Tab:* 750 mg ext-rel

Comment: Alcohol is contraindicated during treatment with oral *metronidazole* and for 72 hours after therapy due to a possible *disulfiram*-like reaction (nausea, vomiting, flushing, headache).

➤ *moxifl oxacin* (C)(G)
    Avelox *Tab:* 400 mg

Comment: *moxifloxacin* is contraindicated <18 years-of-age, and during pregnancy and lactation. Risk of tendonitis or tendon rupture, especially 60 years-of-age and older.

➤ *ofloxacin* (C)(G)
    Floxin *Tab:* 200, 300, 400 mg

Comment: *ofloxacin* is contraindicated <18 years-of-age, and during pregnancy and lactation. Risk of tendonitis or tendon rupture, especially 60 years-of-age and older.

➤ *tinidazole* (not for use in 1st; B in 2nd, 3rd)
    Tindamax *Tab:* 250*, 500*mg

Comment: Alcohol is contraindicated during treatment with oral *tinidazole* and for 72 hours after therapy due to a possible *disulfiram*-like reaction (nausea, vomiting, flushing, headache).

◯ URINARY RETENTION: UNOBSTRUCTIVE

➤ *bethanechol* (C) 10-30 mg tid
    Urecholine *Tab:* 5, 10, 25, 50 mg

Comment: Contraindicated in presence of urinary obstruction. *atropine* 0.4 mg administered SC reverses *bethanechol* toxicity.

◯ URINARY TRACT INFECTION (UTI, CYSTITIS: ACUTE)

URINARY TRACT ANALGESIA

➤ *phenazopyridine* (B)(G) 95-200 mg q 6 hours prn; max 2 days
    Pediatric: not recommended
    AZO Standard, Prodium, Uristat (OTC) *Tab:* 95 mg
    AZO Standard Maximum Strength (OTC) *Tab:* 97.5 mg
    Pyridium, Urogesic *Tab:* 100, 200 mg

ANTI-INFECTIVES: THERAPY IN ADULT FEMALE WITH UNCOMPLICATED UTI

▷ *amoxicillin/clavulanate* (B)(G) 500 mg tid or 875 mg bid x 10 days
> **Augmentin** *Tab:* 250, 500, 875 mg; *Chew tab:* 125, 250 mg (lemon-lime); 200, 400 mg (cherry-banana) (phenylalanine); *Oral susp:* 125 mg/5 ml (banana), 250 mg/5 ml (75, 100, 150 ml) (orange); 200, 400 mg/5 ml (50, 75, 100 ml) (orange) (phenylalanine)
>> *Pediatric:* 40-45 mg/kg/day divided tid x 10 days or 90 mg/kg/day divided bid x 10 days *see pages 556-557 for dose by weight*
> **Augmentin ES-600** *Oral susp:* 600 mg/5 ml (50, 75, 100, 125, 150, 200 ml) (strawberry cream) (phenylalanine) every 12 hours
>> *Pediatric:* <3 months: not recommended; ≥3 months, <40 kg: 90 mg/kg/day in 2 divided doses; ≥40 kg: not recommended
> **Augmentin XR** 2 tabs q 12 hours x 7-10 days
>> *Pediatric:* <16 years: use other forms; ≥16 years: same as adult
>> *Tab:* 1000*mg ext-rel

▷ *ciprofloxacin* (C)
> *Pediatric:* <18 years: not recommended
> **Cipro (G)** *Tab:* 250, 500, 750 mg; *Oral susp:* 250, 500 mg/5 ml (100 ml) (strawberry)
> **Cipro XR** *Tab:* 500, 1000 mg ext-rel
> **ProQuin XR** *Tab:* 500 mg ext-rel
> **Comment:** *ciprofloxacin* is contraindicated <18 years-of-age, and during pregnancy and lactation. Risk of tendonitis or tendon rupture, especially 60 years-of-age and older.

▷ *fosfomycin* (B) 1 pkt in 3-4 oz cold water x 1 dose
> **Monurol** *Single-dose pkts:* 1-3 g (mandarin orange; sucrose)

▷ *levofloxacin* (C) 250 mg once daily x 3 days
> *Pediatric:* <18 years: not recommended
> **Levaquin** *Tab:* 250, 500, 750 mg; *Oral soln:* 25 mg/ml (480 ml) (benzyl alcohol); *Inj conc:* 25 mg/ml for IV infusion after dilution (20, 30 ml single-use vial) (preservative-free); *Premix soln:* 5 mg/ml for IV infusion (50, 100, 150 ml) (preservative-free)
> **Comment:** *levofloxacin* is contraindicated <18 years-of-age, and during pregnancy and lactation. Risk of tendonitis or tendon rupture, especially 60 years-of-age and older.

▷ *norfloxacin* (C) 400 mg once daily x 3 days
> *Pediatric:* <18 years: not recommended
> **Noroxin** *Tab:* 400 mg
> **Comment:** *norfloxacin* is contraindicated <18 years-of-age, and during pregnancy and lactation. Risk of tendonitis or tendon rupture, especially 60 years-of-age and older.

▷ *ofloxacin* (C)(G) 200 mg q 12 hours x 3 days
> *Pediatric:* <18 years: not recommended
> **Floxin** *Tab:* 200, 300, 400 mg
> **Floxin UroPak** *Tab:* 200 mg (6/pck)
> **Comment:** *ofloxacin* is contraindicated <18 years-of-age, and during pregnancy and lactation. Risk of tendonitis or tendon rupture, especially 60 years-of-age and older.

▷ *trimethoprim* (C)(G)
> **Primsol** 100 mg q 12 hours or 200 mg once daily x 10 days

Pediatric: <6 months: not recommended; ≥6 months: 10 mg/kg/day in 2 divided doses x 10 days

Oral soln: 50 mg/5 ml (bubble gum; dye-free, alcohol-free)

Proloprim 100 mg q 12 hours or 200 mg once daily x 10 days
Pediatric: not recommended
Tab: 100, 200 mg

Trimpex 100 mg q 12 hours or 200 mg once daily x 10 days
Pediatric: not recommended
Tab: 100 mg

▶ *trimethoprim/sulfamethoxazole* (D)(G)
Pediatric: <2 months: not recommended; >2 months: 40 mg/kg/day of *sulfamethoxazole* in 2 divided doses bid x 10 days; see page 587 for dose by weight

Bactrim, Septra 2 tabs bid x 10 days
Tab: trim 80 mg/*sulfa* 400 mg*

Bactrim DS, Septra DS 1 tab bid x 10 days
Tab: trim 160 mg/*sulfa* 800 mg*

Bactrim Pediatric Suspension, Septra Pediatric Suspension
Oral susp: trim 40 mg/*sulfa* 200 mg per 5 ml (100 ml) (cherry) (alcohol 0.3%)

Comment: *trimethoprim/sulfamethoxazole* is not recommended in pregnancy or lactation. *CrCl 15-30 mL/min:* reduce dose by 1/2; *CrCl <15 mL/min:* not recommended

ANTI-INFECTIVES: STANDARD REGIMEN FOR UTI

▶ *acetyl sulfisoxazole* (C)(G)
Gantrisin initially 2-4 g in a single or divided doses; then 4-8 g/day in 4-6 divided doses x 7 days
Tab: 500 mg

Gantrisin
Pediatric: <2 months: not recommended; ≥2 months: initial dose 75 mg/kg/day; then 150 mg/kg/day in 4-6 divided doses x 7 days; max 6 g/day
Oral susp: 500 mg/5 ml (4, 16 oz); *Syr:* 500 mg/5 ml (16 oz)

▶ *amoxicillin* (B)(G) 500-875 mg bid or 250-500 mg tid x 7 days
Pediatric: <40 kg (88 lb): 20-40 mg/kg/day in 3 divided doses x 7 days or 25-45 mg/kg/day in 2 divided doses x 7 days; see page 554 for dose by weight

Amoxil *Cap:* 250, 500 mg; *Tab:* 875*mg; *Chew tab:* 125, 200, 250, 400 mg (cherry-banana-peppermint) (phenylalanine); *Oral susp:* 125, 250 mg/5 ml (80, 100, 150 ml) (strawberry); 200, 400 mg/5 ml (50, 75, 100 ml) (bubble gum); *Oral drops:* 50 mg/ml (30 ml) (bubble gum)

Moxatag *Tab:* 775 mg ext-rel

Trimox *Tab:* 125, 250 mg; *Cap:* 250, 500 mg; *Oral susp:* 125, 250 mg/5 ml (80, 100, 150 ml) (raspberry-strawberry)

▶ *amoxicillin/clavulanate* (B)(G) 500 mg tid or 875 mg bid x 10 days
Augmentin *Tab:* 250, 500, 875 mg; *Chew tab:* 125, 250 mg (lemon-lime); 200, 400 mg (cherry-banana) (phenylalanine); *Oral susp:* 125 mg/5 ml (banana), 250 mg/5 ml (75, 100, 150 ml) (orange); 200, 400 mg/5 ml (50, 75, 100 ml) (orange) (phenylalanine)
Pediatric: 40-45 mg/kg/day divided tid x 10 days or 90 mg/kg/day divided bid x 10 days see pages 556-557 for dose by weight

Augmentin ES-600 *Oral susp:* 600 mg/5 ml (50, 75, 100, 125, 150, 200 ml)
(strawberry cream) (phenylalanine) every 12 hours
> *Pediatric:* <3 months: not recommended; ≥3 months, <40 kg: 90 mg/kg/day
> in 2 divided doses; ≥40 kg: not recommended

Augmentin XR 2 tabs q 12 hours x 7-10 days
> *Pediatric:* <16 years: use other forms; ≥16 years: same as adult
> *Tab:* 1000*mg ext-rel

▷ *ampicillin* (B) 500 mg qid x 7-14 days
Pediatric: 50-100 mg/kg/day in 4 divided doses x 7-14 days; *see page 558 for dose by weight*

Omnipen, Principen *Cap:* 250, 500 mg; *Oral susp:* 125, 250 mg/5 ml (100, 150, 200 ml) (fruit)

▷ *carbenicillin* (B) 1-2 tabs qid x 7-14 days
Pediatric: not recommended

Geocillin *Tab:* 382 mg

▷ *cefaclor* (B)(G) 250-500 mg q 8 hours x 10 days; max 2 g/day
Pediatric: <1 month: not recommended; 20-40 mg/kg bid or q 12 hours x 10 days; max 1 g/day; *see page 560 for dose by weight*
Tab: 500 mg; *Cap:* 250, 500 mg; *Susp:* 125 mg/5 ml (75, 150 ml) (strawberry); 187 mg/5 ml (50, 100 ml) (strawberry); 250 mg/5 ml (75, 150 ml) (strawberry); 375 mg/5 ml (50, 100 ml) (strawberry)
Pediatric: <16 years: ext-rel not recommended; ≥16 years: same as adult

Cefaclor Extended Release *Tab:* 375, 500 mg ext-rel

▷ *cefadroxil* (B) 1-2 g in a single or 2 divided doses x 10 days
Pediatric: 30 mg/kg/day in 2 divided doses x 10 days; *see page 561 for dose by weight*
Duricef *Cap:* 500 mg; *Tab:* 1 g; *Oral susp:* 250 mg/5 ml (100 ml); 500 mg/5 ml (75, 100 ml) (orange-pineapple)

▷ *cefixime* (B) 400 mg once daily x 10 days
Pediatric: <6 months: not recommended; 6 months-12 years, <50 kg: 8 mg/kg/day in a single or 2 divided doses x 10 days; >12 years, >50 kg: same as adult; *see page 563 for dose by weight*
Suprax *Tab:* 400 mg; *Cap:* 400 mg; *Oral susp:* 100, 200 mg/5 ml (50, 75, 100 ml) (strawberry)

▷ *cefpodoxime proxetil* (B) 100 mg bid x 7 days
Pediatric: <2 months: not recommended; 2 months-12 years: 10 mg/kg/day (max 400 mg/dose) or 5 mg/kg/day bid (max 200 mg/dose) x 7 days: >12 years: same as adult; *see page 564 for dose by weight*
Vantin *Tab:* 100, 200 mg; *Oral susp:* 50, 100 mg/5 ml (50, 75, 100 mg) (lemon creme)

▷ *cefuroxime axetil* (B)(G) 125-250 mg bid x 7-10 days
Pediatric: <3 months: not recommended; 3 months-12 years: 20-30 mg/kg/day in 2 divided doses x 7-10 days; >12 years: same as adult; *see page 567 for dose by weight*
Ceftin *Tab:* 250, 500 mg; *Oral susp:* 125, 250 mg/5 ml (50, 100 ml) (tutti-frutti)

▷ *cephalexin* (B)(G) 500 mg bid x 7-10 days
Pediatric: 25-50 mg/kg/day in 4 divided doses x 7-10 days; *see page 568 for dose by weight*
Keflex *Cap:* 250, 333, 500, 750 mg; *Oral susp:* 125, 250 mg/5 ml (100, 200 ml) (strawberry)

▷ *ciprofloxacin* (C) 500 mg bid or 1000 mg XR once daily x 3-14 days
Pediatric: <18 years: not recommended

Cipro (G) *Tab:* 250, 500, 750 mg; *Oral susp:* 250, 500 mg/5 ml (100 ml)
(strawberry)
Cipro XR *Tab:* 500, 1000 mg ext-rel
ProQuin XR *Tab:* 500 mg ext-rel
Comment: *ciprofloxacin* is contraindicated <18 years-of-age, and during pregnancy
and lactation. Risk of tendonitis or tendon rupture, especially 60 years-of-age and
older.

▷ *doxycycline* **(D)(G)** 100 mg bid x 7-10 days
Pediatric: <8 years: not recommended; ≥8 years, <100 lb: 2 mg/lb on first day in 2
divided doses, followed by 1 mg/lb/day in a single or 2 divided doses x 7-10 days;
≥8 years, >100 lb: same as adult
   Actilate *Tab:* 75, 150**mg
   Adoxa *Tab:* 50, 75, 100, 150 mg ent-coat
   Doryx *Tab:* 50, 75, 100, 150, 200 mg del-rel
   Monodox *Cap:* 50, 75, 100 mg
   Oracea *Cap:* 40 mg del-rel
   Vibramycin *Tab:* 100 mg; *Cap:* 50, 100 mg; *Syr:* 50 mg/5 ml (raspberry-apple)
   (sulfites); *Oral susp:* 25 mg/5 ml (raspberry)
   Vibra-Tab *Tab:* 100 mg film-coat
Comment: *doxycycline* is contraindicated <8 years-of-age, in pregnancy, and
lactation (discolors developing tooth enamel). A side effect may be photo-
sensitivity (photophobia). Do not give with antacids, calcium supplements, milk or
other dairy, or within two hours of taking another drug.

▷ *enoxacin* **(C)** 200 mg q 12 hours x 7 days
Pediatric: <18 years: not recommended
   Penetrex *Tab:* 200, 400 mg
Comment: *enoxacin* is contraindicated <18 years-of-age, and during pregnancy and
lactation. Risk of tendonitis or tendon rupture, especially 60 years-of-age and older.

▷ *levofloxacin* **(C)** 250 mg once daily x 7-10 days
Pediatric: <18 years not recommended
   Levaquin *Tab:* 250, 500, 750 mg; *Oral soln:* 25 mg/ml (480 ml) (benzyl alcohol);
   Inj conc: 25 mg/ml for IV infusion after dilution (20, 30 ml single-use vial)
   (preservative-free); *Premix soln:* 5 mg/ml for IV infusion (50, 100, 150 ml)
   (preservative-free)
Comment: *levofloxacin* is contraindicated <18 years-of-age, and during pregnancy
and lactation. Risk of tendonitis or tendon rupture, especially 60 years-of-age and
older.

▷ *lomefloxacin* **(C)** 400 mg once daily x 10 days
Pediatric: <18 years: not recommended
   Maxaquin *Tab:* 400 mg
Comment: *lomefloxacin* is contraindicated <18 years-of-age, and during pregnancy
and lactation. Risk of tendonitis or tendon rupture, especially 60 years-of-age and
older.

▷ *minocycline* **(D)(G)** 100 mg q 12 hours x 10 days
Pediatric: <8 years: not recommended; ≥8 years, <100 lb: 2 mg/lb on first day in 2 divided
doses, followed by 1 mg/lb q 12 hours x 9 more days; ≥8 years, >100 lb: same as adult
   Dynacin *Cap:* 50, 100 mg
   Minocin *Cap:* 50, 75, 100 mg; *Oral susp:* 50 mg/5 ml (60 ml) (custard) (sulfites,
   alcohol 5%)

Comment: *minocycline* is contraindicated <8 years-of-age, in pregnancy, and lactation (discolors developing tooth enamel). A side effect may be photosensitivity (photophobia). Do not give with antacids, calcium supplements, milk or other dairy, or within two hours of taking another drug.

▷ *nalidixic acid* (B) 1 g qid x 7-14 days
Pediatric: <3 months: not recommended; >3 months: 25 mg/lb/day in 4 divided doses x 7-14 days
  NegGram *Tab:* 250, 500 mg; 1 g; *Cap:* 250, 500 mg; *Oral susp:* 250 mg/5 ml

▷ *nitrofurantoin* (B)(G)
  Furadantin 50-100 mg qid x 7-10 days
    Pediatric: <1 month: not recommended; ≥1 month: 5-7 mg/kg/day in 4 divided doses x 7-10 days; *see page* 582 *for dose by weight*
    Oral susp: 25 mg/5 ml (60 ml)
  Macrobid 100 mg q 12 hours x 7-10 days
    Pediatric: <12 years: not recommended; ≥12 years: same as adult
    Cap: 100 mg
  Macrodantin 50-100 mg qid x 5-7 days; long-term use 50-100 mg q HS
    Cap: 25, 50, 100 mg

▷ *norfloxacin* (C) 400 mg x 7-10 days
  Pediatric: <18 years: not recommended
    Noroxin *Tab:* 400 mg

Comment: *norfloxacin* is contraindicated <18 years-of-age, and during pregnancy and lactation. Risk of tendonitis or tendon rupture, especially 60 years-of-age and older.

▷ *ofloxacin* (C)(G) 200 mg q 12 hours x 7-10 days
  Pediatric: <18 years: not recommended
    Floxin *Tab:* 200, 300, 400 mg

Comment: *ofloxacin* is contraindicated <18 years-of-age, and during pregnancy and lactation. Risk of tendonitis or tendon rupture, especially 60 years-of-age and older.

▷ *trimethoprim* (C)(G)
  Primsol 100 mg q 12 hours or 200 mg once daily x 10 days
    Pediatric: <6 months: not recommended; ≥6 months: 10 mg/kg/day in 2 divided doses divided q 12 hours x 10 days
    Oral soln: 50 mg/5 ml (bubble gum; dye-free, alcohol-free)
  Proloprim 100 mg q 12 hours or 200 mg once daily x 10 days
    Pediatric: not recommended
    Tab: 100, 200 mg
  Trimpex 100 mg q 12 hours or 200 mg once daily x 10 days
    Pediatric: not recommended
    Tab: 100 mg

▷ *trimethoprim/sulfamethoxazole* (D)(G)
  Pediatric: <2 months: not recommended; ≥2 months: 40 mg/kg/day of *sulfamethoxazole* in 2 divided doses bid x 10 days; *see page* 587 *for dose by weight*
    Bactrim, Septra 2 tabs bid x 10 days
      Tab: trim 80 mg/*sulfa* 400 mg*
    Bactrim DS, Septra DS 1 tab bid x 10 days
      Tab: trim 160 mg/*sulfa* 800 mg*
    Bactrim Pediatric Suspension, Septra Pediatric Suspension
      Oral susp: trim 40 mg/*sulfa* 200 mg per 5 ml (100 ml) (cherry) (alcohol 0.3%)

Comment: *trimethoprim/sulfamethoxazole* is not recommended in pregnancy or lactation. *CrCl 15-30 mL/min:* reduce dose by 1/2; *CrCl <15 mL/min:* not recommended

PARENTERAL THERAPY

▷ *ertapenem* (B) 1 g once daily; *CrCl <30 mL/min:* 500 mg once daily; treat x 10-14 days; may switch to an oral antibiotic after 3 days if warranted; *IV infusion:* administer over 30 minutes; *IM injection:* reconstitute with lidocaine only
  Pediatric: <18 years: not recommended
    Ivanz *Vial:* 1 g pwdr for reconstitution

LONG-TERM PROPHYLACTIC/SUPPRESSION THERAPY

▷ *methenamine hippurate* (C) 1 tab bid
  Pediatric: <6 years: not recommended; ≥6-12 years: 1/2 tab bid
    Hiprex, Urex *Tab:* 1 g

URINARY TRACT ANALGESIC/ANTISPASMODICS

▷ *hyoscyamine* (C)(G)
    Anaspaz 1-2 tabs q 4 hours prn; max 12 tabs/day
      Pediatric: <2 years: not recommended; ≥2-12 years: 0.0625-0.125 mg q 4 hours prn; max 0.75 mg/day; >12 years: same as adult
      Tab: 0.125*mg
    Levbid 1-2 tabs q 12 hours prn; max 4 tabs/day
      Pediatric: <12 years: not recommended; ≥12 years: same as adult
      Tab: 0.375*mg ext-rel
    Levsin 1-2 tabs q 4 hours prn; max 12 tabs/day
      Pediatric: <6 years: not recommended; 6-12 years: 1 tab q 4 hours prn; ≥12 years: same as adult
      Tab: 0.125*mg
    Levsin Drops 1-2 ml q 4 hours prn; max 60 ml/day
      Pediatric: 3.4 kg: 4 drops q 4 hours prn; max 24 drops/day; 5 kg: 5 drops q 4 hours prn; max 30 drops/day; 7 kg: 6 drops q 4 hours prn; max 36 drops/day; 10 kg: 8 drops q 4 hours prn; max 40 drops/day
      Oral drops: 0.125 mg/ml (15 ml) (orange) (alcohol 5%)
    Levsin Elixir 5-10 ml q 4 hours prn
      Pediatric: <10 kg: use drops; 10-19 kg: 1.25 ml q 4 hours prn; 20-39 kg: 2.5 ml q 4 hours prn; 40-49 kg: 3.75 ml q 4 hours prn; >50 kg: 5 ml q 4 hours prn
      Elix: 0.125 mg/5 ml (16 oz) (orange) (alcohol 20%)
    Levsinex SL 1-2 tabs q 4 hours SL or PO; max 12 tabs/day
      Pediatric: 2-12 years: 1 tab q 4 hours; max 6 tabs/day; >12 years: same as adult
      Tab: 0.125 mg sublingual
    Levsinex Timecaps 1-2 caps q 12 hours; may adjust to 1 cap q 8 hours
      Pediatric: 2-12 years: 1 cap q 12 hours; max 2 caps/day; >12 years: same as adult
      Cap: 0.375 mg time-rel
    NuLev dissolve 1-2 tabs on tongue, with or without water, q 4 hours prn; max 12 tabs/day
      Pediatric: <2 years: not recommended; 2-12 years: dissolve 1 tab on tongue, with or without water, q 4 hours prn; max 6 tabs/day

      ODT: 0.125 mg (mint) (phenylalanine)

▷ *methenamine/phenyl salicylate/methylene blue/benzoic acid/atropine sulfate/hyoscyamine* (C)(G) 2 tabs qid prn
    Pediatric: <6 years: not recommended
        Urised *Tab:* meth 40.8 mg/*phenyl salic* 18.1 mg/*meth blue* 5.4 mg/*benz acid* 4.5 mg/*atro sulf* 0.03 mg/*hyoscy* 0.03 mg
        Comment: **Urised** imparts a blue-green color to urine which may stain fabrics.

▷ *methenamine/phenyl salicylate/methylene blue/na phosphate onobasic/hyoscyamine* (C) 1 cap qid prn
    Pediatric: <6 years: not recommended; ≥6 years: same as adult
        Uribel *Cap:* meth 118 mg/*phenyl salic* 36 mg/*meth blue* 10 mg/*naphos mono* 40.8 mg/*hyoscy* 0.12 mg

▷ *methenamine/phenyl salicylate/methylene blue/na biphosphate/hyoscyamine* (C) 1 tab qid prn
    Pediatric: <6 years: not recommended; ≥6 years: same as adult
        Urelle *Cap:* meth 81 mg/*phenyl salic* 32.4 mg/*meth blue* 10.8 mg/*na biphos* 40.8 mg/*hyoscy* 0.12 mg

▷ *phenazopyridine* (B)(G) 95-200 mg q 6 hours prn; max 2 days
    Pediatric: not recommended
        AZO Standard, Prodium, Uristat (OTC) *Tab:* 95 mg
        AZO Standard Maximum Strength (OTC) *Tab:* 97.5 mg
        Pyridium, Urogesic *Tab:* 100, 200 mg
    Comment: *phenazopyridine* imparts an orange-red color to urine which may stain fabrics.

PROPHYLACTIC/SUPPRESSION THERAPY

▷ *methenamine hippurate* (C) 1 g bid
    Pediatric: <6 years: 0.25 g/30 lb qid; 6-12 years: 25-50 mg/kg/day in 2 divided doses <u>or</u> 0.5-1 g bid; >12 years: same as adult
        Hiprex *Tab:* 1 g; *Oral susp:* 500 mg/5 ml (480 ml)

 ## UROLITHIASIS (RENAL CALCULI, KIDNEY STONES)

Acetaminophen for IV Infusion *see Pain page 306*
Oral Prescription NSAIDs *see page 501*
Other Oral Analgesics *see Pain page 308*
Opioids and Other Analgesics *see page 308*

ANTISPASMOTIC

▷ *flavoxate* (B)(G)
        Urispaz 100-200 mg tid-qid

PARENTERAL NARCOTICS

Aid to Stone Passage: Alpha-1A Blockers

▷ *alfuzosin* (B)(G) 10 mg once daily taken immediately after the same meal each day

      UroXatral *Tab:* 10 mg ext-rel
▷ *tamsulosin* (B)(G) initially 0.4 mg once daily; may increase to 0.8 mg once daily after 2-4 weeks if needed
      Flomax *Cap:* 0.4 mg
      Comment: May take **Flomax** 0.4 mg with **Avodart** 0.5 mg once daily as combination therapy.
▷ *buprenorphine* (C)
      Buprenex administer 1-2 mg IM/IV q 3-4 hours prn; may repeat once (up to 0.3 mg) if required, 30 to 60 minutes after initial dose
        Pediatric: 2-12 years: 2-6 mcg/kg IM/IV q 4-6 hours prn
          Amp: 0.3 mg/ml (1 ml)
      Comment: **Buprenex** is approximately equivalent to 10 mg morphine sulfate in analgesic and respiratory depressant effects.
▷ *meperidine* (B; D in 2nd, 3rd)(II)(G) 50-100 mg IM q 3-4 hours prn
      Demerol *Tubex:* 25, 50, 75, 100 mg/ml (2 ml); *Vial:* 25 mg/ml (1 ml); 50 mg/ml (1, 30 ml); 75 mg/ml; (1 ml); 100 mg/ml (1, 20 ml)
        Amp: 25, 50, 75, 100 mg/ml (1 ml)
▷ *morphine sulfate* (C)(II)(G) 10-15 mg q 3-4 hours prn
        Vial: 1 mg/ml (1, 60 ml); 5 mg/ml (1 ml); 8 mg/ml (1 ml); 10 mg/ml (1, 2, 10 ml); 15 mg (1, 20 ml); *Amp:* 8 mg/ml (1 ml); 10 mg/ml (1 ml); 15 mg/ml (1 ml)

PREVENTION OF CALCIUM STONES

▷ *chlorothiazide* (B)(G) 50 mg bid
      Diuril *Tab:* 250*, 500*mg; *Oral susp:* 250 mg/5 ml (237 ml)
▷ *hydrochlorothiazide* (B)(G) 50 mg bid
      Esidrix *Tab:* 25, 50mg
      Microzide *Cap:* 12.5 mg

PREVENTION OF CYSTINE STONES

▷ *penicillamine* (D) 1-4 g/day
      Pediatric: not recommended
        Cuprimine *Cap:* 125, 250 mg
        Depen *Titratable tab:* 250 mg
▷ *potassium citrate* (C)(G) 30 mEq qid
      Umetozolvrocit-K *Tab:* 5, 10, 15 mEq ext-rel
      Comment: *potassium citrate* is contraindicated in hyperkalemia.

PREVENTION OF URIC ACID STONES

▷ *allopurinol* (C)(G) 200-300 mg in 1-3 doses; max 800 mg/day
      Zyloprim *Tab:* 100*, 300*mg
▷ *potassium citrate* (C)(G) 30 mEq qid
      Urocit-K *Tab:* 5, 10, 15 mEq ext-rel
      Comment: *potassium citrate* is contraindicated in hyperkalemia. Encourage patients to limit salt intake and maintain liberal hydration (urine volume should be at least 2 liters/day). Target urine pH is 6.0-7.0 and urine citrate at least 320 mg/day and close to the normal mean of 640 mg/day. Take with food.

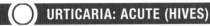 URTICARIA: CHRONIC IDIOPATHIC (CIU)

▷ *hydroxyzine* (C)(G) 25 mg tid prn; max 600 mg/day
  Pediatric: <6 years: 50 mg/day divided qid prn; ≥6 years: 50-100 mg/day divided qid prn; max 600 mg/day
    AtaraxR *Tab:* 10, 25, 50, 100 mg; *Syr:* 10 mg/5 ml (alcohol 0.5%)
    VistarilR *Cap:* 25, 50, 100 mg; *Oral susp:* 25 mg/5 ml (4 oz) (lemon)
Oral Drugs for Allergy, Cough, and Cold Symptoms *see page* 535

URTICARIA: ACUTE (HIVES)

MILD/MODERATE URTICARIA

Oral Drugs for Allergy, Cough, and Cold Symptoms *see page* 535
Topical Corticosteroids *see page* 506
Oral Corticosteroids *see page* 509

SEVERE URTICARIA

Parenteral Antihistamines

▷ *diphenhydramine* (C)(G) 25-50 mg IM immediately; then q 6 hours
  Pediatric: 1.25 mg/kg up to 25 mg IM x 1 dose; then q 6 hours
    Benadryl Injectable *Vial:* 50 mg/ml (1 ml single-use); 50 mg/ml (10 ml multi-dose); *Amp:* 10 mg/ml (1 ml); *Prefilled syringe:* 50 mg/ml (1 ml)

Parenteral Corticosteroids *see page* 511

▷ *epinephrine* (C) 1:1000 0.01 ml/kg SC; max 0.3 ml
  Pediatric: 0.01 mg/kg SC

VAGINAL IRRITATION: EXTERNAL

▷ Replens Vaginal Moisturizer (NE)(OTC) apply as needed; for external use only
  Bottle: 2 oz
▷ Vagisil Intimate Moisturizer (NE)(OTC) apply as needed; for external use only
  Bottle: 2 oz
  Comment: Vagisil has no effect on condom integrity.

VERTIGO

▷ *meclizine* (B)(G) 25-100 mg/day in divided doses
  Pediatric: not recommended
    Antivert *Tab:* 12.5, 25, 50*mg
    Bonine (OTC) *Cap:* 15, 25, 30 mg; *Tab:* 12.5, 25, 50 mg; *Chew tab/Film-coat tab:* 25 mg

Dramamine II (OTC) *Tab:* 25*mg
Zentrip *Strip:* 25 mg orally-disint

◯ VITILIGO

REPIGMENTATION ENHANCEMENT

▷ *methoxsalen* (C) Apply to well-defined area of vitiligo; then expose area to source of UVA (ultraviolet A) <u>or</u> sunlight; initial exposure no more than 1/2 predicted minimal erythemal dose; repeat weekly
Pediatric: <12 years: not recommended
    Oxsoralen *Lotn:* 1% (30 ml)
Comment: *methoxsalen* may only be applied by a health care provider. Do not dispense to patient.
▷ *trioxsalen* (C) 10 mg daily, taken 2-4 hours before ultraviolet light exposure; max 14 days and 28 tabs
Pediatric: <12 years: not recommended
    Trisoralen *Tab:* 5 mg
    Depigmenting Agents *see Hyperpigmentation page* 206

◯ WART: COMMON (VERRUCA VULGARIS)

▷ *salicylic acid* (NE)(G)
    Duo Film (OTC) apply daily-bid; max 12 weeks; *Liq:* 17% (1/2 oz w. applicator)
    Duo Film Patch for Kids (OTC) apply 1 patch q 48 hours; max 12 weeks
    Patch: 40% (18/pck)
    Occlusal HP (OTC) apply daily-bid; max 12 weeks
    Liq: 17% (10 ml w. applicator)
    Wart-Off (OTC) apply one drop at a time to sufficiently cover wart, let dry; repeat 1-2 times daily; max 12 weeks
    Liq: 17% (0.45 oz)

◯ WART: PLANTAR (VERRUCA PLANTARIS)

▷ *salicylic acid* (NE)(G)
    Duo Plant Gel (OTC) apply daily bid; max 12 weeks
    Gel: 17% (1/2 oz)
    Mediplast cut to size of wart and apply; remove q 1-2 days, peel keratin, and reapply; repeat as long as needed
    Occlusal-HP (OTC) apply once daily-bid; max 12 weeks
    Liq: 17% (10 ml w. applicator)
    Wart-Off (OTC) apply one drop at a time to sufficiently cover wart, let dry; repeat 1-2 times daily; max 12 weeks
    Liq: 17% (0.45 oz)
▷ *trichloroacetic acid* (NE) apply after wart is pared and repeat weekly

WART: VENEREAL, HUMAN PAPILLOMAVIRUS (HPV), CONDYLOMA ACUMINATA

Comment: This section contains treatment regimens for genital warts published in the **2015 CDC Sexually Transmitted Diseases Treatment Guidelines** as well as other treatment options. Due to the increased risk of cervical cancer with HPV, Pap smears should be done q 3 months during active disease and then q 3-6 months for the next 2 years.

PATIENT-APPLIED AGENTS

Regimen 1

▷ *imiquimod* (C)
  Pediatric: not recommended
      Aldara (G) rub into lesions before bedtime and remove with soap and water 6-10 hours later; treat 3 times per week; max 16 weeks
        Crm: 5% (12 single-use pkts/carton)
      Zyclara rub into lesions before bedtime and remove with soap and water 8 hours later; treat 3 times per week; max 1 packet per treatment; max 8 weeks
        Crm: 3.75% (28 single-use pkts/carton) (parabens)

Regimen 2

▷ *podofilox 0.5% cream* (C) apply bid (q 12 hours) x 3 days; then discontinue for 4 days; may repeat if needed; max 4 treatment cycles
      Condylox *Soln:* 0.5% (3.5 ml); *Gel:* 0.5% (3.5 g)

Regimen 3

▷ *sinecatechins 15% ointment* (C) apply to each lesion tid for up to 16 weeks
      Veregen *Oint:* 15% (15, 30 g)

PROVIDER-ADMINISTERED AGENTS

Regimen 1

▷ Cryotherapy with liquid nitrogen or cryoprobe; repeat applications every 1-2 weeks as needed

Regimen 2

▷ *trichloroacetic acid (TCA) 80-90%* (C) apply to warts; repeat weekly if needed
Comment: TCA is the preferred treatment during pregnancy. Immediate application of sodium bicarbonate paste following treatment decreases pain.

Regimen 3

▷ *podofilox 0.5% cream* (C) apply bid (q 12 hours) x 3 days; then discontinue for 4 days; may repeat if needed; max 4 treatment cycles
      Condylox *Soln:* 0.5% (3.5 ml); *Gel:* 0.5% (3.5 g)

Regimen 4

▷ *interferon alfa-n3* (C) 0.05 ml injected into base of wart twice weekly for up to 8 weeks; max 0.5 ml/session (20 warts/session)

Alferon N *Vial:* 5 million units/ml (1 ml)

Regimen 5

▷ *interferon alfa-2b* (C) 0.1 ml injected into base of wart three times weekly for up to 3 weeks; max 0.5 ml/session (5 warts/session)

Intron A *Vial:* 1 million units/0.1 ml (0.5, 1 ml)

Regimen 6

▷ Surgical removal either by tangential scissor excision, tangential shave excision, curettage, <u>or</u> electrosurgery

 WHIPWORM (TRICHURIASIS)

ANTHELMINTICS

▷ *albendazole* (C) 400 mg as a single dose; may repeat in 3 weeks; take with a meal
Pediatric: <2 years: 200 mg daily x 3 days; may repeat in 3 weeks; 2-12 years: 400 mg daily x 3 days; may repeat in 3 weeks; >12 years: same as adult

Albenza *Tab:* 200 mg

▷ *mebendazole* (C) chew, swallow, <u>or</u> mix with food; 100 mg bid x 3 days; may repeat in 3 weeks if needed; take with a meal
Pediatric: <2 years: not recommended; ≥2 years: same as adult

Emverm *Chew tab:* 100 mg

Vermox (G) *Chew tab:* 100 mg

▷ *pyrantel pamoate* (C) 11 mg/kg x 1 dose; max 1 g/dose; take with a meal
Pediatric: 25-37 lb: 1/2 tsp x 1 dose; 38-62 lb: 1 tsp x 1 dose; 63-87 lb: 1 tsp x 1 dose; 88-112 lb: 2 tsp x 1 dose; 113-137 lb: 2 tsp x 1 dose; 138-162 lb: 3 tsp x 1 dose; 163-187 lb: 3 tsp x 1 dose; >187 lb: 4 tsp x 1 dose

Antiminth (OTC) *Cap:* 180 mg; *Liq:* 50 mg/ml (30 ml); 144 mg/ml (30 ml); *Oral susp:* 50 mg/ml (60 ml)

Pin-X (OTC) *Cap:* 180 mg; *Liq:* 50 mg/ml (30 ml); 144 mg/ml (30 ml); *Oral susp:* 50 mg/ml (30 ml)

▷ *thiabendazole* (C) 25 mg/kg bid x 7 days; max 1.5 g/dose; take with a meal
Pediatric: same as adult; <30 lb: consult mfr pkg insert; >30 lb: 2 doses/day with meals; 30-50 lb: 250 mg bid with meals; >50 lb: 10 mg/lb/dose bid with meals; max 3g/day

Mintezol *Chew tab:* 500*mg (orange); *Oral susp:* 500 mg/5 ml (120 ml) (orange)

Comment: *thiabendazole* is not for prophylaxis. May impair mental alertness.

 WOUND: INFECTED, NONSURGICAL, MINOR

TETANUS PROPHYLAXIS

Previously Immunized (within previous 5 years)

▷ *tetanus toxoid* vaccine (C) 0.5 ml IM x 1 dose

Vial: 5 Lf units/0.5 ml (0.5, 5 ml); *Prefilled syringe:* 5 Lf units/0.5 ml (0.5 ml)

Not Previously Immunized

see Tetanus *page* 408

TOPICAL ANTI-INFECTIVES

▷ *mupirocin* (B)(G) apply to lesions bid
Pediatric: same as adult
   Bactroban *Oint:* 2% (22 g); *Crm:* 2% (15, 30 g)
   Centany *Oint:* 2% (15, 30 g)

ORAL ANTI-INFECTIVES

▷ *azithromycin* (B) 500 mg x 1 dose on day 1, then 250 mg daily on days 2-5 <u>or</u> 500 mg
daily x 3 days <u>or</u> Zmax 2 g in a single dose
Pediatric: 10 mg/kg x 1 dose on day 1, then 5 mg/kg/day on days 2-5; max 500 mg/
day; *see page 559 for dose by weight*
   Zithromax *Tab:* 250, 500, 600 mg; *Oral susp:* 100 mg/5 ml (15 ml); 200 mg/5 ml
   (15, 22.5, 30 ml) (cherry); *Pkt:* 1 g for reconstitution (cherry-banana)
   Zithromax Tri-pak *Tab:* 3 x 500 mg tabs/pck
   Zithromax Z-pak *Tab:* 6 x 250 mg tabs/pck
   Zmax *Oral susp:* 2 g ext-rel for reconstitution (cherry-banana) (148 mg Na$^+$)
▷ *amoxicillin/clavulanate* (B)(G) 500 mg tid <u>or</u> 875 mg bid x 10 days
   Augmentin *Tab:* 250, 500, 875 mg; *Chew tab:* 125, 250 mg (lemon-lime); 200,
   400 mg (cherry-banana) (phenylalanine); *Oral susp:* 125 mg/5 ml (banana), 250
   mg/5 ml (75, 100, 150 ml) (orange); 200, 400 mg/5 ml (50, 75, 100 ml) (orange)
   (phenylalanine)
      Pediatric: 40-45 mg/kg/day divided tid x 10 days <u>or</u> 90 mg/kg/day divided
      bid x 10 days; *see pages 556-557 for dose by weight*
   Augmentin ES-600 *Oral susp:* 600 mg/5 ml (50, 75, 100, 125, 150, 200 ml)
   (strawberry cream) (phenylalanine) every 12 hours
      Pediatric: <3 months: not recommended; ≥3 months, <40 kg: 90 mg/kg/day
      in 2 divided doses; ≥40 kg: not recommended
   Augmentin XR 2 tabs q 12 hours x 7-10 days
      Pediatric: <16 years: use other forms; ≥16 years: same as adult
      Tab: 1000*mg ext-rel
▷ *cefaclor* (B)(G) 250-500 mg q 8 hours x 10 days; max 2 g/day
Pediatric: <1 month: not recommended; 20-40 mg/kg bid <u>or</u> q 12 hours x 10 days;
max 1 g/day; *see page 560 for dose by weight*
Tab: 500 mg; *Cap:* 250, 500 mg; *Susp:* 125 mg/5 ml (75, 150 ml) (strawberry);
187 mg/5 ml (50, 100 ml) (strawberry); 250 mg/5 ml (75, 150 ml) (strawberry);
375 mg/5 ml (50, 100 ml) (strawberry)
Pediatric: <16 years: ext-rel not recommended
   Cefaclor Extended Release *Tab:* 375, 500 mg ext-rel
▷ *cefadroxil* 1 g/day in 1-2 divided doses x 10 days
Pediatric: 15-30 mg/kg/day in 2 divided doses x 10 days; *see page 561 for dose by
weight*

Duricef *Cap:* 500 mg; *Tab:* 1 g; *Oral susp:* 250 mg/5 ml (100 ml); 500 mg/5 ml (75, 100 ml) (orange-pineapple)

▷ *cefdinir* (B) 300 mg bid <u>or</u> 600 mg daily x 10 days
Pediatric: <6 months: not recommended; 6 months-12 years: 14 mg/kg/day in 1-2 divided doses x 10 days; *see page 562 for dose by weight*
Omnicef *Cap:* 300 mg; *Oral susp:* 125 mg/5 ml (60, 100 ml) (strawberry)

▷ *cefpodoxime proxetil* (B) 400 mg bid x 7-14 days
Pediatric: <2 months: not recommended; 2 months-12 years: 10 mg/kg/day (max 400 mg/dose) <u>or</u> 5 mg/kg/day bid (max 200 mg/dose) x 7-14 days; *see page 564 for dose by weight*
Vantin *Tab:* 100, 200 mg; *Oral susp:* 50, 100 mg/5 ml (50, 75, 100 mg; lemon cream)
Pediatric: see page 564 for dose by weight

▷ *cefprozil* (B) 250-500 mg q 12 hours <u>or</u> 500 mg daily x 10 days
Pediatric: <2 years: not recommended; 2-12 years: 7.5 mg/kg-15 mg/kg q 12 hours x 10 days; >12 years: same as adult; *see page 565 for dose by weight*
Cefzil *Tab:* 250, 500 mg; *Oral susp:* 125, 250 mg/5 ml (50, 75, 100 ml) (bubble gum, phenylalanine)

▷ *cephalexin* (B)(G) 2 g 1 hour before procedure
Pediatric: 50 mg/kg/day in 4 divided doses x 10 days; *see page 568 for dose by weight*
Keflex *Cap:* 250, 333, 500, 750 mg; *Oral susp:* 125, 250 mg/5 ml (100, 200 ml) (strawberry)
Pediatric: see page 568 for dose by weight

▷ *clarithromycin* (C)(G) 500 mg <u>or</u> 500 mg ext-rel for 7-10 days
Pediatric: see page 569 for dose by weight
Biaxin *Tab:* 250, 500 mg
Biaxin Oral Suspension *Oral susp:* 125, 250 mg/5 ml (50, 100 ml) (fruit-punch)
Biaxin XL *Tab:* 500 mg ext-rel

▷ *dirithromycin* (C)(G) 500 mg daily x 7 days
Pediatric: <12 years: not recommended
Dynabac *Tab:* 250 mg

▷ *erythromycin base* (B)(G) 500 mg qid x 14 days
Pediatric: 30-50 mg/kg/day in 2-4 divided doses x 10 days
Ery-Tab *Tab:* 250, 333, 500 mg ent-coat
PCE *Tab:* 333, 500 mg

Comment: *erythromycin* may increase INR with concomitant *warfarin*, as well as increase serum level of *digoxin*, benzodiazepines and statins.

▷ *erythromycin ethylsuccinate* (B)(G) 400 mg qid x 7 days
Pediatric: 30-50 mg/kg/day in 4 divided doses x 7 days; may double dose with severe infection; max 100 mg/kg/day; *see page 574 for dose by weight*
EryPed *Oral susp:* 200 mg/5 ml (100, 200 ml) (fruit); 400 mg/5 ml (60, 100, 200 ml) (banana); *Oral drops:* 200, 400 mg/5 ml (50 ml) (fruit); *Chew tab:* 200 mg wafer (fruit)
E.E.S. *Oral susp:* 200, 400 mg/5 ml (100 ml) (fruit)
E.E.S. Granules *Oral susp:* 200 mg/5 ml (100, 200 ml) (cherry)
E.E.S. 400 Tablets *Tab:* 400 mg

Comment: *erythromycin* may increase INR with concomitant **warfarin**, as well as increase serum level of **digoxin**, benzodiazepines and statins.

▷ *gemifloxacin* (C)(G) 320 mg daily x 5-7 days
  Pediatric: <18 years: not recommended
      Factive *Tab:* 320*mg

Comment: *gemifloxacin* is contraindicated <18 years-of-age, and during pregnancy and lactation. Risk of tendonitis or tendon rupture, especially 60 years-of-age and older.

▷ *levofloxacin* (C) *Uncomplicated:* 500 mg daily x 7 days; *Complicated:* 750 mg daily x 7 days
  Pediatric: <18 years: not recommended
      Levaquin *Tab:* 250, 500, 750 mg

Comment: *levofloxacin* is contraindicated <18 years-of-age, and during pregnancy and lactation. Risk of tendonitis or tendon rupture, especially 60 years-of-age and older.

▷ *loracarbef* (B) 200-400 mg bid x 7 days
  Pediatric: 15 mg/kg/day in 2 divided doses x 7 days; *see page 581 for dose by weight*
      Lorabid *Pulvule:* 200, 400 mg; *Oral susp:* 100 mg/5 ml (50, 100 ml); 200 mg/5 ml (50, 75, 100 ml) (strawberry bubble gum)

▷ *ofloxacin* (C)(G) 400 mg bid x 10 days
  Pediatric: <18 years: not recommended
      Floxin *Tab:* 200, 300, 400 mg

Comment: *ofloxacin* is contraindicated <18 years-of-age, and during pregnancy and lactation. Risk of tendonitis or tendon rupture, especially 60 years-of-age and older.

WRINKLES: FACIAL (CROW'S FEET, FROWN LINES, SMILE LINES)

TOPICAL RETINOIDS

Comment: Wash the affected area with a soap-free cleanser; pat dry and wait 20 to 30 minutes; then apply topical retinoid sparingly to affected area. Use only once daily in the PM. Avoid eyes, ears, nostrils, and mouth.

▷ *adapalene* (C)(G)
  Pediatric: <12 years: not recommended
      Differin *Crm:* 0.1% (15, 45 g); *Gel:* 0.1% (15, 45 g); *Pad:* 0.1% (30/pk; alcohol 30%)
      Differin Solution *Soln:* 0.1% (30 ml; alcohol 30%)

▷ *tazarotene* (X) apply daily at HS
  Pediatric: not recommended
      Avage Cream *Crm:* 0.1% (5, 30 g)
      Tazorac Cream *Crm:* 0.05, 0.1% (15, 30, 60 g)
      Tazorac Gel *Gel:* 0.05, 0.1% (30, 100 g)

▷ *tretinoin* (C) apply daily at HS
  Pediatric: <12 years: not recommended
      Atralin Gel *Gel:* 0.05% (45 g)
      Avita *Crm:* 0.025% (20, 45 g); *Gel:* 0.025% (20, 45 g) **Renova** *Crm:* 0.02% (40 g); 0.05% (40, 60 g)

Retin-A Cream *Crm:* 0.025, 0.05, 0.1% (20, 45 g)
Retin-A Gel *Gel:* 0.01, 0.025% (15, 45 g; alcohol 90%)
Retin-A Liquid *Soln:* 0.05% (alcohol 55%)
Retin-A Micro Gel *Gel:* 0.04, 0.08, 0.1% (20, 45 g)
Tretin-X Cream *Crm:* 0.075% (35 g) (parabens-free, alcohol-free, propylene glycol-free)
Retin-A Micro *Microspheres:* 0.04, 0.1% (20, 45 g)

Comment: Effective for mitigation of fine wrinkles, mottled hyperpigmentation, and tactile roughness of skin. No mitigating effect on deep wrinkles, skin yellowing, lentigines, telangiectasia, skin laxity, keratinocytic atypia, melanocytic atypia, or dermal elastosis. Avoid sun exposure. Cautious use of concomitant astringents, alcohol-based products, sulfur-containing products, salicylic acid-containing products, soap, and other topical agents.

 XEROSIS

MOISTURIZING AGENTS

Aquaphor Healing Ointment (OTC) *Oint:* 1.75, 3.5, 14 oz (alcohol)
Eucerin Daily Sun Defense (OTC) *Lotn:* 6 oz (fragrance-free)
   Comment: **Eucerin Daily Sun Defense** is a moisturizer with SPF 15 sunscreen.
Eucerin Facial Lotion (OTC) *Lotn:* 4 oz
Eucerin Light Lotion (OTC) *Lotn:* 8 oz
Eucerin Lotion (OTC) *Lotn:* 8, 16 oz
Eucerin Original Creme (OTC) *Crm:* 2, 4, 16 oz (alcohol)
Eucerin Plus Creme (OTC) *Crm:* 4 oz
Eucerin Plus Lotion (OTC) *Lotn:* 6, 12 oz
Eucerin Protective Lotion (OTC) *Lotn:* 4 oz (alcohol)
   Comment: **Eucerin Protective** is a moisturizer with SPF 25 sunscreen.
Lac-Hydrin Cream (OTC) *Crm:* 280, 385 g
Lac-Hydrin Lotion (OTC) *Lotn:* 225, 400 g
Lubriderm Dry Skin Scented (OTC) *Lotn:* 6, 10, 16, 32 oz
Lubriderm Dry Skin Unscented (OTC) *Lotn:* 3.3, 6, 10, 16 oz (fragrance-free)
Lubriderm Sensitive Skin Lotion (OTC) *Lotn:* 3.3, 6, 10, 16 oz (lanolin-free)
Lubriderm Dry Skin (OTC) *Lotn:* 2.5, 6, 10, 16 oz (scented); 1, 2.5, 6, 10, 16 oz (fragrance-free)
Lubriderm Bath & Shower Oil (OTC) 1-2 capfuls in bath or rub onto wet skin as needed, then rinse
   Oil: 8 oz
Moisturel apply as needed
   Crm: 4, 16 oz; *Lotn:* 8, 12 oz; *Clnsr:* 8.75 oz

Topical Oil

▷ *fluocinolone acetamide* 0.01% topical oil **(C)**
   Pediatric: <6 years: not recommended; ≥6 years: apply sparingly bid for up to 4 weeks
      Derma-Smoothe/FS Topical Oil apply sparingly tid
      Topical oil: 0.01% (4 oz; peanut oil)

◯ ZOLLINGER-ELLISON SYNDROME

PROTON PUMP INHIBITORS

Comment: If hepatic impairment, or if patient is Asian, consider reducing the PPI dose.

▷ *dexlansoprazole* (B)(G) 30-60 mg daily for up to 4 weeks
   Pediatric: <18 years: not recommended
   Dexilant *Cap:* 30, 60 mg ent-coat del-rel granules; may open and sprinkle on applesauce; do not crush or chew granules
   Dexilant SoluTab *Tab:* 30 mg del-rel orally-disint

▷ *esomeprazole* (B)(OTC)(G) 20-40 mg daily; max 8 weeks; take 1 hour before food; swallow whole or mix granules with food or juice and take immediately; do not crush or chew granules
   Pediatric: <1 year: not recommended; 1-11 years, <20 kg: 10 mg; >20 kg: 10-20 mg once daily; 12-17 years: 20-40 mg once daily; max 8 weeks
   Nexium *Cap:* 20, 40 mg ent-coat del-rel pellets
   Nexium for Oral Suspension *Oral susp:* 10, 20, 40 mg ent-coat del-rel granules/pkt; mix in 2 tblsp water and drink immediately; 30 pkt/carton

▷ *esomeprazole/aspirin* (D) take one dose daily; max 8 weeks; take 1 hour before food
   Yosprala
      Tab: **Yosprala 40/81** *esom* 40 mg/*asa* 81 mg del-rel
      Yosprala 40/325 *esom* 40 mg/*asa* 325 mg del-rel

▷ *lansoprazole* (B)(OTC)(G) 15-30 mg daily for up to 8 weeks; may repeat course; take before eating
   Pediatric: <1 year: not recommended; 1-11 years, <30 kg: 15 mg once daily; >11 years: same as adult
   Prevacid *Cap:* 15, 30 mg ent-coat del-rel granules; swallow whole or mix granules with food or juice and take immediately; do not crush or chew granules; follow with water
   Prevacid for Oral Suspension *Oral susp:* 15, 30 mg ent-coat del- rel granules/pkt; mix in 2 tblsp water and drink immediately; 30 pkt/carton (strawberry)
   Prevacid SoluTab *ODT:* 15, 30 mg (strawberry; phenylalanine)
   Prevacid 24HR *Oral granules:* 15 mg ent-coat del-rel granules; swallow whole or mix granules with food or juice and take immediately; do not crush or chew granules; follow with water

▷ *omeprazole* (C)(OTC)(G) 20-40 mg daily; take before eating; swallow whole or mix granules with applesauce and take immediately; do not crush or chew; follow with water
   Pediatric: <1 year: not recommended; 5-<10 kg: 5 mg daily; 10-<20 kg: 10 mg daily; ≥20 kg: same as adult
   Prilosec *Cap:* 10, 20, 40 mg ent-coat del-rel granules
      Pediatric: <18 years: not recommended
   Prilosec *Tab:* 20 mg del-rel (regular, wild berry)

▷ *pantoprazole* (B) initially 40 mg bid
   Pediatric: not recommended
   Protonix (G) *Tab:* 40 mg ent-coat del-rel

Protonix for Oral Suspension *Oral susp:* 40 mg ent-coat del-rel granules/pkt; mix in 1 tsp apple juice for 5 seconds <u>or</u> sprinkle on 1 tsp apple sauce, and swallow immediately; do not mix in water <u>or</u> any other liquid <u>or</u> food; take approximately 30 minutes prior to a meal; 30 pkt/carton any other liquid <u>or</u> food; take approximately 30 minutes prior to a meal; 30 pkt/carton

▷ *rabeprazole* (B)(OTC)(G) initially 20 mg daily; then titrate; may take 100 mg daily in divided doses <u>or</u> 60 mg bid

Pediatric: <12 years: not recommended; ≥12 years: 20 mg once daily; max 8 weeks

AcipHex *Tab:* 20 mg ent-coat del-rel

SECTION II

APPENDICES

APPENDIX A: FDA PREGNANCY CATEGORIES

Category	Description
A	Controlled studies in women have failed to demonstrate risk to the fetus in the first trimester of pregnancy and there is no evidence of risk in later trimesters.
B	Animal reproduction studies have not demonstrated risk to the fetus, but there are no controlled studies in pregnant women, or animal studies have demonstrated an adverse effect, but controlled studies in pregnant women have not documented risk to the fetus in the first trimester of pregnancy and there is no evidence of risk in later trimesters.
C	Risk to the fetus cannot be ruled out. Animal reproduction studies have demonstrated adverse effects on the fetus (i.e., teratogenic or embryocidal effects or other) but there are no controlled studies in pregnant women or controlled studies in women and animals are not available.
D	There is positive evidence of human fetal risk, but benefits from use by pregnant women may be acceptable despite the potential risk (e.g., if the drug is needed in a life-threatening situation or for a serious disease for which safer drugs cannot be used or are ineffective.
X	Studies in animals or humans have demonstrated fetal abnormalities or there is evidence of fetal risk based on human experience, or both, and the risk of using the drug in pregnant women clearly outweighs any possible benefit. The drug is contraindicated in women who are pregnant or who may become pregnant.

APPENDIX B: U.S. SCHEDULE OF CONTROLLED SUBSTANCES

Schedule	Description
I	High potential for abuse and of no currently accepted medical use. Not obtainable by prescription, but may be legally procured for research, study, or instructional use. (Examples: *heroin, LSD, marijuana, mescaline, peyote*)
II	High abuse potential and high liability for severe psychological or physical dependence potential. Prescription required and cannot be refilled. Prescription must be written in ink or typed and signed. A verbal prescription may be allowed in an emergency by the dispensing pharmacist, but must be followed by a written prescription within 72 hours. Includes opium derivatives, other opioids, and short-acting barbiturates.

(continued)

(*continued*)

Schedule	Description
III	Potential for abuse is less than that for drugs in schedules I and II. Moderate to low physical dependence and high psychological dependence potential. Prescription required. May be refilled up to 5 times in 6 months. Prescription may be verbal (telephone) <u>or</u> written. Includes certain stimulants and depressants not included in the above schedules, and prepararations containing limited quantities of certain opioids.
IV	Lower potential for abuse than Schedule III drugs. Prescription required. May be refilled up to 5 times in 6 months. Prescription may be verbal (telephone) <u>or</u> written.
V	Abuse potential less than that for Schedule IV drugs. Preparations contain limited quantities of certain narcotic drugs. Generally intended for antitussive and anti-diarrheal purposes and may be distributed without a prescription provided that • such distribution is made only by a pharmacist; • not more than 240 ml <u>or</u> not more than 48 solid dosage units of any substance containing opium, nor more than 120 ml <u>or</u> not more than 24 solid dosage units of any other controlled substance may be distributed at retail to the same purchaser in any given 48-hour period without a valid prescription order; • the purchaser is at least 18 years old; • the pharmacist knows the purchaser <u>or</u> requests suitable identification; • the pharmacist keeps an official written record of: name and address of purchaser, name, and quantity of controlled substance purchased, date of sale, initials of dispensing pharmacist. This record is to be made available for inspection and copying by the U.S. officers authorized by the Attorney General; • other federal, state, <u>or</u> local law does not reuire a prescription order. Under jurisdiction of the Federal Controlled Substances Act. Refillable up to 5 times within 6 months.

APPENDIX C: JNC-8* AND ASH** HYPERTENSION EVALUATION AND TREATMENT RECOMMENDATIONS[1]

APPENDIX C.1: BLOOD PRESSURE CLASSIFICATION

Classification	SBP mmHg		DBP mmHg
Normal	<120	<u>and</u>	<80
Prehypertension	120-139	<u>or</u>	80-89

(*continued*)

(*continued*)

Classification	SBP mmHg		DBP mmHg
Hypertension, Stage 1	140-159	or	90-99
Hypertension, Stage 2	≥160	or	≥100

¶Adapted from: PL Detail-Document, Treatment of Hypertension: JNC 8 and More. *Pharmacist's Letter/Prescriber's Letter*, February 2014.

APPENDIX C.2: BLOOD PRESSURE RCOMMENDATIONS

Classification	SBP mmHg	DBP mmHg
Optimal	<120	<80
Normal	<130	<85
High normal	130-139	85-89

APPENDIX C.3: IDENTIFIABLE CAUSES OF HYPERTENSION (JNC-8)

- Obstructive sleep apnea
- Chronic kidney disease
- Primary aldosteronism
- Renovascular disease
- Excess sodium ingestion
- Herbal supplements
- Coarctation of the aorta
- Pheochromocytoma
- Thyroid disease
- Parathyroid disease
- Cushing's syndrome

- *Prescription Drugs:* oral contraceptives, sympathomimetics, venlafaxine, bupropion, clozapine, buspirone, bromocriptine, carbamazepine, metoclopramide
- *Illicit, Over-the-Counter Drugs, and Herbal Products:* excess alcohol consumption, alcohol withdrawal, anabolic steroids, cocaine, cocaine withdrawal, phenylpropanolamine analogs, ephedra alkalois, ergotcontaining herbal products, St. John's wart, nicotine withdrawal

APPENDIX C.4: CVD RISK FACTORS (JNC-8)

- Hypertension
- Obesity (BMI ≥30 kg/m²)
- Dyslipidemia
- Diabetes mellitus
- Cigarette smoking
- Physical inactivity

- Microalbuminuria, GFR <60 mL/min
- Age (men >55 yrs, women >65 yrs)
- Family History of premature CVD (men <55 yrs, women <65 yrs)

APPENDIX C.5: DIAGNOSTIC WORKUP OF HYPERTENSION (JNC-8)

- Assess risk factors and comorbidities
- Reveal identifiable causes of hypertension
- Assess for presence of target organ damage
- History and physical examination

(*continued*)

(continued)

> • Urinalysis, blood glucose, hematocrit, lipid panel, potassium, creatinine, calcium, (*optional* urine albumin/Cr ratio), EKG

APPENDIX C.6: BLOOD PRESSURE MEASUREMENT RECOMMENDATIONS (JNC-8)

> • Blood pressure should be measured after the patient has emptied their bladder and has been seated for 5 minutes with back supported and legs resting on the ground (not crossed)
> • Arm used for measurement should rest on a table, at heart level.
> • Use a sphygmomanometer/stethoscope or automated electronic device (preferred) with the correct size arm cuff
> • Take two readings one to two minutes apart, and average the readings (preferred)
> • Measure blood pressure in both arms at initial valuation; use the higher reading for measurements thereafter
> • Confirm the diagnosis of HTN at a subsequent visit one to four weeks after the first
> • If blood pressure is very high (e.g., systolic 180 mmHg or higher), or timely follow-up unrealistic, treatment can be started after just one set of measurements

APPENDIX C.7: PATIENT-SPECIFIC FACTORS TO CONSIDER WHEN SELECTING DRUG THERAPY(IES) (JNC-8* AND ASH**)

> JNC-8:
> • Nonblack, including those with diabetes: thiazide, CCB, ACEI, or ARB
> • African American, including those with diabetes: thiazide or CCB
> • CKD; regimen should include an ACEI or ARB (including African Americans)
> • Can initiate with two agents, especially if systolic >20 mmHg above goal or diastolic >10 mmHg above goal
> • If goal not reached: stress adherence to medication and lifestyle, increase dose or add a second or third agent from one of the recommended classes
> • Choose a drug outside of the classes recommended above only if these options have been exhausted. Consider specialist referral
>
> ASH:
> • **Nonblack <60 years of age:** *First-line:* ACEI or ARB; *Second-line (add-on):* CCB or thiazide; *Third-line:* CCB plus ACEI or ARB plus thiazide
> • **Nonblack 60 years of age and older:** *First-line:* CCB or thiazide preferred, ACEI, or ARB; *Second-line (add-on):* CCB, thiazide, ACEI, or ARB (don't use ACEI plus ARB); *Third-line:* CCB plus ACEI or ARB plus thiazide
> • **African American:** *First-line:* CCB or thiazide; *Second-line (add-on):* ACEI or ARB. *Third-line:* CCB plus ACEI or ARB plus thiazide

(continued)

(continued)

Comorbidities (ASH):

- **Diabetes:** *First-line:* ACEI or ARB (can start with CCB or thiazide in African Americans); *Second-line:* add CCB or thiazide (can add ACEI or ARB in African Americans); *Third-line:* CCB plus ACEI or ARB plus thiazide
- **CKD:** *First-line:* ARB or ACEI (ACEI for African Americans) *Second-line (add-on):* CCB or thiazide; *Third-line:* CCB plus ACEI or ARB plus thiazide
- **CAD:** *First-line:* BB plus ARB or ACEI; *Second-line (add-on):* CCB or thiazide; *Third-line:* BB plus ARB or ACEI plus CCB plus thiazide
- **Stroke history:** *First-line:* ACEI or ARB; *Second-line:* add CCB or thiazide; *Third-line:* CCB plus ACEI or ARB plus thiazide
- **Heart failure:** ACEI or ARB plus BB plus diuretic plus aldosterone antagonist. Amlodipine can be added for additional BP control (Start with ACEI, BB, diuretic. Can add BB even before ACE-I optimized. Use diuretic to manage fluid.)
- In patients 60 years of age or older who do not have diabetes or chronic kidney disease, the goal blood pressure level is now <150/90 mmHg
- In patients 18 to 59 years of age without major comorbidities, and in patients 60 years of age or older who have diabetes, chronic kidney disease, or both conditions, the new goal blood pressure level is <140/90 mmHg

---

APPENDIX C.8: BLOOD PRESSURE MANAGEMENT CHANGES FROM JNC VII TO JNC-8¶

- First-line and later-line treatments should now be limited to 4 classes of medications: thiazide-type diuretics, calcium channel blockers (CCBs), ACEIs, and ARBs
- Second- and third-line alternatives included higher doses or combinations of ACEIs, ARBs, thiazide type diuretics, and CCBs
- Several medications are now designated as later-line alternatives, including the following:
  - Beta-blockers
  - Alpha-blockers
  - Alpha$_1$/beta-blockers (e.g., carvedilol)
  - Vasodilating beta-blockers (e.g., nebivolol)
  - Central alpha$_2$-adrenergic agonists (e.g, clonidine)
  - Direct vasodilators (e.g., hydralazine)
  - Loop diuretics (e.g., furosemide)
  - Aldosterone antagonists (e.g., spironolactone)
  - Peripherally acting adrenergic antagonists (e.g., reserpine)
- When initiating therapy, patients of African descent without chronic kidney disease should use CCBs and thiazides instead of ACEIs.
- Use of ACEIs and ARBs is recommended in all patients with chronic kidney disease regardless of ethnic background, either as first-line therapy or in addition to first-line therapy.

(continued)

(*continued*)

- ACEIs and ARBs should not be used in the same patient simultaneously.
- CCBs and thiazide-type diuretics should be used instead of ACEIs and ARBs in patients over the age of 75 with impaired kidney function due to the risk of hyperkalemia, increased creatinine, and further renal impairment.

¶Adapted from: PL Detail-Document, Treatment of Hypertension: JNC 8 and More. *Pharmacist's Letter/Prescriber's Letter*, February 2014.

APPENDIX D: ATP-IV TARGET LIPID RECOMMENDATIONS¶

APPENDIX D.1: TARGET TC, TG, HDL-C, NON-HDL-C

Total cholesterol	<200 mg/dL
Triglyceride	<150 mg/dL
High-density lipoprotein (HDL)	>40 mg/dL (male) >50 mg/dL (female)
Non-high-density lipoprotein (Non-HDL-C)	<130 mg/dL; 30 mg/dL above the LDL-C treatment target

¶Adapted from the National Cholesterol Education Program Expert Panel on Detection, Evaluation, and Treatment of High Blood Cholesterol in Adults (Adult Treatment Panel IV, 2012)

APPENDIX D.2: TARGET LDL-C†

Risk Assessment††	LDL Target	Initiate TLC†††	Initiate Drug Therapy
0-1	<160 mg/dL	≥160 mg/dL	≥190 mg/dL (optional at 160-189 mg/dL)
2 or more plus 10-year risk <10%	<130 mg/dL	≥130 mg/dL	≥160 mg/dL
2 or more plus 10-year risk <20%	<130 mg/dL <100 mg/dL optional	≥130 mg/dL	≥130 mg/dL
CHD or CHD risk equivalents 10-year risk >20%	<100 mg/dL <70 mg/dL optional	≥100 mg/dL	≥100 mg/dL

†Treatment decisions based on LDL cholesterol.

††Risk factors include age (men ≥45 years and women ≥55 years).

†††Therapeutic lifestyle changes (e.g., exercise, weight loss, low fat diet).

APPENDIX D.3: NON-HDL-C[¶]

		Non-HDL-C is calculated as total cholesterol minus HDL-C. The addition of non-HDL-C to the Lipid Panel reflects the recognition of this calculated value as a predictive factor in cardiovascular disease based on the National Cholesterol Education III studies. The reference ranges for non-HDL-C are based on National Cholesterol Education III guidelines: Non-HDL-C is thought to be a better predictor of CVD than LDL-C; treatment goal for non-HDL-C is usually 30 mg/dL above the LDL-C treatment target. For example, if the LDL-C treatment goal is <70 mg/dL, the non-HDL-C treatment target would be <100 mg/dL.
Desirable	<130 mg/dL	
Borderline high	139-159 mg/dL	
High	160-189 mg/dL	
Very high	≥190 mg/dL	

[¶]Adapted from the National Cholesterol Education Program Expert Panel on Detection, Evaluation, and Treatment of High Blood Cholesterol in Adults (Adult Treatment Panel IV, 2012).

APPENDIX E: EFFECTS OF SELECTED DRUGS ON INSULIN ACTIVITY

Hyper- and Hypo-glycemic Drug Effects	
Drugs That May Cause Hyperglycemia	Drugs That May Cause Hypoglycemia
Calcium channel blockers	Alcohol
Thiazide diuretics	Beta-blockers
Corticosteroids	MAO inhibitors
Nicotinic acid	Salicylates
Oral contraceptives	NSAIDs
Phenytoin	Warfarin
Sympathomimetics diazoxide	Phenylbutazone

APPENDIX F: GLYCOSYLATED HEMOGLOBIN (HBA1c) AND AVERAGE BLOOD GLUCOSE EQUIVALENT

HbA1c and Average Blood Glucose Equivalent			
HbA1c	GLU	HbA1c	GLU
4%	60 mg/dL	14%	360 mg/dL
5%	90 mg/dL	15%	390 mg/dL
6%	120 mg/dL	16%	420 mg/dL
7%	150 mg/dL	17%	450 mg/dL
8%	180 mg/dL	18%	480 mg/dL
9%	210 mg/dL	19%	510 mg/dL
10%	240 mg/dL	20%	540 mg/dL
11%	270 mg/dL	21%	570 mg/dL
12%	300 mg/dL	22%	600 mg/dL
13%	330 mg/dL	23%	630 mg/dL

APPENDIX G: ROUTINE IMMUNIZATION RECOMMENDATIONS[1]

- Prior to 1 year-of-age, administer IM vaccinations in the vastus lateralis muscle
- After 1 year-of-age, administer vaccinations in the posterolateral upper arm
- Influenza vaccine should be administered annually for all ages ≥6 months of age
- Inactivated vaccines (e.g., pneumococcal, meningococcal, and inactivated influenza vaccines), are generally acceptable and live vaccines are generally avoided, in persons with immune deficiencies or immuneocompromising conditions
- Additional information about routine vaccinations, unknown vaccination status, travel vaccinations, vaccinations in pregnancy, and other vaccines, is available at:
  www.cdc.gov/vaccines/hcp/acip-recs/index.html
  www.cdc.gov/mmwr/preview/mmwrhtml rr6002a1/htm
  wwwnc.cdc.gov/travel/destinations/list
  www.cdc.gov/vaccines/adult/rec-vac/pregnant.html
  www.cdc.gov/flu/protect/vaccine/vaccines/htm
- DTaP (*diphtheria-tetanus-toxoid, acellular pertussis*); minimum age 6 wks
- DTaP should not be administered at or after the 7th birthday
- The 4th dose of DTaP vaccine can be administered as early as age 12 months, provided that the interval between doses 3 and 4 is at least 6 months
- DTaP and IPV should be administered at or before school entry
- HAV (*hepatitis A vaccine*) is recommended for all children at 1 year (12-23 months) of age

(*continued*)

(continued)

- **HAV** 2-dose series should be administered at least 6 months apart
- **HBV** (*hepatitis B vaccine*) is a 3-dose series initiated at birth; administer 2nd dose at 1-2 months; administer the 3rd dose at age 6 months (not before ≥24 weeks)
- **HBV** should be offered to all children who have not received the full series
- Infants born to HVsAG-positive mothers should be tested for HBsAG and antibody to HBsAg after completion of the **HBV** series (at age 9-18 months)
- **Hib** (*hemophilus influenzae* type b conjugate vaccine) minimum age 6 months
- **Hib** is not recommended if age >5 years
- **HPV** (*human papillovirus vaccine*) vaccine should be administered anytime between 11 and 12 years-of-age
- **HPV** is a 3-series vaccine administered months 0, 1, 6; females may recive HPV/4 or HPV/2; males should receive HPV/2
- **HPV** if not previously received at 11 or 12 years-of-age, may be iniitiated at any time between 13 and 26 years-of-age
- **IIV** (*inactivated influenza vaccine*) can be administered >6 months (use age-appropriate formulation), pregnant women, and persons with hives-only allergy to eggs
- **IHD** (*influenza high dose*) (**Fluzone High Dose**) may be recommended to persons ≥65 years of age
- **IPV** (*inactivated poliovirus vaccine*) minimum age 4 weeks
- An all-**IPV** schedule is recommended to eliminate the risk of vaccine-associated paralytic polio (VAPP) associated with **OPV** (*oral poliovirus vaccine*)
- **LAIV** (*live attenuated influenza vaccine*) may be administered intranasally (**FluMist**)
- **Men** (*meningococcal vaccine*) should be administered to all children at the 11-12 year old visit as well as to unvaccinated adolescents 15 years-of-age (usually at high school entry)
- **Men** should be administered to all college freshmen living in dormitories\
- Use MPSV4 for children aged 2-10 years and MCV4 for older children, although MPSV4 is an acceptable alternative for prophylaxis in men
- **MMR** (*mumps-measles-rubella*) should be administered at age 12 months in high-risk areas; if indicated, tuberculin testing can be done at the same visit
- **MMR** should be administered at age 11-12 years unless 2 doses were given after the first birthday; the interval between doses should be at least 4 weeks
- **MMR** adults born <1957 are generally considered immune to measles and mumps; all adults born ≥1957 should have documentation of at least I dose of MMR vaccine unless there is a medical contraindication or laboratory evidence of immunity to each of the 3 disease components; documentation of provider-diagnosed disease is not acceptable evidence of immunity to any of the 3 disease components
- **PCV-13** (*pneumococcal vaccine*) does not replace 23-valent pneumococcal polysaccharide in children age ≥24 months
- **PCV-13** when PCV-13 and PCV-23 are indicated, administer PCV-13 first; do not administer PCV-13 and PCV-23 in the same visit
- **PCV-13** adults ≥65 years-of-age, who have not received PCV-13 or PCV-23, should receive PCV-13 followed by PCV-23 6-12 months later
- **PCV-23** (*pneumococcal vaccine 23 trivalent*) minimum age 6 weeks
- **PCV-23** adults ≥65 years of age, who have received **PCV-23**, but not received PCV-13, should receive. **PCV-13** at least I year later; adults ≥65 years of age, who have not received **PCV-23**, should receive

(continued)

(*continued*)

- **PCV-13** followed by **PCV-23** 6-12 months later
- **RIV** (*recombinant influenza vaccine*; **FluBlok**) may be administered to any adult >18 years-of-age, including pregnant women
- **RIV** does <u>not</u> contain any egg protein; can be administered to anyone with egg allergy at any severity
- Older infants and children previously vaccinated with **PCV** should receive 3 doses (if age 7-11 months), 2 doses (if age 12-23 months) <u>or</u> 1 dose (if age >24 months)
- **Rot** (*rotavirus vaccine*) is a live attenuated oral vaccine for infants age >6 weeks <u>or</u> <32 weeks *only*; administer the 1st dose at 6-12 weeks-of-age; administer 2nd and 3rd doses at 4-10-week intervals for a total of 3 doses
- **Rot** If an incomplete dose is administered, *do <u>not</u>* administer a replacement dose, but continue with the remaining doses in the recommended series
- **Td** (*tetanus-diphtheria vaccine*) should be repeated every 10 years throughout life (<u>or</u> if at-risk injury ≥5 years after previous dose)
- **Td** should <u>*not*</u> be administered until minimum age ≥7 years
- **TdaP** (*tetanus-diphtheria-acellular pertussis*) administer 1 dose to pregnant women during each pregnancy, preferably during 27-36 weeks gestation, regardless of interval since prior Td <u>or</u> TdaP
- **TdaP** persons ≥11 years of age who have <u>not</u> received **Tdap** vaccine <u>or</u> for whom vaccine status is unknown, should receive 1 dose of **TdaP** followed by a **Td** booster every 10 years
- **Var** should be administered to children at age 11-12 years who have <u>not</u> had chicken-pox <u>or</u> who report having had chickenpox but do <u>not</u> have laboratory documentation of immunity
- **Var** If <u>not</u> received between age 11 and 12 years, administer 2 doses at least 4 weeks apart anytime after 12 years-of-age <u>or</u> a 2nd dose if previously only received 1 dose
- **VarZ** (*herpes zoster vaccine*) should be administered in a single dose once at ≥60 years-of-age, whether <u>or</u> <u>not</u> the person reports a prior episode of active herpes zoster infection
- **VarZ** is contraindicated in pregnancy and immune deficiency
- DTaP and IPV can be initiated as early as 4 weeks in areas of high endemicity <u>or</u> outbreak.

¶Adapted from DHHS CDC 2015.

APPENDIX G.1: CONTRAINDICATIONS TO VACCINES¶

All vaccines	Previous anaphylactic reaction to the vaccine Moderate <u>or</u> severe illness with <u>or</u> without fever
TDaP/DTaP, Td	Encephalopathy within 7 days of administration of previous dose
Hib	Previous anaphylactic reaction to the vaccine Moderate <u>or</u> severe illness with <u>or</u> without fever
HBV	Anaphylactic reaction to baker's yeast

(*continued*)

(*continued*)

HAV	Previous anaphylactic reaction to the vaccine Moderate <u>or</u> severe illness with <u>or</u> without fever
Influenza	Allergy to eggs (*except* **FluBlok** which does <u>not</u> contain any egg protein)
IPV	Anaphylactic reaction to neomycin <u>or</u> streptomycin
Pneumococcal	Hypersensitivity to diphtheria toxoid
MMR	Pregnancy, immunodeficiency, anaphylactic reaction to eggs <u>or</u> neomycin
Meningococcal	Encephalopathy within 7 days of administration of previous dose
Rotavirus	<6 months <u>or</u> >32 months
HPV	Pregnancy; pregnancy testing is <u>not</u> required; however, if administered, defer the remaining dose(s) until completion <u>or</u> termination of pregnancy
Varicella	Pregnancy
Herpes zoster	Pregnancy

¶ Adapted from DHHS CDC 2015.

APPENDIX G.2: ROUTE OF ADMINISTRATION AND DOSE OF VACCINES¶

Vaccine	Route	Dose
Single Vaccines		
Diphtheria-Tetanus-Pertussis (DTaP, Dtap, DT)	IM	0.5 ml
Haemophilus influenza type b (Hib)	IM	0.5 ml
Hepatitis A vaccine (HAV)	IM	0.5 ml: age <18 yrs 1.0 ml: age ≥19 yrs
Hepatitis B vaccine (HBV)	IM	0.5 ml: age <18 yrs 1.0 ml: age ≥19 yrs
Human Papillomavirus (HPV)	IM	0.5 ml
Influenza (**Fluzone Intradermal**)	ID	0.5 ml
Influenza, inactivated (IIV), recombinant (RIV)	IM	0.25 ml: age 6-35 months 0.5 ml: age ≥3 yrs
Influenza, live attenuated (LAIV)	NS	0.2 ml; 0.1 ml in each nostril
Meningococcal conjugate	IM	0.5 ml

(*continued*)

(*continued*)

Vaccine	Route	Dose
Meningococcal polysaccharide (MPSV)	SC	0.5 ml
Meningococcal sero group B (Men B)	IM	0.5 ml
Mumps-Measles-Rubella (MMR)	SC	0.5 ml
Pneumococcal conjugate (PCV)	IM	0.5 ml
Pneumococcal polysaccharide (PPSV)	IM/SC	0.5 ml
Polio, Inactivated (IPV)	IM/SC	0.5 ml
Rotavirus (**Rotarix**)	PO	1 ml
Rotavirus (**Rotateq**)	PO	2 ml
Tetanus (Td)	IM	0.5 ml
Varicella	SC	0.5 ml
Herpes Zoster	SC	0.65 ml: age ≥60 yrs
Combination Vaccines		
MMR-Var (**ProQuad**)	SC	0.5 ml: age ≤12 yrs
HBV-HAV (**Twinrix**)	IM	1 ml: >18 yrs
DTaP-HBV-IPV (**Pediarix**)	IM	0.5 ml
DTaP-IPV-Hib (**Pentacel**)	IM	0.5 ml
DTaP-IPV (**Kinrix, Quadracel**)	IM	0.5 ml
Hib-HBV (**Comvax**)	IM	0.5 ml
Hib-MenCY (**MenHibrix**)	IM	0.5 ml

¶ Adapted from DHHS CDC 2015.

APPENDIX G.3: ADVERSE REACTIONS TO VACCINES¶

Vaccine	Signs and Symptoms	Treatment
Inactivated antigens: DTP, Dtap, DTaP, Td, IPV, influenza inactiveted (IIV) recombinant (RIV) Live attenuated viruses: MMR, Meningococcal, rotavirus, varicella, herpes zoster	Local tenderness Erythema Swelling Low-grade fever Drowsiness Fretfulness Decreased appetite Prolonged crying Unusual cry	*acetaminophen* or *ibuprofen* for age and/or weight; *aspirin* and *aspirin*-containing products are contraindicated

¶ Adapted from DHHS CDC 2015.

APPENDIX G.4: MINIMUM INTERVALS BETWEEN VACCINE DOSES¶

Type	#1 to #2	#2 to #3	#3 to #4	#4 to #5
HBV	4 weeks	5 months		
HAV	6 months			
DTaP	4 weeks	4 weeks	6 months	6 months
IPV	4 weeks	4 weeks	4 weeks	
MMR	4 weeks			
Var	4 weeks			
Rotavirus	4 weeks	4 weeks; do not administer >32 weeks of age		
PCV-13	4 weeks (if #1 at age <12 months and current age <24 months); 8 weeks (as last dose if #1 at age >12 months or current age 24-59 months); No more doses needed if healthy and #1 at age ≥24 months	4 weeks if age <12 months; 8 weeks (as last dose if age ≥12 months); No more doses needed if healthy and previous dose at age ≥24 months	8 weeks (as last dose; only necessary for age 12 months to 5 years who received 3 doses before age 12 months)	
Hib	4 weeks (if #1 at age <12 months); 8 weeks (as last dose if #1 at age 12-14 months); No more doses needed if healthy and #1 at age ≥15 months	4 weeks if age 12 months; 8 weeks (as last dose if age ≥12 months); No more doses needed if previous dose at age ≥15 months	8 weeks (as last dose; only necessary for age 12 months to 2 years who received 3 doses before age 12 months)	
HPV	4 weeks	20 weeks (24 weeks after #1		

¶ Adapted from DHHS CDC 2015.

APPENDIX G.5: RECOMMENDED CHILDHOOD IMMUNIZATION SCHEDULE[¶]

Type	Birth	1 month	2 months	4 months	6 months	6-18 months	12-15 months	15-18 months	4-6 years	11-12 years
HBV	•	•								
DTaP			•	•	•				•	
IPV			•	•		•			•	
Hib			•	•	•		•			
Rotavirus			•	•	•					
MMR							•		•	
TDaP										•
Varicella							•		•	
PVC-13			•	•	•		•			
HAV							•	•		
Meningitis										•
HPV•										•••

[¶] Adapted from DHHS CDC 2015.
• Shaded box=immunization due.
••• HPV 3-dose series, months 0, 1, 6.

APPENDIX G.6: RECOMMENDEND CHILDHOOD IMMUNIZATION CATCH-UP SCHEDULE[¶]

Vaccine	Minimum Interval Between Doses			
	#1 to #2	#2 to #3	#3 to #4	#4 to #5
HBV	4 weeks	8 weeks (16 weeks after #1)		
DTaP	4 weeks	4 weeks	6 months	6 months
IPV	4 weeks	4 weeks	4 weeks	
MMR	4 weeks			
Var	4 weeks			
Rotavirus	4 weeks	4 weeks; do not administer >32 weeks of age		
PCV	2 months	2 months	2 months	6-15 months
HPV	4 weeks	20 weeks (24 weeks after #1		

[¶]Adapted from DHHS CDC 2015.

APPENDIX G.7: RECOMMENDED ADULT IMMUNIZATION SCHEDULE[¶]

Type	19-21 yrs	22-26 yrs	27-49 yrs	50-59 yrs	60-65 yrs	≥65 yrs
Influenza	1 dose annually					
HBV	3 dose series: months 0, 1, 6					
Td/TdaP	Substitute Tdap for Td one time; then continue Td once every 10 years					
MMR*	Born >1957: 2 doses					
Varicella*	Without evidence of immunity: 2 doses, 4 weeks apart					
Herpes zoster*					1 time dose	
PVC-13/ PVC-23					1 time dose	
HAV	Single Antigen, 2 doses: months 0, 6-12 (Havrix); 0, 6-18 (Vaqta)					
Meningitis	1 or more doses					

(continued)

(*continued*)

Type	19-21 yrs	22-26 yrs	27-49 yrs	50-59 yrs	60-65 yrs	≥65 yrs
HPV (female)*β	3 doses; months 0, 1, 6					
HPV (male)β	3 doses; months 0, 1, 6					

¶Adapted from DHHS CDC 2015.

*Contraindicated in pregnancy.

βOnly if <u>not</u> previously vaccinated between 11-12 years-of-age.

APPENDIX H: CONTRACEPTIVES: CONTRAINDICATIONS AND RECOMMENDATIONS

- All contraceptives are pregnancy category X
- No non-barrier contraceptives protect against STDs
- **Absolute Contraindication**:
  - HTN >35 years-of-age
  - DM >35 years-of-age
  - LDL-C >160 <u>or</u> TG >250
  - Known <u>or</u> suspected pregnancy
  - Known <u>or</u> suspected carcinoma of the breast
  - Known <u>or</u> suspected carcinoma of the endometrium
  - Known <u>or</u> suspected estrogen-dependent neoplasia
  - Undiagnosed abnormal genital bleeding
  - Cerebral vascular <u>or</u> coronary artery disease
  - Cholestatic jaundice of pregnancy <u>or</u> jaundice with prior use
  - Hepatic adenoma <u>or</u> carcinoma <u>or</u> benign liver tumor
  - Active <u>or</u> past history of thrombophlebitis <u>or</u> thromboembolic disorder
- **Relative Contraindications**
  - Lactation
  - Asthma
  - Ulcerative colitis
  - Migraine <u>or</u> vascular headache
  - Cardiac <u>or</u> renal dysfunction
  - Gestational diabetes, prediabetes, diabetes mellitus
  - Diastolic BP 90 mmHg <u>or</u> greater <u>or</u> hypertension by any other criteria
  - Psychic depression
  - Varicose veins
  - Smoker >35 years-of-age
  - Sickle-cell <u>or</u> sickle-hemoglobin C disease
  - Cholestatic jaundice during pregnancy, active gallbladder disease
  - Hepatitis <u>or</u> mononucleosis during the preceding year

(*continued*)

(*continued*)
- First-order family history of fatal <u>or</u> nonfatal rheumatic CVD <u>or</u> diabetes prior to age 50 years
- Drug(s) with known interaction(s)
- Elective surgery <u>or</u> immobilization within 4 weeks
- Age >50 years
- **Recommendations**
  - Start the first pill on the first Sunday after menses begins. Thereafter, each new pill pack will be started on a Sunday.
  - Take each daily pill in the same 3-hour window (e.g., 9A-12N, 12N-3P; a 4-hour window prior to bedtime is not recommended).
  - If 1 pill is missed, take it as soon as possible and the next pill at the regular time.
  - If 2 pills are missed, take both pills as soon as possible and then two pills the following day. A barrier method should be used for the remainder of the pill pack.
  - If 3 pills are missed before 10th cycle day, resume taking OCs on a regular schedule and take precautions.
  - If 3 pills are missed after the 10th cycle day, discard the current pill pack and begin a new one 7 days after the last pill was taken.
  - If very low-dose OCs are used <u>or</u> if combination OCs are begun after the th day of the menstrual cycle, an additional method of birth control should be used for the first 7 days of OC use.
  - If nausea occurs as a side effect, select an OC with *lower **estrogen*** content.
  - If breakthrough bleeding occurs during the first half of the cycle, select an OC with *higher **progesterone*** content.
  - Symptoms of a serious nature include loss of vision, diplopia, unilateral numbness, weakness, <u>or</u> tingling, severe chest pain, severe pain in left arm <u>or</u> neck, severe leg pain, slurring of speech, and abdominal tenderness <u>or</u> mass.

APPENDIX H.1: 28-DAY ORAL CONTRACEPTIVES

Comment: Beyaz, **Loryna**, **Syeda**, **Safyral**, **Yasmin**, and **Yaz** are contraindicated with renal and adrenal insufficiency. Monitor k^+ level during the first cycle if the patient is at risk for hyperkalemia for any reason. If the patient is taking drugs that increase potassium (e.g., ACEIs, ARBS, NSAIDs, K^+ sparing diuretics), the patient is at risk for hyperkalemia.

Combined Oral Contraceptive	Estrogen (mcg)	Progesterone (mg)
Alesse-21, Alesse-28 (X)(G) *ethinyl estradiol/levonorgestrel*	20	0.1
Altavera (X) *ethinyl estradiol/levonorgestrel*	30	0.15
Apri (X)(G) *ethinyl estradiol/desogestrel*	30	0.15
Aranelle (X)(G) *ethinyl estradiol/norethindrone*	35	0.5 1 0.5

(*continued*)

(*continued*)

Combined Oral Contraceptive	Estrogen (mcg)	Progesterone (mg)
Aviane (X)(G) *ethinyl estradiol/levonorgestrel*	20	0.1
Balziva (X)(G) *ethinyl estradiol/norethindrone*	35	0.4
Beyaz (X)(G) *ethinyl estradiol/drospirenone* plus *levomefolate calcium* 0.451 mcg (28 tabs)	20	3
Blisovi 24Fe (X)(G) *ethinyl estradiol/norethindrone* plus *ferrous fumarate* 75 mg (4 tabs)	20	1
Brevicon-21, Brevicon-28 (X)(G) *ethinyl estradiol/norethindrone*	35	0.5
Camrese (X) *ethinyl estradiol/levonorgestrel*	30 10	0.15
Camrese Lo (X) *ethinyl estradiol/levonorgestrel*	20 10	0.1
Cesia (X)(G) *ethinyl estradiol/desogestrel*	25 25 25	0.1 0.125 0.15
Cryselle (X)(G) *ethinyl estradiol/norgestrel*	30	0.3
Cyclessa (X)(G) *ethinyl estradiol/desogestrel*	25 25 25	0.1 0.125 0.15
Demulen 1/35-21, Demulen 1/35-28 (X) (G) *ethinyl estradiol/ethynodiol diacetate*	35	1
Demulen 1/50-21, Demulen 1/50-28 (X) (G) *ethinyl estradiol/ethynodiol diacetate*	50	1
Desogen (X)(G) *ethinyl estradiol/desogestrel diacetate*	30	0.15
Enpresse (X)(G) *ethinyl estradiol/levonorgestrel*	30 40 30	0.05 0.075 0.125

(*continued*)

(*continued*)

Combined Oral Contraceptive	Estrogen (mcg)	Progesterone (mg)
Estrostep Fe (X) *ethinyl estradiol/norethindrone* plus *ferrous fumarate* 75 mg	20 30 35	1 1 1
Femcon Fe (X)(G) *ethinyl estradiol/norethindrone* plus *ferrous fumarate* 75 mg	35	0.4
Generess Fe Chew tab (X)(G) *ethinyl estradiol/norethindrone* plus *ferrous fumarate* 75 mg	25	0.8
Genora (X)(G) *ethinyl estradiol/norethindrone*	35 35 35	0.5 1 0.5
Gianvi (X)(G) *ethinyl estradiol/drospirenone*	20	3
Gildess 1.5/30 (X)(G) *ethinyl estradiol/norethindrone*	30	1.5
Introvale (X) *ethinyl estradiol/levonorgestrel*	30	0.15
Jenest-28 (X) *ethinyl estradiol/norethindrone*	35 35	0.5 1
Jolessa (X)(G) *ethinyl estradiol/levonorgestrel*	30	0.15
Junel 1/20 (X)(G) *ethinyl estradiol/norethindrone*	20	1
Junel 1.5/30 (X)(G) *ethinyl estradiol/norethindrone*	30	1.5
Junel Fe 1/20 (X)(G) *ethinyl estradiol/norethindrone* plus *ferrous fumarate* 75 mg	20	1
Junel Fe 1.5/30 (X)(G) *ethinyl estradiol/norethindrone* plus *ferrous fumarate* 75 mg	30	1.5
Kaitlib Fe Chew Tab (X)(G) *ethinyl estradiol/norethindrone* plus *ferrous fumarate* 75 mg	25	0.8

(*continued*)

(continued)

Combined Oral Contraceptive	Estrogen (mcg)	Progesterone (mg)
Kariva (X)(G) *ethinyl estradiol/desogestrel*	20 10	0.15 0.15
Kelnor 1/35 (X)(G) *ethinyl estradiol/ethynodiol diacetate*	35	1
Leena (X) *ethinyl estradiol/norethindrone*	35 35 35	0.5 1 0.5
Lessina 28 (X)(G) *ethinyl estradiol/levonorgestrel*	20	0.1
Levlen 21, Levlen 28 (X)(G) *ethinyl estradiol/levonorgestrel*	30	0.15
Levlite 28 (X)(G) *ethinyl estradiol/levonorgestrel*	20	0.1
Levora-21, Levora-28 (X)(G) *ethinyl estradiol/levonorgestrel*	30	0.15
Loestrin 21 1/20 (X)(G) *ethinyl estradiol/norethindrone*	20	1
Loestrin 21 1.5/30 (X)(G) *ethinyl estradiol/norethindrone*	30	1.5
Loestrin Fe 1/20 (X)(G) *ethinyl estradiol/norethindrone* plus *ferrous fumarate* 75 mg	20	1
Loestrin Fe 1.5/30 (X)(G) *ethinyl estradiol/norethindrone* plus *ferrous fumarate* 75 mg (4 tabs)	30	1.5
Loestrin 24 Fe (X)(G) *ethinyl estradiol/norethindrone* plus *ferrous fumarate* 75 mg (4 tabs)	20	1
Lo Loestrin Fe (X) *ethinyl estradiol/norethindrone* plus *ferrous fumarate* 75 mg (2 tabs)	10	1
Lomedia 24 Fe (X)(G) *ethinyl estradiol/norethindrone* plus *ferrous fumarate* 75 mg	20	1
Lo/Ovral-21, Lo/Ovral-28 (X)(G) *ethinyl estradiol/norgestrel*	30	0.3

(continued)

(*continued*)

Combined Oral Contraceptive	Estrogen (mcg)	Progesterone (mg)
Loryna (X) *ethinyl estradiol/drospirenone*	20	3
Low-Ogestrel-21, **Low-Ogestrel-28 (X)(G)** *ethinyl estradiol/norgestrel*	30	0.3
Lutera (X)(G) *ethinyl estradiol/levonorgestrel*	20	0.1
Lybrel (X) *ethinyl estradiol/levonorgestrel*	20	0.09
Mibelas 24 FE (X)(G) *ethinyl estradiol/norethindrone* plus *ferrous fumarate 75 mg*	20	1
Microgestin 1/20 (X)(G) *ethinyl estradiol/norethindrone*	20	1
Microgestin Fe 1/20 (X)(G) *ethinyl estradiol/norethindrone* plus *ferrous fumarate 75 mg*	20	1
Microgestin 1.5/30 (X)(G) *ethinyl estradiol/norethindrone*	30	1.5
Microgestin Fe 1.5/30 (X)(G) *ethinyl estradiol/norethindrone* plus *ferrous fumarate 75 mg*	30	1.5
Mircette (X)(G) *ethinyl estradiol/desogestrel diacetate*	20 10	0.15
Minastrin 24 FE (X)(G) *ethinyl estradiol/norethindrone* plus *ferrous fumarate 75 mg*	20	1
Modicon 0.5/35-28 (X)(G) *ethinyl estradiol/norethindrone*	35	0.5
MonoNessa (X)(G) *ethinyl estradiol/norgestimate*	35	0.25
Natazia (X)(G) *estradiol valerate/dienogest*	30 20 20 10	— 2 3 —

(*continued*)

(*continued*)

Combined Oral Contraceptive	Estrogen (mcg)	Progesterone (mg)
Necon 0.5/35-21, Necon 0.5/35-28 (X)(G) *ethinyl estradiol/norethindrone*	35	0.5
Necon 1/35-21, Necon 1/35-28 (X)(G) *ethinyl estradiol/norethindrone*	35	0.5
Necon 10/11-21, Necon 10/11-28 (X)(G) *ethinyl estradiol/norethindrone*	35 35	0.5 1
Necon 1/50-21, Necon 1/50-28 (X)(G) *mestranol/norethindrone*	50	1
Nelova 0.5/35-21, Nelova 0.5/35-28 (X)(G) *ethinyl estradiol/norethindrone*	35	0.5
Nelova 1/35-21, Nelova 1/35-28 (X)(G) *ethinyl estradiol/norethindrone*	35	1
Nelova 10/11-21, Nelova 10/11-28 (X)(G) *ethinyl estradiol/norethindrone*	35 35	0.5 1
Nelova 1/50-21, Nelova 1/50-28 (X)(G) *mestranol/norethindrone*	50	1
Neocon 7/7/7 (X)(G) *ethinyl estradiol/norethindrone*	35 35 35	0.5 0.75 1
Nordette-21, Nordette-28 (X)(G) *ethinyl estradiol/levonorgestrel*	30	0.15
Norinyl 1+35-21, Norinyl 1+35-28 (X)(G) *ethinyl estradiol/norethindrone*	35	1
Norinyl 1+50-21, Norinyl 1+50-28 (X)(G) *mestranol/norethindrone*	50	1
Nortrel 0.5/35 (X)(G) *ethinyl estradiol/norethindrone*	35	0.5
Nortrel 1/35-21, Nortrel 1/35-28 (X)(G) *ethinyl estradiol/norethindrone*	35	1
Nortrel 7/7/7-28 (X)(G) *ethinyl estradiol/norethindrone*	35 35 35	0.5 0.75 1
Ocella (X)(G) *ethinyl estradiol/drospirenone*	30	3

(*continued*)

(continued)

Combined Oral Contraceptive	Estrogen (mcg)	Progesterone (mg)
Ortho-Cept 28 (X)(G) *ethinyl estradiol/desogestrel*	30	0.15
Ortho-Cyclen 28 (X)(G) *ethinyl estradiol/norgestimate*	35	0.25
Ortho-Novum 1/35-21, Ortho-Novum 1/35-28 (X)(G) *ethinyl estradiol/norethindrone*	35	1
Ortho-Novum 1/50-21, Ortho-Novum 1/50-28 (X)(G) *mestranol/norethindrone*	50	1
Ortho-Novum 7/7/7-28 (X)(G) *ethinyl estradiol/norethindrone*	35 35 35	0.5 0.75 1
Ortho-Novum 10/11-28 (X) *ethinyl estradiol/norethindrone*	35 35	0.5 1
Ortho Tri-Cyclen 21, Ortho Tri-Cyclen 28 (X)(G) *ethinyl estradiol/norgestimate*	35 35 35	0.18 0.215 0.25
Ortho Tri-Cyclen Lo (X)(G) *ethinyl estradiol/norgestimate*	25 25 25	0.18 0.215 0.25
Ovcon 35 Fe (X)(G) *ethinyl estradiol/norethindrone plus ferrous fumarate* 75 mg (4 tabs)	35	0.4
Ovcon 50-28, Ovcon 50-28 (X)(G) *ethinyl estradiol/norethindrone*	50	1
Ovral-21, Ovral-28 (X)(G) *ethinyl estradiol/norgestrel*	50	0.5
Portia (X)(G) *ethinyl estradiol/levonorgestrel*	30	0.15
Previfem (X) *ethinyl estradiol/norgestimate*	35	0.25
Quasense (X) *ethinyl estradiol/levonorgestrel*	30	0.15

(continued)

(*continued*)

Combined Oral Contraceptive	Estrogen (mcg)	Progesterone (mg)
Reclipsen (X)(G) *ethinyl estradiol/desogestrel* plus *ferrous fumarate* 75 mg (4 tabs)	30	0.15
Safyral (X) *ethinyl estradiol/drospirenone* plus *levomefolate calcium* 0.451 mg	30	3
Sprintec 28 (X)(G) *ethinyl estradiol/norgestimate*	35	0.25
Syeda (X) *ethinyl estradiol/drospirenone*	30	3
Tarina Fe 1/20 (X)(G) *ethinyl estradiol/norethindrone* plus *ferrous fumarate* 75 mg (7 tabs)	20	1
Taytulla Fe 1/20 (X)(G) (Softgel caps) *ethinyl estradiol/norethindrone* plus *ferrous fumarate* 75 mg (4 Softgel caps)	20	1
Tilia Fe (X)(G) *ethinyl estradiol/norethindrone* plus *ferrous fumarate* 75 mg (7 tabs)	20 30 35	1 1 1
Tri-Legest 21 (X)(G) *ethinyl estradiol/norethindrone*	20 30 35	1 1 1
TriLegest Fe (X)(G) *ethinyl estradiol/norethindrone* plus *ferrous fumarate* 75 mg (7 tabs)	20 30 35	1 1 1
Tri-Levlen 21, Tri-Levlen 28 (X)(G) *ethinyl estradiol/levonorgestrel*	30 40 30	0.05 0.075 0.125
Tri-Lo-Estarylla (X)(G) *ethinyl estradiol/norgestimate*	25 25 25	0.18 0.215 0.25
Tri-Lo-Sprintec (X)(G) *ethinyl estradiol/norgestimate*	25 25 25	0.18 0.215 0.25

(*continued*)

(*continued*)

Combined Oral Contraceptive	Estrogen (mcg)	Progesterone (mg)
TriNessa (X)(G) *ethinyl estradiol/norgestimate*	35 35 35	0.18 0.215 0.25
Tri-Norinyl 21, Tri-Norinyl 28 (X)(G) *ethinyl estradiol/norethindrone*	35 35 35	0.5 1 0.5
Triphasil-21, Triphasil-28 (X)(G) *ethinyl estradiol/levonorgestrel*	30 40 30	0.050 0.075 0.125
Tri-Previfem (X)(G) *ethinyl estradiol/norgestimate*	35 35 35	0.18 0.215 0.25
Tri-Sprintec (X)(G) *ethinyl estradiol/norgestimate*	35 35 35	0.18 0.215 0.25
Trivora (X)(G) *ethinyl estradiol/levonorgestrel*	30 40 30	0.05 0.075 0.125
Velivet (X)(G) *ethinyl estradiol/desogestrel*	25 25 25	0.1 0.125 0.15
Yasmin (X)(G) *ethinyl estradiol/drospirenone*	30	3
Yaz (X)(G) *ethinyl estradiol/drospirenone*	20	3
Zovia 1/35E-28 (X)(G) *ethinyl estradiol/ethynodiol diacetate*	35	1
Zovia 1/50E-28 (X)(G) *ethinyl estradiol/ethynodiol diacetate*	50	1

APPENDIX H.2: EXTENDED-CYCLE ORAL CONTRACEPTIVES

91 Day
▶ *ethinyl estradiol/levonorgestrel* (X) 1 tab daily x 91 days; repeat (no tablet-free days)
    Ashlyna (G) *Tab: levnorgest* 15 mcg/*eth est* 30 mcg (84) + *eth est* 10 mcg (7)
    (91 tabs/pck)
    Jolessa (G) *Tab: levonorgest* 15 mcg/*eth est* 30 mcg (84) + inert tabs (7m91 tabs/pck)
    LoSeasonique *Tab: levnorgest* 0.1 mcg/*eth est* 20 mcg (84) + *eth est* 10 mcg (7)
    (91 tabs/pck)

(*continued*)

(continued)

> **Quartette (G)** *Tab: levonorgest* 15 mcg/*eth est* 30 mcg (84) + *eth est* 10 mcg (7) (91 tabs/pck)
> **Quasense (G)** *Tab: levonorgest* 15 mcg/*eth est* 30 mcg (84) + inert tabs (7) (91 tabs/pck)
> **Seasonale (G)** *Tab: levonorgest* 15 mcg/*eth est* 30 mcg (84) + inert tabs (7) (91 tabs/pck)
> **Seasonique (G)** *Tab: levnorgest* 15 mcg/*eth est* 30 mcg (84) + *eth est* 10 mcg (7) (91 tabs/pck)

365 Day
> ▶ *ethinyl estradiol/levonorgestrel* (X) 1 tab daily x 28 days; repeat (no tablet-free days)
> **Lybrel** *Tab: levnorgest* 0.09 mcg/*eth est* 20 mcg (28 tabs/pck)

APPENDIX H.3: PROGESTERONE-ONLY ORAL CONTRACEPTIVES ("MINI-PILL")

Brand	Progesterone	Mcg
Comment: Take progestin-only pills at the same time each day (within a 3-hour time window). If a pill is missed, another method of contraception should be used for the remainder of the pill pack.		
Camila	*norethindrone* (X)(G)	35
Errin	*norethindrone* (X)(G)	35
Jolivette	*norethindrone* (X)(G)	35
Micronor	*norethindrone* (X)(G)	35
Nora-BE	*norethindrone* (X)(G)	35
Nor-QD	*norethindrone* (X)(G)	35
Ovrette	*norgestrel* (X)	7.5

APPENDIX H.4: INJECTABLE CONTRACEPTIVES

H.4.1: Injectable Progesterone

90 Days
Comment: Administer first dose within 5 days of onset of normal menses, within 5 days postpartum if not breastfeeding, or at 6 weeks postpartum if breastfeeding exclusively. Do not use for >2 years unless other methods are inadequate.

> ▶ *medroxyprogesterone* (X)(G)
> **Depo-Provera** 150 mg deep IM q 3 months
> *Vial:* 150 mg/ml (1 ml); *Prefilled syringe:* 150 mg/ml
> **Depo-SubQ** 104 mg SC q 3 months
> *Prefilled syringe:* 104 mg/ml (0.65 ml) (parabens)

APPENDIX H.5: TRANSDERMAL CONTRACEPTIVE

Ethinyl Estradiol/Norelgestromin
Comment: Apply the transdermal patch to the abdomen, buttock, upper-outer arm, or upper torso. *Do* not apply the transdermal patch to the breast. Rotate the site (however, may use the same anatomical area).

▷ *ethinyl estradio/norelgestromin* **(X)(G)** apply one patch once weekly x 3 weeks; then 1 patch-free week; then repeat sequence
  Ortho Evra
    Transdermal patch: eth est 20 mcg/*norel* 150 mcg per day (1, 3/pck)

APPENDIX H.6: CONTRACEPTIVE VAGINAL RINGS

Ethinyl Estradiol/Etonogestrel
Comment: The vaginal ring should be inserted prior to, or on 5th day, of the menstrual cycle. Use of a backup method is recommended during the first week. When switching from oral contraceptives, the vaginal ring should be inserted anytime within 7 days after the last active tablet and no later than the day a new pill pack would have been started (no back up method is needed). If the ring is accidently expelled for less than 3 hours, it should be rinsed with cool to lukewarm water and reinserted promptly. If ring removal lasts for more than 3 hours, an additional contraceptive method should be used. If the ring is lost, a new ring should be inserted and the regimen continued without alteration.

▷ *etonogestrel/ethinyl estradiol* **(X)** insert 1 ring vaginally and leave in place for 3 weeks; then remove for 1 ring-free week; then repeat
  NuvaRing
    Vag ring: eth est 15 mcg/*eton* 120 mcg per day (1, 3/pck)

APPENDIX H.7: SUBDERMAL CONTRACEPTIVES

Comment: Implants must be inserted within 7 days of the onset of menses. A complete physical examination is required annually. Remove if pregnancy, thromboembolic disorder including thrombophlebitis, jaundice, visual disturbances. Not for use by patients with hypertension, diabetes, hyperlipidemia, impaired liver function, epilepsy, asthma, migraine, depression, cardiac or renal insufficiency, thromboembolic disorder including thrombophlebitis, pro-longed immobilization, or who are smokers.

▷ *etonogestrel* **(X)** implant rod subdermally in the upper inner non-dominant arm; remove and replace at the end of 3 years
  Implanon, Nexplanon
    Implantable rod: 68 mg implant for subdermal insertion (w. insertion device; latex-free)

(continued)

(continued)

> ▷ *levonorgestrel* (X) implant rods subdermally in the upper inner nondominant arm; remove and replace at the end of 5 years
> > **Norplant**
> > > *Implantable rods:* 6-36 mg implants (total 216 mg) for subdermal insertion (1 kit w. sterile supplies)

APPENDIX H.8: INTRAUTERINE CONTRACEPTIVES

Comment: Indicated in women who have had at least one child and who are in a stable, mutually monogamous relationship. Reexamine after menses within 3 months (recommend 4-6 weeks) to check placement.

> ▷ *levonorgestrel* (X)
> > **Kyleena** *IUD:* 19.5 mg (replace at least every 5 years)
> > **Liletta** *IUD:* 52 mg (replace at least every 3 years)
> > **Mirena** *IUD:* 52 mg (replace at least every 5 years)
> > **Skyla** *IUD:* 13.5 mg (replace at least every 3 years)

APPENDIX H.9: EMERGENCY CONTRACEPTION

Comment: Emergency contraception must be started within 72 hours after unprotected intercourse following a negative urine hCG pregnancy test. If vomiting occurs within 1 hour of taking a dose, repeat the dose.

> ▷ *ethinyl estradiol/levonorgestrel* (X) 2 tabs as soon as possible after unprotected intercourse <u>or</u> contraceptive failure, then 2 more 12 hours after first dose
> *Pediatric:* premenarchal: not applicable
> > **Preven**
> > > *Tab: eth est* 50 mcg/*lev* 250 mcg (4/pck) + *Pregnancy test:* 1 hCG home pregnancy test
> > **Yuzpe Regimen**
> > > *Tab: eth est* 50 mcg/*lev* 250 mcg (4/pck)

> ▷ *levonorgestrel* (X)(OTC)(G)
> **Comment:** <17 years of age (prescription required; ≥17 years of age (OTC)
> *Pediatric:* premenarchal: not applicable
> > **My Way** take 1 tab as soon as possible, within 72 hours, after unprotected sex <u>or</u> suspected contraceptive failure
> > > *Tab:* 1.5 mg
> > **Plan B One Step** take 1 tab as soon as possible, within 72 hours, after unprotected sex <u>or</u> suspectedcontraceptive failure
> > > *Tab:* 1.5 mg
> > **EContra EZ** take 1 tab within 72 hours after unprotected sex <u>or</u> suspected contraceptive failure
> > > *Tab:* 1.5 mg

(continued)

(*continued*)

> ▷ **ulipristal** (X)
> *Pediatric:* premenarchal: not applicable
> **ella** 1 tab as soon as possible within 120 hours (5 days) after unprotected
> intercourse <u>or</u> contraceptive failure; may repeat dose if vomiting occurs
> within 3 hours
> *Tab:* 30 mg

APPENDIX I: ANESTHETIC AGENTS FOR LOCAL INFILTRATION AND DERMAL/MUCOSAL MEMBRANE APPLICATION

Agents and Indications	
Brand/*generic*	Indication(s)
AnaMantle HC *lidocaine 3%/hydrocortisone 0.5%*	Local anesthetic/steroid; for hemorrhoids, pruritus ani, anal fissure
Decadron Phosphate with Xylocaine *dexamethasone 4 mg/lidocaine 10 mg/ ml (5 ml)*	Local anesthetic/steroid; infiltration by injection
Dyclone *dyclonine 0.5%, 0.1%*	Local anesthetic; infiltration by injection
Duranest (B) *etidocaine 1% (30 ml)* **Duranest (B) w. Epinephrine** *Inj: etido 1.5%/epi 1:200,000 (30 ml)* *Dental Cartridge: etido 1.5%/epi 1:200,000 (1.8 ml)*	Nerve block and local anesthetic; mouth, pharynx, larynx, trachea, esophagus, anogenital area, urethra Local anesthetic: dental procedures
Ela-Max 4% Cream (B) *lidocaine 4%* **Ela-Max 5% Cream (B)** *lidocaine 5%*	Local dermal anesthetic and for anorectal irritation and pain
Emla Cream (B) (5, 30 g) **Emla Anesthetic Disc (B)** (2 discs/box) *lidocaine 2.5%/prilocaine 2.5%*	Local dermal anesthetic; preparation for phlebotomy, PIV starts, injections
Flector Patch (C/D) (30/box) *diclofenac epolamine 180 mg*	Local dermal NSAID analgesic
Exparel (B) *Vial:* 13.3 mg/ml (20 ml) *bupivacaine liposome 1.3% susp for inj*	Surgical site injection for postop pain management

(*continued*)

(*continued*)

Agents and Indications	
Brand/*generic*	**Indication(s)**
LidaMantle (B) cream (1, 2 oz) **LidaMantle (B)** lotion (177 ml) **Lidoderm** cream **(B)** (85 g) *lidocaine 3%* **Lidoderm (B)(G)** adhesive patch (10 cm x14 cm; 30/box) *lidocaine 5%*	Local dermal anesthetic lotion, cream, and adhesive patch
Ophthaine (B) (15 ml) *proparacaine 0.5% ophthalmic solution*	Ophthalmic anesthetic for examination/ removal of foreign body (eye)
Pliaglis Cream (B) (30 g) *lidocaine 7%/tetracaine 7%*	Local dermal anesthetic for superficial dermatological procedures
Qutenza (B) (1, 2 patches, each *with 50 g tube of cleansing gel*) *capsaicin 8% patch*	Local dermal NSAID analgesic for postherpetic neuralgia
Synera Topical Patch (B) (2, 10/pck) *lidocaine 70 mg/tetracaine 70 mg*	Local dermal anesthetic for venous access or skin lesion removal
Tetracaine Ophthalmic Solution (B) (15 ml) *proparacaine 0.5% ophthalmic solution*	Ophthalmic anesthetic for examination/removal of foreign body (eye)
Xylocaine Jelly (B) (5, 10, 20, 30 ml) *lidocaine 2% aqueous*	For procedures of the urethra, painful urethritis, and endotracheal intubation
Xylocaine Ointment (B) (3.5, 35 g) *lidocaine 5% water miscible*	For procedures of the urethra, painful urethritis, and endotracheal intubation
Xylocaine Topical Solution (B) (100 ml) *lidocaine 2% solution* **Xylocaine Viscous (B)** (50 ml) *lidocaine 2% viscous solution*	Anesthetic for the nasal and oropharyngeal mucosa and the proximal portions of the GI tract
Zingo *lidocaine monohydrate 0.5 mg*	Hand-held, needle-free device, helium-powered delivery system that numbs site in 1-3 minutes delivers 0.5 mg sterile lidocaine HCL monohydrate sterile lidocaine HCL pwdr for intradermal injection for the management of venous access pain

(*continued*)

(*continued*)

Agents and Indications	
Brand/*generic*	Indication(s)
Zostrix (B) (0.7, 1.5, 3 oz) *capsaicin 0.025% cream* **Zostrix HP (B)** (1, 2 oz) *capsaicin 0.075% emollient cream*	Local dermal NSAID analgesic

APPENDIX J: ORAL PRESCRIPTION NSAIDs

Comment: NSAIDs should be taken with food to decrease gastric upset. Dosing of NSAIDs should be scheduled rather than PRN for maximal benefit. NSAIDs are contraindicated with sulfonamide or *aspirin* allergy, 3rd trimester pregnancy (causes premature closure of the ductus arteriosus), and coronary artery bypass graft (CABG) surgery. Concomitant use of *misoprostol* (**Cytotec**) with NSAIDs reduces gastric upset and potential for ulceration; however, *misoprostol* is pregnancy category X. Administration of *misoprostol* in pregnancy can cause spontaneous abortion, premature birth, birth defects, and uterine rupture (beyond the 8th week of pregnancy). NSAIDs and *warfarin* (**Coumadin**) are synergistic. With all patients, use the lowest effective dose for the shortest time necessary. NSAIDs should be taken with food to reduce the risk of gastrointestinal adverse side effects (GIASE).

GI ADVERSE SIDE EFFECTS:
(+) MILD; (++) FREQUENT; (+++) MORE FREQUENT/SEVERE

▷ *celecoxib* (C/D)(G)(+) 100 mg twice daily or 200 mg once daily or 200 mg twice daily or 400 mg once daily; <50 kg, start at lowest dose
Pediatric: <2 years: not recommended; ≥2 years, >10<25 kg: 50 mg twice daily; ≥25 kg: 100 mg once daily
   Celebrex
      Cap: 50, 100, 200, 400 mg

▷ *diclofenac sodium* (D)(+++)
Pediatric: not recommended
      Dyloject administer 37.5 mg IV bolus over 15 seconds q 6 hours; max 150 mg/day
         Vial: 37.5 mg/ml (25/box)
      Pennsaid 1% in 10 drop increments, dispense and rub into front, side, and back of knee: usually 40 drops (40 mg) qid
         Topical soln: 1.5% (150 ml)

(*continued*)

(continued)

Pennsaid 2% apply 2 pump actuations (40 mg) and rub into front, side, and
back of knee bid
Topical soln: 2% (20 mg/pump actuation; 112 g)
Solaraze Gel apply to affected areas bid
Gel: 3% (30 mg (100 g)
Voltaren 50 mg bid <u>or</u> qid <u>or</u> 75 mg bid <u>or</u> 25 mg qid with an additional 25
mg at HS if necessary
Tab: 25, 50, 75 mg ent-coat
Voltaren XR 100 mg once daily; rarely, 100 mg bid may be used
Tab: 100 mg ext-rel
Zorvolex 35 mg tid
Gelcap: 18, 35 mg ext-rel

▷ *diclofenac potassium* (C/D)(G)(+++) 50 mg tid <u>or</u> qid <u>or</u> 25 mg tid <u>or</u> qid and may
add 25 mg at HS
Pediatric: not recommended
Cataflam
Tab: 50 mg
Zipsor
Gel cap: 25 mg

▷ *diclofenac sodium* plus *misoprostol* (X)(++)
Pediatric: not recommended
Arthrotec
Tab: 50, 75 mg

▷ *diflunisal* (C/D)(G)(+++) initially 1 g as a single dose followed by 500 mg q 8-12
hours <u>or</u> 500 mg as a single dose followed by 250 mg q 8-12 hours
Pediatric: <12 years: not recommended
Dolobid
Tab: 500*mg

▷ *etodolac* (C/D)(G)(+)
Pediatric: not recommended
Lodine initially 600 mg to 1 g/day in 2-3 divided doses; usual max 1 g/day in
divided doses; may increase to 1.2 g/day when needed
Tab: 400, 500 mg; *Cap:* 200, 300 mg
Lodine XL 400 mg to 1 g once daily; max 1.2 g/day
Tab: 400, 500, 600 mg ext-rel

▷ *fenoprofen* (B/D)(++) 300-600 mg tid-qid; max 3.2 g/day
Pediatric: not recommended
Nalfon
Tab: 200 mg

▷ *flurbiprofen* (B/D)(G)(++) 200-300 mg/day in 2-4 divided doses; max single dose
100 mg; reduce dosage for renal impairment
Pediatric: not recommended
Ansaid
Tab: 50, 100 mg

(continued)

(*continued*)

➤ **ibuprofen/famotidine** (B/D)(++) 1 tab 3 times daily; swallow whole; use lowest effective dose for the shortest duration
Pediatric: not recommended
> **Duexis**
> > *Tab: ibu* 800 mg/*fam* 26.6 mg

➤ **indomethecin** (B/D)(G)(+++) 75-100 mg daily in 3-4 divided doses; max 200 mg/day
Pediatric: <14 years: not recommended
> **Indocin**
> > *Cap:* 25, 50 mg; *Rectal supp:* 50 mg; *Oral susp:* 25 mg/5 ml; *Vial:* 1 mg pwdr for reconstitution and IV infusion
> **Indocin SR**
> > *Cap:* 75 mg ext-rel
> **Tivorbex**
> > *Cap:* 20, 40 mg

➤ **ketoprofen** (C/D)(G)(++) 75 mg tid <u>or</u> 50 mg qid; max 300 mg/day
Pediatric: <18 years: not recommended
> **Orudis**
> > *Cap:* 50, 75 mg
> **Oruvail**
> > *Cap:* 100, 150, 200 mg ext-rel

➤ **ketorolac tromethamine** (C/D)(G)(+++)
Pediatric: <17 years: not recommended
> **Sprix** *17-64 years:* 1 spray each nostril (total dose 31,5 mg) every 6-8 hours prn; max 4 doses/24 hours (total daily dose 126 mg); *≥65 years, renal impairment* <u>or</u> *<50 kg:* 1 spray in one nostril (total dose 15.75 mg) every 6-8 hours prn; max 4 doses/24 hours (63 mg); discard used bottle after 24 hours
> > *Nasal spray:* 15.75 mg/100 mcl nasal spray (8 sprays, 1.7 g)
> **Toradol** 60 mg as a single IM dose; max 30 mg as a single IV dose; may administer 30 mg IV and 30 mg IM as a single dose; oral dosing is indicated <u>*only*</u> as continuation therapy to IM <u>or</u> IV dosing; oral formulation should <u>*never*</u> be administered as an initial dose; initiate oral dosing at 20 mg followed by 10 mg q 4-6 hours prn; max oral dosing 40 mg/day; >65 years, initiate oral dosing at 10 mg followed by 10 mg q 4-6 hours prn; max 40 mg/day; the combined duration of IV/IM/PO dosing is not to exceed 5 days
> > *Tab:* 10 mg; *Inj* 15, 30, 60 mg/ml

➤ **magnesium chol salicylate** (C/D)(G)(+)
Pediatric:
> **Trilisate**
> > *Tab:* 10 mg

➤ **meclofenamate sodium** (B/D)(G)(++) 50-100 mg q 4-6 hours <u>or</u> 300-400 mg/day in 3-4 equal doses; max 400 mg/day
Pediatric: <14 years: not recommended
> **Meclofen**
> > *Cap:* 50, 100 mg

(*continued*)

(continued)

> ▷ **mefenamic acid** (C)(G)(++) 500 mg once; then, 250 mg q 6 hours
> *Pediatric:* <14 years: not recommended
>   **Ponstel**
>   *Cap:* 250 mg

> ▷ **meloxicam** (C/D)(G)(+) 7.5 mg once daily; max 15 mg/day; hemodialysis max
> 7.5 mg/day
> *Pediatric:* <2 years: not recommended; ≥2 years: 0.125 mg/kg; max 7.5 mg once
> daily
>   **Mobic**
>   *Tab:* 7.5, 15 mg; *Oral susp:* 7.5 mg/5 ml (100 ml) (raspberry)
>   **Relafen**
>   *Tab:* 500, 750 mg

> ▷ **nabumetone** (C/D)(G)(+) 1-2 g/day in a single dose <u>or</u> 2 divided doses; max 2 g/
> day; <50 kg, max 1 g/day
> *Pediatric:* not recommended

> ▷ **naproxen** (B)(G)(++) 275-550 mg twice daily <u>or</u> 275 mg every 6-8 hours; max 1.375
> g first day; then, max 1.1 g/day; acute gout: 825 mg once, then 275 mg every 8 hours
> *Pediatric:* <2 years: not recommended; ≥2 years: 5 mg/kg bid; max 15 mg/kg/day
> has been used; use suspension
>   **Naprosyn**
>   *Tab:* 250, 375, 500 mg
>   **Naprosyn Suspension**
>   *Oral susp:* 125 mg/5 ml

> ▷ **naproxen/esomeprazole (as magnesium trihydrate)** (C/D)(++)(G) one 375/20
> <u>or</u> one 500/20 tab twice daily; take at least 30 minutes before meals; take lowest
> effective dose
> *Pediatric:* <18 years: not recommended
>   **Vimovo 375/20**
>   *Tab: nap* 375 mg/*eso* 20 mg
>   **Vimovo 500/20**
>   *Tab: nap* 500 mg/*eso* 20 mg

> ▷ **oxaprozin** (C/D)(++) 1.2 g once daily; max 1.8 g <u>or</u> 26 mg/kg daily, whichever is
> less, in divided doses; low body weight, milder disease, <u>or</u> on dialysis: initially 600
> mg once daily; max 1.2 g daily
> *Pediatric:* <6 years: not recommended; 6-16 years, 21-31 kg: 600 mg daily;
> 32-54 kg: 900 mg once daily; ≥55 kg: 1.2 g once daily
>   **Daypro** *Tab:* 600*

> ▷ **piroxicam** (C/D)(G)(+++) 20 mg once daily
> *Pediatric:* not recommended
>   **Feldene**
>   *Cap:* 10, 20 mg
> **Comment:** Because of the long half-life, steady state blood levels of **piroxicam** are
> not reached for 7-12 days. Therefore, there is a progressive response over several
> weeks.

(continued)

(*continued*)

➤ *salsalate* (C/D)(G)(+) 1.5 g bid <u>or</u> 1 g tid
   Pediatric: not recommended
     Disalcid
       Tab: 500*, 750*mg; *Cap:* 500 mg

➤ *sulindac* (B/D)(G)(+++) 150-200 mg bid; max 400 mg/day; usually x 7-14 days
   Pediatric: not recommended
     Clinoril
       Tab: 150*, 200*mg
     Tolectin DS
       Cap: 400 mg
     Tolectin 600
       Tab: 600 mg film-coat

➤ *tolmetin* (C/D)(G)(+++) initially 400 mg tid; usual range 600 mg to 1.8 g/day in divided doses; max 1,800 mg/day
   Pediatric: <2 years: not recommended; ≥2 years: 20 mg/kg divided tid to qid; usual range 15-30 mg/kg/day divided tid to qud: max 30 mg/kg/day
     Tolectin *Tab:* 200*mg

➤ *nabumetone* (C/D)(G)(+) 1-2 g/day in a single dose <u>or</u> 2 divided doses; max 2 g/day; <50 kg, max 1 g/day
   Pediatric: not recommended

➤ *naproxen* (B)(G)(++) 275-550 mg bid <u>or</u> 275 mg q 6-8 hours; max 1.375 g first day, then, max 1.1 g/day; *Acute gout attack:* 825 mg once, then 275 mg every 8 hours
   Pediatric: <2 years: not recommended; ≥2 years: 5 mg/kg bid; max 15 mg/kg/day has been used; use suspension
     Naprosyn
       Tab: 250, 375, 500 mg
     Naprosyn Suspension
       Oral susp: 125 mg/5 ml

➤ *naproxen/esomeprazole (as magnesium trihydrate)* (C/D)(++)(G) 1 x 375/20 <u>or</u> 1 x 500/20 tab bid; take at least 30 minutes before meals; take lowest effective dose
   Pediatric: <18 years: not recommended
     Vimovo 375/20
       Tab: nap 375 mg/*eso* 20 mg
     Vimovo 500/20
       Tab: nap 500 mg/*eso* 20 mg

➤ *oxaprozin* (C/D)(++) 1.2 g once daily; max 1.8 g <u>or</u> 26 mg/kg daily, whichever is less, in divided doses; *Low body weight, milder disease,* <u>or</u> *on dialysis:* initially 600 mg once daily; max 1.2 g daily
   Pediatric: <6 years: not recommended; 6-16 years, 21-31 kg: 600 mg once daily; 32-54 kg: 900 mg once daily; ≥55 kg: 1.2 g once daily
     Daypro
       Tab: 600*

(*continued*)

(continued)

> ▷ **piroxicam** (C/D)(G)(+++) 20 mg once daily
>   *Pediatric:* not recommended
>   **Feldene**
>   *Cap:* 10, 20 mg
>
> Comment: Because of the long half-life, steady state blood levels of *piroxicam* are not reached for 7-12 days. Therefore, there is a progressive response over several weeks.
>
> ▷ **salsalate** (C/D)(G)(+) 1.5 g bid or 1 g tid
>   *Pediatric:* not recommended
>   **Disalcid**
>   *Tab:* 500*, 750*mg; *Cap:* 500 mg
>   **Tolectin 600**
>   *Tab:* 600 mg film-coat

APPENDIX K: TOPICAL CORTICOSTEROIDS BY POTENCY

Comment: All topical, oral, and parenteral corticosteroids are pregnancy category C. Use with caution in infants and children. Steroids should be applied sparingly and for the shortest time necessary. Do not use in the diaper area. Do not use an occlusive dressing. Systemic absorption of topical corticosteroids can induce reversible hypothalamic-pituitary-adrenal (HPA) axis suppression with the potential for clinical glucocorticoid insufficiency.

Potency guide:
- Face: Low potency
- Ears/scalp margin: Intermediate potency
- Eyelids: Hydrocortisone in ophthalmic ointment base 1%
- Chest/back: Intermediate potency
- Skin folds: Low potency

Generic	Brand/Formulation/ Frequency	Strength/Volume
Low Potency		
alclometasone dipropionate (C)	**Aclovate** Crm bid-tid **Aclovate** Oint bid-tid	0.05% (15,45, 60 g) 0.05% (15,45, 60 g)
fluocinolone acetonide (C)	**Synalar** Crm bid-qid	0.025% (15, 60 g)
hydrocortisone base or *acetate* (C)(G)	**Anusol-HC** Crm bid-qid **Hytone** Crm bid-qid **Hytone** Oint bid-qid **Hytone** Lotn bid-qid	2.5% (30 g) 1% (1, 2 oz) 1% (1 oz) 1% (2 oz)

(continued)

(*continued*)

Generic	Brand/Formulation/ Frequency	Strength/Volume
	Hytone Crm bid-qid	2.5% (1, 2 oz)
	Hytone Oint bid-qid	2.5% (1 oz)
	Hytone Lotn bid-qid	2.5% (1 oz)
	U-cort Crm bid-qid	1% (7, 28, 35 g)
triamcinolone acetonide (C)(G)	**Kenalog** Crm bid-qid	0.025% (15, 80 g)
	Kenalog Lotn bid-qid	0.025% (60 ml)
	Kenalog Oint bid-qid	0.025% (15, 60, 80 g)
Intermediate Potency		
betamethasone valerate (C)(G)	**Luxiq** Foam bid	0.12% (100 g)
clocortolone pivalate (C)	**Cloderm** Crm bid	
desonide (C)(G)	**Desonate** Gel/Formulation bid-tid	0.05% (15, 60 g)
	DesOwen Crm bid-tid	0.05% (15, 60 g)
	DesOwen Lotn bid-tid	0.05% (2, 4 fl oz)
	DesOwen Oint bid-tid	0.05% (15, 60 g)
	Tridesilon Crm bid-qid	0.05% (15, 60 g)
	Tridesilon Oint bid-qid	0.05% (15, 60 g)
	Verdeso Foam	
desoximetasone (C)(G)	**Topicort**-LP Emol Crm bid	0.05% (15, 60 g, 4 oz)
fluocinolone acetonide (C)(G)	**Capex** Shampoo	0.01% (4 oz)
	Derma-Smoothe/FS Oil tid	0.01% (4 oz)
	Derma-Smoothe/FS Shampoo	0.01% (4 oz)
	Synalar Crm bid-qid	0.025% (15, 30, 60 g)
	Synalar Oint bid-qid	0.025% (15, 60 g)
flurandrenolide (C)	**Cordran-SP** Crm bid to tid	0.025% (30, 60 g)
	Cordran Oint bid-tid	0.025% (30, 60 g)
	Cordran-SP Crm bid-tid	0.05% (15, 30, 60 g)
	Cordran Lotn bid-tid	0.05% (15, 60 ml)
	Cordran Oint bid-tid	0.05% (15, 30, 60 g)
fluticasone propionate (C)(G)	**Cutivate** Oint bid	0.005% (15, 30, 60 g)
	Cutivate Crm qd-bid	0.05% (15, 30, 60 g)
	Cutivate Lotn qd-bid	0.05%

(*continued*)

(*continued*)

Generic	Brand/Formulation/Frequency	Strength/Volume
hydrocortisone probutate (C)	**Pandel** Crm qd-bid	0.1% (15, 45 g)
hydrocortisone butyrate (C)(G)	**Locoid** Crm bid-tid **Locoid** Oint bid-tid **Locoid** Soln bid-tid	0.1% (15, 45 g) 0.1% (15, 45 g) 0.1% (30, 60 ml)
hydrocortisone valerate (C)(G)	**Westcort** Crm bid-tid **Westcort** Oint bid-tid	0.2% (15, 45, 60, 120 g) 0.2% (15, 45, 60 g)
mometasone furoate (C)	**Elocon** Crm qd **Elocon** Lotn qd **Elocon** Oint qd	0.1% (15, 45 g) 0.1% (30, 60 ml) 0.1% (15, 45 g)
prednicarbate	**Dermatop** Emol Crm bid **Dermatop** Oint bid	0.1% (15, 60 g)
triamcinolone acetonide (C)(G)	**Kenalog** Crm bid-tid **Kenalog** Lotn bid-tid **Kenalog** Emul Spray bid-tid	0.1% (15, 60, 80 g) 0.1% (60 ml) 0.2% (63, 100 g)
High Potency		
amcinonide (C)(G)	Crm bid-tid Lotn bid Oint bid	0.1% (15, 30, 60 g) 0.1% (20, 60 ml) 0.1% (15, 30, 60 g)
Betamethasone dipropionate (C)	**Sernivo Spray** Emul Spray bid	0.05% (60, 120 ml)
betamethasone dipropionate, augmented (C)	**Diprolene AF** Emol Crm qd-bid **Diprolene** Lotn qd-bid	0.05% (15, 50 g) 0.05% (30, 60 ml)
desoximetasone (C)(G)	**Topicort** Gel bid **Topicort** Emol Crm bid **Topicort** Oint bid	0.05% (15, 60 g) 0.25% (15, 60 g) 0.25% (15, 60 g)
diflorasone diacetate (C)	**Psorcon e** Emol Crm bid **Psorcon e** Emol Oint qd-tid	0.05% (15, 30, 60 g) 0.05% (15, 30, 60 g)
fluocinonide (C)	**Lidex** Crm bid-qid **Lidex** Gel bid-qid **Lidex** Oint bid-qid **Lidex** Soln bid-qid **Lidex-E** Emol Crm bid-qid	0.05% (15, 30, 60, 120 g) 0.05% (15, 30, 60 g) 0.05% (15, 30, 60, 120 g) 0.05% (20, 60 ml) 0.05% (15, 30, 60 g)

(*continued*)

(*continued*)

Generic	Brand/Formulation/Frequency	Strength/Volume
Flurandrenolide (C)	**Cordan** Oint bid-tid **Cordan** Crm bid-tid	0.05% (15, 30, 60 g) 0.025% (30, 60, 120 g) 0.05% (15, 30, 60, 120 g)
halcinonide (C)	**Halog** Crm bid-tid **Halog** Oint bid-tid **Halog** Soln bid-tid **Halog-E** Emol Crm qd-tid	0.1% (15, 30, 60, 240 g) 0.1% (15, 30, 60, 120 g) 0.1% (20, 60 ml) 0.1% (15, 30, 60 g)
triamcinolone acetonide (C)(G)	**Kenalog** Crm bid-tid	0.5% (20 g)
Super High Potency		
betamethasone dipropionate, augmented (C)	**Diprolene** Oint qd-bid **Diprolene** Gel qd-bid	0.05% (15, 50 g) 0.05% (15, 50 g)
clobetasol propionate (C)(G)	**Clobex** Shampoo daily **Clobex** Spray bid **Cormax** Oint bid **Cormax** Scalp App **Olux** Foam **Olux E** Foam **Temovate** Crm bid **Temovate** Gel bid **Temovate** Oint bid **Temovate** Scalp App bid **Temovate-E** Emol Crm bid	0.05% (4 oz) 0.05% (2, 4.5 oz) 0.05% (15, 45 g) 0.05% (15, 45 g) 0.05% (50, 100 g) 0.05% (50, 100 g) 0.05% (15, 30, 45, 60 g) 0.05% (15, 30, 60 g) 0.05% (15, 30, 45, 60 g) 0.05% (25, 50 ml) 0.05% (15, 30, 60 g)
fluocinonide (C)	**Vanos** Oint qd-tid	0.1% (30, 60, 120 g)
flurandrenolide (C)	**Cordran** Tape q 12 hours	4 mcg/sq cm (roll of 3"x 80")
halobetasol propionate (C)	**Ultravate** Crm qd-bid **Ultravate** Oint qd to bid	0.05% (15, 45 g) 0.05% (15, 45 g)

 APPENDIX L: ORAL CORTICOSTEROIDS

Comment: Systemic corticosteroids increase glucose intolerance, reduce the action of insulin and oral hypoglycemic agents, reduce adrenal cortex activity, decrease immunity, mask signs of infection, impair wound healing, suppress growth in

(*continued*)

(*continued*)

children, and promote osteoporosis, fluid retention, and weight gain. Use systemic steroids with caution, using the lowest possible dose to affect clinical response, and withdraw (wean) gradually in tapering doses to avoid adrenal insufficiency. The American Academy of Rheumatology (AAR) recommends the following daily doses for anyone on a chronic systemic corticosteroid regimen: Calcium 1,200-1,500 mg/day and vitamin D 800-1,000 IU/day.

▷ *betamethasone* (C)(G) initially 0.6-7.2 mg daily
    Pediatric: same as adult
        Celestone *Tab:* 0.6 mg; *Syr:* 0.6 mg/5 ml (120 ml)

▷ *cortisone* (D)(G) initially 25-300 mg daily or every other day
    Pediatric: not recommended
        Cortone Acetate *Tab:* 25 mg

▷ *xamethasone* (C)(G) initially 0.75-9 mg/day
    Pediatric: same as adult
        Decadron *Tab:* 0.5*, 0.75*, 4*mg; *Syr:* 0.5 mg/5 ml (100 ml)
        Decadron 5-12 Pak *Tabs:* 0.75*mg (12/pck)

▷ *hydrocortisone* (C)(G) 20-240 mg daily
    Pediatric: 2-8 mg/day
        Cortef *Tab:* 5, 10, 20 mg; *Oral susp:* 10 mg/5 ml
        Hydrocortone *Tab:* 10 mg

▷ *methylprednisolone* (C)(G) 4-48 mg/day
    Pediatric: same as adult
        Medrol *Tab:* 2*, 4*, 8*, 16*, 24*, 32*mg
        Medrol Dosepak *Dosepak:* 4*mg tabs (21/pck)

▷ *prednisolone* (C)(G) initially 5-60 mg/day in 1-2 doses x 3-5 days
    Pediatric: 0.14-2 mg/kg/day in 3-4 doses x 3-5 days
        Flo-Pred *Susp:* 5, 15 mg/5 ml
        Orapred *Soln:* 15 mg/5 ml (grape) (dye-free, alcohol 2%)
        Orapred ODT *Tab:* 10, 15, 30 mg orally disintegrating (grape)
        Pediapred *Soln:* 5 mg/5 ml (raspberry, sugar-, alcohol-, dye-free)
        Prelone *Syr:* 15 mg/5 ml
        Comment: Flo-Pred does not require refrigeration or shaking prior to use.

▷ *prednisone* (C)(G) initially 5-60 mg/day in 1-2 doses x 3-5 days
    Pediatric: 0.14-2 mg/kg/day in 3-4 doses x 3-5 days
        Deltasone *Tab:* 2.5*, 5*, 10*, 20*, 50*mg

▷ *prednisone (delayed release)* (C) initially 5-60 mg/day in 1-2 doses x 3-5 days
    Pediatric: 0.14-**2 mg**/kg/day in 3-4 doses x 3-5 days
        RAYOS *Tab:* 1, 2, 5 mg del-rel

▷ *triamcinolone* (C)(G) initially 4-48 mg/day in 1-2 doses x 3-5 days
    Pediatric: 0.14-2 mg/kg/day in 3-4 doses x 3-5 days
        Aristocort *Tab:* 4*mg
        Aristocort Forte *Susp:* 40 mg/ml (benzoyl alcohol)
        Aristocort Aristopak *Tab:* 4*mg (16/pck)

APPENDIX M: PARENTERAL CORTICOSTEROID THERAPY

Comment: Systemic glucocorticosteroids increase glucose intolerance, reduce the action of insulin and oral hypoglycemic agents, reduce adrenal cortex activity, decrease immunity, mask signs of infection, impair wound healing, suppress growth in children, and promote osteoporosis, fluid retention, and weight gain. Use systemic steroids with caution, using the lowest possible dose to affect clinical response, and withdraw (wean) gradually in tapering doses to avoid adrenal insufficiency. The American Academy of Rheumatology (AAR) recommends the following daily doses for anyone on a chronic systemic corticosteroid regimen: Calcium 1,200-1,500 mg/day and vitamin D 800-1,000 IU/day.

▷ *betamethasone* (C)(G)
  Celestone 0.5-9 mg IM/IV x 1 dose
    Vial: 3 mg/ml (10 ml)
  Celestone Soluspan 0.5-9 mg IM/IV x 1 dose; usual IM dose 6 mg
    Vial: 6 mg/ml (10 ml)

▷ *cortisone* (D)(G) 20-300 mg IM
  Pediatric: not recommended
    Cortone Acetate *Vial:* 50 mg/ml (10 ml)

▷ *dexamethasone* (C)(G) initially 0.5-9 mg IM/IV daily
  Dalalone D.P. *Vial:* 16 mg/ml (1, 5 ml)
  Decadron *Vial:* 4, 24 mg/ml for IM use (5 ml, sulfites)
  Decadron-LA *Vial:* 8 mg/ml (1, 5 ml)

▷ *hydrocortisone* (C)(G) initially 100-500 mg IM/IV daily
  Pediatric: 2-8 mg/kg loading dose (max 250 mg); then 8 mg/kg/day
    Hydrocortone *Vial:* 50 mg/ml (5 ml)
    Solu-Cortef *Vial:* 100 mg (2 ml); 250 mg (2 ml); 500 mg (4 ml); 1 g (8 ml)

▷ *hydrocortisone phosphate* (C)(G) for IM, IV, and SC injection
    Hydrocortone *Vial:* 50 mg/ml (2 ml)

▷ *methylprednisolone* (C)(G) 40-120 mg IM/week for 1-4 weeks
    Depo-Medrol *Vial:* 20 mg/ml (5 ml); 40 mg/ml (5, 10 ml); 80 mg/ml (5 ml)

▷ *methylprednisolone sodium succinate* (C)(G) 10-40 mg IV initially; then, IM <u>or</u> IV
  Pediatric: 1-2 mg/kg loading dose; then 1.6 mg/kg/day in divided doses at least 6 hours apart
    Solu-Medrol *Vial:* 40 mg (1 ml), 125 mg (2 ml), 500 mg (4 ml); 1 g (8 ml); 2 g (8 ml)

▷ *triamcinolone* (C)(G) 40 mg IM/week
    Aristocort *Vial:* 25 mg/ml (5 ml)
    Aristocort Forte *Vial:* 40 mg/ml (1, 5 ml)*(do not administer IV)*
    Aristospan *Vial:* 5 mg/ml (5 ml); 20 mg/ml (1, 5 ml)
    TAC-3 *Vial:* 3 mg/ml (5 ml) for intralesional and intradermal use

Injectable Corticosteroid/Anesthetic

▷ *dexamethasone/lidocaine* (C) 0.1-0.75 ml into painful area
    Decadron Phosphate with Xylocaine *Vial: dexa* 4 mg/*lido* 10 mg per ml (5 ml)

APPENDIX N: INHALATIONAL CORTICOSTEROID THERAPY

Comment: Inhaled glucocorticosteroids are indicated for the long-term control of asthma. Inhaled corticosteroids are not indicated for exercise induced asthma <u>or</u> for relief of acute symptoms (i.e., "rescue"). Low doses are indicated for mild persistent asthma, medium doses are indicated for moderate persistent asthma, and high doses are reserved for severe cases. Titrate to lowest effective dose. To reduce the potential for adverse effects with inhalers, the patient should use a spacer <u>or</u> holding chamber and rinse the mouth and spit after every inhalation treatment. Linear growth should be monitored in children. When inhaled doses exceed 1000 mcg/day, consider supplements of calcium (1-1.5 g/day), vitamin D (400 IU/day), and *estrogen* replacement therapy for postmenopausal women.

▷ *beclomethasone* (C)

    Beclovent 2 inhalations tid-qid <u>or</u> 4 inhalations bid; max 20 inhalations/day
        Pediatric: <6 years: not recommended; 6-12 years: 1-2 inhalations tid-qid <u>or</u> 4 inhalations bid; max 10 inhalations/day
        Inhaler: 42 mcg/actuation (6.7 g, 80 inh); 16.8 g (200 inh)
    Qvar *Previously using only bronchodilators:* initiate 40-80 mcg bid; max 320 mcg/day; *Previously using an inhaled corticosteroid:* initiate 40-160 mcg bid; max 320 mcg/day; *Previously taking a systemic corticosteroid:* attempt to wean off the systemic drug after approximately 1 week after initiating Qvar
        Pediatric: not recommended
        Inhaler: 40, 80 mcg/actuation metered-dose aerosol w. dose counter (8.7 g, 120 inh) (CFC-free)
    Vanceril 2 inhalations tid to qid <u>or</u> 4 inhalations bid
        Pediatric: <6 years: not recommended; 6-12 years: 1-2 inhalations tid to qid
        Inhaler: 42 mcg/actuation (16.8 g, 200 inh)
    Vanceril Double Strength 2 inhalations bid
        Pediatric: <6 years: not recommended; 6-12 years: 1-2 inhalations bid; >12 years: same as adult
        Inhaler: 84 mcg/actuation (12.2 g, 120 inh)

▷ *budesonide* (B)(G)

    Pulmicort Respules use turbuhaler
        Pediatric: <12 months: not recommended; ≥12 months to 8 years: *Previously using only bronchodilators:* initiate 0.5 mg/day once daily <u>or</u> in 2 divided doses; may start at 0.25 mg/day; *Previously using inhaled orticosteroids:* initiate 0.5 mg/day daily <u>or</u> in 2 divided doses; max 1 mg/day; *Previously using oral orticosteroids:* initiate 1 mg/day daily <u>or</u> in 2 divided doses
        Inhal susp: 0.25 mg/2 ml (30/box)
    Pulmicort Turbuhaler 1-2 inhalations bid; *Previously on oral corticosteroids:* 2-4 inhalations bid
        Pediatric: <6 years: not recommended; ≥6 years: 1-2 inhalations bid
        Turbuhaler: 200 mcg/actuation (200 inh)

(continued)

(continued)

> *flunisolide* (C)(G)

AeroBid, AeroBid M initially 2 inhalations bid; max 8 inhalations/day
Pediatric: <6 years: not recommended; 6-15 years: 2 inhalations bid; ≥16 years: same as adult
Inhaler: 250 mcg/actuation (7 g, 100 inh)

> *fluticasone* (C)(G)

Flovent HFA initially 88 mcg bid; if previously using an inhaled corticosteroid, initially 88-220 mcg bid; if previously taking an oral corticosteroid, initially 880 mcg/day
Pediatric: use **Rotadisk**: initially 50-88 mcg inh bid; <4 years: not recommended; 4-11 years: initially 50-88 mcg bid; >11 years: initially 100 mcg bid; if previously using an inhaled corticosteroid, initially 100-200 mcg bid; *Previously taking an oral corticosteroid;* initially 1000 mcg bid
Inhaler: 44 mcg/actuation (7.9 g, 60 inh; 13 g, 120 inh); 110 mcg/actuation (13 g, 120 inh); 220 mcg/actuation (13 g, 120 inh)
Rotadisk 50 mcg/actuation (60 blisters/disk); 100 mcg/actuation (60 blisters/disk); 250 mcg/actuation (60 blisters/disk)

> *mometasone furoate* (C) *Previously using a bronchodilator* or *inhaled corticosteroid:* 220 mcg q PM or bid; max 440 mcg q PM or 220 mcg bid; *Previously using an oral corticosteroid:* 440 mcg bid; max 880 mcg/day
Pediatric: <12 years: not recommended
Asmanex Twisthaler
Inhaler: 220 mcg/actuation (6.7 g, 80 inh); 16.8 g (200 inh)

◯ APPENDIX O: ORAL ANTIARRHYTHMIA DRUGS

Antiarrhythmics by Classification With Dose Forms		
Brand/*generic* Pregnancy Category	**Class/Indication(s)**	**Dose Form(s)**
Betapace *sotalol* (B)	*Class:* Class II and III Antiarrhythmic *Indications:* Documented life-threatening ventricular arrhythmias	*Tab:* 80*, 120*, 160*, 240*mg
Betapace AF *sotalol* (B)	*Class:* Class II and III Antiarrhythmic *Indications:* Maintenance of normal sinus rhythm in patients with highly symptomatic atrial fibrillation or atrial flutter who are currently in sinus rhythm	*Tab:* 80*, 120*, 160*mg
Calan *verapamil* (C)(G)	*Class:* Calcium Channel Blocker *Indications:* Control (with *digitalis*) of ventricular rate in patients with chronic atrial fibrillation or atrial flutter; prophylaxis of repetitive paroxysmal supraventricular tachycardia	*Tab:* 40, 80*, 120*mg

(continued)

(continued)

Antiarrhythmics by Classification With Dose Forms		
Brand/*generic* **Pregnancy Category**	**Class/Indication(s)**	**Dose Form(s)**
Cordarone *amiodarone* (D)(G)	*Class:* Class III Antiarrhythmic *Indications:* Documented life threatening recurrent refractory ventricular fibrillation <u>or</u> hemodynamically unstable ventricular tachycardia	*Tab:* 200*mg
Quinidex *quinidine sulfate* (C) (G)	*Class:* Class I Antiarrhythmic *Indications:* Atrial and ventricular arrhythmias	*Tab:* 300 mg ext-rel
Inderal *propranolol* (C)(G) **Inderal XL** *propranolol* ext-rel (C)(G) **InnoPran XL** *Propranolol* ext-rel (C)	*Class:* Beta-Blocker *Indications:* Atrial and ventricular arrhythmias; tachyarrhythmias due to *digitalis* intoxication; reduce mortality and risk of reinfarction in stabilized patients after myocardial infarction	*Tab:* 10*, 20*, 40*, 60*, 80*mg *Cap:* 60, 80, 120, 160 mg sust-rel *Cap:* 80, 120 mg ext-rel
Mexitil *mexiletine* (C)	*Class:* Class IB Antiarrhythmic *Indications:* Documented life-threatening ventricular arrhythmias	*Cap:* 150, 200, 250 mg
Multaq *dronedarone* (C)	*Class:* IB Antiarrhythmic *Indications:* Paroxysmal <u>or</u> persistent atrial fibrillation <u>or</u> atrial flutter	*Tab:* 400 mg
Norpace *disopyramide* (C)	*Class:* Class I Antiarrhythmic *Indications:* Documented life threatening ventricular arrhythmias	*Cap:* 100, 150 mg
Procanbid *procainamide* (C)(G)	*Class:* Class IA Antiarrhythmic *Indications:* Life threatening ventricular arrhythmias	*Tab:* 500, 1000 mg ext-rel
Quinaglute *quinidine gluconate* (C)(G)	*Class:* Class I Antiarrhythmic *Indications:* Atrial and ventricular arrhythmias	*Tab:* 324 mg ext-rel

(continued)

(continued)

Antiarrhythmics by Classification With Dose Forms		
Brand/*generic* Pregnancy Category	Class/Indication(s)	Dose Form(s)
Rythmol *propafenone* (C)(G)	*Class:* Class IC Antiarrhythmic *Indications:* Documented lifethreatening ventricular arrhythmias; prolonged recurrence of paroxysmal atrial fibrillation and/<u>or</u> atrial flutter <u>or</u> paroxysmal supraventricular tachycardia associated with disabling symptoms in patients without structural heart disease	*Tab:* 150*, 225*, 300*mg *Cap:* 225, 325, 425 mg ext-rel
Sectral *acebutolol* (B)(G)	*Class:* Beta-Blocker *Indications:* Ventricular arrhythmias	*Cap:* 200, 400 mg
Sotylize *sotalol* (B)	*Class:* Class II and III Antiarrhythmic *Indications:* Documented life threatening ventricular arrhythmias, and highly symptomatic AF/AF	*Oral soln:* 5 mg/ml
Tambocor *flecainide acetate* (C)(G)	*Class:* Class IC Antiarrhythmic *Indications:* Documented life threatening ventricular arrhythmias; paroxysmal atrial fibrillation <u>and/or</u> atrial flutter <u>or</u> paroxysmal supraventricular tachycardia in patients without structural heart disease	*Tab:* 50, 100*, 150* mg
Tenormin *atenolol* (C)(G)	*Class:* Beta-Blocker *Indications:* Reduce mortality and in stabilized patients after myocardial infarction	*Tab:* 25, 50, 100 mg *Inj:* 5 mg/ml (10 ml) for IV adminis-tration
timolol maleate (C) (G)	*Class:* Beta-Blocker *Indications:* Reduce mortality and in stabilized patients after myocardial infarction	*Tab:* 5, 10*, 20*mg

(continued)

(continued)

Antiarrhythmics by Classification With Dose Forms		
Brand/*generic* Pregnancy Category	Class/Indication(s)	Dose Form(s)
dofetilide (C)(G)	*Class:* Class III Antiarrhythmic *Indications:* Maintenance of normal sinus rhythm in patients with atrial fibrillation or atrial flutter of >1 week duration who were converted to normal sinus rhythm (only for highly symptommatic patients); conversion to normal sinus rhythm	*Cap:* 125, 250, 500 mcg
Tonocard *tocainide* (C)(G)	*Class:* Class I Antiarrhythmic *Indications:* Documented lifethreatening ventricular arrhythmias	*Tab:* 400*, 600*mg
Toprol XL *metoprolol* (C)(G)	*Class:* Beta-Blocker *Indications:* Ischemic, hypertensive, or cardiomyopathic heart failure	*Tab:* 25*, 50*, 100*, 200*mg

APPENDIX P: ORAL ANTINEOPLASIA DRUGS

Antineoplastics With Classification With Dose Forms		
Brand/*generic* Pregnancy Category	Class/Indications	Dose Forms
Alkeran *melphalan* (D)	Alkylating Agent	*Tab:* 2*mg
Arimidex *anastrozole* (D)	Aromatase Inhibitor	*Tab:* 1 mg
Aromasin *exemestane* (D)	Aromatase Inactivator	*Tab:* 25 mg
Arranon *nelarabine* (D)	Nucleoside Analog	*Vial:* 250 mg for IV infusion
Casodex *Bicalutamide* (X)	Antiandrogen	*Tab:* 50 mg
Cytoxan *Cyclophosphamide* (D)	Alkylating Agent	*Tab:* 25, 50 mg

(continued)

(*continued*)

Antineoplastics With Classification With Dose Forms		
Brand/*generic* Pregnancy Category	Class/Indications	Dose Forms
Eligard *leuprolide acetate* (**X**)	GnRH Analogue	*Inj:* 7.5 mg ext-rel per monthly SC injection
Eulexin *flutamide* (**D**)	Antiandrogen	*Cap:* 125 mg
Faslodex *fulvestrant* (**D**)(**G**)	Estrogen Receptor Antagonist	*Prefilled syringe for IM inj:* 50 mg/ml (2.5, 5 ml/syringe)
Femara *letrozole* (**D**)	Aromatase Inhibitor	*Tab:* 2.5 mg
Gleevec *imatinib mesylate* (**D**)	Signal Transduction Inhibitor	*Cap:* 100 mg
Hydrea *hydroxyurea* (**D**)(**G**)	Substituted Urea	*Cap:* 500 mg
Iressa *gefitinib* (**D**)	Epidermal Growth Factor receptor tyrosine kinase inhibitor	*Tab:* 250 mg
Leukeran *chlorambucil* (**D**)(**G**)	Alkylating Agent	*Tab:* 2 mg
Leupron *leuprolide* (**X**)	GnRH Analogue	*Susp for IM inj:* 1 mg (daily); 7.5 mg depot (monthly); 22.5 mg depot (every 3 months); 30 mg depot (every 4 months)
Megace, Megace Oral Suspension, Megace ES, *megestrol acetate* (**D**) (**G**)	Progestin	*Tab:* 20*, 40*mg; *Susp:* 40 mg/ml; ES concentrate: 125 mg/ml, 625 mg/5 ml
Nexavar *sorafenib* (**D**)	Multikinase Inhibitor	*Tab:* 200 mg
Nolvadex *tamoxifen citrate* (**D**) (**G**)	Antiestrogen	*Tab:* 10, 20 mg

(*continued*)

(continued)

Antineoplastics With Classification With Dose Forms		
Brand/*generic* **Pregnancy Category**	**Class/Indications**	**Dose Forms**
Tarceva *erlotinib* (D)	Kinase Inhibitor	*Tab:* 25, 100, 150 mg
Velcade *bortezomib* (D)	Proteasome Inhibitor	*Vial:* 3.5 mg (pwdr for IV injection after reconstitution)
Viadur *leuprolide acetate* (X)	GnRH Analogue	*SC implant:* 65 mg depot (replace every 12 months)
Xeloda *capecitabine* (D)	Fluoropyrimidine (prodrug of *5-fluorouracil*)	*Tab:* 150, 500 mg
Zoladex *goserelin acetate* (D)	GnRH Analogue	*SC implant:* 3.6 mg depot (28 days), 10.8 mg depot (3-month)
Zometa *zoledronic acid* (D)	Bisphosphonate	*Vial:* 4 mg pwdr for reconstitution for IV infusion, single dose

APPENDIX Q: ORAL AND DEPOT ANTIPSYCHOSIS DRUGS

ANTIPSYCHOSIS DRUGS WITH DOSE FORMS

Comment: Patients receiving an antipsychosis agent should be monitored closely for the following adverse side effects: neuroleptic malignant syndrome, extrapyramidal reactions, tardive dyskinesia, blood dyscrasias, anticholinergic effects, drowsiness, hypotension, photosensitivity, retinopathy, and lowered seizure threshold. Use lower doses for elderly or debilitated patients. Prescriptions should be written for the smallest practical amount. Foods and beverages containing alcohol are contraindicated for patients receiving psychotropic drug therapy.

➤ *aripiprazole* (C)(G)
  Abilify *Tab:* 2, 5, 10, 15, 20, 30 mg; *Oral soln:* 1 mg/ml (150 ml; orange crèam; parabens)
  Abilify Discmelt *Tab:* 15 mg orally disintegrating (vanilla) (phenylalanine)
  Abilify Maintena *Vial:* 300, 400 mg ext-rel pwdr for IM injection after reconstitution; 300, 400 mg single dose prefilled dual chamber syringes w. supplies

(continued)

(*continued*)

▷ *asenapine* (C)
    Saphris *SL tab:* 2.5, 5, 10 mg

▷ *brexpizole* (C)
    Rexulti *Tab:* 0.25, 0.5, 1, 2, 3, 4 mg

▷ *bupropion* (C)
    Forfivo XL *Tab:* 450 mg ext-rel

▷ *cariprazine* (NE)
    Vraylar *Cap:* 1.5, 3, 4.5, 6 mg

▷ *chlorpromazine* (C)(G)
    Thorazine *Tab:* 10, 25, 50, 100, 200 mg; *Cap:* 30, 75, 150 mg sust-rel; *Syr:* 10 mg/5 ml (4 oz, orange-custard); *Vial/Amp:* 25 mg/ml (1, 2 ml) (sulfites)

▷ *clozapine* (B)(G)
    Clozapine ODT (G) *ODT:* 150, 200 mg
    Clozaril (G) *Tab:* 25*, 100* mg; *ODT:* 150, 200 mg
    FazaClo ODT (G) *ODT:* 12.5, 25, 100, 150, 200 mg (phenylalanine)
    Versacloz *Oral susp:* 50 mg/ml (100 ml)

▷ *fluphenazine* (C)(G)
    Prolixin *Tab:* 1, 2.5, 5*, 10 mg (tartrazine); *Conc:* 5 mg/ml (4 oz w. calib dropper) (alcohol 14%); *Elix:* 5 mg/ml (2 oz w. calib dropper) (alcohol 14%); *Vial:* 25 mg/ml (10 ml)

▷ *fluphenazine decanoate* (C)(G)
    Prolixin Decanoate *Vial:* 25 mg/ml (5 ml) (benzyl alcohol)

▷ *fluphenazine* (C)(G)
    Prolixin Ethanate *Vial:* 25 mg (5 ml) (benzyl alcohol)

▷ *fluphenazine decanoate* (C)(G)
    Prolixin Decanoate *Vial:* 25 mg/ml (5 ml) (benzyl alcohol)

▷ *haloperidol* (B)(G)
    Haldol *Tab:* 0.5*, 1*, 2*, 5*, 10*, 20 mg

▷ *iloperidone* (C)
    Fanapt *Tab:* 1, 2, 4, 6, 8, 10, 12 mg

▷ *loxapine* (C)
    Adasuve *Oral inhal pwdr:* 10 mg single-use disposable inhaler (5/box)

▷ *lurasidone* (B)
    Latuda *Tab:* 20, 40, 80 mg

▷ *olanzapine fumarate* (C)(G)
    Zyprexa *Tab:* 2.5, 5, 7.5, 10, 15, 20 mg
    Zyprexa Zydis *ODT:* 5, 10, 15, 20 mg (phenylalanine)

(*continued*)

> *paliperidone* (C)(G)
>   **Invega** *Tab:* 3, 6, 9 mg ext-rel
>   **Invega** Sustenna *Prefilled syringe:* 39, 78, 117, 156, 234 mg ext-rel suspension
>   w. needle
>   **Invega** Trinza *Prefilled syringe:* 273, 410, 546, 819 mg ext-rel suspension
>
> *prochlorperazine* (C)(G)
>   **Compazine** *Tab:* 5, 10 mg; *Cap:* 10, 15 mg susrel; *Syr:* 5 mg/5 ml (4 oz; fruit);
>   *Supp:* 2.5, 5, 25 mg
>
> *quetiapine* (C)(G)
>   **Seroquel** *Tab:* 25, 100, 200, 300 mg
>   **Seroquel XR** *Tab:* 50, 150, 200, 300, 400 mg ext-rel
>
> *risperidone* (C)(G)
>   **Risperdal** *Tab:* 0.25, 0.5, 1, 2, 3, 4 mg; *Soln:* 1 mg/ml (30 ml w. pipette);
>   *Consta (Inj):* 25, 37.5, 50 mg
>   **Risperdal M-Tabs** *M-tab:* 0.5, 1, 2, 3, 4 mg orally-disint (phenylalanine)
>
> *thioridazine* (C)(G) *Tab:* 10, 25, 50, 100 mg
>
> *trifluoperazine* (C)(G)
>   **Stelazine** *Tab:* 1, 2, 5, 10 mg; *Conc:* 10 mg/ml; (2 oz w. calib dropper (ba-
>   nana-vanilla) (sulfites); *Vial:* 2 mg/ml (10 ml)
>
> *ziprasidone* (C)(G)
>   **Geodon** *Cap:* 20, 40, 60, 80 mg

⬭ APPENDIX R: ORAL ANTICONVULSANT DRUGS

ANTICONVULSANT DRUGS WITH DOSE FORMS

> *brivaracetam* (C)
>   **Briviact** *Tab:* 10, 25, 50, 75, 100 mg; *Oral soln:* 10 mg/ml (300 ml); *Vial:* 50 mg/
>   5 ml single-dose for IV inj
> *carbarbamazepine* (D)(G)
>   **Carbatrol** *Cap:* 200, 300 mg ext-rel
>   **Equetro** *Cap:* 100, 200, 300 mg ext-rel
>   **Tegretol** *Tab:* 100*, 200*mg; *Chew tab:* 100*mg
>   **Tegretol Suspension** *Oral susp:* 100 mg/5 ml (450 ml) (citrus vanilla) (sorbitol)
>   **Tegretol-XR** *Tab:* 100, 200, 400 mg ext-rel
>
> *clobazam* (C)(IV)
>   **Onfi** *Tab:* 10*, 20*mg
>   **Onfi Oral Suspension** *Oral susp:* 2.5 mg/ml (120 ml w. 2 dosing syringes)
>   (berry)

(*continued*)

(continued)

▷ *clonazepam* (D)(IV)(G)
    Clonazepam ODT *ODT:* 0.125, 0.25, 0.5, 1, 2, oral-dis
    Klonopin *Tab:* 0.5*, 1, 2 mg

▷ *diazepam* (D)(IV)(G)
    Diastat *Rectal gel delivery system:* 2.5 mg
    Diastat AcuDial *Rectal gel delivery system:* 10, 20 mg
    Valium *Tab:* 2*, 5*, 10*mg
    Valium Injectable *Vial:* 5 mg/ml (10 ml); *Amp:* 5 mg/ml (2 ml); *Prefilled syringe:* 5 mg/ml (5 ml)
    Valium Intensol *Conc oral soln:* 5 mg/ml (30 ml w. dropper) (alcohol 19%)
    Valium Oral Solution *Oral soln:* 5 mg/5 ml (500 ml) (winter green-spice)

▷ *divalproex sodium* (D)(G)
    Depakene *Cap:* 250 mg; *Syr:* 250 mg/5 ml (16 oz)
    Depakote *Tab:* 125, 250, 500 mg
    Depakote ER *Tab:* 250, 500 mg ext-rel
    Depakote Sprinkle *Cap:* 125 mg

▷ *eslicarbazepine* (C)
    Aptiom *Tab:* 200*, 400, 600*, 800* mg

▷ *ezogabine* (C)
    Potiga *Tab:* 50, 200, 300, 400 mg

▷ *felbamate* (C)(G)
    Felbatol *Tab:* 400*, 600*mg
    Felbatol Oral Suspension *Oral susp:* 600 mg/5 ml (4, 8, 32 oz)
    Peganone *Tab:* 250, 500 mg

▷ *bapentin* (C)
    Horizant *Tab:* 300, 600 ext-rel
    Neurontin (G) *Cap:* 100, 300, 400 mg; *Tab:* 600*, 800*mg
    Neurontin Oral Solution *Oral soln:* 250 mg/5 ml (480 ml) (strawberry-anise)

▷ *lacosamide* (C)(V)(G)
    Vimpat *Tab:* 50, 100, 150, 200 mg; *Oral soln:* 10 mg/ml (200, 465 ml); *Vial:* 10 mg/ml soln for IV infusion, single-use (20 ml)

▷ *lamotrigine* (C)(G)
    Lamictal *Tab:* 25*, 100*, 150*, 200*mg
    Lamictal Chewable Dispersible Tab *Chew tab:* 2, 5, 25, 50 mg (black current)
    Lamictal ODT *ODT:* 25, 50, 100, 200 mg oral-dis
    Lamictal XR *Tab:* 25, 50, 100, 200, 250, 300 mg ext-rel

▷ *levetiracetam* (C)
    Elepsia *Tab:* 1000, 1500 mg ext-rel
    Keppra *Tab:* 250*, 500*, 750*, 1000*mg
    Keppra Oral Solution *Oral soln:* 100 mg/ml (16 oz) (grape) (dye-free)
    Keppra XR *Tab:* 500, 750 mg ext-rel
    Levitiracetam IV (G) *Premixed:* 500, 1,000, 1,500 mg for IV infusion (100 ml)

(continued)

▷ *mephobarbital* (D)(II)
  Mebaral *Tab:* 32, 50, 100 mg

▷ *methsuximide* (C)
  Celontin Kapseals *Cap:* 150, 300 mg

▷ *oxcarbazepine* (C)(G)
  Trileptal *Tab:* 150, 300, 600 mg; *Oral susp:* 300 mg/5 ml (lemon) (alcohol)
  Oxtella XR *Tab:* 150, 300, 600 mg ext-rel

▷ *perampanel* (C)(III)
  Fycompa *Tab:* 2, 4, 6, 8, 10, 12 mg
  Fycompa Oral Suspension *Oral susp:* 0.5 mg/ml (340 ml w. dosing syringe)

▷ *phenytoin* (D)(G), *primidone* (D)(G)
  Dilantin *Cap:* 30, 100 mg ext-rel
  Dilantin Infatabs *Chew tab:* 50 mg
  Dilantin Oral Suspension *Oral susp:* 125 mg/5 ml (237 ml) (alcohol 6%)
  Phenytek *Cap:* 200, 300 mg ext-rel

▷ *pregabalin* (C)(V)
  Lyrica *Cap:* 25, 50, 75, 100, 200, 225, 300 mg
  Lyrica Oral Solution *Oral soln:* 20 mg/ml

▷ *primidone* (C)
  Mysoline *Tab:* 50*, 250*mg
  Mysoline Oral Solution *Oral susp:* 250 mg/5 ml (8 oz)

▷ *rufinamide* (C)(G)
  Banzel *Tab:* 200*, 400*mg
  Banzel Oral Solution *Susp:* 40 mg/ml (orange) (lactose-free, gluten-free, dye-free)

▷ *tiagabine* (C)(G)
  Gabitril *Tab:* 2, 4, 12, 16 mg

▷ *topiramate* (D)(G)
  Topamax *Tab:* 25, 50, 100, 200 mg
  Topamax Sprinkle Caps *Cap:* 15, 25, 50 mg
  Trokendi XR *Cap:* 100, 200 mg ext-rel
  Qudexy *Tab:* 25, 50, 100, 150, 200 mg ext-rel
  Qudexy XR *Cap:* 25, 50, 100, 150, 200 mg ext-rel

▷ *vigabatrin* (C)
  Sabril *Tab:* 500 mg
  Sabril for Oral Solution 500 mg/pkt pwdr for reconstitution

▷ *zonisamide* (C)
  Zonegran *Cap:* 25, 50, 100 mg

(continued)

APPENDIX S: ORAL ANTI-HIV DRUGS WITH DOSE FORMS

Aptivus (C) *tipranavir*

Gel cap: 250 mg (alcohol); *Oral soln:* 100 mg/ml (95 ml w. dosing syringe) (Vit E 116 IU/ml) (buttermint-butter, toffee)

Comment: *valganciclovir* is indicated for the treatment of AIDS-related cytomegalovirus (CMV) retinitis.

Atripla (D) *efavirenz/emtricitabine/tenofovir disoproxil*

Tab: efa 600 mg/*emtri* 200 mg/*teno diso* 300 mg

Combivir (C)(G) *lamivudine/zidovudine*

Tab: aba/lami 150/*zido* 300 mg

Complera (B) *emtricitabine/tenofovir disoproxil fumarate/ rilpivirine*

Tab: emtri 200 mg/*teno diso* 300 mg/*rilpiv* 25 mg

Crixivan (C) *indinavir sulfate*

Cap: 100, 200, 333, 400 mg

Cytovene (C)(G) *ganciclovir*

Cap: 250, 500 mg; *Vial:* 50 mg/ml single-dose (500 mg, 10 ml)

Descovy (D) *emtricitabine/tenofovir alafenamide/rilpivirine*

Tab: emtri 200 mg/*teno ala* 25 mg

Edurant (B) *rilpivirine*

Tab: 25 mg

Emtriva (B) *emtricitabine*

Cap: 200 mg; *Oral soln:* 10 mg/ml (170 ml) (cotton candy)

Epivir (C)(G) *lamivudine*

Tab: 150*, 300*mg; *Oral soln:* 10 mg/ml (240 ml) (strawberry-banana) (sucrose 3 g/15 ml)

Epzicom (B) *abacavir sulfate/lamivudine*

Tab: aba 600 mg/*lami* 300 mg

(*continued*)

(*continued*)

Evotaz (B) *atazanavir/cobicistat*

Tab: ataz 300/*cobi* 150 mg

Fortovase (B) *aquinavir*

Soft gel cap: 200 mg

Fuzeon (B) *enfuvirtide*

Vial: 90 mg/ml pwdr for SC inj after reconstitution (1 ml, 60 vials/kit) (preservative-free)

Genvoya (B) *elvitegravir/cobicistat/emtricitabine/tenofovir alafenamide (TAF)*

Tab: elv 150 mg/*cob* 150 mg/*emtri* 200 mg/*teno alafen* 10 mg

Intelence (C) *etravirine*

Tab: 25*, 100, 200 mg

Invirase (B) *saquinavir mesylate*

Hard gel cap: 200 mg

Isentress (C) *raltegravir (potassium)*

Tab: 400 mg film-coat; *Chew tab:* 25, 100*mg (orange-banana) (phenylalanine); *Oral susp:* 100 mg/pkt pwdr for oral susp (banana)

Kaletra (C) *lopinavir plus ritonavir*

Cap: lopin 100 mg/*riton* 25 mg, *lopin* 200 mg/*riton* 50 mg; *Oral soln: lopin* 80 mg/*riton* 20 mg per ml (160 ml w. dose cup) (cotton candy) (alcohol 42%)
Hard gel cap: 200 mg

Lexiva (C)(G) *fosamprenavir*

Tab: 700 mg; *Oral soln:* 50 mg/ml (grape, bubble gum) (peppermint)

Norvir (B) *ritonavir*

Soft gel cap: 100 mg (alcohol); *Oral soln:* 80 mg/ml (8 oz) (peppermint-caramel) (alcohol)

Odefsey (D) *emtricitabine/rilivirine/tenofovir alafenamide*

Tab: emtri 200 mg/*rilpiv* 25 mg/*tenof alafen* 25 mg

Prezcobix (B) *darunavir/cobicistat*

Tab: daru 800/*cobi* 150 mg

(*continued*)

(continued)

Prezista (C) *darunavir*

Tab: 75, 150, 600, 800 mg; *Oral susp:* 100 mg/ml (200 ml) (strawberry cream)

Rescriptor (C) *delavirdine mesylate*

Tab: 100, 200 mg

Retrovir (C)(G) *zidovudine*

Tab: 300 mg; *Cap:* 100 mg; *Syr:* 50 mg/5 ml (240 ml) (strawberry); *Vial:* 10 mg/ml (20 ml vial for IV infusion) (peservative-free)

Reyataz (B) *atazanavir*

Cap: 100, 150, 200, 300 mg

Selzentry (B) *maraviroc*

Tab: 150, 300 mg

Stribild (B) *elvitegravir/cobicistat/emtricitabine/tenofovir diso-proxil fumarate*

Tab: elv 150 mg/*cob* 150 mg/*emtri* 200 mg/*teno diso fumar* 300 mg

Sustiva (C) *efavirenz*

Tab: 75, 150, 600, 800 mg; *Cap:* 50, 200 mg

Tivicay (B) *dolutegavir*

Tab: 50 mg

Triumeq (C) *abacavir sulfate/dilutegravir/lamivudine*

Tab: aba 600 mg/*dilu* 50 mg/*lami* 300 mg

Trizivir (C)(G) *abacavir sulfate/lamivudine/zidovudine*

Tab: aba 300 mg/*lami* 150 mg/*zido* 300 mg

Truvada (B) *emtricitabine/tenofovir disoproxil fumarate*

Tab: emt 100 mg/*teno 150 mg,* 133 mg/*teno* 200 mg, *emt* 167 mg/*teno* 250 mg, *emt* 200 mg/*teno* 300 mg

Valcyte (C)(G) *valganciclovir*

Tab: 450 mg

Videx EC (C)(G) *didanosine*

Cap: 125, 200, 250, 400 mg ent-coat del-rel; *Chew tab:* 25, 50, 100, 150, 200 mg (mandarin orange; buffered with calcium carbonate and magnesium hydroxide, phenylalanine); *Pwdr for oral soln:* 2, 4 g (120, 240 ml)

(continued)

(continued)

Videx Pediatric Pwdr for Oral Solution (C) *didanosine*

 Pwdr for oral soln: 2, 4 g (120, 240 ml)

Viracept (B) *nelfinavir mesylate*

 Tab: 250, 625 mg; *Pwdr for oral soln:* 50 mg/g (144 g) (phenylalanine)

Viramune (C)(G) *nevirapine*

 Tab: 200*mg; *Oral susp:* 50 mg/5 ml (240 ml)

Viramune XR (C) *nevirapine*

 Tab: 100, 400 mg ext-rel

Viread (C) *tenofovir disoproxil fumarate*

 Tab: 150, 200, 250, 300 mg; *Oral pwdr:* 40 mg/1 g pwdr (60 g w. dosing scoop)

Vistide (C) *cidofovir*

 Inj: 75 mg/ml (5 ml vials for IV infusion) (preservative free)

Comment: *cidofovir* is indicated for the treatment of AIDS-related cytomegalovirus (CMV) retinitis.

Vitekta (C) *elvitegravir*

 Inj: 75 mg/ml (5 ml vials for IV infusion) (preservative free)

Comment: *cidofovir* is indicated for the treatment of AIDS-related cytomegalovirus (CMV) retinitis.

Zerit (C)(G) *stavudine*

 Cap: 15, 20, 30, 40 mg; *Oral soln:* 1 mg/ml pwdr for reconstitution (200 ml) (fruit) (dye-free)

Ziagen (C)(G) *abacavir sulfate*

 Tab: 300*mg; *Oral soln:* 20 mg/ml (240 ml) (strawberry-banana) (parabens, propylene glycol)

◯ APPENDIX T: COUMADIN (WARFARIN)

T.1: COUMADIN TITRATION AND DOSE FORMS

▷ *warfarin* (X)(G) dosage initially 2-5 mg/day; usual maintenance 2-10 mg/day; adjust dosage to maintain INR in therapeutic range:
 Venous thrombosis: 2.0-3.0

(continued)

(continued)

> *Atrial fibrillation*: 2.0-3.0
> *Post MI*: 2.5-3.5
> *Mechanical and bioprosthetic heart valves:* 2.0-3.0 for 12 weeks after valve insertion, then 2.5-3.5 long-term
> *Pediatric:* not recommended <18 years
> **Coumadin** *Tab:* 1*, 2*, 2.5*, 3*, 4*, 5*, 6*, 7.5*, 10* mg
> **Coumadin for Injection** *Vial:* 2 mg/ml (2.5 ml)
> Comment: **Coumadin for Injection** is for peripheral IV administration only.

T.2: COUMADIN OVER-ANTICOAGULATION REVERSAL

> ➤ *phytonadione (vitamin K)* (G) 2.5-10 mg PO or IM; max 25 mg
> **AquaMEPHYTON**
> *Vial:* 1 mg/0.5 ml (0.5 ml); 10 mg/ml (1, 2.5, 5 ml)
> **Mephyton**
> *Tab:* 5 mg

T.3: AGENTS THAT INHIBIT COUMADIN'S ANTICOAGULATION EFFECTS

Increase Metabolism	Decrease Absorption	Other Mechanism(s)
azathioprine	azathioprine	coenzyme Q10
carbamazepine	cholestyramine	estrogen
dicloxacillin	colestipol	griseofulvin
ethanol	sucralfate	oral contraceptives
griseofulvin		ritonavir
nafcillin		spironolactone
pentobarbital		trazodone
phenobarbital		vitamin C (high
phenytoin		dose)
primidone		vitamin K
rifabutin		
rifampin		

⭕ APPENDIX U: LOW MOLECULAR WEIGHT HEPARINS

Comment: Administer by subcutaneous injection *only*, in the abdomen, and rotate sites. Avoid concomitant drugs that affect hemostasis (e.g., oral anticoagulants and platelet aggregation inhibitors, including *aspirin*, NSAIDs, *dipyridamole*, *sulfinpyrazone*, *ticlopidine*). Pediatrics not recommended.

(continued)

(*continued*)

> *ardeparin* (C)
>> **Normiflo** *Soln for inj:* 5,000 anti-Factor Xa U/0.5 ml; 10,000 anti-Factor Xa U/0.5 ml (sulfites, parabens)

> *dalteparin* (B)
>> **Fragmin** *Prefilled syringe:* 2500 IU/0.2 ml, 5000 IU/0.2 ml (10/box) (preservative-free); *Multi-dose*
>> *vial:* 1,000 IU/ml (95,000 IU, 9.5 ml) (benzyl alcohol)

> *danaparoid* (B)
>> **Orgaran** *Amp:* 750 anti-Xa units/0.6 ml (0.6 ml, 10/box); *Prefilled syringe:* 750 anti-Xa units/0.6 ml (0.6 ml, 10/box) (sulfites)

> *enoxaparin* (B)(G)
>> **Lovenox** *Prefilled syringe:* 30 mg/0.3 ml, 40 mg/0.4 ml, 60 mg/0.6 ml, 80 mg/0.8 ml (100 mg/ml)
>> (preservative-free); *Vial:* 100 mg/ml (3 ml)

> *tinzaparin* (B)
>> **Innohep** *Vial:* 20,000 *anti-Factor Xa* IU/ml (2 ml) (sulfites, benzyl alcohol)

APPENDIX V: FACTOR XA INHIBITOR THERAPY

FACTOR XA INHIBITOR THERAPY

> *apixaban* (C) 5 mg bid; reduce to 2.5 mg bid if any two of the following: ≥80 years, ≤60 kg, serum Cr ≥1.5
> *Pediatric:* not recommended
>> **Eliquis** *Tab:* 2.5, 5 mg
>> Comment: **Eloquis** is indicated to reduce the risk of stroke and systemic embolism in patients with nonvalvular atrial fibrillation (NVAF).

> *edoxaban* (C) transition to and from **Savaysa**; assess CrCl prior to initiation: *NVAF CrCl >50 mL/min:* 60 mg once daily; *CrCl 15-50 mL/min:* 30 mg once daily *DVT/PE CrCl >50 mL/min:* 60 mg once daily following initial parental anticoagulant; *CrCl 15-50 mL/min, <60 kg, or concomitant Pgp inhibitors:* 30 mg once daily
> *Pediatric:* not established
>> **Savaysa** *Tab:* 15, 30, 60 mg
>> Comment: **Savaysa** is indicated to reduce the risk of stroke and systemic embolism in patients with nonvalvular atrial fibrillation (NVAF), treatment of DVT and pulmonary embolism (PE) following 5-10 days of initial therapy with with parenteral anticoagulant. Not for use in persons with NVAF with CrCl >95 mL/min.

> *fondaparinux* (B) Administer SC; administer first dose no earlier than 6-8 hours after hemostasis is achieved, start warfarin usually within 72 hours of last dose of *fondaparinux*

(*continued*)

(continued)

Post-op: 2.5 mg once daily x 5-9 days
Hip/Knee Replacement: once daily x 11 days
Hip Fracture: once daily x 32 days
Abdominal Surgery: once daily x 10 days
Prophylaxis: do not use <50 kg
Treatment: once daily for at least 5 days until INR=2-3 (usually 5-9 days); max 26 days; <50 kg: 5 mg; 50-100 kg: 7.5 mg; >100 kg: 10 mg
Pediatric: not established

Arixtra *Soln for SC inj:* 2.5 mg/0.5 ml, 5 mg/0.4 ml, 7.5 mg/0.6 ml, 10 mg/ 0.8 ml *prefilled syringe* (10/box) (preservative-free)

▷ **prasugrel (B)** *Loading dose:* 60 mg once in a single-dose; *Maintenance:* 10 mg once daily; *<60 kg:* consider 5 mg once daily; take with aspirin 75-325 mg once daily
Pediatric: not recommended

Effient *Tab:* 5, 10 mg

Comment: *Effient* is indicated to reduce the risk of thrombotic cardiovascular events in persons with acute coronary syndrome (ACS) who aret to be managed with percutaneous coronary intervention (PCI) including unstable angina, non-ST elevation myocardial infarction (NSTEMI) and STEMI. Do not start if active pathological bleeding (e.g., peptic ulcer, intracranial hemorrhage), prior TIA or stroke, or if patient likely to undergo urgent CABG. Discontinue 7 days before surgery and if TIA or stroke occurs.

▷ **rivaroxaban (C)** take with food
Treatment of DVT or PE: 15 mg twice daily for the first 21 days; then 20 mg once daily
Reduction in risk of DVT or PE recurrence: 20 mg once daily with the evening meal; *CrCl <30 mL/min:* avoid
Prophylaxis of DVT: take 6-10 hours after surgery when hemostasis established, then 20 mg once daily with the evening meal; *CrCl 30-50 mL/min:* 10 mg; *CrCl <30 mL/min:* avoid; discontinue if acute renal failure develops; monitor closely for
blood loss
Hip: treat for 35 days; *Knee:* treat for 12 days
Nonvalvular AF: take once daily with the evening meal; *CrCl >50 mL/min:* 20 mg; *CrCl 15-50 mL/min:* 15 mg; *CrCl >15 mL/min:* avoid
Pediatric: not recommended

Xarelto *Cap:* 10, 15, 20 mg

Comment: **Xarelto** is indicated to reduce the risk of stroke and systemic embolism in nonvalvular atrial fibrillation (AF), to treat deep vein thrombosis (DVT) and pulmonary embolism (PE), to reduce the risk of recurrence of DVT and/or PE following 6 months treatment for DVT and/ or PE, and prophylaxis of DVT which may lead to PE in patients undergoing knee or hip replacement surgery. **Xarelto** eliminates the need for bridging with heparin or lmwh; no need for routine monitoring of INR or other coagulation parameters; no need for dose adjustments for age, weight, or gender; no known dietary restrictions. Switching from **warfarin** or other anticoagulant, see mfr pkg insert.

(continued)

APPENDIX W: DIRECT THROMBIN INHIBITOR THERAPY

▷ *aspirin* (D) single dose once daily
Pediatric: not established
    Durlaza *Cap:* 162.5 mg 24-hr ext-rel (30, 90/bottle)
    Comment: Presently there is only one reversal agent for this drug class.
idarucizumab (**Praxbind**) is a specific reversal agent for dabigatran (**Pradaxa**).
It is a humanized monoclonal antibody fragment (Fab) that binds to
dabigatran and its acylglucuronide metabolites with higher affinity than the
binding affinity of dabigatran to thrombin, neutralizing its anticoagulant
effects.

IDARUCIZUMAB REVERSAL AGENT: HUMANIZED MONOCLONAL ANTIBODY FRAGMENT (FAB)

▷ *idarucizumab* (NE) administer 5 g (2 vials) IV drip <u>or</u> push; administer within 1
hour of removal from vial
Pediatric: not established
    Praxbind *Vial:* 2.5 g/50 ml, single-use (preservative-free)
    Comment: Presently, there is inadequate human and animal data to assess
risk of *idarucizumab* (**Praxbind**) use in pregnancy. Risk/benefit should be
considered prior to use.

▷ *dabigatran etexilate mesylate* (C) swallow whole; *CrCl >30 mL/min:* 150 mg bid;
CrCl 15-30 mL/min: 75 mg twice daily; *CrCl <15 mL/min:* not recommended
Pediatric: not recommended
    Pradaxa *Cap:* 75, 150 mg
    Comment: **Pradaxa** is indicated to reduce the risk of stroke and systemic
embolism in nonvalvular AF, DVT prophylaxis, PE prophylaxis in patients
who have undergone hip replacement surgery, treatment of DVT and PE in
patients who have been treated with a parenteral anticoagulant for 5-10 days,
and to reduce the risk of recurrent DVT and PE in patients who have been
previously treated. **Pradaxa** is contraindicated in patients with a mechanical
prosthetic heart valve.

▷ *desirudin (recombinant hirudin)* (C) 15 mg SC every 12 hours, preferably in the
abdomen <u>or</u> thigh, starting up to 5-15 minutes before surgery (after induction of
regional block anesthesia, if used); may continue for 9-12 days post-op; *CrCl <60
mL/min:* reduce dose (see mfr pkg insert)
Pediatric: not recommended
    Iprivask *Pwdr for SC inj after reconstitution:* 15mg/single-use vial (10/box)
(preservative-free, diluent contains mannitol)
    Comment: **Iprivask** is indicated for DVT prophylaxis in patients
undergoing hip replacement surgery. It is not interchangeable with other
hirudins.

(*continued*)

APPENDIX X: PLATELET AGGREGATION INHIBITOR THERAPY

▷ *cilostazol* (B) 100 mg bid
  Pediatric: not recommended
     Pletal *Tab:* 50, 100 mg
     Comment: **Pletal** is an (antiplatelet/vasodilator [PDE III inhibitor])

▷ *clopidogrel* (B) 75 mg once daily
  Pediatric: not recommended
     Plavix *Tab:* 75, 300 mg
     Comment: **Plavix** is indicated for the reduction of atherosclerotic events
     in recent MI or stroke, established PAD, non-ST-segment elevation acute
     coronary syndrome (unstable angina/non-STEMI), or STEMI.

▷ *dipyridamole* (B)(G) 75-100 mg qid
  Pediatric: not recommended
     Persantine *Tab:* 25, 50, 75 mg
  Comment: *dipyridamole* is indicated as an adjunct to oral anticoagulants after
  cardiac valve replacement surgery to prevent thromboembolism.

▷ *dipyridamole/aspirin* (B)(G) swallow whole; one cap bid
  Pediatric: not recommended
     Aggrenox *Cap: dipyr* 200 mg/*asa* 25 mg

▷ *pentoxifylline* (C) [hemorrheologic (xanthine)]
  Pediatric: not recommended
     Trental *Tab:* 400 mg sust-rel

▷ *prasugrel* (C)
  Pediatric: not recommended
     Effient *Tab:* 5, 10 mg
     Comment: **Effient** is indicated to reduce the risk of cardiovascular events in
     patients with acute coronary syndrome (ACS) who are to be managed with
     percutaneous coronary intervention (unstable angina or non-STEMI), and
     STEMI when managed with either primary or delayed PCI.

▷ *ticagrelor* (C) initiate 180 mg loading dose once in a single dose with aspirin 325
  mg loading dose in a single dose; maintenance 90 mg twice daily with aspirin
  75-100 mg once daily; ACS patients may start *ticagrelor* after a loading dose of
  clopidogrel
     Brilinta *Tab:* 90 mg
  Comment: **Effient** is indicated to reduce the risk of cardiovascular events
  in patients with acute coronary syndrome (ACS) (unstable angina, Non-ST
  elevation (NSTEMI), myocardial infarction, or STEMI).

▷ *ticlopidine* (B) 250 mg bid
  Pediatric: not recommended
     Ticlid *Tab:* 250 mg

(continued)

(*continued*)

> Comment: **Ticlid** is indicated to reduce the risk of thrombotic stroke in
> selected patients intolerant of aspirin.

APPENDIX Y: PROTEASE-ACTIVATED RECEPTOR-1 (PAR-1) INHIBITOR THERAPY

▷ *vorapaxar* (B) administer 2.08 mg once daily; use with *aspirin* or *clopidogrel*
  Pediatric: not established
  Zontivity *Tab:* 2.08 mg (equivalent to 2.5 mg vorapaxar sulfate)
  Comment: **Zontivity** is indicated to reduce thrombotic cardiovascular events
  in patients with a history of myocardial infarction or with peripheral arterial
  disease (PAD). Contraindicated with active pathological bleeding (e.g., peptic
  ulcer, intra-cranial hemorrhage), prior TIA or stroke. Not recommended
  with severe hepatic impairment.

APPENDIX Z: PRESCRIPTION PRENATAL VITAMINS

Comment: It is recommended that prenatal vitamins be started at least 3 months
prior to conception to improve preconception nutritional status, and continued
throughout pregnancy and the postnatal period, in lactating and nonlactating
women, and throughout the childbearing years.

▷ **CitraNatal 90 DHA** take 1 tab* and 1 DHA cap daily
  Tab: thiamine 3 mg, riboflavin 3.4 mg, niacinamide 20 mg, pyridoxine HCL 20
  mg, folic acid 1 mg, Vit C 120 mg, Vit D$_3$ 400 IU, Vit E 30 IU, calcium (as citrate)
  160 mg, copper (as oxide) 2 mg, iodine (as potassium iodide) 150 mcg, iron (as
  carbonyl) 90 mg, zinc (as oxide) 25 mg, docusate sodium 50 mg
  Cap: docosahexaenoic acid (DHA) 300 mg

▷ **CitraNatal Assure** take 1 tab and 1 DHA cap daily
  Tab: thiamine 3 mg, riboflavin 3.4 mg, niacinamide 20 mg, pyridoxine HCL 25 mg,
  folic acid 1 mg, Vit C 120 mg, Vit D$_3$ 400 IU, Vit E 30 IU, calcium (as citrate) 125
  mg, copper (as oxide) 2 mg, iodine (as potassium oxide) 150 mcg, iron (as carbonyl
  and ferrous gluconate) 35 mg, zinc (as oxide) 25 mg, docusate sodium 50 mg
  Cap: docosahexaenoic acid (DHA) 300 mg

▷ **CitraNatal B-Calm** take 1 tab every 8 hours; begin with tab #1.
  Tab: pyridoxine HCL 25 mg, folic acid 1 mg, Vit C 120 mg, Vit D$_3$ 400 IU, calci-
  um (as citrate) 120 mg, iron (as carbonyl) 20 mg
  Tab: pyridoxine 25 mg
  Comment: **Citranatal B-Calm** may be used as an adjunct treatment to help
  minimize pregnancy-related nausea and vomiting.

(*continued*)

(*continued*)

▷ **CitraNatal DHA** take 1 tab and 1 DHA cap daily
Tab: thiamine 3 mg, riboflavin 3.4 mg, niacinamide 20 mg, pyridoxine HCL 20 mg, folic acid 1 mg, Vit C 120 mg, Vit D₃ 400 IU, Vit E 30 IU, calcium (as citrate) 125 mg, copper (as oxide) 2 mg, iodine (as potassium oxide) 150 mcg, iron (as carbonyl and gluconate) 27 mg, zinc (as oxide) 25 mg, docusate sodium 50 mg
Cap: docosahexaenoic acid (DHA) 250 mg

▷ **CitraNatal Harmony** take 1 gelcap daily
Gelcap: pyridoxine HCL 25 mg, folic acid 1 mg, Vit D₃ 400 IU, Vit E 30 IU, calcium (as citrate) 104 mg, iron (as carbonyl and ferrous fumarate) 27 mg, docusate sodium 50 mg, docosahexaenoic acid (DHA) 260 mg

▷ **CitraNatal Rx** take 1 tab* and 1 DHA cap daily
Tab: thiamine 3 mg, riboflavin 3.4 mg, niacinamide 20 mg, pyridoxine HCL 20 mg, folic acid 1 mg, Vit C 120 mg, Vit D₃ 400 IU, Vit E 30 IU, calcium (as citrate) 125 mg, copper (as oxide) 2 mg, iodine (as potassium iodide) 150 mcg, iron (as carbonyl and gluconate) 27 mg, zinc (as oxide) 25 mg, docusate sodium 50 mg

▷ **Duet DHA Balanced** take 1 tab and 1 gelcap daily
Tab: Vit A (as beta carotene) 2800 IU, thiamine 1.5 mg, riboflavin 2 mg, niacinamide 20 mg, pyridoxine HCL 50 mg, Vit B₁₂ 12 mcg, folic acid 1 mg, Vit C 120 mg, Vit D₃ 640 IU, Vit E 15 IU, calcium (as carbonate) 215 mg, iron (as polysaccharide iron complex and sodium iron EDTA, Ferrazone) 25 mg, copper (as oxide) 1.8 mg, magnesium (as oxide) 25 mg, zinc (as oxide) 25 mg, iodine (as potassium iodide) 210 mcg, selenium 65 mcg, choline (as bartrate) 55 mg
Gelcap: omega 3 fatty acids 267 mg (includes docosahexaenoic acid [DHA], eicosapentaenoic acid [EPA], alpha-linolenic acid [ALA], docasapentaeoic acid [DPA]) (gelatin, gluten-free)

▷ **Duet DHA Complete** take 1 tab and 1 gelcap daily
Tab: Vit A (as beta carotene) 3000 IU, thiamine 1.8 mg, riboflavin 4 mg, niacinamide 20 mg, pyridoxine HCL 50 mg, Vit B₁₂ 12 mcg, folic acid 1 mg, Vit C 120 mg, Vit D₃ 800 IU, Vit E 3 mg, calcium (as carbonate) 230 mg, iron (as polysaccharide iron complex and sodium iron EDTA, ferrazone) 27 mg, copper (as oxide) 2 mg, magnesium (as oxide) 25 mg, zinc (as oxide) 25 mg, iodine 220 mcg
Gelcap: omega 3 fatty acids ≥430 mg (as docosahexaenoic acid (DHA) ≥295 mg, as other omega-3 fatty acids ≥135 mg (eicosapentaenoic acid (EPA), docasapentaenoic acid (DHA) (gluten-free)

▷ **Natachew** take 1 chew tab daily
Chew tab: Vit A 1000 IU (as beta carotene), thiamine 2 mg, riboflavin 3 mg, niacinamide 20 mg, pyridoxine HCL 10 mg, B₁₂ 12 mcg, folic acid 1 mg, Vit C 120 mg, Vit D₃ 400 IU, Vit E 11 IU, iron (as ferrous fumarate) 29 mg (wildberry)

▷ **Natafort** take 1 tab daily
Tab: Vit A 1000 IU (as acetate and beta carotene), thiamine 2 mg, riboflavin 3 mg, niacinamide 20 mg, pyridoxine HCL 10 mg, B₁₂ 12 mcg, folic acid 1 mg, Vit C 120 mg, Vit D₃ 400 IU, Vit E 11 IU, iron (as carbonyl and sulfate) 60 mg

(*continued*)

(*continued*)

▷ **Neevo DHA** take 1 cap daily
Cap: l-methylfolate (as Metafolin) 1.3 mg, thiamin1.4 mg, riboflavin 1.4 mg, niacinamide 18 mg, pyridoxine HCL 25 mg, B12 1 mg, Vit C 85 mg, Vit D3, 5 mcg, Vit E 15 IU, calcium (as carbonate) 110 mg, iron (ferrous fumarate) 27 mg, iodine (as potassium iodide) 220 mcg, magnesium (as oxide) 60 mg, docosahexaenoic acid (DHA, vegetarian source (algal oil) 581.92 mg (soy, gelatin, sorbitol, glycerin)
Comment: **Neevo DHA** is indicated as a nutritional supplement during pregnancy, and the prenatal and postnatal periods, in women with dietary needs for the biologically active form of folate, who are at risk for hyperhomocys-teinemia, impaired folic acid absorption, <u>and/or</u> impaired folic acid metabolism due to 667C >T mutations in the MTHFR gene.

▷ **Nexa Plus** take 1 cap daily
Cap: pyridoxine HCL 25 mg, folic acid 1.25 mg, Vit C 28 mg, Vit D3 800 IU, Vit E 30 IU, biotin 250 mcg, calcium (as carbonate [158 mg] + docusate calcium [2 mg] 160 mg, iron (as ferrous fumarate) 29 mg, docosahexaenoic acid (DHA, plant-based source [algal oil]) 350 mg (soy)

▷ **Nexa Select** take 1 softgel cap daily
Softgel cap: pyridoxine HCL 25 mg, folic acid 1.25 mg, Vit C 28 mg, Vit D3 800 IU, Vit E 30 IU, calcium (as phosphate) 160 mg, iron (as ferrous fumarate) 29 mg, docosahexaenoic acid (DHA) plant-based source (algal oil) 325 mg, docusate sodium 55 mg (soy)

▷ **Prenate AM** take 1 tab daily
Tab: pyridoxine HCL 75 mg, folate (as folic acid 400 mcg + Quatrefolic 1.1 mg [equivalent to 600 mcg folic acid]) 1 mg, Vit B12 12 mcg, calcium (as carbonate) 200 mg, ginger extract 500 mg, lingon-berry 25 mg

▷ **Prenate Chewable** take 1 chew tab daily
Chew tab: pyridoxine HCL 10 mg, Vit B12 125 mcg, calcium (as carbonate) 500 mg, Vit D3 300 IU, biotin 280 mcg, boron amino acid chelate 250 mcg, folate (as Quatrefolic) 1 mg, magnesium (as oxide) 50 mg, blueberry extract 25 mg (Dutch chocolate)

▷ **Prenate DHA** take 1 gel cap daily
Gelcap: pyridoxine HCL 26 mg, folate (as folic acid) 400 mcg + Quatrafolic 1.1 mg [equivalent to 600 mcg folic acid]) 1 mg, Vit B12 13 mcg, Vit C 90 mg, Vit D3 220 IU, Vit E 10 IU, calcium (as carbonate) 145 mg, iron (as ferrous fumarate) 28 mg, magnesium (as oxide) 50 mg, docosahexaenoic acid (DHA) 300 mg (fish oil, soy, gelatin)

▷ **Prenate Elite** take 1 gel cap daily
Gelcap: Vit A (as beta-carotene) 2600 IU, thiamine 3 mg, riboflavin 3.5 mg, pyridoxine HCl 21 mg, niacinamide 21 mg, pantothenic acid 6 mg, folate (as folic acid 400 mcg + Quatrefolic 1.1 mg [equivalent to 600 mcg folic acid]) 1 mg, Vit B12 13 mcg, Vit C 75 mg, Vit D3 450 IU, Vit E 10 IU, calcium (as carbonate) 100 mg, iron (as ferrous fumarate) 27 mg, magnesium (as oxide) 25 mg, copper (as oxide) 1.5 mg, iodine 150 mcg, iron (as ferrous fumarate) 26 mg, zinc (as oxide) 15 mg

(*continued*)

(continued)

▷ **Prenate Enhance** take 1 gel cap daily
Gelcap: pyridoxine HCL 25 mg, folate (as folic acid 400 mcg + Quatrefolic 1.1 mg [equivalent to 600 mcg folic acid]) 1 mg, Vit B12 12 mcg, Vit C 85 mg, Vit D3 1000 IU, Vit E 10 IU, biotin 500 mcg, calcium (as carbonate + Formical) 155 mg, iodine (as potassium) 150 mcg, iron (as ferrous fumarate) 28 mg, magnesium (as oxide) 50 mg, docosahexaenoicacid (DHA) 400 mg (soy, gelatin)

▷ **Prenate Essential** take 1 gel cap daily
Gelcap: pyridoxine HCL 26 mg, folate (as folic acid 400 mcg + Quatrefolic 1.1 mg [equivalent to 600 mcg folic acid]) 1 mg, Vit B12 13 mcg, Vit C 90 mg, Vit D3 220 IU, Vit E 10 IU, biotin 280 mcg, calcium (as carbonate) 145 mg, iodine (as potassium iodide) 150 mcg, iron (as ferrous fumarate) 29 mg, magnesium (as oxide) 50 mg, docosahexaenoic acid (DHA) 300 mg, eicosapentaenoic acid (EPA) 40 mg (fish oil, soy, gelatin)

▷ **Prenate Mini** take 1 gel cap daily
Gelcap: pyridoxine HCL 26 mg, folate (as folic acid) 400 mcg + Quatrefolic 1.1 mg [equivalent to 600 mcg folic acid]) 1 mg, Vit B12 13 mcg, Vit C 60 mg, Vit D3 220 IU, Vit E 10 IU, calcium (as carbonate) 100 mg, iron (as carbonyl iron) 29 mg, iodine (as potassium iodide) 150 mcg, biotin 280 mcg, magnesium (as oxide) 25 mg, docosahexaenoic acid (DHA) 300 mg, blueberry extract 25 mg (fish oil, soy, gelatin)

▷ **Prenate Restore** take 1 gel cap daily
Gelcap: pyridoxine HCL 25 mg, folate (as folic acid 400 mcg + Quatrefolic 1.1 mg [equivalent to 600 mcg folic acid]) 1 mg, Vit B12 12 mcg, Vit C 85 mg, Vit D3 1000 IU, Vit E 10 IU, biotin 500 mcg, calcium (as carbonate + Formical) 155 mg, iron (as ferrous fumarate) 27 mg, magnesium (as oxide) 45 mg, docosahexaenoic acid (DHA) 400 mg, *Bacillus coagulans* 150 million CFU (as lactospore) 10 mg (soy, gelatin)

▷ **Prenexa** take 1 gel cap daily
Gelcap: pyridoxine HCL 25 mg, folic acid 1.25 mg, Vit C 28 mg, Vit D3 400 IU, Vit E 30 IU, calcium (as phosphate) 160 mg, iron (as ferrous fumarate) 27 mg, docosahexaenoic acid (DHA) plant-based source (algal oil) 300 mg, docusate sodium 55 mg (soy)

APPENDIX AA: ORAL PRESCRIPTION DRUGS FOR THE MANAGEMENT OF ALLERGY, COUGH, AND COLD SYMPTOMS

Oral prescription drugs for the management of allergy symptoms, cough, and symptoms of the common cold are listed in alphabetical order by brand name.

Legend:	*acriv*	*acrivastine*
	benzo	*benzonatate*

(continued)

(*continued*)

	brom	*brompheniramine*
	carb	*carbinoxamine*
	carbeta	*carbetapentane*
	chlor	*chlorpheniramine*
	cod	*codeine*
	cypro	*cyproheptadine*
	deslorat	*desloratadine*
	dexchlo	*dexchlorphenirimine*
	dextro	*dextromethorphan*
	diphen	*diphenhydramine*
	hydrox	*hydroxyzine*
	guaiac	*potassium guaiacosulfonate*
	guaif	*guaifenesin*
	homat	*homatropine*
	hydro	*hydrocodone*
	hydrox	*hydroxyzine*
	levocetir	*levocetirizine*
	meth	*methscopolamine*
	phenyle	*phenylephrine*
	prometh	*promethazine*
	pseud	*pseudoephedrine*
	pyril	*pyrilamine tannate*

▷ **Allerex (C)** 1 AM tab in the morning and 1 PM tab in the evening prn
Pediatric: not recommended
AM tab: meth 2.5 mg/*pseud* 120 mg ext-rel; *PM tab: meth* 2.5 mg/*chlor* 8 mg/
phenyle 10 mg* ext-rel (*Dose Pack 20:* 10 AM tabs+10 PM tabs; *Dose Pack 60:*
30 AM tabs+30 PM tabs)

(*continued*)

(*continued*)

▷ **Allures-D (C)** 1 tab q 12 hours prn
Pediatric: not recommended
Tab: meth 2.5 mg/*pseud* 120 mg ext-rel

▷ **Allerex DF (C)** 1 AM tab in the morning and 1 PM tab in the evening prn
Pediatric: not recommended
AM tab: meth 2.5 mg/*chlor* 4 mg/*PM tab: meth* 2.5 mg/*chlor* 8 mg* (*Dose Pack 20:*
10 AM tabs+10 PM tabs; *Dose Pack 60:* 30 AM tabs+30 PM tabs)

▷ **Allerex PE (C)** 1 AM tab in the morning and 1 PM tab in the evening prn
Pediatric: not recommended
AM tab: meth 2.5 mg/*phenyle* 40 mg/*PM tab: meth* 8 mg/*phenyle* 10 mg* (*Dose Pack
20:* 10 AM tabs+10 PM tabs; *Dose Pack 60:* 30 AM tabs+30 PM tabs)

▷ **Allerex Suspension (C)** 15 ml q 12 hours prn
Pediatric: <6 years: not recommended; 6-12 years: 2.5-5 ml q 12 hours prn;
>12 years: same as adult
Susp: chlor 3 mg/*phenyle* 7.5 mg ext-rel (raspberry)

▷ **Atarax (B)(G)** 25 mg tid <u>or</u> qid prn
Pediatric: <2 years: not recommended; 2-6 years: 6.25 mg q 4-6 hours prn;
6-12 years: 12.5-25 mg q 4-6 hours prn; >12 years: same as adult
Tab: hydrox 10, 25, 50, 100 mg; *Syr:* 10 mg/5 ml (alcohol 0.5%)

▷ **Bromfed DM (C)(G)** 2 tsp q 4 hours prn: max 6 doses/day
Pediatric: <2 years: not recommended; 2-6 years: 1/2 tsp q 4 hours prn;
>6-12 years: 1
tsp q 4 hours prn; max 6 doses/day; >12 years: same as adult
Susp: brom 2 mg/*pseudo* 30 mg/*dextro* 10 mg per 5 ml (butterscotch; alcohol
0.95%)

▷ **Bromfed DM Sugar-Free (C)(G)** 2 tsp q 4 hours prn: max 6 doses/day
Pediatric: <2 years: not recommended; 2-6 years: 1/2 tsp q 4 hours prn; 6-12 years: 1
tsp q 4 hours prn; >12 years: same as adult
Max 6 doses/day
Susp: brom 2 mg/*pseudo* 30 mg/*dextro* 10 mg per 5 ml (butterscotch; alcohol
0.95%)

▷ **Clarinex (C)** 1 tab daily prn
Pediatric: <6 years: not recommended; ≥6 years: ½-1 tab once daily
Tab: deslorat 5 mg

▷ **Clarinex RediTabs (C)** 5 mg daily prn
Pediatric: <6 years: not recommended; 6-12 years: 2.5 mg once daily; >12 years:
same as adult
ODT: deslorat 2.5, 5 mg (tutti-frutti; phenylalanine)

▷ **Clarinex Syrup (C)** 1 tab daily prn
Pediatric: <6 months: not recommended; 6-11 months: 1 mg (2 ml) daily prn;
1-5 years: 1.25 mg (2.5 ml) daily prn; 6-11 years: 2.5 mg (5 ml) daily prn; ≥12 years:
5 mg (10 ml) daily prn
Tab: deslorat 0.5 mg per ml (4 oz)(tutti-frutti; phenylalanine)

▷ **Duratuss AC 12 (C)** 1-2 tsp q 12 hours prn
Pediatric: <2 years: not recommended; 2-6 years: 1/2 tsp q 12 hrs prn; >6 years: 1
tsp q 12 hours prn; >6 years: same as adult
Susp:diphen 12.5 mg/*dextro* 15 mg/*phenyle* 15 mg per 5 ml (strawberry banana;
sugar-free, alcohol-free, phenylalanine)

(*continued*)

(*continued*)

▷ **Duratuss DM (C)** 1 tsp q 4 hours prn
Pediatric: <2 years: not recommended; 2-6 years: 1/4 tsp q 4 hrs prn; >6 years: ½ tsp q 4 hours prn
Susp: dextro 25 mg/*guaif* 225 mg per 5 ml (grape) (sugar-free, alcohol-free)

▷ **Duratuss DM 12 (C)** 1-2 tsp q 12 hours prn; max 6 tabs/day
Pediatric: <2 years: not recommended; 2-6 years: 1/2 tsp q 12 hrs prn; >6 years: ½-1 tsp q 12 hours prn; >6 years: same as adult
Susp: dextro 15 mg/*guaif* 225 mg per 5 ml (grape; sugar-free, alcohol-free)

▷ **Flowtuss Oral Solution (C)(II)(G)** 1-2 tsp q 4-6 hours prn; max 6 tsp/24 hours
Pediatric: <6 years: not recommended; 6-12 years: 1/2 tsp q 4-6 hours prn; max 15 ml/day; >12 years: same as adult
Oral soln: hydro 2.5 mg/guaif 200 mg per 5 ml (black raspberry)
Comment: *hydrocodone* is known to be excreted in human milk.

▷ **Hycodan (C)(III)** 1 tab q 4-6 hours prn; max 6 tabs/day
Pediatric: <6 years: not recommended; 6-12 years: 1/2 tab q 4-6 hours prn; max 3 tabs/day; >12 years: same as adult
Tab: hydro 5 mg/*homat* 1.5 mg
Comment: *hydrocodone* is known to be excreted in human milk.

▷ **Hycodan Syrup (C)(II)(G)** 1 tsp q 4-6 hours prn
Pediatric: <6 years: not recommended; 6-12 years: 1/2 tsp q 4-6 hours prn; max 15 ml/day; >12 years: same as adult
Syr: hydro 5 mg/*homat* 1.5 mg per 5 ml
Comment: *hydrocodone* is known to be excreted in human milk.

▷ **Hycofenix Oral Solution (C)(II)** 1 tsp q 4-6 hours prn
Pediatric: <6 years: not recommended; 6-12 years: 1/2 tsp q 4-6 hours prn; max 15 ml/day; >12 years: same as adult
Oral soln: hydro 2.5 mg/pseudo 30 mg/quaf 200 mg per 5 ml (black raspberry)
Comment: *hydrocodone* is known to be excreted in human milk.

▷ **Obredon Oral Solution (C)(II)** 10 ml q 4-6 hours prn cough; max 60 ml/day
Pediatric: <18 years: not recommended
Oral soln: hydro 2.5 mg/*guaif* 200 mg per 5 ml
Comment: **Obredon** is indicated only for short term treatment of cough due to the common cold. **Obredon** is not indicated for persistent or chronic cough such as occurs with smoking, asthma, chronic bronchitis, or emphysema, or where cough is accompanied by excessive phlegm. Use with caution in patients with diabetes, thyroid disease, Addison's disease, BPH or urethral stricture, and asthma. **Obredon** is contraindicated with paralytic ileus, anticholinergics, TCAs, and within 14 days of an MAOI. *hydrocodone* is known to be excreted in human milk. There is no FDA-approved generic form of *hydrocodone/guaifenesin.*

▷ **Palgic (C)** 4 mg daily prn; max 24 mg/day in divided doses 6-8 hours apart
Pediatric: <2 year: not recommended; 2-3 years: 2 mg tid or qid prn or 0.2-0.4 mg/kg/day divided tid or qid; 3-6 years: 2-4 mg daily prn or 0.2-0.4 mg/kg/day divided tid or qid; >6 years: same as adult
Tab: carb 4*mg; *Syr: carb* 4 mg per 5 ml (bubble gum)

▷ **Periactin (B)(G)** initially 4 mg tid prn, then adjust as needed; usual range 12-16 mg/day; max 32 mg/day

(*continued*)

(*continued*)

Pediatric: <2 years: not recommended; 2-6 years: 2 mg 2-3 times/day: max 12 mg daily; 7-14 years: 4 mg 2-3 times/day: max 16 mg daily; >14 years: same as adult
Tab: cypro 4*mg; *Syr:* cypro 2 mg per 5 ml

➤ **Prolex-DH (C)(III)** 1-1½ tsp qid prn
Pediatric: <3 years: not recommended; 3-6 years: 1/4-1/2 tsp qid prn; ≥6-12 years: 1/2-1 tsp qid prn; >12 years: same as adult
Liq: hydro 4.5 mg/pot guaiac 300 mg per 5 ml (tropical fruit punch; alcohol-free, sugar-free)

➤ **Phenergan (C)(G)** 25 mg po or rectally tid ac and HS prn
Pediatric: <2 years: not recommended; >2 years: 0.5 mg/lb or 6.25-25 mg po or rectally tid; ≥12 years: same as adult
Tab: 12.5*, 25*, 50 mg; *Syr:* prom 6.25 mg per 5 ml; *Syr fortis:* prom 25 mg per 5 ml; *Rectal supp:* prom 12.5, 25, 50 mg

➤ **Promethazine DM (C)(V)(G)** 1 tsp q 4-6 hours prn
Pediatric: <6 years: not recommended; 6-12 years: ½-1 tsp q 4-6 hours prn; >12 years: same as adult
Syr: prometh 6.25 mg/dex 15 mg per 5 ml (alcohol 7%)
Comment: Contraindicated with asthma.

➤ **Promethazine VC (C)(V)(G)** 1 tsp q 4-6 hours prn; max 30 ml/day
Pediatric: 2-6 years: 1.25 ml q 4-6 hours prn; max 7.5 ml/day; 6-12 years: 2.5 ml q 4-6 hours prn; max 15 ml/day; >12 years: same as adult
Syr: prometh 6.25 mg/phenyle 5 mg per 5 ml (alcohol 7%)
Comment: Contraindicated with asthma.

➤ **Promethazine VC w. Codeine (C)(V)(G)** 1 tsp q 4-6 hours prn; max 30 ml/day
Pediatric: <6 years: not recommended; 6-12 years: ½-1 tsp q 4-6 hours prn; max 30 ml/day; >12 years: same as adult
Syr: prometh 6.25 mg/phenyle 5 mg/cod 10 mg per 5 ml (alcohol 7%)
Comment: Contraindicated with asthma.

➤ **Promethazine w. Codeine (C)(V)(G)** 1 tsp q 4-6 hours prn
Pediatric: <6 years: not recommended; 6-12 years: ½-1 tsp q 4-6 hours prn; >12 years: same as adult
Liq: prometh 6.25 mg/cod 10 mg per 5 ml (alcohol 7%)
Comment: Contraindicated with asthma.

➤ **Rynatan (C)** 1-2 tabs q 12 hours prn
Pediatric: not recommended
Tab: chlor 9 mg/phenyle 25 mg

➤ **Rynatan Pediatric Suspension (C)**
Pediatric: <2 years: not recommended; 2-6 years: ½-1 tsp q 12 hours prn; >6-12 years: 1-2 tsp q 12 hours prn; >12 years: same as adult
Susp: chlor 4.5 mg/phenyle 5 mg

➤ **Ryneze (C)** 1 tab q 12 hours prn
Pediatric: <6 years: not recommended; 6-12 years: 1/2 tab q 12 hours prn; >12 years: same as adult
Tab: chlor 8 mg/meth 2.5 mg

(*continued*)

(*continued*)

▷ **Robitussin AC (C)(III)(G)** 2 tsp q 4 hours prn; max 60 ml/day
  Pediatric: <2 years: not recommended; 2-6 years: 1/4-1/2 tsp q 4 hours prn;
  6-12 years: 1 tsp q 4 hours prn; >12 years: same as adult
  Liq: cod 10 mg/*guaif* 100 mg per 5 ml

▷ **Rondec Syrup (C)(G)** 1 tsp qid prn; max 30 ml/day
  Pediatric: <2 years: not recommended; 2-5 years: 1/4 tsp q 4-6 hours prn; max
  7.5 ml/day; 6-11 years: 1/2 tsp q 4-6 hours prn; max 15 ml/day; >11 years: same
  as adult
  Syr: phenyle 12.5 mg/*chlor* 4 mg per 5 ml (bubblegum; sugar-free, alcohol-free)

▷ **Semprex-D (B)** 1 cap q 4-6 hours prn; max 4 doses/day
  Pediatric: not recommended
  Cap: acriv 8 mg/*pseud* 60 mg

▷ **Tanafed DMX (C)(G)** 2-4 tsp q 12 hours prn
  Pediatric: <2 years: not recommended; 2-6 years: ½-1 tsp q 12 hours prn;
  6-12 years: 1-2 tsp q 12 hours prn
  Susp: dexchlor 2.5 mg/*pseud* 75 mg/*dextro* 25 mg per 5 ml (cotton candy,
  alcohol-free)

▷ **Tessalon Caps (C)** 100-200 mg tid prn; max 600 mg/day
  Pediatric: <10 years: not recommended; ≥10 years: same as adult
  Cap: benzo 200 mg
  Comment: Swallow whole. Do not suck or chew.

▷ **Tessalon Perles (C)** 100-200 mg tid prn; max 600 mg/day
  Pediatric: <10 years: not recommended; ≥10 years: same as adult
  Perles: benzo 100 mg
  Comment: Swallow whole. Do not suck or chew.

▷ **Tussi-12 D Tablets (C)** 1-2 tabs q 12 hours prn
  Pediatric: <6 years: use susp; 6-11 years: ½-1 tab q 12 hours prn; >11 years: same
  as adult
  Tab: carbeta 60 mg/*pyril* 40 mg/*phenyle* 10*mg

▷ **Tussi-12 D S (C)** 1-2 tsp q 12 hours prn
  Pediatric: <2 years: individualize; 2-6 years: ½-1 tsp q 12 hours prn; 6-12 years:
  1-2 tsp q 12 hours prn; >12 years: same as adult
  Liq: carbeta 30 mg/*pyril* 30 mg/*phenyle* 5 mg per 5 ml (strawberry-currant;
  tartrazine)

▷ **TussiCaps 5 mg/4 mg (C)(III)** 2 caps q 12 hours prn; max 4 caps/day
  Pediatric: <6 years: not recommended; 6-11 years: 1 cap q 12 hours prn; max 2 caps/
  day; >11 years: same as adult
  Cap: hydro 5 mg/*chlor* 4 mg ext-rel (alcohol)

▷ **TussiCaps 10 mg/8 mg (C)(III)** 1 cap q 12 hours prn; max 2 caps/day
  Pediatric: not recommended
  Cap: hydro 10 mg/*chlor* 8 mg ext-rel (alcohol)

▷ **Tussionex (C)(III)** 1 tsp q 12 hours prn
  Pediatric: <6 years: not recommended; >6 years: same as adult; 6-12 years: ½ tsp
  q 12 hours prn; >12 years: same as adult
  Susp: hydro 10 mg/*chlor* 8 mg per 5 ml ext-rel

(*continued*)

(*continued*)

▷ **Tussi-Organidin DM NR Liquid (C)(III)** 5 ml q 4 hours prn; max 40 ml/day
Pediatric: <6 months: not recommended; 6-23 months: 0.6 ml q 4 hours prn; max
3.7 ml/day; 2-5 years: 1.25 ml q 4 hours prn; max 7.5 ml/day; 6-11 years: 2.5 ml
q 4 hours prn; max 15 ml/day; ≥12 years: same as adult
Liq: dextro 10 mg/*guaif* 300 mg per 5 ml (grape; sugar-free, alcohol-free)
▷ **Tussi-Organidin NR (C)(V)** 1 tsp q 4 hours prn; max 40 ml/day
Pediatric: <2 years: not recommended; 2 years: 1.5 ml q 4-6 hours prn; max 6 ml/
day; 3 years: 1.75 ml q 4-6 hours prn; max 7 ml/day; 4 years: 2 ml q 4-6 hours prn;
max 8 ml/day; 5 years: 2.25 ml q 4-6 hours prn; max 9 ml/day; 6-11 years: 2.5 ml
q 4 hours prn; max 20 ml/day; ≥12 years: same as adult
Liq: cod 10 mg/*guaif* 300 mg per 5 ml (grape; sugar-free, alcohol-free)
▷ **Tuzistra XR (C)(III)** 1-2 tsp q 12 hours prn; max 20 ml/day
Pediatric: <18 years: not recommended
Liq: cod 14.7 mg/*chlor* 2.8 mg per 5 ml (cherry)
▷ **Vistaril (C)(G)** 25 mg tid or qid prn
Pediatric: <6 years: 50 mg/day prn; 6-12 years: 50-100 mg daily prn; >12 years: same
as adult
Cap: hydrox 25, 50, 100 mg; *Susp: hydrox* 25 mg/5 ml (lemon)
▷ **Xyzal, Xyzal Oral Solution (B)** 2.5-5 mg in the evening prn
CrCl 30-50 mL/min: 2.5 mg every other day
CrCl 10-30 mL/min: 2.5 mg twice weekly
CrCl <10 mL/min or hemodialysis: contraindicated
Pediatric: <6 months: not recommended; 6 months to 5 years: max 1.25 mg once
daily in the PM prn; 6-11 years: max 2.5 mg once daily in the PM prn; ≥12 years:
same as adult
Tab: levocetir 5*mg film-coat; *Oral soln: levocetir* 0.5 mg/ml (150 ml)

APPENDIX BB: SYSTEMIC ANTI-INFECTIVE DRUGS

Comment:
- Adverse effects of aminoglycosides include nephrotoxicity and ototoxicity.
- Use cephalosporins with caution in persons with penicillin allergy due to potential cross allergy.
- Sulfonamides are contraindicated with sulfa allergy and G6PD deficiency. A high fluid intake is indicated during sulfonamide therapy.
- Tetracyclines should be taken on an empty stomach to facilitate absorption. Tetracyclines should not be taken with milk.
- Tetracyclines are contraindicated during pregnancy and breastfeeding, and in children <8 years of age, due to the risk of developing tooth enamel discoloration.
- Systemic quinolones and fluoroquinolones are contraindicated in pregnancy and children <18 years of age due to the risk of joint dysplasia.

(*continued*)

(continued)

Anti-infectives by Class With Dose Forms		
Generic Name	Brand Name	Dose Form/Volume
Amebicide		
chloroquine phosphate (C)	**Aralen**	*Tab:* 500 mg; *Inj:* 50 mg/ml (5 ml)
iodoquinol (C)	**Yodoxin**	*Tab:* 210, 650 mg
metronidazole (**not for use in 1st; B in 2nd, 3rd**)(G)	**Flagyl**	*Tab:* 250*, 500* mg
	Flagyl 375	*Cap:* 375 mg
	Flagyl ER	*Tab:* 750 mg ext-rel
tinidazole (C)	**Tindamax**	*Tab:* 250*, 500* mg
Antihelmintic		
albendazole (C)(G)	**Albenza**	*Tab:* 200 mg
mebendazole (C)(G)	**Emverm, Vermox**	*Chew tab:* 100 mg
	Pin-X	*Cap:* 180 mg; *Liq:* 50 mg/ml (30 ml); 144 mg/ml (30 ml); *Oral susp:* 50 mg/ml (30 ml)
Antifungal		
atovaquone (C)	**Mepron**	*Susp:* 750 mg/5ml (210 ml)
clotrimazole (B)(G)	**Mycelex Troche**	10 mg (70, 40/bottle)
fluconazole (C)(G)	**Diflucan**	*Tab:* 50, 100, 150, 200 mg; *Oral susp:* 10, 40 mg/ml (35 ml) (orange)
griseofulvin, microsize (C)	**Grifulvin V**	*Tab:* 250, 500 mg; *Oral susp:* 125 mg/5 ml (120 ml) (alcohol 0.02%)
	Gris-PEG	*Tab:* 125, 250 mg
itraconazole (C)	**Sporanox**	*Cap:* 100 mg; *Soln:* 10 mg/ml (150 ml); *Pulse Pack:* 100 mg caps (7/pck)
ketoconazole (C)(G)	**Nizoral**	*Tab:* 200 mg
nystatin (C)(G)	**Mycostatin**	*Pastille:* 200,000 units/pastille (30 pastilles/pck); *Oral susp:* 100,000 units/ml (60 ml w. dropper)
terbinafine (B)(G)	**Lamisil**	*Tab:* 250 mg
vorconazole (D)(G)	**Vfend**	*Tab:* 50, 200 mg
Antimalarial		
atovaquone/ proguanil (C)	**Malarone**	*Tab: atov* 250 mg/*proq* 100 mg
	Malarone Pediatric	*Tab: atov* 62.5 mg/*proq* 25 mg

(continued)

(*continued*)

Anti-infectives by Class With Dose Forms		
Generic Name	Brand Name	Dose Form/Volume
chloroquine (C)(G)	Aralen	*Tab:* 500 mg; *Amp:* 50 mg/ml (5 ml)
doxycycline (D)(G)	Actilate	*Tab:* 75, 150**mg
	Adoxa	*Tab:* 50, 75, 100, 150 mg ent-coat
	Doryx	*Cap:* 100 mg; *Tab:* 50, 75, 100, 150, 200 mg
	Monodox	*Cap:* 50, 75, 100 mg
	Oracea	*Cap:* 40 mg del-rel
	Vibramycin	*Cap:* 50, 100 mg; *Syr:* 50 mg/5 ml (raspberry-apple) (sulfites); *Oral susp:* 25 mg/5 ml (raspberry)
	Vibra-Tab	*Tab:* 100 mg film-coat
hydroxychloroquine (C)(G)	Plaquenil	*Tab:* 200 mg
mefloquine (C)	Lariam	*Tab:* 250 mg
Antiprotozoal/Antibacterial		
metronidazole (**not for use in 1st; B in 2nd, 3rd**)(G)	Flagyl, Protostat	*Tab:* 250*, 500* mg
	Flagyl 375	*Cap:* 375 mg
	Flagyl ER	*Tab:* 750 mg ext-rel
tinidazole (C)	Tindamax	*Tab:* 250*, 500*mg
Antiviral (for HIV-specific antiviral drugs see page 523)		
acyclovir (C)(G)	Zovirax	*Cap:* 200 mg; *Tab:* 400, 800 mg; *Oral susp:* 200 mg/5 ml (banana)
amantadine (C)(G)	Symmetrel	*Tab:* 100 mg; *Syr:* 50 mg/5ml (16 oz) (raspberry)
famciclovir (B)	Famvir	*Tab:* 125, 250, 500 mg
lamivudine (C)	Epivir-HBV	*Tab:* 100 mg; *Oral soln:* 5 mg/ml (240 ml) (strawberry-banana)
oseltamivir (C)	Tamiflu	*Cap:* 75 mg

(*continued*)

(*continued*)

Anti-infectives by Class With Dose Forms		
Generic Name	Brand Name	Dose Form/Volume
rimantadine (C)	**Flumadine**	*Tab:* 100 mg
valacyclovir (B)	**Valtrex**	*Tab:* 500 mg; 1 g
zanamivir	**Relenza**	*Tab: lami* 150/*zido* 300 mg
Antitubercular		
ethambutol (EMB) (B)(G)	**Myambutol**	*Tab:* 100, 400*mg
isoniazid (INH) (C)(G)	*generic only*	*Tab:* 100, 300*mg; *Syr:* 50 mg/5 ml; *Inj:* 100 mg/ml
pyrazinamide (PZA) (C)	*generic only*	*Tab:* 500*mg
rifampin (C)(G)	**Priftin**	*Tab:* 150 mg
	Rifadin	*Cap:* 150, 300 mg
rifampin/isoniazid (C)	**Rifamate**	*Cap: rif* 300 mg/*iso* 150 mg
rifampin/isoniazid/ pyrazinamide (C)	**Rifater**	*Tab: rif* 120 mg/*iso* 50 mg/*pyr* 300 mg
Aminoglycoside		
amikacin (C)	**Amikin**	*Vial:* 500 mg, 1 g (2 ml)
gentamicin (C)(G)	**Garamycin**	*Vial:* 20, 80 mg/2 ml
streptomycin (D)(G)	**Streptomycin**	*Amp:* 1 g/2.5 ml or 400 mg/ml (2.5 ml)
Cephalosporin		
First Generation Cephalosporin		
cefadroxil (B)	**Duricef**	*Cap:* 500 mg; *Tab:* 1 g; *Oral susp:*250 mg/5 ml (100 ml); 500 mg/5 ml (75, 100 ml) (orange-pineapple)
cefazolin (B)	**Ancef, Zolicef**	*Vial:* 500 mg; 1, 10 g
cephalexin (B)	**Keflex**	*Cap:* 250, 333, 500, 750 mg; *Oral susp:*125, 250 mg/5 ml (100, 200 ml)

(*continued*)

(*continued*)

Anti-infectives by Class With Dose Forms		
Generic Name	Brand Name	Dose Form/Volume
Second Generation Cephalosporin		
cefaclor (B)(G)	generic only	*Tab:* 500 mg; *Cap:* 250, 500 mg; *Susp:* 125 mg/5 ml (75, 150 ml) (strawberry); 187 mg/5 ml (50, 100 ml) (strawberry); 250 mg/5 ml (75, 150 ml) (strawberry); 375 mg/5 ml (50, 100 ml) (strawberry)
	Cefaclor Extended Release	*Tab:* 375, 500 mg ext-rel
cefamandole (B)	Mandol	*Vial:* 1, 2 g
cefotetan (B)	Cefotan	*Vial:* 1, 2 g
cefoxitin (B)	Mefoxin	*Vial:* 1, 2 g
cefprozil (B)	Cefzil	*Tab:* 250, 500 mg; *Oral susp:* 125, 250 mg/5 ml (50, 75, 100 ml) (bubble gum) (phenylalanine)
ceftaroline (B)	Teflaro	*Vial:* 400, 600 mg
cefuroxime axetil (B)	Ceftin	*Tab:* 250, 500 mg; *Oral susp:* 125, 250 mg/5 ml (50, 100 ml) (tutti-frutti)
cefuroxime sodium (B)(G)	Zinacef	*Vial:* 750 mg; 1.5 g
loracarbef (B)	Lorabid	*Pulvule:* 200, 400 mg; *Oral susp:* 100 mg/5 ml (50, 100 ml); 200 mg/5 ml (50, 75, 100 ml) (strawberry bubble gum)
Third Generation Cephalosporin		
cefoperazone (B)	Cefobid	*Vial:* 1, 2 g pwdr for reconstitution
cefotaxime (B)	Claforan	*Vial:* 500 mg; 1, 2 g pwdr for reconstitution
cefpodoxime (B)	Vantin	*Tab:* 100, 200 mg; *Oral susp:* 50, 100 mg/5 ml (50, 75, 100 ml) (lemon creme)
ceftazidime (B)	Ceptaz	*Vial:* 1, 2 g pwdr for reconstitution
	Fortaz	*Vial:* 500 mg; 1, 2 g pwdr for reconstitution
	Tazicef	*Vial:* 1, 2 g pwdr for reconstitution
	Tazidime	*Vial:* 1, 2 g pwdr for reconstitution

(*continued*)

(*continued*)

Anti-infectives by Class With Dose Forms		
Generic Name	Brand Name	Dose Form/Volume
ceftazidime/ avibactam (B)	Avycaz	*Vial:* 2.5 g pwdr for reconstitution
ceftibuten (B)	Cedax	*Cap:* 400 mg; *Oral susp:* 90 mg/5 ml (30, 60, 90, 120 ml); 180 mg/5 ml (30, 60, 120 ml) (cherry)
Third/Fourth Generation Cephalosporin		
cefdinir (B)	Omnicef	*Cap:* 300 mg; *Oral susp:* 125 mg/5 ml (60, 100 ml) (strawberry)
cefditoren pivoxil (C)	Spectracef	*Tab:* 200 mg
cefepime (B)	Maxipime	*Vial:* 1 g pwdr for reconstitution
cefixime (B)	Suprax	*Tab/Cap:* 400 mg; *Oral Susp:* 100 mg/ 5 ml (50, 75, 100 ml)(strawberry)
ceftaroline (B)	Teflaro	*Vial:* 400, 600 mg
ceftriaxone (B)(G)	Rocephin	*Vial:* 250, 500 mg; 1, 2 g
cytolozane/ tazobactam (B)	Zerbaxa	*Vial:* 1.5 g pwdr for reconstitution
Fluoroquinolone and Quinolone		
First-Generation Quinolone		
enoxacin (C)	Penetrex	*Tab:* 200, 400 mg
Second-Generation Fluoroquinolone		
ciprofloxacin (C) (G)	Cipro	*Tab:* 250, 500, 750 mg; *Oral susp:* 250, 500 mg/5 ml (100 ml) (strawberry) *IV conc:* 10 mg/ml after dilution (20, 40 ml); *IV premix:* 2 mg/ml (100, 200 ml)
	Cipro XR	*Tab:* 500, 1000 mg ext-rel
	ProQuin XR	*Tab:* 500 mg ext-rel
lomefloxacin (C)	Maxaquin	*Tab:* 400 mg
norfloxacin (C)(G)	Noroxin	*Tab:* 400 mg
ofloxacin (C)(G)	Floxin	*Tab:* 200, 300, 400 mg

(*continued*)

(*continued*)

Anti-infectives by Class With Dose Forms		
Generic Name	Brand Name	Dose Form/Volume
Third-Generation Fluoroquinolone		
levofloxacin (C)(G)	Levaquin	*Tab:* 250, 500, 750 mg
Fourth-Generation Fluoroquinolone		
gemifloxacin (C)(G)	Factive	*Tab:* 320*mg
moxifloxacin (C) (G)	Avelox	*Tab:* 400 mg
Ketolide		
telithromycin (C)	Ketek	*Tab:* 300, 400 mg
Macrolide		
azithromycin (B)	Zithromax	*Tab:* 250, 500, 600 mg; *Pkt:* 1 g for reconstitution (cherry-banana)
	ZithPed Syr	*Oral susp:* 100 mg/5 ml, (15 ml); 200 mg/5 ml (15, 22.5, 30 ml) (cherry)
	Zithromax Tri-Pak	*Tab:* 3 x 500 mg tabs/pck
	Zithromax Z-Pak	*Tab:* 6 x 250 mg tabs/pck
	Zmax	Pkt: 2 g for reconstitution (cherry-banana)
clarithromycin (C)(G)	Biaxin	*Tab:* 250, 500 mg; *Oral susp:* 125, 250 mg/5 ml (50, 100 ml)(fruit punch)
	Biaxin XL	*Tab:* 500 mg ext-rel
dirithromycin (C)(G)	*generic only*	*Tab:* 250 mg
erythromycin base (B)(G)	Ery-Tab	*Tab:* 250, 333, 500 mg ent-coat
	PCE	*Tab:* 333, 500 mg
erythromycin estolate (B)(G)	Ilosone	*Pulvule:* 250 mg; *Tab:* 500 mg; *Liq:* 125, 250 mg/5 ml (100 ml)
erythromycin ethylsuccinate (B)(G)	E.E.S.	*Tab:* 400 mg; *Oral susp:* 200 mg/5 ml (100, 200 ml) (cherry); 200, 400 mg/5 ml (100 ml)(fruit)
	EryPed	*Oral susp:* 200 mg/5 ml (100, 200 ml) (fruit); 400 mg/5 ml (60, 100, 200 ml) (banana); *Oral drops:* 200, 400 mg/5 ml (50 ml) (fruit); *Chew tab:* 200 mg wafer (fruit)

(*continued*)

(*continued*)

Anti-infectives by Class With Dose Forms		
Generic Name	Brand Name	Dose Form/Volume
erythromycin stearate (B)(G)	**Erythrocin**	*Film tab:* 250, 500 mg
Penicillin		
amoxicillin (B)(G)	**Amoxil**	*Cap:* 250, 500 mg; *Tab:* 500, 875* mg; *Chew tab:* 125, 200, 250, 400 mg (cherry-banana-peppermint) (phenylalanine); *Oral susp:*125, 250 mg/ml (80, 100, 150 ml) (bubble gum); 200, 400 mg/5ml (50, 75, 100 ml) (bubble gum); *Oral drops:* 50 mg/ml (30 ml) (bubble gum)
	Moxatag	*Tab:* 775 mg ext-rel
	Trimox	*Cap:* 250, 500 mg; *Oral susp:* 125, 250 mg/5ml (80, 100, 150 ml) (raspberry-strawberry)
amoxicillin/ clavulanate (B)(G)	**Augmentin**	*Tab:* 250, 500, 875 mg; *Chew tab:* 125, 250 mg (lemon lime); 200, 400 mg (cherry-banana; phenylalanine); *Oral susp:* 125 mg/5 ml (banana), 250 mg/5 ml (orange) (75, 100, 150 ml); 200, 400 mg/5ml (50, 75, 100 ml) (orange)
	Augmentin ES-600	*Oral susp:* 600 mg/5 ml (50, 75, 100, 125, 150, 200 ml) (strawberry cream) (phenylalanine)
	Augmentin XR	*Tab:* 1000*mg ext-rel
ampicillin (B)(G)	**Omnipen**	*Cap:* 250, 500 mg; *Oral susp:* 125, 250 mg/ml (100, 150, 200 ml)
	Principen	*Cap:* 250, 500 mg; *Syr:* 125, 250 mg/5 ml
ampicillin/ sulbactam (B)(G)	**Unasyn**	*Vial:* 1.5, 3 g
carbenicillin (B)	**Geocillin**	*Tab:* 382 mg film-coat
dicloxacillin (B)(G)	**Dynapen**	*Cap:* 125, 250, 500 mg; *Oral susp:* 62.5 mg/5 ml (80, 100, 200 ml)

(*continued*)

(*continued*)

Anti-infectives by Class With Dose Forms		
Generic Name	Brand Name	Dose Form/Volume
ertapenem (B)	Ivanz	*Vial:* 1 g pwdr for reconstitution
meropenem (B)(G)	Merrem	*Vial:* 500 mg; 1 g pwdr for reconstitution (sodium 3.92 mEq/g)
penicillin G benzathine (B)(G)	Bicillin LA, Bicillin C-R	*Cartridge-needle unit:* 600,000 million units (1 ml); 1.2 million units (2 ml); 2.4 million units (4 ml)
	Permapen	*Prefilled syringe:* 1.2 million units
penicillin G procaine (B)(G)	*generic only*	*Prefilled syringe:* 1.2 million units
penicillin v potassium (B)(G)	Pen-Vee K	*Tab:* 250, 500 mg; *Oral soln:* 125 mg/5 ml (100, 200 ml); 250 mg/5 ml (100, 150, 200 ml)
piperacillin/ tazobactam (B)(G)	Zosyn	*Vial:* 2, 3, 4 g pwdr for reconstitution
Sulfonamide		
sulfamethoxazole (B/D)(G)	Gantrisin Pediatric	*Oral susp:* 500 mg/5 ml; *Syr:* 500 mg/5 ml
trimethoprim (C) (G)	Primsol	*Oral soln:* 50 mg/5 ml (bubble gum) (dye-free, alcohol-free)
	Trimpex	*Tab:* 100 mg
	Proloprim	*Tab:* 100, 200 mg
trimethoprim/ sulfamethoxazole (C)(G)	Bactrim, Septra	*Tab: trim* 80 mg/*sulfa* 400 mg*
	Bactrim DS, Septra DS	*Tab: trim* 160 mg/*sulfa* 800 mg*; *Oral susp: trim* 40 mg/*sulfa* 200 mg per 5 ml (100 ml) (cherry) (alcohol 0.3%)
Tetracycline		
demeclocycline (D)	Declomycin	*Tab:* 300 mg
doxycycline (D)(G)	Adoxa	*Tab:* 50, 100 mg ent-coat
	Doryx	*Cap:* 100 mg
	Monodox	*Cap:* 50, 100 mg

(*continued*)

(*continued*)

Anti-infectives by Class With Dose Forms		
Generic Name	Brand Name	Dose Form/Volume
doxycycline (D)(G)	Vibramycin	*Cap:* 50, 100 mg; *Syr:* 50 mg/5 ml; (raspberry) (sulfites); *Oral susp:* 25 mg/5 ml (raspberry-apple); *IV conc: doxy* 100 mg/*asc acid* 480 mg after dilution; *doxy* 200 mg/*asc acid* 960 mg after dilution
	Vibra-Tab	*Tab:* 100 mg film-coat
minocycline (D)(G)	Dynacin	*Cap:* 50, 100 mg
	Minocin	*Cap:* 50, 100 mg; *Oral susp:* 50 mg/5 ml (60 ml) (custard) (sulfites, alcohol 5%); *Vial:* 100 mg soln for inj:
tetracycline (D)(G)	Achromycin V	*Cap:* 250, 500 mg
	Sumycin	*Tab:* 250, 500 mg; *Oral susp:* 125 mg/5 ml (fruit) (sulfites)
Macrolide/Sulfisoxazole		
erythromycin ethylsuccinate/ sulfisoxazole (C)(G)	Pediazole	*Oral susp: eryth* 200 mg/*sulf* 600 mg per 5 ml (100, 150, 200 ml) (strawberry-banana)
Miscellaneous		
aztreonam (B)	Cayston	*Vial:* 75 mg pwdr for reconstitution (preservative-free)
chloramphenicol (C)(G)	Chloromycetin	*Vial:* 1 g
clindamycin (B)(G)	Cleocin	*Cap:* 75 (tartrazine), 150 (tartrazine), 300 mg; *Oral susp:* 75 mg/5 ml (100 ml) (cherry); *Vial:* 150 mg/l (2, 4 ml) (benzyl alcohol)
dalbavancin (C)	Dalvance	*Vial:* 500 mg pwdr for IV infusion (preservative-free)
daptomycin (B)(G)	Cubicin	*Vial:* 500 mg pwdr for reconstitution
doripenem (B)	Doribax	*Vial:* 500 mg pwdr for reconstitution
fosfomycin (B)	Monurol	*Sachet:* 3 g single-dose (mandarin orange; sucrose)

(*continued*)

(*continued*)

Anti-infectives by Class With Dose Forms		
Generic Name	Brand Name	Dose Form/Volume
imipenem/cilastatin (C)(G)	Primaxin	*Vial: imip* 500 mg/*cila* 500 mg; *imip* 750 mg/*cila* 750 mg pwdr for reconstitution
lincomycin (B)(G)	Lincocin	*Vial:* 300 mg/ml (10 ml)
linezolid (C)(G)	Zyvox	*Tab:* 400, 600 mg; *Oral susp:* 100 mg/5 ml (orange) (phenylalanine); *IV:* 2 mg ml (100, 200, 300 ml)
meropenem (B)	Merrem	*Vial:* 500 mg; 1 g (sodium 3.92 mEq/g)
nitrofurantoin (B) (G)	Furadantin	*Oral susp:* 25 mg/5 ml (60 ml)
	Macrobid	*Cap:* 100 mg
	Macrodantin	*Cap:* 25, 50, 100 mg
quinupristin/ dalfopristin (B)	Synercid	*Vial:* 150 mg/350 mg, 180 mg/420 mg
tygecycline (D)(G)	Tygacil	*Vial:* 50 mg pwdr for reconstitution
rifaximin (C)	Xifaxan	*Tab:* 200, 550 mg
telavancin (C)	Vibativ	*Vial:* 250, 750 mg pwdr for reconstitution for IV infusion (preservative-free)
vancomycin (C)(G)	Vancocin	*Cap:* 125, 250 mg; *Vial:* 500 mg, 1 g pwdr for reconstitution for IV infusion

APPENDIX CC.1: *ACYCLOVIR* (ZOVIRAX SUSPENSION)

Weight												
Pounds	15	20	25	30	35	40	45	50	55	60	65	70
Kilograms	6.8	9	11.4	13.6	15.9	18.2	20.5	22.7	25	27.3	29.5	31.8
Single Dose (ml)/Frequency/Strength/5-Day Volume (ml)												
20 mg/kg/d ml/dose qid	3.5	4.5	5.5	6.5	8	9	10	11.5	12.5	13.5	14.5	16
mg/5ml	200	200	200	200	200	200	200	200	200	200	200	200
Volume (ml)	70	90	110	130	160	180	200	230	250	270	290	320

Zovirax Oral Suspension <2 years: not recommended; >2 years, <40 kg: 20 mg/kg dosed qid x 5 days; ≥2 years, >40 kg: 800 mg dosed qid x 5 days; *Oral susp:* 200 mg/5 ml (banana).

APPENDIX CC.2: *AMANTADINE* (SYMMETREL SYRUP)

Weight												
Pounds	15	20	25	30	35	40	45	50	55	60	65	70
Kilograms	6.8	9	11.4	13.6	15.9	18.2	20.5	22.7	25	27.3	29.5	31.8
Single Dose (ml)/Frequency/Strength/10-Day Volume (ml)												
4 mg/kg/d ml/dose bid	3	4	5	6	7	8	9	10	11	12	13	14
mg/5ml	50	50	50	50	50	50	50	50	50	50	50	50
Volume (ml)	30	40	50	60	70	80	90	100	110	120	130	140
8 mg/lb/d ml/dose bid	6	8	10	12								
mg/5ml	50	50	50	50								
Volume (ml)	60	80	100	60								

Symmetrel Suspension (C)(G) **Symmetrel** <1 year: not recommended; 1-8 years: max 150 mg/day; 9-12 years: 2 tsp bid; >12 years: 100 mg bid or 200 mg once daily; *Syr:* 50 mg/5 ml (raspberry).

APPENDIX CC.3: *AMOXICILLIN* (AMOXIL SUSPENSION, TRIMOX SUSPENSION)

Weight

Pounds	15	20	25	30	35	40	45	50	55	60	65	70
Kilograms	6.8	9	11.4	13.6	15.9	18.2	20.5	22.7	25	27.3	29.5	31.8
Single Dose (ml)/Frequency/Strength/10-Day Volume (ml)												
20 mg/kg/d ml/dose tid	2	2.5	3	3.5	4	5	5.5	6	7	7.5	8	9
mg/5ml	125	125	125	125	125	125	125	125	125	125	125	125
Volume (ml)	60	75	90	105	120	150	165	180	210	225	240	270
30 mg/kg/d ml/dose tid	3	3.5	2.5	3	3	3.5	4	4.5	5	5.5	6	6.5
mg/5ml	125	125	250	250	250	250	250	250	250	250	250	250
Volume (ml)	90	105	75	90	90	105	120	135	150	165	180	195
40 mg/kg/d ml/dose bid	5	7	4.5	5	6	7	8	9	10	11	12	13
mg/5ml	125	125	250	250	250	250	250	250	250	250	250	250
Volume (ml)	100	140	90	100	120	140	160	180	200	220	240	250
45 mg/kg/d ml/dose bid	4	2.5	3	4	4.5	5	6	6.5	7	7.5	8.5	9

(continued)

APPENDIX CC.3: *AMOXICILLIN* (AMOXIL SUSPENSION, TRIMOX SUSPENSION) (*continued*)

mg/5ml	200	400	400	400	400	400	400	400	400	400	400	400
Volume (ml)	80	50	60	80	90	100	120	130	140	150	170	180
90 mg/kg/d ml/dose bid	8	5	6	7	9	10	12	13	14	15	17	18
mg/5ml	200	400	400	400	400	400	400	400	400	400	400	400
Volume (ml)	160	100	120	140	180	200	240	260	280	300	340	360

<40 kg (88 lb): 20-30 mg/kg/day in 3 divided doses or 40-90 mg/kg/day in 2 divided doses; >40 kg: same as adult.

Amoxil Suspension (B)(G) 125, 250 mg/5ml (80, 100, 150 ml) (strawberry); 200, 400 mg/5 ml (50, 75, 100 ml) (bubble gum).

Trimox Suspension (B)(G) 125, 250 mg/5 ml (80, 100, 150 ml) (raspberry-strawberry).

APPENDIX CC.4: *AMOXICILLIN/CLAVULANATE* (AUGMENTIN SUSPENSION)

Weight												
Pounds	15	20	25	30	35	40	45	50	55	60	65	70
Kilograms	6.8	9	11.4	13.6	15.9	18.2	20.5	22.7	25	27.3	29.5	31.8
Single Dose (ml)/Frequency/Strength/10-Day Volume (ml)												
40 mg/kg/d ml/dose bid	5.5	7	4.5	5.5	6.5	7	8	9	10	11	12	13
mg/5ml	125	125	250	250	250	250	250	250	250	250	250	250
Volume (ml)	110	140	90	110	130	140	160	180	200	220	240	260
45 mg/kg/d ml/dose bid	3	4	5	6	7	8	9	10	11.5	12.5	13.5	14.5
mg/5ml	250	250	250	250	250	250	250	250	250	250	250	250
Volume (ml)	60	80	100	120	140	160	180	200	230	250	270	290
45 mg/kg/d ml/dose bid	4	2.5	3	4	4.5	5	6	6.5	7	7.5	8.5	9
mg/5ml	200	400	400	400	400	400	400	400	400	400	400	400
Volume (ml)	80	50	60	80	90	100	120	130	140	150	170	180
90 mg/kg/d ml/dose bid	4	5	6.5	8	9	10	11.5	13	14	15.5	16.5	18
mg/5ml	400	400	400	400	400	400	400	400	400	400	400	400
Volume (ml)	80	100	130	160	180	200	240	260	280	300	340	360

Augmentin Suspension (B)(G) 40-45 mg/kg/day divided tid or 90 mg/kg/day divided bid; 125mg/5 ml (75, 100, 150 ml) (banana), 250 mg/5 ml (75, 100, 150 ml) (orange); 200, 400 mg/5 ml (50, 75, 100 ml) (orange-raspberry) (phenylalanine).

APPENDIX CC.5: *AMOXICILLIN/CLAVULANATE* (AUGMENTIN ES 600 SUSPENSION)

Weight												
Pounds	15	20	25	30	35	40	45	50	55	60	65	70
Kilograms	6.8	9	11.4	13.6	15.9	18.2	20.5	22.7	25	27.3	29.5	31.8
Single Dose (ml)/Frequency/Strength/10-Day Volume (ml)												
40 mg/kg/d ml/dose bid	1	1.5	2	2	2.5	3	3.5	4	4	4.5	5	5
mg/5ml	600	600	600	600	600	600	600	600	600	600	600	600
Volume (ml)	30	40	40	40	50	60	70	80	80	90	100	100
45 mg/kg/d ml/dose bid	1.25	1.5	2	2.5	3	3.5	4	4.5	5	5	5.5	6
mg/5ml	600	600	600	600	600	600	600	600	600	600	600	600
Volume (ml)	25	30	40	50	60	70	80	90	100	100	110	120
90 mg/kg/d ml/dose bid	2.5	3.5	4	5	6	7	8	8.5	9.5	10	11	12
mg/5ml	600	600	600	600	600	600	600	600	600	600	600	600
Volume (ml)	50	70	80	100	120	140	160	170	190	200	220	240

Augmentin ES 600 Suspension (B) <3 months: not recommended; ≥3 months, <40 kg: 90 mg/kg/day in 2 divided doses; ≥40 kg: not recommended; 600 mg/5 ml (50, 75, 100, 125, 150, 200 ml) (strawberry cream) (phenylalanine).

APPENDIX CC.6: *AMPICILLIN* (OMNIPEN SUSPENSION, PRINCIPEN SUSPENSION)

Weight												
Pounds	15	20	25	30	35	40	45	50	55	60	65	70
Kilograms	6.8	9	11.4	13.6	15.9	18.2	20.5	22.7	25	27.3	29.5	31.8
Single Dose (ml)/Frequency/Strength/10-Day Volume (ml)												
50 mg/kg/d ml/dose q6h	3.5	4.5	3	3.5	4	4.5						
mg/5ml	125	125	250	250	250	250						
Volume (ml)	140	180	120	140	160	180						
100 mg/kg/d ml/dose q6h	3.5	4.5	6	7	8	9						
mg/5ml	250	250	250	250	250	250						
Volume (ml)	140	180	240	280	320	360						

Omnipen Suspension, Principen Suspension (B)(G) >20 kg: 250–500 mg q 6 h 125, 250 mg/5 ml (100, 150, 200 ml) (fruit).

APPENDIX CC.7: *AZITHROMYCIN* (ZITHROMAX SUSPENSION, ZMAX SUSPENSION)

Weight									
Pounds	11	22	33	44	55	66	77	88
Kilograms	5	10	15	20	25	30	35	40
Single Dose (ml)/Frequency/Strength/Volume (ml)									
3 Day Regimen									
10 mg/kg qd	2.5	5	7.5	5	6	7.5	9	10
mg/5ml	100	100	100	200	200	200	200	200
Volume (ml)	7.5	15	22.5	15	18	22.5	27	30
5 Day Regimen									
10 mg/kg qd									
Day 1	2.5	5	7.5	5	6	7.5	7.5	10
Days 2–5	1.25	2.5	4	2.5	3	4	4	5
mg/5ml	100	100	100	200	200	200	200	200
Volume (ml)	10	15	23.5	15	18	23.5	23.5	30

Zithromax ES 600 Suspension (B)(G) 100 mg/5 ml (15 ml), 200 mg/5 ml (15 ml), 200 mg/5 ml (15, 22.5, 30 ml) (cherry-vanilla-banana).

APPENDIX CC.8: *CEFACLOR* (CECLOR SUSPENSION)

Weight												
Pounds	15	20	25	30	35	40	45	50	55	60	65	70
Kilograms	6.8	9	11.4	13.6	15.9	18.2	20.5	22.7	25	27.3	29.5	31.8
Single Dose (ml)/Frequency/Strength/10-Day Volume (ml)												
20 mg/kg/d ml/dose tid	2	2.5	3	3.5	4	5	5.5	6	7	7.5	8	8.5
mg/5ml	125	125	125	125	125	125	125	125	125	125	125	125
Volume (ml)	60	75	90	105	120	150	165	180	210	225	240	255
20 mg/kg/d ml/dose tid	1.5	1.5	2	2.5	3	3	4	4	4.5	5	5.5	6
mg/5ml	187	187	187	187	187	187	187	187	187	187	187	187
Volume (ml)	45	45	60	75	90	90	105	120	135	150	165	180
40 mg/kg/d ml/dose tid	2	2.5	3	3.5	4	5	5.5	6	6.5	7	8	8.5
mg/5ml	250	250	250	250	250	250	250	250	250	250	250	250
Volume (ml)	60	75	90	105	120	150	165	180	195	210	240	255
40 mg/kg/d ml/dose tid	1.5	1.5	2	2.5	3	3	3.5	4	4.5	5	5	5.5
mg/5ml	375	375	375	375	375	375	375	375	375	375	375	375
Volume (ml)	45	45	60	75	90	90	105	120	135	150	150	165

Ceclor Suspension (B) <6 months: not recommended; 125, 250 mg/5 ml (75, 150 ml) (strawberry); 187, 375 mg/5ml (50, 100 ml) (strawberry).

APPENDIX CC.9: *CEFADROXIL* (DURICEF SUSPENSION)

Weight												
Pounds	15	20	25	30	35	40	45	50	55	60	65	70
Kilograms	6.8	9	11.4	13.6	15.9	18.2	20.5	22.7	25	27.3	29.5	31.8
Single Dose (ml)/Frequency/Strength/10-Day Volume (ml)												
30 mg/kg/d ml/dose bid	2	3	3.5	4	5	5.5	6	7	7.5	8	9	9.5
mg/5ml	250	250	250	250	250	250	250	250	250	250	250	250
Volume (ml)	40	60	75	80	100	110	120	140	150	160	180	190
30 mg/kg/d ml/dose qd	2	3	3.5	4	5	5.5	6	7	7.5	8	9	9.5
mg/5ml	500	500	500	500	500	500	500	500	500	500	500	500
Volume (ml)	20	30	35	40	50	55	60	70	75	80	90	95

Duricef Suspension (B) 250 mg/5 ml (100 ml) (orange-pineapple); 500 mg/5ml (75, 100 ml) (orange-pineapple).

APPENDIX CC.10: *CEFDINIR* (OMNICEF SUSPENSION)

Weight

Pounds	15	20	25	30	35	40	45	50	55	60	65	70
Kilograms	6.8	9	11.4	13.6	15.9	18.2	20.5	22.7	25	27.3	29.5	31.8

Single Dose (ml)/Frequency/Strength/10-Day Volume (ml)

	15	20	25	30	35	40	45	50	55	60	65	70
7 mg/kg/d ml/dose bid	2	2.5	3	4	4.5	5	6	6.5	7	7.5	8	9
mg/5ml	125	125	125	125	125	125	125	125	125	125	125	125
Volume (ml)	40	50	60	80	90	100	120	130	140	150	160	180
14 mg/kg ml/dose bid	4	5	6	8	9	10	12	13	14	15	16	18
mg/5ml	125	125	125	125	125	125	125	125	125	125	125	125
Volume (ml)	40	50	60	80	90	100	120	130	140	150	160	180

Omnicef Suspension (B) <6 months: not recommended; 125 mg/5 ml (60, 100 ml) (strawberry).

APPENDIX CC.11: *CEFIXIME* (SUPRAX ORAL SUSPENSION)

Weight												
Pounds	15	20	25	30	35	40	45	50	55	60	65	70
Kilograms	6.8	9	11.4	13.6	15.9	18.2	20.5	22.7	25	27.3	29.5	31.8
Single Dose (ml)/Frequency/Strength/10-Day Volume (ml)												
8 mg/kg/d ml/dose bid	1.3	1.8	2.2	2.5	3.1	3.5	4	4.5	5	5.5	6	6.5
mg/5ml	100	100	100	100	100	100	100	100	100	100	100	100
8 mg/kg/d ml/dose qd	2.7	3.6	4.5	5.5	6.3	7.2	8.2	9	10	11	12	13
mg/5ml	100	100	100	100	100	100	100	100	100	100	100	100
Volume (ml)	27	36	45	55	65	70	80	90	100	110	120	130

Supra Oral Suspension (B)(G) <6 months: not recommended; 100 mg/5 ml (50, 75, 100 ml) (strawberry).

APPENDIX CC.12: CEFPODOXIME PROXETIL (VANTIN SUSPENSION)

Weight

Pounds	15	20	25	30	35	40	45	50	55	60	65	70
Kilograms	6.8	9	11.4	13.6	15.9	18.2	20.5	22.7	25	27.3	29.5	31.8

Single Dose (ml)/Frequency/Strength/10-Day Volume (ml)

	15	20	25	30	35	40	45	50	55	60	65	70
5 mg/kg/d ml/dose bid	3.5	4.5	5.5	7	8	9	10	11	12.5	13.5	15	16
mg/5ml	50	50	50	50	50	50	50	50	50	50	50	50
Volume (ml)	70	90	110	140	160	180	200	220	250	270	300	320
5 mg/kg/d ml/dose bid	2	2	3	3.5	4	4.5	5	5.5	6	7	7.5	8
mg/5ml	100	100	100	100	100	100	100	100	100	100	100	100
Volume (ml)	40	40	60	70	80	90	100	110	120	140	150	160

Vantin Suspension (B) <2 months: not recommended; 50, 100 mg/5 ml (50, 75, 100 ml) (lemon-crème).

APPENDIX CC.13: *CEFPROZIL* (CEFZIL SUSPENSION)

Weight												
Pounds	15	20	25	30	35	40	45	50	55	60	65	70
Kilograms	6.8	9	11.4	13.6	15.9	18.2	20.5	22.7	25	27.3	29.5	31.8
Single Dose (ml)/Frequency/Strength/10-Day Volume (ml)												
7.5 mg/kg/d ml/dose bid	2	3	3.5	4	5	5.5	6	7	7.5	4	4.5	5
mg/5ml	125	125	125	125	125	125	125	125	125	250	250	250
Volume (ml)	40	60	70	80	100	110	120	140	150	80	90	100
15 mg/kg/d ml/dose bid	2	3	3.5	4	5	5	6	7	7.5	8	9	9.5
mg/5ml	250	250	250	250	250	250	250	250	250	250	250	250
Volume (ml)	40	60	70	80	100	100	120	140	150	160	180	190
20 mg/kg/d ml/dose qd	3	3.5	4.5	5.5	6.5	7	8	9	10	11	12	13
mg/5ml	250	250	250	250	250	250	250	250	250	250	250	250
Volume (ml)	60	70	90	110	130	140	160	180	200	220	240	260

Cefzil Suspension (B) ≤6 months: not recommended; 2–12 years: 7.5–20 mg/kg bid >12 years: same as adult, 250–500 mg bid or 500 mg once daily; 125, 250 mg/5 ml (50, 75, 100 ml) (bubble gum) (phenylalanine).

APPENDIX CC.14: *CEFTIBUTEN* (CEDAX SUSPENSION)

Weight												
Pounds	15	20	25	30	35	40	45	50	55	60	65	70
Kilograms	6.8	9	11.4	13.6	15.9	18.2	20.5	22.7	25	27.3	29.5	31.8
Single Dose (ml)/Frequency/Strength/10-Day Volume (ml)												
9 mg/kg/d ml/dose qd	3.5	4.5	6	7	8	9	10	11.5	12.5	13.5	15	16
90 mg/5ml	90	90	90	90	90	90	90	90	90	90	90	90
Volume (ml)	35	45	60	70	80	90	100	115	125	135	150	160
9 mg/kg/d ml/dose qd	1.75	2.3	3	3.5	4	4.5	5	5.4	6.2	6.6	7.5	8
180 mg/5ml	180	180	180	180	180	180	180	180	180	180	180	180
Volume (ml)	20	25	30	35	40	45	50	55	60	65	70	80

Cefzil Suspension (B) 90 mg/5 ml (30, 60, 90, 120 ml) (cherry); 180 mg/5ml (30, 60, 120 ml) (cherry).

APPENDIX CC.15: *CEFUROXIME AXETIL* (CEFTIN SUSPENSION)

Weight												
Pounds	15	20	25	30	35	40	45	50	55	60	65	70
Kilograms	6.8	9	11.4	13.6	15.9	18.2	20.5	22.7	25	27.3	29.5	31.8
Single Dose (ml)/Frequency/Strength/10-Day Volume (ml)												
20 mg/kg/d ml/dose bid	2.5	3.5	4.5	3	3	3.5	4	4.5	5	5.5	6	6.5
mg/5ml	125	125	125	250	250	250	250	250	250	250	250	250
Volume (ml)	50	70	90	60	60	70	80	90	100	110	120	130
30 mg/kg/d ml/dose bid	2	3	3.5	4	5	5.5	6	7	7.5	8	9	9.5
mg/5ml	250	250	250	250	250	250	250	250	250	250	250	250
Volume (ml)	40	60	70	80	100	110	120	140	150	160	180	190

Ceftin Suspension (B) 125, 250 mg/5 ml (50, 100 ml) (tutti-frutti).

APPENDIX CC.16: *CEPHALEXIN* (KEFLEX SUSPENSION)

Weight												
Pounds	15	20	25	30	35	40	45	50	55	60	65	70
Kilograms	6.8	9	11.4	13.6	15.9	18.2	20.5	22.7	25	27.3	29.5	31.8
Single Dose (ml)/Frequency/Strength/10-Day Volume (ml)												
25 mg/kg/d ml/dose tid	1	1.5	2	2	3	3	3.5	4	4	4.5	5	5
mg/5ml	125	125	125	125	125	125	125	125	125	125	125	125
Volume (ml)	30	45	60	60	90	90	105	120	120	135	150	150
25 mg/kg/d ml/dose qid	1	1	1.5	2	2	2.5	2.5	3	3	3.5	4	4
mg/5ml	250	250	250	250	250	250	250	250	250	250	250	250
Volume (ml)	40	40	60	80	80	100	100	120	120	140	160	160
50 mg/kg/d ml/dose tid	2	3	4	4.5	5	6	7	7.5	8	9	10	10.5
mg/5ml	250	250	250	250	250	250	250	250	250	250	250	250
Volume (ml)	60	90	120	135	150	180	210	225	240	270	300	315
50 mg/kg/d ml/dose qid	2	2	3	3.5	4	4.5	5	6	6	7	7.5	8
mg/5ml	250	250	250	250	250	250	250	250	250	250	250	250
Volume (ml)	80	80	120	140	160	180	200	240	240	280	300	320

Keflex Suspension (B)(G) <2 months: not recommended; 125, 250 mg/5 ml (100, 200 ml) (strawberry).

APPENDIX CC.17: *CLARITHROMYCIN* (BIAXIN SUSPENSION)												
Weight												
Pounds	15	20	25	30	35	40	45	50	55	60	65	70
Kilograms	6.8	9	11.4	13.6	15.9	18.2	20.5	22.7	25	27.3	29.5	31.8
Single Dose (ml)/Frequency/Strength/10-Day Volume (ml)												
7.5 mg/kg/d ml/dose bid	2	3	3.5	4	5	5.5	6	7	7.5	8	9	10
mg/5ml	125	125	125	125	125	125	125	125	125	125	125	125
Volume (ml)	40	60	70	80	100	110	120	140	150	160	180	200
7.5 mg/kg/d ml/dose bid	1	1.5	2	2	2.5	3	3	3.5	4	4	4.5	5
mg/5ml	250	250	250	250	250	250	250	250	250	250	250	250
Volume (ml)	20	30	40	40	50	60	60	70	80	80	90	100

Biaxin Suspension (B) <6 months: not recommended; 125, 250 mg/5 ml (50, 100 ml) (fruit-punch).

APPENDIX CC.18: *CLINDAMYCIN* (CLEOCIN PEDIATRIC GRANULES)

Weight

Pounds	15	20	25	30	35	40	45	50	55	60	65	70
Kilograms	6.8	9	11.4	13.6	15.9	18.2	20.5	22.7	25	27.3	29.5	31.8

Single Dose (ml)/Frequency/Strength/10-Day Volume (ml)

	15	20	25	30	35	40	45	50	55	60	65	70
8 mg/kg/d ml/dose tid	1	1.5	2	2.5	3	3	3.5	4	4.5	5	5	5.5
mg/5ml	75	75	75	75	75	75	75	75	75	75	75	75
Volume (ml)	30	45	60	75	90	90	105	120	135	150	150	165
16 mg/kg/d ml/dose tid	2.5	3	4	5	5.5	6.5	7	8	9	9.5	10.5	11
mg/5ml	75	75	75	75	75	75	75	75	75	75	75	75
Volume (ml)	75	90	120	150	165	105	210	240	270	285	315	330

Cleocin Pediatric Granules (B)(G) 75 mg/5 ml (100 ml) (cherry).

APPENDIX CC.19: *DICLOXACILLIN* (DYNAPEN SUSPENSION)

Weight												
Pounds	15	20	25	30	35	40	45	50	55	60	65	70
Kilograms	6.8	9	11.4	13.6	15.9	18.2	20.5	22.7	25	27.3	29.5	31.8
Single Dose (ml)/Frequency/Strength/10-Day Volume (ml)												
12.5 mg/kg/d ml/dose qid	2	2.5	3	3.5	4	4.5	5	6	6	7	7.5	8
mg/5ml	62.5	62.5	62.5	62.5	62.5	62.5	62.5	62.5	62.5	62.5	62.5	62.5
Volume (ml)	80	100	120	140	160	180	200	240	240	280	300	320
25 mg/kg/d ml/dose qid	3.5	4.5	6	7	8	9	10	11.5	12.5	13.5	15	16
mg/5ml	62.5	62.5	62.5	62.5	62.5	62.5	62.5	62.5	62.5	62.5	62.5	62.5
Volume (ml)	140	180	240	280	320	360	400	460	500	540	600	640

Dynapen Suspension (B)(G) 6.25 mg/5 ml (80, 100 ml) (raspberry-strawberry).

APPENDIX CC.20: *DOXYCYCLINE* (VIBRAMYCIN SYRUP/SUSPENSION)

Weight												
Pounds	15	20	25	30	35	40	45	50	55	60	65	70
Kilograms	6.8	9	11.4	13.6	15.9	18.2	20.5	22.7	25	27.3	29.5	31.8
Single Dose (ml)/Frequency/Strength/10-Day Volume (ml)												
1 mg/lb/d ml/dose qd	1.5	2	2.5	3	3.5	4	4.5	5	5.5	6	6.5	7
50 mg/5ml	50	50	50	50	50	50	50	50	50	50	50	50
Volume (ml)	15	20	25	30	35	40	45	50	55	60	65	70
1 mg/lb/d ml/dose qd	3	4	5	6	7	8	9	10	11	12	13	14
25 mg/5ml	25	25	25	25	25	25	25	25	25	25	25	25
Volume (ml)	30	40	50	60	70	80	90	100	110	120	130	140

Vibramycin Syrup (B)(G) <8 years: not recommended; double dose first day; 50 mg/5 ml (80, 100, ml) (raspberry-apple) (sulfites).

Vibramycin Suspension (B)(G) <8 years: not recommended; double dose first day; 25 mg/5 ml (80, 100, ml) (raspberry).

APPENDIX CC.21: *ERYTHROMYCIN ESTOLATE* (ILOSONE SUSPENSION)

Weight												
Pounds	15	20	25	30	35	40	45	50	55	60	65	70
Kilograms	6.8	9	11.4	13.6	15.9	18.2	20.5	22.7	25	27.3	29.5	31.8
Dose/Volume (10 days) in ml												
10 mg/kg/d ml/dose bid	3	3.5	4.5	5.5	6	7	8	9	10	5.5	6	6.5
mg/5ml	125	125	125	125	125	125	125	125	125	250	250	250
Volume (ml)	60	70	90	110	120	140	160	180	200	110	120	130
15 mg/kg/d ml/dose bid	4	5.5	7	8	9.5	5.5	6	7	7.5	8	9	9.5
mg/5ml	125	125	125	125	125	250	250	250	250	250	250	250
Volume (ml)	80	110	140	160	190	110	120	140	150	160	180	190
20 mg/kg/d ml/dose bid	3	3.5	4.5	5.5	6.5	7	8	9	10	11	12	13
mg/5ml	250	250	250	250	250	250	250	250	250	250	250	250
Volume (ml)	60	70	90	110	120	140	160	180	200	220	240	260
25 mg/kg/d ml/dose bid	3.5	4.5	5.5	7	8	9	10	11.5	12.5	13.5	15	16
mg/5ml	250	250	250	250	250	250	250	250	250	250	250	250
Volume (ml)	70	90	110	140	160	180	200	230	250	280	300	320

Ilosone Suspension (B)(G) 125, 250 mg/5 ml (100 ml).

APPENDIX CC.22: *ERYTHROMYCIN ETHYLSUCCINATE* (E.E.S. SUSPENSION, ERY-PED DROPS/SUSPENSION)

Weight												
Pounds	15	20	25	30	35	40	45	50	55	60	65	70
Kilograms	6.8	9	11.4	13.6	15.9	18.2	20.5	22.7	25	27.3	29.5	31.8
Single Dose (ml)/Frequency/Strength/10-Day Volume (ml)												
30 mg/kg/d ml/dose qid	1.5	2	2	2.5	3	3.5	4	4	4.5	5	5.5	6
mg/5ml	200	200	200	200	200	200	200	200	200	200	200	200
Volume (ml)	60	80	80	100	120	140	160	160	180	200	220	240
30 mg/kg/d ml/dose qid			1	1.5	1.5	2	2	2	2.5	2.5	3	3
mg/5ml			400	400	400	400	400	400	400	400	400	
Volume (ml)			60	60	80	80	80	100	100	120	120	
50 mg/kg/d ml/dose qid	2	3	3.5	4.5	5	5.5	6.5	7	8	8.5	9	10
mg/5ml	200	200	200	200	200	200	200	200	200	200	200	200

(continued)

APPENDIX CC.22: *ERYTHROMYCIN ETHYLSUCCINATE (E.E.S. SUSPENSION, ERY-PED DROPS/SUSPENSION) (continued)*

Volume (ml)	80	120	140	180	200	220	260	280	320	340	360	400
50mg/kg/d ml/dose qid	1	1.5	2	2	2.5	3	3	3.5	4	4.5	4.5	5
mg/5ml	400	400	400	400	400	400	400	400	400	400	400	400
Volume (ml)	40	60	80	80	100	120	140	140	160	180	180	200

Ery-Ped Drops/Suspension (B)(G) 200 mg/5 ml (100, 200 ml; fruit); 400 mg/5 ml (60, 100, 200 ml) (banana); Oral drops: 200, 400 mg/5 ml (50 ml) (fruit).

E.E.S. Suspension (B)(G) 200 mg/5 ml, 400 mg/5 ml (100 ml) (fruit).

E.E.S. Granules (B)(G) 200 mg/5 ml (100, 200 ml) (cherry).

APPENDIX CC.23: *ERYTHROMYCIN/SULFAMETHOXAZOLE (ERYZOLE, PEDIAZOLE)*

Weight												
Pounds	15	20	25	30	35	40	45	50	55	60	65	70
Kilograms	6.8	9	11.4	13.6	15.9	18.2	20.5	22.7	25	27.3	29.5	31.8
Single Dose (ml)/Frequency/Strength/10-Day Volume (ml)												
10 mg/kg/d ml/dose bid	3	4	5	6	6.5	7.5	8.5	9.5	10	11	12	13.5
mg/5ml	200	200	200	200	200	200	200	200	200	200	200	200
Volume (ml)	90	120	150	180	200	225	255	285	300	330	360	400

Eryzole (C)(G) <2 months: not recommended; *eryth* 200 mg/*sulf* 600 mg/5 ml (100, 150, 200, 250 ml).

Pediazole (C)(G) <2 months: not recommended; *eryth* 200 mg/*sulf* 600 mg/5 ml (100, 150, 200 ml) (strawberry-banana).

APPENDIX CC.24: *FLUCONAZOLE* (DIFLUCAN SUSPENSION)

Weight

Pounds	15	20	25	30	35	40	45	50	55	60	65	70
Kilograms	6.8	9	11.4	13.6	15.9	18.2	20.5	22.7	25	27.3	29.5	31.8

Single Dose (ml)/Frequency/Strength/21-Day Volume (ml)

3 mg/kg/d ml/dose qd	2	3	3.5	4	5	5.5	6	7	7.5	8	9	9.5
mg/ml	10	10	10	10	10	10	10	10	10	10	10	10
Volume (ml)	44	66	77	88	110	121	132	154	165	176	198	209
6 mg/kg/d ml/dose qd	4	5.5	2	2	2.5	3	3	3.5	4	4	4.5	5
mg/ml	10	10	40	40	40	40	40	40	40	40	40	40
Volume (ml)	88	121	44	44	55	66	66	77	88	88	99	110

Diflucan Suspension (B)(G) double-dose first day; 10, 40 mg/5 ml (35 ml) (orange).

APPENDIX CC.25: *FURAZOLIDONE* (FUROXONE LIQUID)

Weight												
Pounds	15	20	25	30	35	40	45	50	55	60	65	70
Kilograms	6.8	9	11.4	13.6	15.9	18.2	20.5	22.7	25	27.3	29.5	31.8
Single Dose (ml)/Frequency/Strength/7-Day Volume (ml)												
5 mg/kg/d ml/dose qid	2.5	3.5	4	5	6	7	8	8.5	9.5	10	11	12
mg/15 ml	50	50	50	50	50	50	50	50	50	50	50	50
Vol	100	140	160	200	240	280	320	340	380	400	440	480

Furoxone Liquid (C)(G) double-dose first day; 50 mg/15 ml (35 ml).

APPENDIX CC.26: *GRISEOFULVIN, MICROSIZE* (GRIFULVIN V SUSPENSION)

Weight												
Pounds	15	20	25	30	35	40	45	50	55	60	65	70
Kilograms	6.8	9	11.4	13.6	15.9	18.2	20.5	22.7	25	27.3	29.5	31.8
Single Dose (ml)/Frequency/Strength/30-Day Volume (ml)												
5 mg/lb/d ml/dose day	3	4	5	6	7	8	9	10	11	12	13	14
mg/5ml	125	125	125	125	125	125	125	125	125	125	125	125
Volume (ml)	90	120	150	180	210	240	270	300	330	360	390	420

Grifulvin V Suspension (C)(G) double-dose first day; 125 mg/5 ml (120 ml) (orange) (alcohol 0.02%).

APPENDIX CC.27: ITRACONAZOLE (SPORANOX SOLUTION)

Weight												
Pounds	15	20	25	30	35	40	45	50	55	60	65	70
Kilograms	6.8	9	11.4	13.6	15.9	18.2	20.5	22.7	25	27.3	29.5	31.8
Single Dose (ml)/Frequency/Strength/7-Day Volume (ml)												
5 mg/kg/d ml/dose qd	3.5	4.5	6	7	8	9	10	11.5	12.5	14	15	16
mg/ml	10	10	10	10	10	10	10	10	10	10	10	10
Volume (ml)	25	32	42	49	56	63	70	71	88	98	105	112

Sporanox V Solution (C)(G) double-dose first day; 10 mg/ml (150 ml) (cherry-caramel).

APPENDIX CC.28: *LORACARBEF* (LORABID SUSPENSION)

Weight

	15	20	25	30	35	40	45	50	55	60	65	70
Pounds	15	20	25	30	35	40	45	50	55	60	65	70
Kilograms	6.8	9	11.4	13.6	15.9	18.2	20.5	22.7	25	27.3	29.5	31.8

Single Dose (ml)/Frequency/Strength/10-Day Volume (ml)

	15	20	25	30	35	40	45	50	55	60	65	70
15 mg/kg/d ml/dose bid	2.5	3.5	4	5	3	3.5	4	4	5	5	5.5	6
mg/5ml	100	100	100	100	200	200	200	200	200	200	200	200
Volume (ml)	50	70	80	100	60	70	80	80	100	100	110	120
30 mg/kg/d ml/dose bid	2.5	3.5	4	5	6	7	8	8.5	9.5	10	11	12
mg/5ml	200	200	200	200	200	200	200	200	200	200	200	200
Volume (ml)	50	70	80	100	120	140	160	170	190	200	220	240

Lorabid Suspension **(B)** 100 mg/5 ml (50, 100 ml) (strawberry bubble gum); 200 mg/5 ml (50, 75, 100 ml) (strawberry bubble gum).

APPENDIX CC.29: *NITROFURANTOIN* (FURADANTIN SUSPENSION)

Weight												
Pounds	15	20	25	30	35	40	45	50	55	60	65	70
Kilograms	6.8	9	11.4	13.6	15.9	18.2	20.5	22.7	25	27.3	29.5	31.8
Single Dose (ml)/Frequency/Strength/10-Day Volume (ml)												
5 mg/kg ml/dose qid	1.5	2.5	3	3.5	4	4.5	5	5.5	6	7	7.5	8
mg/5 ml	25	25	25	25	25	25	25	25	25	25	25	25
Volume (ml)	60	100	120	140	160	190	200	220	240	280	300	320

Furadantin Suspension (B)(G) 25 mg/5 ml (60 ml).

APPENDIX CC.30: *PENICILLIN V POTASSIUM* (PEN-VEE K SOLUTION, VEETIDS SOLUTION)

Weight												
Pounds	15	20	25	30	35	40	45	50	55	60	65	70
Kilograms	6.8	9	11.4	13.6	15.9	18.2	20.5	22.7	25	27.3	29.5	31.8
Single Dose (ml)/Frequency/Strength/10-Day Volume (ml)												
25 mg/kg/d ml/dose qid	2	2.5	3	3.5	4	4.5	5	5.5	6	7	7.5	8
mg/5ml	125	125	125	125	125	125	125	125	125	125	125	125
Volume (ml)	80	90	120	140	160	180	200	220	240	280	300	320
25 mg/kg/d ml/dose qid	1	1	1.5	2	2	2.5	2.5	3	3	3.5	4	4
mg/5ml	250	250	250	250	250	250	250	250	250	250	250	250
Volume (ml)	40	40	60	80	80	100	100	120	120	140	160	160
50 mg/kg/d ml/dose qid	2	2.5	3	3.5	4	4.5	5	6	6.5	7	7.5	8
mg/5ml	250	250	250	250	250	250	250	250	250	250	250	250
Volume (ml)	80	100	120	140	160	180	200	240	260	280	300	320

Pen-Vee K Solution (B)(G) 125 mg/5 ml (100, 200 ml), 250 mg/5 ml (100, 150, 200 ml).

Veetids Solution (B)(G) 125, 250 mg/5 ml (100, 200 ml).

APPENDIX CC.31: *RIMANTADINE* (FLUMADINE SYRUP)

Weight												
Pounds	15	20	25	30	35	40	45	50	55	60	65	70
Kilograms	6.8	9	11.4	13.6	15.9	18.2	20.5	22.7	25	27.3	29.5	31.8
Single Dose (ml)/Frequency/Strength/10-Day Volume (ml)												
5 mg/kg/d ml/dose qd	3.5	4.5	6	7	8	9	10	11.5	12.5	13.5	15	16
mg/5ml	50	50	50	50	50	50	50	50	50	50	50	50
Volume (ml)	35	45	60	70	80	90	100	115	125	135	150	160

Flumadine Syrup (B) >10 years: same as adult; 50 mg/5 ml (2, 8, 16 oz) (raspberry).

APPENDIX CC.32: *TETRACYCLINE* (SUMYCIN SUSPENSION)

Weight

Pounds	15	20	25	30	35	40	45	50	55	60	65	70
Kilograms	6.8	9	11.4	13.6	15.9	18.2	20.5	22.7	25	27.3	29.5	31.8

Single Dose (ml)/Frequency/Strength/10-Day Volume (ml)

	15	20	25	30	35	40	45	50	55	60	65	70
25 mg/kg/d ml/dose qid	1.5	2.5	3	3.5	4	4.5	5	6	6.5	7	7.5	8
mg/5ml	125	125	125	125	125	125	125	125	125	125	125	125
Volume (ml)	60	100	120	140	160	180	200	240	260	280	300	320
50 mg/kg/d ml/dose qid	3.5	4.5	6	7	8	9	10	11.5	12.5	13.5	15	16
mg/5ml	125	125	125	125	125	125	125	125	125	125	125	125
Volume (ml)	140	180	240	280	320	360	400	460	500	540	600	640

Sumycin Suspension (D)(G) <8 years: not recommended; 125 mg/5 ml (100, 200 ml) (fruit) (sulfites).

APPENDIX CC.33: *TRIMETHOPRIM* (PRIMSOL SUSPENSION)

Weight												
Pounds	15	20	25	30	35	40	45	50	55	60	65	70
Kilograms	6.8	9	11.4	13.6	15.9	18.2	20.5	22.7	25	27.3	29.5	31.8
Single Dose (ml)/Frequency/Strength/10-Day Volume (ml)												
5 mg/kg/d ml/dose bid	3.5	4.5	6	7	8	9	10	11.5	12.5	13.5	15	16
mg/5ml	50	50	50	50	50	50	50	50	50	50	50	50
Volume (ml)	70	90	120	140	160	180	200	230	250	270	300	320

Primsol Suspension (C)(G) 50 mg/5 ml (50 mg/5 ml) (bubble gum) (dye-free, alcohol-free).

APPENDIX CC.34: *TRIMETHOPRIM/SULFAMETHOXAZOLE* (BACTRIM SUSPENSION, SEPTRA SUSPENSION)

Weight												
Pounds	15	20	25	30	35	40	45	50	55	60	65	70
Kilograms	6.8	9	11.4	13.6	15.9	18.2	20.5	22.7	25	27.3	29.5	31.8
Single Dose (ml)/Frequency/Strength/10-Day Volume (ml)												
10 mg/kg/d ml/dose bid	2	2	3	3.5	4	4.5	5	5.5	6	7	7.5	8
mg/5ml	200	200	200	200	200	200	200	200	200	200	200	200
Volume (ml)	40	40	60	70	80	90	100	110	120	140	150	160
20 mg/kg/d ml/dose bid	4	4	6	7	8	9	10	11	12	14	15	16
mg/5ml	200	200	200	200	200	200	200	200	200	200	200	200
Volume (ml)	80	80	120	140	160	180	200	220	240	280	300	320

Bactrim Pediatric Suspension, Septra Pediatric Suspension (C)(G) *trim* 40 mg/*sulfa* 200 mg/5 ml (100 ml) (cherry) (alcohol 0.3%).

APPENDIX CC.35: *VANCOMYCIN* (VANCOCIN SUSPENSION)

Weight												
Pounds	15	20	25	30	35	40	45	50	55	60	65	70
Kilograms	6.8	9	11.4	13.6	15.9	18.2	20.5	22.7	25	27.3	29.5	31.8
Single Dose (ml)/Frequency/Strength/10-Day Volume (ml)												
40 mg/kg/d ml/dose tid	2	2.5	3	3.5	4.5	5	5.5	6	7	7.5	8	8.5
mg/5ml	250	250	250	250	250	250	250	250	250	250	250	250
Volume (ml)	60	75	90	105	135	150	165	180	210	225	240	255
40 mg/kg/d ml/dose qid	1.5	2	2.5	3	3	3.5	4	4.5	5	5.5	6	6.5
mg/5ml	250	250	250	250	250	250	250	250	250	250	250	250
Volume (ml)	60	80	100	120	120	140	160	180	200	220	240	260
40 mg/kg/d ml/dose tid	1	1	1.5	2	2	2.5	3	3	3.5	3.5	4	4
mg/6ml	500	500	500	500	500	500	500	500	500	500	500	500
Volume (ml)	30	30	45	60	60	75	90	90	105	105	120	120
40 mg/kg/d ml/dose qid	1	1	1.5	1.5	1.5	2	2	2.5	2.5	3	3	3.5
mg/6ml	500	500	500	500	500	500	500	500	500	500	500	500
Volume (ml)	40	40	60	60	60	80	80	100	100	120	120	140

Vancomycin Suspension (C)(G).

RESOURCES

Advance for Nurse Practitioners
  http://nurse-practitioners.advanceweb.com

Advanced Practice Education Associates
  www.apea.com

American Association of Nurse Practitioners
  www.aanp.org

American Academy of Pediatrics (AAP)
  http://aapexperience.org

American College of Cardiology. Then and now: ATP III vs. IV: Comparison of ATP III and ACC/AHA guidelines.
  http://www.acc.org/latest-in-cardiology/articles/2014/07/18/16/03/then-and-now-atp-iii-vs-iv

American Diabetes Association (ADA), Professional Diabetes Resources Online
  http://professional.diabetes.org/content/clinical-practice-recommendations/?loc=rp-slabnav

American diabetes association standards of medical care. *Diabetes Care 2016, 38*(Suppl. 1).
  http://care.diabetesjournals.org/content/38/Supplement_1

American Family Physician
  http://www.aafp.org/online/en/home.html

American Geriatrics Society 2015 Beers Criteria Update Expert Panel. (2015). American geriatrics society 2015 updated Beers Criteria for potentially inappropriate medication use in older adults. *Journal of the American Geriatrics Society, 63*(11), 2227–2246.

American Headache Society
  www.americanheadachesociety.org

American Pain Society
  http://americanpainsociety.org/

American Pharmacists Association. (2015). *Pediatric and neonatal dosage handbook: A universal resource for clinicians treating pediatric and neonatal patients* (22nd ed.). Hudson, OH: Lexicomp.

CDC: Morbidity and Mortality Weekly Report (MMWR)
  http://www.cdc.gov/mmwr/mmwr_wk.html

CDC 2015 Sexually Transmitted Diseases Treatment Guidelines
http://www.cdc.gov/std/tg2015/default.htm

Centers for Disease Control and Prevention
www.cdc.gov

Centers for Disease Control and Prevention. (2016). *Facts about ADHD*.
www.cdc.gov/ncbddd/adhd/facts.html

Chow, A. W., Benninger, M. S., Brook, I., Brozek, J. L., Goldstein, E. J., Hicks, L. A., . . .
File, T. M., Jr., Infectious Disease Society of America. (2012). IDSA clinical practice
guideline for acute and bacterial rhinosinusitis in children and adults. *Clinical Infectious
Diseases, 54*(8), e72–e112.

Clinician Reviews
http://www.clinicianreviews.com

Consultant 360
http://www.consultant360.com/home

Daily Med: NIH. US Library of Medicine
https://dailymed.nlm.nih.gov/dailymed/index.cfm

Domino, F. J., Baldor, R. A., Golding, J., & Stephens, M. B. *The 5-minute clinical consult
standard 2016*. Philadelphia, PA: Wolters Kluwer.

DRUGS.COM
www.drugs.com

DRUGS at FDA: FDA Approved Drug Products
http://www.accessdata.fda.gov/scripts/cder/drugsatfda/index.cfm

Engorn, B., & Flerlage, J. (Eds.). (2015). *The Harriet Lane handbook: A handbook for
pediatric house officers* (20th ed.). Philadelphia, PA: Elsevier.

epocrates
https://online.epocrates.com/drugs

eMPR: Monthly Prescribing Reference (new FDA approved products, new generics,
new drug withdrawals, safety alerts)
http://www.empr.com

FDA: Recalls, Market Withdrawals, and Safety alerts
http://www.fda.gov/Safety/Recalls/default.htm

Gilbert, D. N., Chambers, H. F., Eliopoulos, G. M., Saag, M. S., & Pavla, A. T. (2016). *The
Sanford guide to antimicrobial therapy, 2016*. Sperryville, VA: Antimicrobial Therapy.

Handbook of Antimicrobial Therapy (20th ed.). (2015). New Rochelle, NY: The Medical Letter.

International Diabetes Federation (IDF) Clinical Practice Guidelines
http://www.idf.org/guidelines

James, P. A., Oparil, S., Carter, B. L., Cushman, W. C., Dennison-Himmelfarb, C., Handler, J., . . . Ortiz, E. (2014). 2014 evidence-based guidelines for the management of high blood pressure in adults: Report from the panel members appointed to the eighth joint national committee (JNC 8). *Journal of the American Medical Association, 311*(5), 507–520.

JNC 8 Guideline Summary. *Pharmacist's Letter/Prescriber's Letter*
https://www.scribd.com/doc/290772273/JNC-8-guideline-summary

Journal of the American Academy of Nurse Practitioners
https://www.aanp.org/publications/jaanp

Journal of the American Medical Association (JAMA) Internal Medicine
http://archinte.jamanetwork.com/journal.aspx

Journal of the American Geriatrics Society
http://onlinelibrary.wiley.com/journal/10.1111/(ISSN)1532-5415

Lieberthal, A. S., Carroll, A. E., Chonmaitree, T., Ganiats, T. G., Hoberman, A., Jackson, M. A., . . . Tunkel, D. E. (2013). The diagnosis and management of acute otitis media. *Pediatrics, 131*(3), e964–e999.

Mandell, L. A. Wunderink, R. G., Anzueto, A., Bartlett, J. G., Campbell, G. D., Dean, N. C., . . . Whitney, C. G. (2007). Infectious diseases society of America/American Thoracic Society consensus guidelines on the management of community-acquired pneumonia in adults. *Clinical Infectious Diseases, 44*(Suppl. 2), S27–S72.
https://enp-network.s3.amazonaws.com/NPA_Long_Island/pdf/Pneumonia.pdf

McMillan, J. A., Lee, C. K. K., Siberry, G. K., & Carroll, K. C. (2013). *The Harriet Lane handbook of pediatric antimicrobial therapy*. Philadelphia, PA: Elsevier Saunders.

MedlinePlus
https://www.nlm.nih.gov/medlineplus/ency/article/000165.htm

MedPage Today
http://www.medpagetoday.com

Medscape
http://www.medscape.com

National Academy of Medicine
http://nam.edu

National Cholesterol Education Program Expert Panel on Detection, Evaluation, and Treatment of High Blood Cholesterol in Adults (Adult Treatment Panel IV, 2012).
http://circ.ahajournals.org/content/circulationaha/106/25/3143.full.pdf

National Heart Lung and Blood Institute (NHLBI)
http://www.nhlbi.nih.gov

New England Journal of Medicine (NEJM) Journal Watch General Medicine
http://www.jwatch.org/general-medicine

Pharmacist's Letter
www.pharmacistsletter.com

Physician's Desk Reference (PDR)
http://www.pdr.net

Prescriber's Letter
http://prescribersletter.therapeuticresearch.com/pl/sample.aspx?cs=&s=PRL&AspxAutoDetectCookieSupport=1

Psychopharmacology
http://link.springer.com/journal/213

Reference for Interpretation of Hepatitis C Virus (HCV) Test Results
www.cdc.gov/hepatitis

RxLIST
http://www.rxlist.com/script/main/hp.asp

RxLIST: Drugs A-Z
http://www.rxlist.com/drugs/alpha_a.htm

Sanford Guide Web Edition
https://webedition.sanfordguide.com

Solutions for Safer ER/LA Opioid Prescribing in a New Era of Health Care. American Nurses Credentialing Center, Post Graduate Institute of Medicine
www.cmeuniversity.com

The American Congress of Obstetrics and Gynecology (ACOG)
http://www.acog.org

The American Geriatric Society
http://www.americangeriatrics.org

The Handbook of Antimicrobial Therapy (20th ed.). The Medical Letter

The Journal for Nurse Practitioners
www.elsevier.com/locate/tjnp

The Medical Letter on Drugs and Therapeutics (subscription)
http://secure.medicalletter.org

The Nurse Practitioner Journal
www.tnpj.com

Third Report of the National Cholesterol Education Program (NCEP) Expert Panel on Detection, Evaluation, and Treatment of High Blood Cholesterol in Adults (Adult Treatment Panel III) final report.
http://www.ncbi.nlm.nih.gov/pubmed/12485966

Treatment Guidelines [Annual Volume]: The Medical Letter

Updated CDC guidance: Superbugs threaten hospital patients. *Medscape Education Clinical Briefs* (March 31, 2016).
http://www.medscape.org/viewarticle/859361?nlid=105320_2713&src=wnl_cmemp_160523_mscpedu_nurs&impID=1106718&faf=1

U.S. Pharmacist Weekly Newsletter
http://www.uspharmacist.com

Wald, E. R., Applegate, K. E., Bordley, C., Darrow, D. H., Glode, M. P., Marcy, S. M., . . . Weinberg, S. T., American Academy of Pediatrics. (2013). Clinical practice guidelines for the diagnosis and management of acute bacterial sinusitis in children 1 to 18 years. *Pediatrics, 132*(1), e262–280.
http://www.ncbi.nlm.nih.gov/pubmed/23796742

WebMD: Drugs and Medications A to Z. Latest Drug News
http://www.webmd.com/drugs

FDA Pregnancy Category	DEA Schedule	Drug	Page Numbers
C		*auranofin*, **Ridaura**	378
C		**Auvi-Q**, *epinephrine*	14, 402
X		**Avage**, *tazarotene*	7, 150, 207, 254, 366, 464
D		**Avalide**, *irbesartan/ hydrochlorothiazide*	218
B		*avanafil*, **Stendra**	140, 372
C		**Avandamet**, *rosiglitazone/ metformin*	436
C		**Avandaryl**, *rosiglitazone/ glimeperide*	437
C		**Avandia**, *rosiglitazone*	434, 436
D		**Avapro**, *irbesartan*	213
A		**Aveeno**, *oatmeal colloid*	111–113
C		**Avelox**, *moxifloxacin*	62, 75, 338, 345, 395, 400, 449, 547
X		**Aviane**, *ethinyl estradiol/ levonorgestrel*	488
C		**Avita**, *tretinoin*	7, 150, 207, 254, 464
X		**Avodart**, *dutasteride*	45
C		**Avonex**, *interferon beta-1a*	270
B		**Avycaz**, *ceftazidime/avibactam*	546
C		**Axert**, *almotriptan*	168
C		**Axid, Axid AR**, *nizatidine*	153, 327
X	III	**Axiron**, *testosterone*	406
X		**Aygestin**, *norethindrone*	14, 138, 266
D		**Azasan**, *azathioprine*	378
B		**AzaSite**, *azithromycin*	89

FDA Pregnancy Category	DEA Schedule	Drug	Page Numbers
D		*azathioprine*, Azasan, Imuran	378
B		*azelaic acid*, Azelex, Finacea, Optivar	3, 5
C		*azelastine*, Astelin, Astepro Nasal Spray	384, 386
B		Azelex, *azelaic acid*	3, 5
D		*azilsartan medoxomil*, Edarbi	213
B		*azithromycin*, AzaSite, Zithromax, Zithromax Tri Pak, max	42, 60, 71–73, 76, 79, 82, 83, 89, 93, 94, 160, 161, 165, 234, 258, 302, 332, 333, 334, 339, 340, 342, 343, 346, 348, 389–392, 397, 418–419, 443, 448, 462, 547
C		Azmacort, *triamcinolone acetonide*	30
B		AZO, AZO Standard Extra Strength, AZO Urinary Pain Relief/AZO Urinary Pain Relief Maximum Strength, *phenazopyridine*	244, 245, 373, 449, 456
C		Azopt, *brinzolamide*	156
D		Azor, *amlodipine/olmesartan medoxomil*	222
B		*aztreonam*, Azactam, Cayston	550
B/D		Azulfidine, Azulfidine EN-Tabs, *sulfasalazine*	101, 379, 446
C		Babylax, *glycerin suppository*	137
NE		*bacillus athracis immune globulin intravenous (human)*, Anthrasil	20
C		*bacitracin*, Bacitracin Ophthalmic	89

FDA Pregnancy Category	DEA Schedule	Drug	Page Numbers
C		Blephamide Liquifilm, Blephamide S.O.P., *sulfacetamide/prednisolone*	92
C		Blocadren, *timolol*	171, 209
B		*boceprevir*, Victrelis	186
B		Bonine, *meclizine*	252, 262, 269, 278, 459
C		Boniva, *ibandronate (as monosodium monohydrate)*	297, 305
C	III	Bontril, *phendimetrazine*	283
D		*bortezomib*, Velcade	518
X		Brevicon-21, Brevicon-28, *ethinyl estradiol/norethindrone*	488
C		*brexpiprazole*, Rexulti	110
B		*brimonidine*, Alphagan	156
C		*brinzolamide*, Azopt	156
C		*brivaracetam*, Briviact	520
C		Briviact, *brivaracetam*	520
C		Bromfed DM, *brompheniramine/ dextromethorphan*	537
B		*bromocriptine*, Cycloset, Parlodel	322, 442
C		Brovana, *arformoterol*	33–34
B		*budesonide*, Entocort EC, Pulmicort Respules, Pulmicort Flexhaler, Rhinocort, Rhinocort Aqua, Uceris	29, 101, 383, 445, 512
D		Bufferin, *aspirin/magnesium carbonate/magnesium oxide bumetanide*	145
C	III	Bunavail, *buprenorphine/ naloxone*	290

FDA Pregnancy Category	DEA Schedule	Drug	Page Numbers
C		*entacapone*, **Comtan**	324
C		*entecavir*, **Baraclude**	183
C		**Entocort EC**, *budesonide*	101, 445
D		**Entresto**, *sacubitril/valsartan*	177
B		**Entyvio**, *vedolizumab*	101, 102, 447
D		**Epaned**, *enalapril*	175, 212
NE		**Epanova**, *omega 3-acid ethyl esters*	126, 225
NE		**Epclusa**, *sofosbuvir/velpatasvir*	187
C		**Epiduo Gel**, *adapalene/benzoyl peroxide*	7
C		**Epi-E-Zpen**, *epinephrine*	14, 402
C		*epinastine*, **Elestat**	87
C		*epinephrine*, **Adrenaclick, Adrenalin, Auvi-Q, Epi-E-Zpen, EpiPen, EpiPen Jr, Twinject**	14, 402
C		**EpiPen, EpiPen Jr**, *epinephrine*	14, 402
C		**Epivir, Epivir-HBV**, *lamivudine, 3TC*	183, 197, 523, 543
B		*eplerenone*, **Inspra**	177, 216
C		**Epogen**, *epoetin alpha*	15
C		*epoetin alpha*, **Epogen, Procrit**	15
D		*eprosartan*, **Teveten**	213
C		**Epzicom**, *abacavir/lamivudine*	202, 523
D	IV	**Equagesic**, *meprobamate/aspirin*	273
D		**Equetro**, *carbamazepine*	47–48, 51, 520
C		*ergoloid*, **Hydergine, Hydergine LC, Hydergine Liquid**	12
D		*erlotinib*, **Tarceva**	518
X		**Errin**, *norethindrone*	496
C		**Ertaczo**, *sertaconazole*	414

FDA Pregnancy Category	DEA Schedule	Drug	Page Numbers
C	II	**Fentora,** *fentanyl transmucosal unit*	315
A		**Feosol,** *ferrous sulfate*	16
A		**Fergon,** *ferrous gluconate*	16
A		**Fer-In-Sol,** *ferrous sulfate*	16
C		*fesoterodine fumarate,* **Toviaz**	237
C		**Fetzima,** *levomilnacipran*	106–107
B		**Feverall,** *acetaminophen*	144
B		**Fexmid,** *cyclobenzaprine*	147, 272
C		**Fibercon,** *calcium polycarbophil*	95, 119
C		**Fibricor,** *fenofibrate*	129, 225
B		**Finacea,** *azelaic acid*	3, 5
C		*finafloxacin,* **Xtoro**	299
X		*finasteride,* **Propecia, Proscar**	45, 239
C		*fingolimod,* **Gilenya**	270
C	III	**Fioricet with Codeine,** *butalbital/acetaminophen/ caffeine/codeine*	174
D	II	**Fiorinal,** *butalbital/aspirin/ caffeine*	174, 308
D	III	**Fiorinal with Codeine,** *butalbital/aspirin/caffeine/ codeine*	174, 308
D/B		**Flagyl, Flagyl 375, Flagyl ER,** *metronidazole*	13, 43, 101–102, 124, 155, 327, 364, 392, 421, 449, 542, 543
C		**Flarex,** *fluorometholone acetate*	86
C		**Flector Patch,** *diclofenac epolamine*	27, 275, 308, 330, 353, 499

FDA Pregnancy Category	DEA Schedule	Drug	Page Numbers
B		*golimumab,* Simponi	367, 370, 380
X		*goserelin,* Zoladex	138, 518
C		Gralise, *gabapentin*	116, 147, 351, 375
B		*granisetron,* Kytril, Sancuso	280
NE		*granisetron,* Sustol	280
C		Grifulvin V, *griseofulvin (microsized)*	286, 409, 411, 413, 414, 542, 579
C		*griseofulvin (microsized),* Gris-PEG	286, 409, 411, 413, 414, 542, 579
C		Gris-PEG, *griseofulvin (microsized)*	286, 409, 411, 413, 414, 542, 579
C		*guanabenz*	216
C		*guanethidine,* Ismelin	216
B		*guanfacine,* Intuniv, Tenex	40, 216
B		Gynazole-1, *butoconazole*	70
B		Gyne-Lotrimin, Gyne-Lotrimin-3, *clotrimazole*	70
D		Habitrol, *nicotine transdermal system*	417
C		*halcinonide,* Halog	509
X	IV	Halcion, *triazolam*	22, 147, 243
C		Haldol, *haloperidol*	104, 519
C		Haldol Decanoate, *haloperidol decanoate*	519
C		*halobetasol propionate,* Ultravate	509
C		Halog, *halcinonide*	509
C		*haloperidol,* Haldol	104, 519
C		*haloperidol decanoate,* Haldol Decanoate	519
X		Halotestin, *fluoxymesterone*	406

FDA Pregnancy Category	DEA Schedule	Drug	Page Numbers
B		**Hyal,** *sodium hyaluronate*	294
B		**Hyalgan,** *sodium hyaluronate*	294, 381
C	II	**Hycet,** *hydrocodone bitartrate/ acetaminophen*	309
C	II	**Hycodan, Hycodan Syrup,** *hydrocodone/homatropine*	538
C		**Hydergine, Hydergine LC, Hydergine Liquid,** *ergoloid*	12
C		*hydralazine*	19, 217
D		**Hydrea,** *hydroxyurea*	517
B		*hydrochlorothiazide,* **Esidrix, Microzide**	133, 177, 210, 457
C	II	*hydrocodone bitartrate,* **Hysingla ER, Vantrela ER, Zohydro ER**	309
C		*hydrocortisone,* **Anusol-HC, Cortaid, Cortef, Cortifoam, Hydrocortone, Hytone, Proctocort, Texacort**	181, 445, 506
C		*hydrocortisone acetate,* **U-Cort**	507
C		*hydrocortisone butyrate,* **Locoid**	508
C		*hydrocortisone phosphate,* **Hydrocotone Phosphate**	511
C		*hydrocortisone probutate,* **Pandel**	508
C		*hydrocortisone retention enema,* **Cortenema**	445
C		*hydrocortisone sodium succinate,* **Solu-Cortef**	511
C		*hydrocortisone valerate,* **Westcort**	508
C		**Hydrocortone,** *hydrocortisone*	510, 511
C		**Hydrocotone Phosphate,** *hydrocortisone phosphate*	511

FDA Pregnancy Category	DEA Schedule	Drug	Page Numbers
C		*mesoridazine*, **Serentil**	104
C	II	**Metadate CD, Metadate ER**, *methylphenidate*	39, 277
C		**Metaglip**, *glipizide/metformin*	435
C		**Metamucil**, *psyllium*	95
NE		**Metanx**, *L-methylfolate calcium (as metafolin)/pyridoxyl 5-phosphate/methylcobalamin*	115, 205, 444
C		*metaproterenol*, **Alupent**	32, 36
B		*metaxalone*, **Skelaxin**	272
B		*metformin*, **Fortamet, Glucophage, Glucophage XR, Glumetza, Riomet**	434
B		*methadone*, **Dolophine**	288, 311
C	II	*methamphetamine*, **Desoxyn**	39, 277, 283
C		*methazolamide*, **Neptazane**	159
C		*methenamine hippurate*, **Hiprex**	455, 456
D		*methimazole*, **Tapazole**	224
C		*methocarbamol*, **Robaxin**	273
X		*methotrexate*, **Rheumatrex, Trexall**	251, 350, 379
C		*methoxsalen*, **Oxsoralen, Oxsoralen Ultra**	459
C		*methscopolamine bromide*, **Pamine, Pamine Forte**	98, 249
C		*methylcellulose*, **Citrucel**	95
B		*methyldopa*, **Aldomet**	216
C	II	**Methylin, Methylin ER**, *methylphenidate*	39, 277
B		*methylnaltrexone bromide*, **Relistor**	291

FDA Pregnancy Category	DEA Schedule	Drug	Page Numbers
B		**Propine**, *dipivefrin*	158
C		*propranolol*, **Inderal LA, InnoPran XL**	18, 44, 171, 209, 220, 224, 268, 514
NE		*propylene glycol*, **Systane Balance**	126
D		*propylthiouracil, ptu*, **Propyl-Thyracil**	224
D		**Propyl-Thyracil**, *propylthiouracil, ptu*	224
C		**ProQuin XR**, *ciprofloxacin*	20, 21, 57, 76, 82, 122, 124, 165, 347, 361, 362, 374, 388, 392, 394, 443, 450, 452–453, 546
X	IV	**ProSom**, *estazolam*	243
X		**Proscar**, *finasteride*	45, 239
D		**ProStep**, *nicotine transdermal system*	417
B		**Protonix**, *pantoprazole*	154, 329, 466
C		**Protopic**, *tacrolimus*	112, 353, 363
C		*protriptyline*, **Vivactil**	108–109, 117, 352, 355, 424
C		**Proventil, Proventil HFA**, *albuterol*	31–32, 35–36
X		**Provera**, *medroxyprogesterone*	14, 137, 266
C		**Provigil**, *modafinil*	275, 400, 401
C		**Prozac, Prozac Weekly**, *fluoxetine*	25, 50, 65–66, 106, 172–173, 285, 319, 359–360
B		**Prudoxin**, *doxepin*	112, 352, 363
C		**Psorcon, Psorcon E**, *diflorasone diacetate*	508
C		*psyllium*, **Metamucil**	95

FDA Pregnancy Category	DEA Schedule	Drug	Page Numbers
B		**Pulmicort Flexhaler, Pulmicort Respules,** *budesonide*	29, 101, 434, 500
D		**Pylera,** *metronidazole/ tetracycline/bismuthsubcitrate*	180
C		**Pyrazinamide,** *pyrazinamide*	424, 544
C		*pyrazinamide,* **Pyrazinamide**	424, 544
C		*pyrazolopyrimidines,* **Zaleplon**	148, 242
C		*pyrantel pamoate,* **Pin-X**	193–194, 337, 387, 409, 421, 461, 542
C		*pyrethrins,* **RID**	325
B		**Pyridium,** *phenazopyridine*	244, 246, 373, 450, 456
C		**QNASL,** *beclomethasone dipropionate*	383
X	IV	**Qsymia,** *phentermine/topiramate*	283–284
C		**Qualaquin,** *quinine sulfate*	253, 260
X		**Quartette,** *ethinyl estradiol/ levonorgestrel*	496
X		**Quasense,** *ethinyl estradiol/ levonorgestrel*	493, 496
C		**Qudexy, Qudexy XR,** *topiramate*	522
C		**Questran, Questran Light,** *cholestyramine*	120–121, 130
B		*quetiapine fumarate,* **Seroquel, Seroquel XR**	49, 53, 104, 356, 520
C	II	**QuilliChew XR, Quillivant XR,** *methylphenidate*	39–40
D		*quinapril,* **Accupril**	176, 212
C		*quinine sulfate,* **Qualaquin**	253, 259–260
C		**Quixin,** *levofloxacin ophthalmic solution*	90

FDA Pregnancy Category	DEA Schedule	Drug	Page Numbers
C		*sulconazole*, Exelderm, Extina	410, 412, 414, 416
C		*sulfacetamide*, Bleph-10, Cetamide, Isopto Cetamide, Klaron	58, 90, 403
B/D		*sulfasalazine*, Azulfidine, Azulfidine EN-Tabs	101, 379, 446
C		*sulfinpyrazone*, Anturane	163
B/D		*sulfisoxazole*, Gantrisin	451, 549
C/D		*sulindac*, Clinoril	505
C		*sumatriptan*, Alsuma Injectable, Imitrex, Imitrex Injectable, Imitrex Nasal Spray, Onzetra Xsail, Sumavel DosePro, Zecuity Transdermal, Zembrace SymTouch	168–169
D		Sumycin, *tetracycline*	6, 27, 58, 62, 193, 256, 259, 348, 365, 387, 392, 400, 550, 585
B		Suprax Oral Suspension, *cefixime*	60, 302, 335, 391, 394, 419, 443, 452, 546, 563
C	IV	Suprenza ODT, *phentermine*	283
C		Surfak, *docusate calcium*	96
C		Surmontil, *trimipramine*	109, 117, 352, 355, 424
C		Sustiva, *efavirenz*	198, 525
X		Syeda, *ethinyl estradiol/drospirenone*	494
C		Symbicort, *budesonide/formoterol*	34
C		Symbyax, *olanzapine/fluoxetine*	50, 108
C		Symlin, Symlin Pen, *pramlintide*	428

FDA Pregnancy Category	DEA Schedule	Drug	Page Numbers
C		**Tanafed DMX,** *dexchlorpheniramine/ pseudoephedrine/ dextromethorphan*	540
C	II	*tapentadol,* **Nucynta, Nucynta ER**	331
D		**Tapazole,** *methimazole*	224
D		**Tarceva,** *erlotinib*	518
X		**Tarina,** *ethinyl estradiol/ norethindrone*	494
D		**Tarka,** *trandolapril/verapamil*	221
C		**Tasmar,** *tolcapone*	324
C		*tavaborole,* **Kerydin**	287
X		**Taytulla,** *estradiol/norethindrone*	494
X		*tazarotene,* **Avage, Tazorac**	7, 150, 207, 254, 366, 464
B		**Tazicef,** *ceftazidime*	545
B		**Tazidime,** *ceftazidime*	545
X		**Tazorac,** *tazarotene*	7, 150, 207, 254, 367, 464
C		**Tecfidera,** *dimethyl fumarate*	269
D		**Teczem,** *enalapril/diltiazem*	221
C		*tedizolid,* **Sivextro**	75, 345
B		**Teflaro,** *ceftaroline fosamil*	74, 235, 344, 545, 546
D		**Tegretol, Tegretol XR,** *carbamazepine*	48, 51–52, 422 520
D		**Tekamlo,** *aliskiren/amlodipine*	222
D		**Tekturna,** *aliskiren*	216
D		**Tekturna HCT,** *aliskiren/ hydrochlorothiazide*	221

FDA Pregnancy Category	DEA Schedule	Drug	Page Numbers
C	IV	**Ultram, Ultram ER** *tramadol*	115, 175, 188, 191, 314, 331, 354
C		**Ultrase MT,** *pancrelipase*	318
C		**Ultravate,** *halobetasol propionate*	509
B		**Unasyn,** *ampicillin/sulbactam*	537
NE		*undecylenic acid,* **Desenex**	402
C		**Uniphyl,** *theophylline*	36, 65
D		**Uniretic,** *moexipril/ hydrochlorothiazide*	217
A		**Unithroid,** *levothyroxine*	233
D		**Univasc,** *moexipril*	212
C		*unoprostone isopropyl,* **Rescula**	159
NE		**Uptravi,** *selexipag*	371
C		*urea cream,* **Carmol 40, Keratol 40**	396
C		**Urecholine,** *bethanechol*	239, 449
C		**Urelle,** *methenamine/phenyl salicylate/methylene blue/ sodiumbiphosphate/hyoscyamine*	456
C		**Urised,** *methenamikne/ sodium phosphate monobasic/ phenylephrine salicylate/ methyleneblue/hyoscyamine sulfate*	245, 456
B		**Uristat,** *phenazopyridine*	244, 246, 373, 450, 456
C		**Urocit-K,** *potassium citrate*	458
B		**Urogesic,** *phenazopyridine*	244, 246, 373, 450, 456
B		**UroXetral,** *alfuzosin*	45, 457
B		*ursodiol,* **Actigall**	46, 80

FDA Pregnancy Category	DEA Schedule	Drug	Page Numbers
C		**Zovirax,** *acyclovir*	78, 190, 191, 543, 552
B		**Zuplenz,** *ondansetron*	281, 359
NE		**Zurampic,** *lesinurad*	163
C		**Zyban,** *bupropion hydrochloride*	417
C		**Zyclara,** *imiquimod*	9, 460
C	II	**Zydone,** *hydrocodone/ acetaminophen*	310
C		**Zyflo, Zyflo CR,** *zileuton*	28, 382
C		**Zylet,** *tobramycin/loteprednol*	92
C		**Zyloprim,** *allopurinol*	162, 457
C		**Zymar,** *gatifloxacin*	89
C		**Zymaxid,** *gatifloxacin*	89
C		**Zyprexa, Zyprexa Zudis,** *olanzapine*	104, 356, 519
C		**Zyvox,** *linezolid*	75, 345, 399, 551